Advancing Your Career

Concepts of Professional Nursing

Sixth Edition

Advancing Your Career

Concepts of Professional Nursing

Sixth Edition

Rose Kearney-Nunnery, PhD, RN

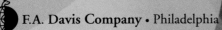
F.A. Davis Company • Philadelphia

F. A. Davis Company
1915 Arch Street
Philadelphia, PA 19103
www.fadavis.com

Printed in the United States of America

Last digit indicates print number: 10 9 8 7 6 5 4 3

Acquisitions Editor: Susan Rhymer
Director of Content Development: Darlene D. Pedersen
Content Project Manager: Echo K. Gerhart
Electronic Product Manager: Kate Crowley
Design and Illustration Manager: Carolyn O'Brien

As new scientific information becomes available through basic and clinical research, recommended treatments and drug therapies undergo changes. The author(s) and publisher have done everything possible to make this book accurate, up to date, and in accord with accepted standards at the time of publication. The author(s), editors, and publisher are not responsible for errors or omissions or for consequences from application of the book, and make no warranty, expressed or implied, in regard to the contents of the book. Any practice described in this book should be applied by the reader in accordance with professional standards of care used in regard to the unique circumstances that may apply in each situation. The reader is advised always to check product information (package inserts) for changes and new information regarding dose and contraindications before administering any drug. Caution is especially urged when using new or infrequently ordered drugs.

Kearney-Nunnery, Rose, author, editor.
  Advancing your career : concepts of professional nursing / Rose Kearney-Nunnery. — Sixth edition.
    p. ; cm.
  Includes bibliographical references and index.
  ISBN 978-0-8036-4203-4
  I. Title.
  [DNLM: 1. Nursing. 2. Career Mobility. WY 16.1]
  RT82
  610.7306'9–dc23
                                                    2015014170

Preface

The nursing profession has undergone major changes in the past decades, and the pace of change seems to accelerate daily. We are redefining practice and basing this practice on evidence of efficacy. We have moved from a position of defending nursing as a profession to our current pivotal role in healthcare. Focusing on human beings in their respective environments with unique healthcare needs that are addressed through nursing care is vitally important with our rapidly expanding knowledge base and the dynamic changes continually occurring in healthcare. In essence, our quest in our nursing roles is to expand knowledge, become involved within the profession and in interdisciplinary healthcare, utilize evidence-based practice and expanding technologies, and broaden the vision of professional practice.

This book is directed to the RN student returning to school. The intent is to provide you, the practicing RN, with professional concepts to advance your practice. These concepts build on your prior nursing education, and their application will greatly enhance your professional practice and growth. The aim is to engage you intellectually in an ongoing professional dialogue and journey with your peers, colleagues, and instructors; broaden your professional development; and build on your pre-existing knowledge and experiences. You are challenged to delve further into professional education and conceptual practice. The book is written for the adult learner with the characteristics of self-direction, prior experiences, applicability to practice, and motivation to meet the challenge to expand his or her knowledge base.

The sixth edition has been updated and is divided into three sections. As with the previous editions, each chapter contains chapter objectives, key terms, key points, chapter exercises to assist in meeting each of the chapter objectives, references, online references, and bibliographical sources. Interactive exercises have been updated and are provided on an Intranet site to truly engage the adult learner progressing through the content. The Intranet site also houses a clinical scenario bank, glossary of terms, important Internet links, discussion sections, and online lessons in presentation graphics with interactive challenges and Web links.

In Section I, the professional bases for nursing practice are introduced. This discussion is the start of *Advancing Your Practice*. Chapter 1 focuses on the characteristics of nursing as a profession and as a unique professional discipline. A focus on the core competencies for all healthcare professionals challenges both professional and interdisciplinary practice. As a first step in your educational pursuit, you are challenged to review your learner characteristics to enhance your educational experience. Next, you focus on your concept of the profession via an analysis of your personal perspectives of professional nursing as a philosophy statement.

From a view of professional practice, Section I continues with a focus on theory as the basis for practice in Chapter 2. Dr. Jacqueline Fawcett addresses how unique nursing knowledge has evolved and been applied to individuals, families, and groups in Chapter 3. A discussion of health, illness, and holism in Chapter 4 delves further into models of health and illness with a focus on cultural and literacy considerations. Section I concludes with a review of the research process and the necessity for the application of evidence-based practice in Chapter 5. Use of known and evolving knowledge replaces tradition as healthcare focuses on guidelines and documented evidence for efficacy of care.

Section II examines selected critical abilities in professional nursing practice. The first of these critical components addresses communication skills, as vital to professional practice and in constant need of refinement. The content is presented by Dr. Lynne Ornes in Chapter 6, with a discussion of communication models, essential ingredients of effective communication, nonverbal communication forms, and specific communication techniques, including communication skills for interdisciplinary and interprofessional practice. Along with effective communication, critical thinking is essential to professional nursing practice. In Chapter 7, Dr. Genevieve M. Bartol discusses aspects of critical thinking in nursing, along with further development of critical thinking and analysis skills. Effective communication and critical thinking are required in collaborative practice situations. Chapter 8 focuses on working with groups, including the characteristics and roles of groups and group leaders and the skills needed for collaboration, coordination, negotiation, and dealing with conflict and difficult people. The next critical component for professional practice is the teaching and learning process. Included in Chapter 9 is a discussion of learning theories and learning readiness, along with information on writing behavioral objectives, teaching skills and methods, and evaluating outcomes, while the Intranet lesson focuses on helping patients locate reliable Web sources.

Leadership and management skills are essential in professional practice, especially in organizational settings. Chapter 10 looks at organizational characteristics and presents the skills needed for effectively managing and leading in organizational settings, including a discussion of selected theories and delegation principles. Organizations continue to redefine themselves, so effectively dealing with change is critical. Chapter 11 includes theories on change and innovation, along with the characteristics of change agents for change in individuals, families, groups, and organizations. Section II concludes with Chapter 12, which examines ethical principles and making ethical decisions focusing on informed consent, advanced directives, the persistive vegetative state, organ procurement and donation, genomics, and impaired practice.

Section III starts with a focus on quality and safety in Chapter 13 and the national initiatives that have driven this process. Theoretical models for quality are discussed, along with strategies for continuous quality improvement, safety, and efficacy in the healthcare environment. In Chapter 14, the focus is on population health. The progress of the Healthy People initiatives in the United States is presented, along with the current focus on social determinants of health. Special populations that are highlighted include the aging population, minorities, and those living in rural areas. In Chapter 15, we look at one of the core competencies for healthcare professionals, the use of informatics. Health information systems in the clinical setting are discussed, along with the implementation of the electronic health record. Informatics competencies for nurses, informatics nurses, and informatics specialists are described in this evolving specialty in the discipline.

Quality care includes a focus on healthcare economics and policy, as presented in Chapter 16. Policy and the associated costs are changing dramatically as we focus on safe, effective, and equitable care for individuals and groups. Stemming from a focus on healthcare policy are the political advocacy skills needed by the politically active nurse in Chapter 17. These skills include both understanding the legislative process and promoting policy improvements for the health of individuals and groups.

We conclude with a look at the reality of the healthcare issues addressed throughout the book and the challenges to be addressed by nursing professionals in the future. In Chapter 18, Sister Rosemary Donley addresses healthcare reform and the issues debated in both legislative and professional areas that have major implications for the healthcare of the nation and global communities, with initiatives for the profession. The final chapter discusses challenges for your professional future in terms of expanding your vision and planning for the future. Topics include a look at the practice environment and the call for change, greater collaboration, and demonstration of competence. You will be challenged to take the lead and demonstrate involvement in the profession for improved care and healthcare initiatives that meet the needs of the population, considering economics, quality initiatives, and demonstration of effective outcomes.

This book is intended to advance your professional practice and continued professional development through further education. Your personal characteristics of self-motivation, a thirst for information, and commitment to your patients and the profession will be enhanced as you develop a more conceptual and visionary approach to professional nursing practice.

—Rose Kearney-Nunnery

Contributors

Genevieve M. Bartol, RN, EdD

Independent Mental Health Care Professional
Greensboro, North Carolina

Chapter 7 Contributor

Sister Rosemary Donley, PhD, APRN, BC, FAAN

Professor, Jacques Laval Endowed Chair for
Justice for Vulnerable Populations
Duquesne University
Pittsburgh, Pennsylvania

Chapter 18 Contributor

Francoise Dunefsky, MS, RN, NEA-BC

President and CEO, Gateway Community
Industries, Inc.
Port Ewen, New York

Chapter 13 Contributor

Jacqueline Fawcett, PhD, FAAN

University of Massachusetts at Boston
Boston, Massachusetts

Chapter 3 Contributor

William A. Himmelsbach, MPH, FACHE

Health Care CEO (Retired)
Okatie, South Carolina

Chapter 16 Contributor

Lynne Ornes, PhD, MS, RN

University of South Carolina Beaufort
Bluffton, South Carolina

Chapter 6 contributor

Reviewers

Pier A. Broadnax, PhD, RN
University of the District of Columbia
Washington, District of Columbia

Dawn M. Goodolf, PhD, RN
Moravian College
Bethlehem, Pennsylvania

Sandy Halford, MSN, RN
East Tennessee State University
Johnson City, Tennessee

April D. Matthia, PhD, RN, CNE
University of North Carolina Wilmington
Wilmington, North Carolina

Beth Norton, DNP, RN, CNE
Northwest Florida State College
Niceville, Florida

Jeanne Tucker, RN, MSN, HSAD, CHES
Patty Hanks Shelton School of Nursing
Abilene, Texas

Acknowledgments

Numerous people have been a large part of this continuing process. Friends and colleagues have more than tolerated my preoccupation with the profession. My respect is extended to all of my professional colleagues across the country for the opportunities they provided for reflection, discussion, and debate. I extend particular thanks to all of the contributors, past and present, who have shared their expertise and insights. Joanne DaCunha merits particular credit for the completion of this project and all prior editions through her encouragement, assistance, and belief in the potential for our profession. And the ongoing efforts of Echo K. Gerhart from F.A. Davis have been invaluable. My ongoing appreciation continues for my late husband, Jimmie E. Nunnery, for his support and encouragement with prior editions, and much sage advice from his political background that contributed to the chapter on politics.

As a final note, I cannot describe the endless encouragement from my professional colleagues, friends, and students, all of whom added to this challenge for the nursing profession to focus on change in the future. And to all who give to the consumers of nursing care, my endless and enduring respect.

—Rose Kearney-Nunnery

Contents

Professional Bases for Practice

INTRODUCTION

This section introduces the professional bases for nursing practice to start the discussion of *Advancing Your Practice*. Chapter 1, "Your Professional Identity," focuses on the characteristics of professional nursing as a profession and as a unique professional discipline. A focus on the core competencies for all healthcare professionals challenges both professional and interdisciplinary practice. As a first step in your educational pursuit, you are challenged to review your learner characteristics to enhance your educational experience. Next, you focus on your concept of the profession and an analysis of your personal perspectives of professional nursing as a philosophy statement.

From a view of professional practice, Section I continues with a focus on theory as the basis for practice in Chapter 2, "Theory As the Basis for Practice." And then we continue with how unique nursing knowledge has evolved and been applied to the consumers of nursing in Chapter 3, "Evolution and Use of Formal Nursing Knowledge." As you will learn in Chapter 4, "Health, Illness, and Holism," holistic practice delves further into models of health and illness with a focus on cultural and literacy considerations.

Section I concludes with Chapter 5, "Evidence-Based Practice," which presents a review of the research process and the necessity of the application of evidence-based practice in professional nursing. Use of known and evolving knowledge replaces tradition as healthcare focuses on guidelines and documented evidence for efficacy of care.

● Rose Kearney-Nunnery

1 Your Professional Identity

The past cannot be changed.
The future is yet in your power.

Mary Pickford, 1893–1979

Chapter Objectives

On completion of this chapter, the reader will be able to:

1. Relate the attributes of a profession to professional nursing practice.
2. Relate the core competencies for health professionals to professional nursing practice.
3. Describe the consumers of professional nursing practice.
4. Discuss responsibility and accountability in professional nursing practice.
5. Discuss the formal and informal educational expectations for professional nursing practice, including essential curricular elements.
6. Consider personal learning attributes, including learning style, time management, and appropriate use of resources.
7. Develop a personal philosophy of professional nursing.

Key Terms

Theory
Paradigm
Metaparadigm
Human Beings
Environment
Health
Nursing
Authority
Community Sanction
Code of Ethics
Professional Culture
Professional Development

Professional Organizations
Ethics
Educational Background
Core Competencies
Evidence-Based Practice and
    Research
Quality of Practice
Communication
Leadership
Collaboration
Professional Practice
    Evaluation

Self-Regulation
Resource Utilization
Environmental Health
Roles
Learning
Knowledge
Skill
Ability
Learning Style
Resources
Philosophy

As a registered nurse (RN) student pursuing an advanced degree in nursing, you must reevaluate personal and collegial perspectives on what truly constitutes professional practice. You are at a gateway for advancing your practice and building a professional commitment. To advance in your professional career, you must broaden and build on your knowledge base. This involves Mezirow's (1991, 2000) theory of adult development and education as transformative learning. This theory proposes that the adult learns in one of four ways:

● By elaborating existing frames of reference
● By learning new frames of reference
● By transforming points of view
● By transforming habits of mind (Mezirow, 2000, p. 19)

Building on your knowledge base and your personal frame of reference, you will be adding and developing new perspectives. This process promotes critical analysis and will allow you as the adult learner to transform your views in new ways, and create new ways of approaching the world and professional practice. Learning occurs through reflection and interpretation to understand perceptions of the self and the world. This transformation provides an ongoing process in both personal and professional development.

From the professional standpoint, armed with technical skills and expertise in the practice setting, we chart a course into the conceptual components that embody and expand professional practice. As a start, consider the concepts that characterize both a profession in general and professional nursing practice specifically.

CHARACTERISTICS OF A PROFESSION

Greenwood (1957) developed a classic work on professionalism in which he proposed five characteristics of a profession:

● Systematic Theory and Knowledge Base
● Authority
● Community Sanction
● Code of Ethics
● Professional Culture

These attributes were then applied to the social work discipline to defend its professional status, but they are applicable to any profession, including professional nursing practice.

Systematic Theory and Knowledge Base

Each profession is guided by systematic theory on which its knowledge base is built. The skills of professional nurses are not trial and error but are supported by a fund of knowledge that has been organized into an internally consistent system that is our theoretical basis for practice. This system includes theoretical foundations unique to the profession as well as those adapted from other scientific disciplines.

Kerlinger and Lee (2000) define a **theory** as "a set of interrelated constructs (concepts), definitions, and propositions that present a systematic view of phenomena by specifying relations among variables, with the purpose of explaining and predicting the phenomena" (p. 11). This theory base is also referred to as the paradigm used by professionals or the practitioners in a particular scientific community.

Kuhn (1970) has provided us with the well-established definition of a **paradigm** as "universally recognized scientific achievements that, for a time, provide model problems and solutions to a community of practitioners" (p. vii). The paradigm consists of the beliefs and the belief system shared by members of a particular scientific community. When the paradigm is no longer useful in explaining, practicing, and conducting research in that community, the paradigm shifts and a new belief structure is promoted, adopted, and used by its members.

The paradigm is merely the phenomenon of concern that guides nursing practice. In Chapter 3, Fawcett proposes that *conceptual model* and *paradigm* are interchangeable terms relative to the phenomena of nursing. Various nursing paradigms or conceptual models are currently used in practice. The selection is based on the belief structure of the particular nursing community—for example, care of people who are chronically ill and need major assistance with health needs versus the wellness initiatives applicable in occupational settings. The paradigm is determined by the type of nursing, because it meets the health needs of a particular group in a certain environment or setting.

The **metaparadigm** is the overall concern of nursing common to each nursing model, whether a conceptual model/paradigm or formal theory. Fawcett (1995, 2000, 2005) and Fawcett and DeSanto-Madeya (2013) have described the following four requirements for a discipline's metaparadigm: identity, inclusiveness, neutrality, and internationality. First, the metaparadigm must provide an identity for the profession that is distinctly different from that of others. Second, the metaparadigm must address all phenomena of interest to the profession in a manageable and understandable manner. Third, the metaparadigm must be neutral, so that all smaller practice paradigms can fit under the umbrella metaparadigm. And, finally, the metaparadigm must be "global in scope and substance" (Fawcett and DeSanto-Madeya, 2013, p. 4) to represent the profession across national, social, cultural, and ethnic boundaries. With that in mind, the metaparadigm of professional nursing incorporates four concepts:

● *Human beings* represent the individual, family, group, or community receiving care, each with unique characteristics.
● The *environment* comprises the physical, social, cultural, spiritual, and emotional climate or setting(s) in which the person lives, works, plays, and interacts.
● *Health* is the focus for the particular type of nursing and specific care provisions needed.
● *Nursing* is defined by its activities, goals, and services.

In any area of professional nursing practice, we can evaluate who the person is as the patient or recipient of nursing care, where the person and the caregiver are seen and influenced by others, why the person needs professional nursing care, and how the professional nurse functions as a provider or manager of care. These concepts are present whether the patient is the frail elder in an acute care setting, the expanding family in a birthing center, or an employee group in an occupational setting. Investigate these concepts specific to your own practice setting for an initial view of the systematic theory and knowledge base of your disciplinary paradigm. Look at how the "patient" is defined in the environmental context. And consider the health actions: Are they perceived as emerging, maintaining, enhancing, or perhaps palliative? Now, how do the nursing actions address patients, in their environment, to meet the concept of health?

Authority

The next characteristic of a professional is authority, as viewed by the patient. This **authority** occurs through education and experience, which give the professional the knowledge and skills to make professional judgments. The patient perceives the professional as having the knowledge and expertise to assist the patient in meeting some need. The professional is therefore viewed as an authority in the area, and his or her judgments are trusted. Authority is the basis for the competence the patient perceives and the patient-professional relationship.

In the nurse-patient relationship, the nurse is perceived as the authority figure, whether providing a selected care technique or filling an informational need. The competence and skill demonstrated justify the patient's trust in the professional nurse. Benner (1984) has described the following five levels of competency in clinical nursing practice: novice, advanced beginner, competent, proficient, and expert (p. xvii). The higher the levels of competence or expertise patients perceive in any profession, the greater trust or authority they place in the practitioners of that profession. Patients and their significant others who see nurses as experts in providing needed healthcare view the profession as having more authority in healthcare judgments. On the basis of this perception of authority, society grants the profession and its practitioners certain rights, privileges, and responsibilities.

Community Sanction

Society grants each profession certain powers and obligations to practice the specific profession. *Nursing's Policy Statement: The Essence of the Profession* (American Nurses Association [ANA], 2010a) attributes professional nursing's authority to a social contract with the community. The professional community is responsible for ensuring safe and effective practice within the discipline. Professional and legal regulation of nursing practice as a **community sanction** occurs through statutes, rules and regulations, definition of practice, and expectations for practitioners. Powers for entry and continuity in the profession are granted through licensure and professional practice parameters dictated in the state practice acts. These laws define a specific practice and provide regulatory powers at the state level for the board, licensing of professionals and protection of title (e.g., RN or APRN), general practice standards, approvals for educational programs, and disciplinary procedures.

Definition of practice and specific practice standards are further specified within the professional community through major nursing associations. The American Nurses Association (ANA) has specified a variety of practice standards for the profession, both general and specific to certain practice areas. The ANA has prepared several specialty standards documents jointly with the particular specialty organization to reflect the expectations for specialized professional practice. These standards, which signify the sanction by the community of the nursing profession, are authoritative statements by which nurses practicing within the role, population, and specialty describe duties they are expected to competently perform and may be used as evidence of the standard of care governing the given context of nursing practice (ANA, 2010b, p. 2).

The publication *Nursing: Scope and Standards of Practice* (ANA, 2010b), for example, prescribes standards of practice and standards of professional performance. Standards of practice address safe and competent practice in general or specialty practice and use of the nursing process with the actions of assessment, diagnosis, outcome identification, planning, implementation, and evaluation (ANA, 2010b). Standards of professional performance are expected professional roles and behaviors, including ethics, education, evidence-based practice and research, quality of practice, communication, leadership, collaboration, professional practice evaluation, resource utilization, and environmental health (ANA, 2010b).

Further standards of specialty practice are provided through the certification process with specialized education, testing, and ongoing learning requirements. Practice standards and expectations have also been developed by the applicable specialty organizations. Check the Web sites listed in Appendix A for standards of practice expected in selected specialty practice areas.

Another area in which the community grants a profession certain privileges on the basis of professional knowledge and expertise is in the education process of future clinicians and practitioners. Educational programs are both approved at the individual state level, as by the Board of Nursing, and accredited at the national level, as by the Commission on Collegiate Nursing Education (CCNE). Development, implementation, and evaluation of the organization, curriculum, faculty, students, graduates, facilities, and program resources are important considerations within the accreditation and reaccreditation process. The job of establishing and evaluating these standards falls to the professional accrediting groups. Here again, the profession is granted the power by the community and has the responsibility to provide the community with practitioners who are appropriately educated for safe and effective practice.

ONLINE CONSULT

American Nurses Association at
http://www.nursingworld.org
American Association of Colleges of Nursing
http://www.aacn.nche.edu

Educational programs are also guided by professional nursing standards. The American Association of Colleges of Nursing (AACN) has specified educational standards for nursing programs at the baccalaureate, master's, and doctoral levels. These essential curricular elements serve as core elements for the educational programs and delineate expected outcomes for the nursing programs by educational level (AACN, 2011, p. 3). Consider the differences in the essentials for baccalaureate and master's nursing education listed in Box 1.1. Further information on and description of these expected curricular elements can be found on the AACN website at http://www.aacn.nche.edu/education-resources/essential-series.

Confidentiality of patient information is one of the most important professional privileges. Professional nursing enjoys this privilege and conscientiously guards the confidentiality of patient information. As discussed in relation to ethical codes, confidentiality is a major consideration in professional nursing practice.

Code of Ethics

A professional abides by a certain **code of ethics** applicable to the practice area. Developed within the profession, the code addresses general ethical practice issues as well as professional personal and practice values, and colleague relationships. The ANA's *Code of Ethics for Nurses* is the ethical standard for professional nursing practice. It embodies both formal and informal ethical codes. The Code is non-negotiable in any setting . . . . [and expresses] the values, virtues, and obligations that shape, guide, and inform nursing as a profession" (ANA,

2015, p. vii). The interpretative statements promote understanding for appropriate application of the code of ethics in professional practice. Adherence to this specific code may be regulated in your state's practice act. To view the ANA Code of Ethics with Interpretative Statements, go online to http://nursingworld.org/codeofethics. However, there are other ethical codes, including the International Council of Nurses (ICN) *Code of Ethics for Nurses* (2012), which presents four elements associated with nurses: people, practice, the profession, and coworkers. In addition, for each of the elements, the roles of practitioners and managers, educators and researchers, and national nursing associations are illustrated. Achieving professional status requires ethical standards for expected behaviors with patients, colleagues, and other professionals.

Professional Culture

The fifth characteristic of a profession is a professional culture. Greenwood (1957) described **professional culture** as the formal and informal groups represented in the profession. *Formal groups* refer to the organizational systems in which the professionals practice, the educational institutions

> ### ONLINE CONSULT
> ANA Code of Ethics for Nurses with Interpretative Statements at
> **http://www.nursingworld.org/codeofethics**
> ICN Code of Ethics for Nurses at
> **http://www.icn.ch/icncode.pdf**

BOX 1.1 **The AACN Essentials for Collegiate Nursing Programs**

1.1 **The AACN Essentials for Collegiate Nursing Education**
   The Essentials of Baccalaureate Education for Professional Nursing Practice (AACN, 2008)
   I. Liberal Education for Baccalaureate Generalist Nursing Practice
   II. Basic Organizational and Systems Leadership for Quality Care and Patient Safety
   III. Scholarship for Evidence-based Practice
   IV. Information Management and Application of Patient Care Technology
   V. Healthcare Policy, Finance, and Regulatory Environments
   VI. Interprofessional Communication and Collaboration for Improving Patient Health Outcomes
   VII. Clinical Prevention and Population Health
   VIII. Professionalism and Professional Values
   IX. Baccalaureate Generalist Nursing Practice
   The Essentials of Master's Education in Nursing (AACN, 2011)
   I. Background for Practice from Sciences and Humanities
   II. Organizational and Systems Leadership
   III. Quality Improvement and Safety
   IV. Translating and Integrating Scholarship into Practice
   V. Informatics and Healthcare Technologies
   VI. Health Policy and Advocacy
   VII. Interprofessional Collaboration for Improving Patient and Population Health Outcomes
   VIII. Clinical Prevention and Population Health for Improving Health
   IX. Master's-Level Nursing Practice

Source: Reprinted with permission from the American Association of Colleges of Nursing, *Essentials Series*, © 2011, 2008 (http://www.aacn.nche.edu/education-resources/essential-series).

that provide for basic and continued learning, and the professional associations. *Informal groups* are the collegial settings that provide for collaboration, stimulation, and sharing of mutual values. These informal groups exist within each formal group, providing further professional, collegial inclusiveness. These groups and the unique culture of nursing are reinforced in the *Code of Ethics for Nurses.*

Organizational systems in which professional nursing is practiced are diverse and multidimensional. As you will see in later chapters, hospital and home health agency settings are complex parts of a larger system. Professional nursing practice provides a unique culture with the values and norms expected of its practitioners. Organizational philosophies and mission statements provide information on the expressed culture of these settings. Further expression of the professional culture is apparent in the behaviors of professional nurses who practice in these settings.

Formal educational settings for professional nursing practice occur in institutions of higher learning with liberal and specialized learning requirements. In addition, values and norms for continued learning and competency in practice are transmitted as expectations for professional practice. Beyond basic educational practice, **professional development** is provided through continuing education and specialty preparation and continual competency as a professional.

Professional organizations or associations are a major component of the culture of professional nursing practice, but they vary in purpose or mission and membership. The purpose of some professional organizations, such as the ANA or the Canadian Nurses Association, is to represent the profession on a national basis. Specialty groups, with a more specific focus, promote education, skills, standards, and perhaps certification opportunities for a particular segment of the profession—for example, the American Association of Critical-Care Nurses. Each organization has a unique philosophy or mission directed at professional nursing practice.

Professional organizations communicate values and norms in official publications, position statements, and specified practice standards. These organizations promote professional parameters for clinical practice, education, administration, and research. They provide educational opportunities and foster expansion of the knowledge base of individual professionals and the discipline in general. Some organizations focus specifically on the science of the profession. Their purpose is to promote the scholarly aspects of the profession and to build professional and leadership skills through education, publications, and conferences. A more global view of practice can be seen in many professional organizations as they reach out to influence public policy. In addition, professional organizations often collaborate with each other on vital issues that enhance the impact and the influence to the professional and public communities.

Consider the organizations that represent professional nursing practice and education listed in Table 1.1. The ANA and its state and territorial associations focus mainly on the profession as an entity, with concern for the health of society as well as the welfare of professional nurses through standards, official position statements, political action initiatives, and certification options for specialty practice. Specific to an area of specialty practice, the American Association of Critical-Care Nurses, with its worldwide membership, is the largest specialty organization. Also more globally, the International Council of Nurses (ICN) is composed of professional associations from over 130 countries, including the ANA. The American Association of Colleges of Nursing focuses on collegiate education, serving member schools with baccalaureate and higher-degree programs through educational standards, programs, policies, research, accreditation, and legislative initiatives directed at high-quality professional education. This organization has published documents identifying educational essentials important for the various nursing education programs. The National League for Nursing (NLN) has individual and agency membership for educational institutions and focuses on excellence in nursing education from practical nursing to graduate education. The National Council of State Boards of Nursing is composed of the member regulatory boards for the 50 states, the District of Columbia, and four U.S. territories as well as international regulatory bodies for nursing as associate members. Sigma Theta Tau, the international honor society for nursing, has a distinctly scientific focus. This organization promotes knowledge development through research, dissemination of scientific information, technology, education, interdisciplinary collaboration, and adaptability for the improvement of the health of people worldwide.

A comprehensive listing of professional organizations and their Web site addresses is located in Appendix A and on the Intranet site. In addition, useful links to additional resources may be discovered within these sites. Just one word of caution: Web site addresses change, as do physical addresses. Try to update your Internet "favorites" listing regularly with any changes and add new sites that you have found useful.

PROFESSIONALISM IN NURSING

We have viewed the profession of nursing according to general attributes. However, consider the specific attributes of the practice professionals specified as standards for professional performance: ethics, education, evidence-based practice and research, quality of practice, communication, leadership, collaboration, professional practice evaluation, resource utilization, and environmental health (ANA, 2010b). In subsequent chapters we will consider specifics on legal and ethical issues, education, evidence-based practice, quality of practice, communication, leadership, and environmental health. But, look further at the following expectations of professional nurses that are guideposts for your professional development.

Ethics

Adherence to a code of **ethics** is expected in any profession. As discussed previously, the *Code of Ethics for Nurses with Interpretative Statements* (ANA, 2015) provides the broad guidelines. It is the responsibility of the practicing professional to know these guidelines and practice in

TABLE 1.1

Characteristics of Professional Organizations

Organization	Focus, Mission, and Membership
American Nurses Association (ANA) and associated constituent state associations and organizational affiliate members Founded 1897 http://www.nursing world.org	**Focus**: Professional nursing **Mission**: "Nurses advancing our profession to improve health for all" (ANA, 2014, p. 1). **Membership**: Individual membership; professional nurses at the state level obtain national membership.
American Association of Colleges of Nursing (AACN) Founded 1969 http://www.aacn.nche.edu	**Focus**: Collegiate nursing education **Mission**: The AACN "serves the public interest by setting standards, providing resources, and developing the leadership capacity of member schools to advance nursing education, research, and practice" (AACN, 2014, p. 1). **Membership**: Deans and directors of member schools with baccalaureate and higher-degree nursing programs
American Association of Critical-Care Nurses (AACN) Founded 1969 http://www.aacn.org	**Focus**: Specialty care **Mission**: "Patients and their families rely on nurses at the most vulnerable times of their lives. Acute and critical care nurses rely on AACN for expert knowledge and the influence to fulfill their promise to patients and their families. AACN drives excellence because nothing less is acceptable" (AACN, 2014, p. 1). **Membership**: Individual membership
International Council of Nurses (ICN) Founded 1899 http://www.icn.ch	**Focus**: Nursing internationally **Mission**: The ICN's mission is "to represent nursing worldwide, advancing the profession and influencing health policy" (ICN, 2013, p. 1). **Membership**: National nurses' associations representing nurses in more than 130 countries
National Council of State Boards of Nursing (NCSBN) Founded 1978 (previously a component of the ANA) http://www.ncsbn.org	**Focus**: Nursing regulation and public protection **Mission**: The NCSBN "provides education, service, and research through collaborative leadership to promote evidence-based regulatory excellence for patient safety and public protection" (NCSBN, 2014, p. 1). **Membership**: All state boards of nursing in the 50 states, the District of Columbia, American Samoa, Guam, Northern Mariana Islands, and the Virgin Islands.
National League for Nursing (NLN) and associated constituent leagues Founded 1952 http://www.nln.org	**Focus**: Nursing education and community health **Mission**: The NLN "promotes excellence in nursing education to build a strong and diverse nursing workforce" to advance the nation's health (NLN, 2013, p. 1). **Membership**: Individuals, Schools of Nursing, Associate Agency membership
Sigma Theta Tau International Honor Society of Nursing and member chapters Founded 1922 http://www.nursingsociety.org	**Focus**: Nursing scholarship (international) **Mission**: Sigma Theta Tau's mission is "advancing world health and celebrating nursing excellence in scholarship, leadership, and service" (Sigma Theta Tau, 2014, p. 1). **Membership**: Individuals are invited to membership in chartered chapters with selection criteria as baccalaureate or higher-degree students, faculty members, or community leaders.

Note: Reference citations in table are excerpts from online resources of the respective nursing organizations.

accordance with the code. In 1993, Miller and associates reported that most professional nurse respondents did not have a copy of the ethical code, and many were unfamiliar with the document (p. 293). This problem occurred with the 1985 *Code of Ethics*. The question then becomes, how many nurses are aware of the 2001 revision and the current code revised in 2015? To meet this criterion of professionalism, nursing professionals need to demonstrate greater knowledge and understanding of the official ethical code. Periodic review of the ethical provisions and their interpretative statements is an important responsibility for all professional nurses. This is especially true when the roles of nurses or patients change, but it is also important for nurses to appreciate fully their professional responsibilities, challenges, and talents when roles are stable.

Ethical considerations also involve personal and interpersonal actions, beyond those directly related to the individual situation, as with autonomy and self-regulation. Autonomy means independent judgment and self-governing within the scope of one's practice, which changes in response to people's healthcare needs. As key professionals in organizational settings, nurses make the time and commitment to ensure that high-quality care and standards are present and upheld. This involves critical analysis, communication, collaboration, and leadership. Important concepts in this area are professional responsibility and accountability. In the *Code of Ethics for Nurses*, responsibility is defined as "an obligation to perform required professional activities at a level commensurate with one's education and in compliance with applicable laws and standards . . ." (ANA, 2015, p. 45) whereas, accountability is being answerable to self and others for one's own choices, decisions and actions as measured against a standard . . ." such as the Code (ANA, 2015, p. 41). Nurses are accountable to both themselves and their patients for good clinical judgment and quality care. However, as we will see in later chapters, accountability is also extended to the broader population as the profession demonstrates involvement in social policy.

Educational Background

The **educational background** required for professional practice is specified to ensure safe and effective practice. In nursing, the basic education required for entry into the profession varies, with differences among baccalaureate, associate degree, diploma education, and even entry-level graduate programs. But within each type of educational program, curricula and requirements are guided by general standards, and, as stated in two of the four key elements of the IOM (2011) *Future of Nursing: Advancing Health, Leading Change* report, nurses should practice to the full extent of their education and achieve higher levels of education.

Although a school's curriculum is developed by its faculty members, certain standards are required for an educational program. Nursing curricula must contain essential content and hours as required by state boards of nursing, higher education boards, professional associations, and national accrediting bodies. Consumers of nursing care can be confused by the different educational routes leading to the title of registered nurse. Numerous studies have reviewed the various health professions, their regulatory bodies, educational program requirements, and workforce needs with respect to the changing healthcare system. Consumer confusion and overlapping scopes of practice are key issues that must be addressed. Ongoing clarification of these areas among professionals and consumers of nursing will have a beneficial effect on the view of nursing as a profession and of individual nurses as true professionals. However, some skills do cross professional boundaries and are important considerations in collaborative practice.

A 2003 report from the Institute of Medicine following a Health Professions Education Summit led to the identification of five **core competencies** (Box 1.2) that are required of all health professions to advance a vision for the education of all health professionals "to deliver patient-centered care as members of an interdisciplinary team, emphasizing evidence-based practice, quality improvement approaches, and informatics" (Greiner & Knebel, 2003, p. 45). To address these competencies in nursing education programs, curricula must be constantly evaluated for currency, content, and practice opportunities. For example, most nurses will agree that providing patient-centered care is a component of our nursing programs. However, we need to assess carefully whether all programs foster interdisciplinary and evidence-based practice focused on quality improvement and the use of informatics.

Beyond the basic education, competent practice requires ongoing learning, continuing education, and continued competency. These attributes are crucial to safe, effective, and ethical professional practice. Ongoing improvement and knowledge are the goals of continuing education, which is required for relicensure in some states and recertification in specialty areas. But continuing education involves more than obtaining required credits, in-service hours, and formal degrees. Remaining current with ideas presented in the nursing and scientific literature is an important component of continued competency as a professional and to incorporate evidence-based information into practice.

The Internet has made remaining current on issues of concern to the profession more convenient. Yet, a word of caution is in order: It is important to evaluate the source of information and its validity. Consider whether the information is provided by an organization, an agency, or an individual's own Web site and personal perspective.

Identifying your own learning and developmental needs is an expectation and a continual process for competent professional practice. In essence, continuing education for competency involves self-assessment, ongoing learning, and self-evaluation. The focus is on discovery, as in baccalaureate and graduate education. Ongoing learning means that your mind is challenged every day with new ideas, building on a professional knowledge base and skills. Opportunities for continuing education abound through a variety of formal programs as well as through professional journals and online resources. Many professional organizations have special online services for their

---

BOX 1.2 Core Competencies for Health Professionals

- Provide patient-centered care
- Work in interdisciplinary teams
- Employ evidence-based practice
- Apply quality improvement
- Utilize informatics

Source: Greiner, A. C., & Knebel, E. (eds.). (2003). *Health professions education: A bridge to quality.* Washington, DC: Institute of Medicine (p. 48). Permission to reproduce material copyrighted by National Academies Press.

members, such as reviews of current literature and care products, bookstores, continuing education programs, e-mail lists, and online discussion forums. Publishers also have online resources with special discounts, e-mail updates, associated Web sites, discussion groups, and interactive continuing education offerings. The ongoing challenge is developing new knowledge, and it is the responsibility of the professional to maintain currency for the specific practice area and to document his or her professional efforts and progress.

Evidence-Based Practice and Research

Nursing research is much more than leading or participating in a research study. We now look to the core competency of **evidence-based practice and research** to guide the way we practice. Greiner and Knebel (2003) define evidence-based practice as the integration of the best research with clinical expertise and the patient's values for optimum care, as well as participation in learning and research activities (pp. 45–46). As found in the interpretive statements of the *Code for Nurses*, "All nurses must participate in the advancement of the profession through the knowledge development, evaluation, dissemination, and application to practice" (ANA, 2015, p. 27).

Involvement in research—whether by using findings, participating in an investigation, protecting human subjects, or searching the literature for demonstrated innovations in practice—is a characteristic of professionalism in nursing. It adds to our knowledge base, enhances our practice, promotes improved outcomes for our patients and fosters practice based on evidence of efficacy rather than tradition or trial and error. Collaborating with others and sharing new knowledge is critical in this process. We will focus further on evidence-based practice and research in Chapter 5.

Quality of Practice

The effectiveness of nursing care to address appropriate and measurable patient outcomes is an expectation of the professional nurse. In addition, recall that improvement in the **quality of practice** is a core competency of all health professionals. It is not just a matter of determining whether a nursing intervention was appropriate and effectively addressed the healthcare need. Now, questions are raised on further improvements that can be made based on the evidence presented in the current case and through documented evidence of practice effectiveness. Quality improvement is the goal for making refinements in practice that are based on efficacy and efficiency. Efficacy in meeting the patient outcomes is not sufficient for professional practice. The activities must be acceptable for the patient population in addressing our metaparadigm concepts of human beings, health, environment, and nursing. The patient is the focus, and efficiency is a vital consideration to preserve resources, both personal resources (such as energy of both the patient and the nurse) and the material and physical healthcare resources in the environment. So, the question becomes, how can practice in the future be made safer and more effective? This question can lead to innovative and changed practices for improved patient outcomes, considering human needs, the environment, the concept of health, and care techniques and technologies.

Communication

Effective **communication** has long been a focus and characteristic of professional nursing. In a subsequent chapter, we will review this important content, as it is an area that needs constant reevaluation in different situations and with different individuals. And effective communication skills are essential with patients as well as nursing colleagues and other members of the healthcare team. Consider communication as more than a verbal encounter with another individual, but rather an interaction involving all the interpersonal and cultural facets. Appropriate verbal messages must be communicated into the plan of care, be documented appropriately, be shared through a variety of channels and media, and lead to quality improvements for the care of patients. Dissent, debate, conflict, and negotiation are natural outcomes and, again, must focus on quality healthcare. And think further about evolving technologies, as in the case of telehealth, with patients and providers interacting at a distance. Effective communication skills are in constant refinement for the professional nurse who is on the front line managing and leading the team for quality patient outcomes. We will consider refinement of interpersonal and professional communication skills in Chapter 6.

Leadership

Leadership is an expectation for the professional nurse, both in the practice setting and in the profession. Nurses must project a positive image and the vision and actions needed for effective patient outcomes on a daily basis and in an effective working environment. Managing care effectively and leading others in the process is more than a job requirement but also a commitment to patients, colleagues, and the profession. And leadership extends beyond the care environment to involvement in the institution or agency, as with shared governance or committee involvement, and in the profession at large.

Nurses also assume leadership positions in the community, through service activities using their unique knowledge, skills, and abilities. Nurses are well equipped and talented in this area because of their orientation of service to patients and society at large. Nurses frequently lead health-promoting activities in their employment role, their professional community, and among their families and acquaintances. Consider how residents in a defined community always seem to know who the nurses in the area are and how frequently those nurses are approached with questions or requests to become involved in projects or serve on committees. Also consider how nurses reach out to others with information on healthcare issues or ideas to foster wellness in their communities. This vision of the community also leads to involvement in healthcare policy and changes needed for improved health status and outcomes in the community.

Collaboration

Each of the standards of professional performance requires **collaboration** in practice. The ANA Standard of Performance on Collaboration includes the patient and the patient's significant others, and other healthcare providers in the plan of care (ANA, 2010b). Professional interactions and behaviors should be ethical and patient-centered, based on the information and needs of the colleagues who influence patients and on the quality of practice. These interactions require good communication and leadership skills focused on effective practice and quality outcomes. The healthcare team is focused on the patient and promoting positive outcomes, which do not occur in isolation by the efforts of one individual. This professional performance standard requires that colleagues assist each other and include the patient in the plan of care to promote long-term positive outcomes. Trust, openness, knowledge, skills, various professional abilities, and commitment are necessary parts of all interactions toward this aim of safe and effective patient-centered care.

Professional Practice Evaluation

The *Scope and Standards of Practice* (ANA, 2010b) specifies practice competencies in this area as the application of current "professional practice standards and guidelines, relevant statutes, rules, and regulations" (p. 59). **Professional practice evaluation** requires self-regulation by both the professional and the profession that sets the standards. The ANA's *Nursing's Policy Statement: The Essence of the Profession* (2010a) describes **self-regulation** as both personal accountability for the knowledge base for practice and participation in the peer review process (pp. 30–32). Professional responsibility and accountability involve upholding quality standards as well as developing and critically analyzing those standards and the outcomes. The regulation of nursing practice includes both self-regulation beyond a limited job description and professional regulation through the defined scope of practice, further education, certification, and adherence to the code of ethics.

Professionals are responsible and answerable to patients and their significant others for nursing care outcomes. And performance feedback from patients as well as professional colleagues should be included in a practice evaluation. Nurses are actively involved in supervising, delegating, and evaluating others. But reflection on professional performance assists in practice improvement as an important component of the peer review process, as part of an annual performance evaluation. The peer review process is a time for professional development for both the reviewer and the person being evaluated. The process is a learning opportunity and much more than a checklist and narrative comment provided on an annual basis.

Resource Utilization

Recall the concept of efficiency related to quality care. Innovative and changed practices for improved patient outcomes must address human needs, the environment, the concept of health, and care techniques and technologies. Identification, procurement, and the judicious use of healthcare resources are requirements of the professional role. The *Scope and Standards of Practice* (ANA, 2010b) describes **resource utilization** as not only the appropriate use of resources but also the assurance that nursing care be "safe, effective, and financially responsible" (p. 60). The focus continues to be on outcomes and the vital role of the nurse in promoting successful outcomes. In the healthcare environment, the focus is on safety and obtaining appropriate resources, supplies, and care provision. However, understanding cost factors and patient concerns and resources is essential. And think further than resources in the healthcare environment, especially when assisting the patient and family to prepare for care in the home and community. Will they have sufficient resources at home for safe healthcare practices? This includes the knowledge for safety at home and the value for the treatments needed, as well as the financial resources to obtain needed medication or treatment. Think about the individual with asthma and whether he or she will, in the long term, have short-term rescue and controller medications, the understanding for proper use and care, and the environmental adjustments needed for successful management of this chronic condition. The professional nurse is concerned with safe and effective care beyond the treatment facility with a focus on human beings, the environment, and health as part of effective nursing care for positive outcomes.

Environmental Health

With nursing's focus on the centrality of the environment in individuals' health and care, concerns over safety and health risks require constant attention and vigilance. Health professionals and consumers of healthcare were alarmed by the release of reports from the Institute of Medicine (IOM) of the National Academies on the high incidence of medical errors. These reports started in 1998 and led to ongoing efforts for improving patient safety, in both the hospital and community settings. The IOM is a nonprofit organization designed to provide science-based advice as a public service. The 2001 report from the IOM, *Crossing the Quality Chasm*, proposed ten rules for quality healthcare in the 21st century (Box 1.3). The six overall aims—that care should be safe, effective, patient-centered, timely, efficient, and equitable—underlie these ten rules (Corrigan et. al, 2001).

Patient safety and effectiveness of outcomes have become major national objectives and have directed additional attention to nursing, especially since the release of the landmark IOM report in 2011 on the *Future of Nursing: Leading Change, Advancing Health*. Research by the Agency for Healthcare Research and Quality (AHRQ) continues to expand the knowledge base on how the quality of the healthcare workplace affects the quality of the healthcare provided, especially in the areas of workload and working conditions, effects of stress and fatigue, reduction of adverse events, and the organizational climate and culture. Patient outcomes are viewed and investigated, along with nursing-sensitive indicators and factors that promote safe and effective practice.

Nurses play an essential role in their constant attention to the environment and the factors that could place patients

BOX 1.3	Rules for the 21st Century Health System

- Care is based on continuous healing relationships.
- Care is customized according to patient needs and values.
- The patient is the source of control.
- Knowledge is shared, and information flows freely.
- Decision making is evidence-based.
- Safety is a system property.
- Transparency is necessary.
- Needs are anticipated.
- Waste is continuously decreased.
- Cooperation among clinicians is a priority.

Source: Corrigan, M.S., Donaldson, M.S., Kohn, L.Y., Maguire, S.K., & Pike, K.C. (2001). *Crossing the quality chasm: A new health system for the 21st century.* Washington, DC: National Academy Press (pp. 61–62). Permission to reproduce material copyrighted by National Academies Press.

at risk. These include product defects, risky or improper medication practices, environmental artifacts like noise, and any other potential hazards. Attention to the environment for care to be safe, effective, patient-centered, timely, efficient, and equitable, and application of these ten rules, are the means for promoting environmental health.

Fulfilling the characteristics described in standards of professional performance is the challenge to you in your educational pursuit and your daily practice in nursing. Professionalism is an attribute in constant refinement. The degree to which professionals demonstrate professionalism in nursing is apparent in their professional practice and how they define nursing. But, have you prepared all your resources for this ongoing professional development?

RETURNING TO SCHOOL

This is a time to celebrate the talents you bring with you to your continuing knowledge development. It is a time for discovery, reflection, and professional development. You have had many experiences in educational settings. Unlike a child in school, the adult learner brings a wealth of experiences to the learning environment. Experiences of the adult learner may be varied, but they occurred in a certain environment or context and have meaning to the individual. To understand this meaning requires careful examination of your situation.

First, consider the reasons why you have returned to school. You may think that the recognition for your work or the pay differential on your career ladder is the reason. These may be considerations, but you are embarking on a journey of professional development that will further your knowledge, skills, and abilities compared with a quick fix to a limiting situation. You will be facing challenges of competing roles and addressing priorities in time management.

Competing Roles

As an adult, you are already engaged in multiple roles. **Roles** are organized behavioral patterns and expectations.

VandenBos (2013) defines a role as "a coherent set of behaviors expected of an individual in a specific position within a group or social setting" (p. 503). Now consider the multiple roles and positions in your unique circumstance.

You are probably employed as a registered nurse. The expectations for your work are written in the state law for practice and in the job description at your place of employment. There are also the less formal expectations of your supervisors and colleagues at work. However, there are many role opportunities in professional nursing. The American Association of Colleges of Nursing (AACN, 2008) has identified three primary roles of the baccalaureate-prepared generalist nurse: provider of care, designer/manager/coordinator of care, and member of the profession. Clinical nurse leaders (CNLs) also function as generalists in nursing practice but are prepared at the master's level in nursing. CNLs practice in an advanced generalist role and are providers and managers of care to individuals and cohorts of patients anywhere healthcare is delivered (AACN, 2014, pp. 1–2). Advanced practice nurses (APRNs) are prepared at the graduate level in nursing within one of four roles and function in a population foci specialty area as a nurse practitioner, clinical nurse specialist, nurse anesthetist, or nurse midwife. Nurses prepared at the master's or doctoral levels in nursing also function in role specialties or specialized advanced nursing positions such as nursing education, administration, informatics, research, public health, and policy analyst (ANA, 2010a). The *Scope and Standards of Practice* (ANA, 2010c) describes the importance to the profession of these specialized advanced nursing positions for the continued expansion of those areas of nursing practice that intersect with another body of knowledge but have a direct influence on nursing practice and support the care provided to patients by other RNs (p. 18).

Your future practice will be in one of these multiple roles of RN. However, your current situation has another role: adult learner. And this new role of student will influence your current career and personal roles. For example, how are your coworkers and supervisors reacting about your return to school? Consider the apparent and hidden behaviors, all of which have an impact on your progress. Align yourself with positive influences and try not be drawn into negativity.

Consider also your varied personal roles. You are also a member of a family—whether it is an extended family with intergenerational considerations, a single partnership, a single-parent family, or even a social or religious group. Your roles and responsibilities for caregiving occur by virtue of your membership in this unique group. You may be a parent concerned about your child's progress in elementary school or your teenager's involvement with a particular social group in high school. You may be living close to extended family members or be isolated by miles or situations. These are all considerations of your unique situation as an RN pursuing additional education.

You have now thought about both your family and work-related roles and responsibilities. Now, what about you? What are your deeply held wishes and desires—personal, career-related, and family-inspired? This is where competition and conflict can occur. Think about the questions posed in Box 1.4 and add others that apply to your personal situation. You made the right decision to return to school. Now relax and prepare. Plan to streamline your life (work, school, and family) and prepare for dealing with your competing roles and responsibilities. This situation is another form of multitasking—a more complex one than encountered in daily practice. You are advancing your career and professional practice through additional learning and building on your knowledge, skills, and abilities.

Learning As Empowerment

Learning is the perception and assimilation of the information presented to us in a variety of ways. Learning leads to knowledge and encompasses the following characteristics:

- Perception of new information
- Reaction to the information
- Ability to recall or repeat the information
- Understanding as rejection or acceptance of the information
- Use of the information in a similar situation
- Critical analysis of the information
- Incorporation of the information into the value system
- Use of the information in various situations and combinations

An increasing complexity emerges here as the learner moves from receiving and recalling information through understanding, application, analysis, and evaluation, to the point of creating new applications.

There are also three domains, or categories, of learning: affective, cognitive, and psychomotor. The affective domain includes attitudes, feelings, and values—for example, how you feel about returning to school. Your perception and value of the positive effects on your life will influence your progress. The cognitive domain involves knowledge and thought processes within an individual's intellectual ability. This cognitive domain involves your understanding of the information received about pathophysiology, theory, and the other areas for knowledge acquisition. The psychomotor domain is probably the one you are most comfortable with. This domain involves the processing and demonstration of behaviors, as with the performance of a skill like changing a dressing or starting an IV infusion.

Learning activities can be very different for the three domains, but continued learning leads to empowerment. Remember, to achieve a lasting change in observed behavior (psychomotor domain), the value of that change (affective domain) and the intellectual capacity to understand and process the information for behavioral changes (cognitive domain) must first be present. What are some of your individual learning needs?

Building Knowledge, Skills, and Abilities

Your plan for professional practice should be tailored to your situation and learning needs, taking into account your knowledge, skills, and abilities. **Knowledge** is the accumulation of appropriate information through learning and experience. **Skill** is the ability to retrieve this knowledge through mental and psychomotor activities and apply it appropriately to a situation. **Ability** refers to your competence and proficiency in the demonstration of that knowledge and skill. Your personal plan needs to address your knowledge, skills, and abilities for success in your nursing program. Consider the particular factors in your own situation.

First, look at your educational goals. Think about your timeline for program completion and determine whether adjustments may be needed to accommodate additional time commitments. Given your personal timeline, consider the factors that will promote your success. Consider the time required for the program. If you are employed, what adjustments to your schedule will need to be made? Do you have to factor in travel for classes or library research? Some nursing programs require a certain number of courses arranged in a specific semester plan with classes, labs or clinical, online activities, and library research. What

---

BOX 1.4 What Are Your Competing and Multiple Roles?

- Will your employer adjust your work schedule for you to attend class or use the library?
- How did your coworkers react (CNAs, LPNs, RN peers, supervisors, others) when they found out you were taking this course?
- Have you taken the prerequisite courses, such as statistics, for the nursing program?
- What study materials do you have readily available?
- How are your computer skills?
- What expectations do your partner, family, or child(ren) have for your returning to school: high/low/none? Are they supportive or unsupportive?
- What are your expectations?
- What will you do to ensure you have the time needed for each of your roles?
- Do you have resources for childcare, if needed?
- If needed, did you apply for tuition assistance through your employer or at the college?
- Do you have any outstanding loans? Are they a worry?
- Do you have reliable transportation to get to work as well as to classes?
- Did taking this course seem like a good plan at the time but now you are having second thoughts?
- Others?

is your computer access and how are your skills with presentation graphics and attaching files? Have you completed some of the prerequisite work? And what about other courses required in the program—have you plotted them into your timeline?

There may be areas in which you want to do some enhancement work. Consider your resources and materials for review. Your program may offer review or tutorial requirements to allow you to refresh certain content areas or to learn about areas that were not known at the time of your program, such as genetics and genomics competencies. If review opportunities are available, take advantage of them and take them seriously. Review and refreshment opportunities can add to your supply of personal knowledge, skills, and abilities.

Look further at your present job. Will the schedule permit you to stay in that job, perhaps on a reduced schedule, or will you need to find another job? How will your peers at work react to you once you are really progressing through the program? You may experience unanticipated reactions, including hostility.

Another consideration is unanticipated costs. You may be evaluating the cost of tuition, books, and materials, but what about additional travel to a clinical site, reduced salary due to a reduced working schedule, and added costs for childcare and perhaps prepared meals? Is your tuition assistance available only after you have successfully completed a course? Are there delays that must be factored into your plan? What other costs will be unique to your situation?

Now, consider your family and significant others. What support systems are available, and what other ones may be needed by you and your family members? You need to differentiate educational commitments that are required during a semester from family activities that can become prominent during semester breaks. This may be the opportunity to have a "family meeting" to discuss the situation. Nurses often do not like to ask for help, but perhaps family members can be enlisted to take on some of the household chores. You may get to a point down the road when your son or daughter scolds you, telling you that you had better get *your* school work done before you can play!

Your own health is also a consideration. Remember, to effectively care for others, you must take good care of yourself. All of this requires prioritization of needs, roles, activities, and, especially, time management skills.

ADDRESSING TIME MANAGEMENT

Now look at your time management skills. What do you do well and what can be further developed? Identify your "time wasters" and your "time enhancers." Much reflection on your part will be involved in this activity—it is not a one-size-fits-all situation. You are unique as is your environment and the people around you. Someone once asked me how I had the time to do a particular activity. My first response was "I make the time." Then I thought about it and added, "I get up an hour earlier, and that seems to work best." It's all about reflecting on the activity and planning ahead, as with a dressing change, to set aside the time and have all the materials at hand. Remember, no one has yet figured out how to add more minutes to the day. So, within any given 24-hour period, you must determine the most efficient use of time. Look at the factors identified in Box 1.5. Depending on your roles and unique situation, you will likely need to add other factors for effective time management, whether at work, at home, at school, in the library, or online. Be honest and realistic, but do not get lost in the details.

Your Learning Style

Learning styles and associated inventories have been discussed with varied research for over 50 years in an attempt to improved teaching and learning outcomes. (See Box 1.6.) The research and discussion continue as we seek to understand better how individuals acquire meaning and knowledge. Increasingly we are concerned with the active involvement of the learner in the process. Your **learning style** is simply the ways you best perceive, think, organize, use, and retain knowledge. To understand this concept, merely recall colleagues in the same learning environment—those who take a lot notes, those who just listen, and those who make notes or drawings on what they interpret the message in the lecture to be. Understanding differences in learning styles can help teachers and learners make more informed decisions

---

BOX 1.5   Factors to Consider for Efficient Time Management

Family
- Meals
- Homework
- Laundry
- Relationships
- Social obligations

Work
- Work schedule
- Hours and fatigue
- Coworkers and colleagues
- Practices to refine
- Scope of practice

School/College
- Costs
- Transportation
- Learning needs
- Course requirements
- Academic schedule and timeline

Personal
- Health and fitness
- Hope and aspirations
- Spirituality
- Knowledge, skills, and abilities
- Individual needs

Myers-Briggs Inventory

The Myers-Briggs Inventory is used widely in education and business applications. A classification system of four scales identifies 16 personality types that can be further classified for learning preferences:

- Introversion—Extroversion
- Sensing—Intuition
- Thinking—Feeling
- Judging—Perceptive

Source: Myers & Briggs Foundation. (2014). MBTI basics. Retrieved from http://www.myersbriggs.org/my-mbti-personality-type/mbti-basics/

about which learning activities will be useful or productive to them as individuals and as members of learning groups or communities.

Individuals with different learning styles vary in their preferences for how they absorb and assimilate information:

- visual learning (reading or watching)
- auditory learning (listening or talking)
- kinesthetic learning (doing or participating)

For example, some learners are highly visual in the way they perceive information and derive meaning. For these learners, a structured lecture with few visual aids is a less desirable learning environment than one enhanced by visual aids. Others learn better through the written word, by either reading or taking notes. Learners who are highly auditory in their learning preference derive greater meaning from just listening to the information. One of the exercises at the end of this chapter is the identification of your particular learning style.

The learning environment for health professionals has changed. The explosion of knowledge that continues on a daily basis no longer allows for the memorization of discrete facts. Health professionals must understand the underlying concepts, discover new information, reflect on applications, and apply relevant knowledge to their situation. Reflection and critical analysis are important parts of this process. The learner is now active in the process, no longer considering the teacher as the "sage on the stage" but rather as the facilitator of learning. You, as the learner, are the active one, seeing how information fits with facts and perceptions. Recall that in Mezirow's (2000) view of transformative learning, adults learn by elaborating existing frames of reference, learning new frames of reference, transforming points of view, or transforming habits of mind (p. 19). Building on your knowledge base and your personal frame of reference, you will learn new perspectives. This process will further allow you as the adult learner to transform your views, and create new ways of approaching the world and nursing practice.

Learning occurs through reflection and interpretation to understand perceptions of the self and the world. But you also need to identify and organize your resources.

GARNERING RESOURCES

Consider the resources that you will need to assist you as a student. Perhaps the initial things that come to mind are books, a stethoscope, a computer, and perhaps a car to get to a class meeting or clinical site. Look beyond supplies and reliable transportation. **Resources** are tools or means of support. Consider those things and people that can help you study, prepare assignments, succeed on examinations, and thrive in your education.

Studying

Once you understand your learning style, you can look to the resources needed to capitalize on your assets. Remember, once you know your style, you will still be in a group with individuals with varying styles, including the instructor. If you learn best through participation in discussions, you may want to find a compatible study group. But a word of caution: Study groups are not for everyone and can be time wasters if the group is not focused, compatible, and committed to ground rules of preparing on the topic prior to the meeting. In addition, some individuals are more solitary and need to think about something for a while and work it out in their frame of reference before being put on the spot in a discussion.

Your environment is another area you need to carefully consider, with regard to where you best think and concentrate. Do you prefer a completely quiet environment or soft background music? Think about what helps you to understand information and see relationships. Do you have a favorite place in the house, either a cozy corner or a clean kitchen table after the children are in bed? Maybe it is in a special chair with the cat in your lap. Or perhaps it is at the library where additional resources are available without other distractions. Again, you must determine your best environment to concentrate and be open to new information.

Preparing Assignments

This is an area feared by many returning students, as they face a blank piece of paper or computer screen. First, write or type the expectation. It may help to see it isolated from the distraction of other course expectations and grading criteria. Make sure you have sufficient access to a reliable computer for document preparation, sending and receiving e-mail, accessing the Internet, and preparing presentation graphics. Competing with your spouse or children for time online does not count! Locate the dictionary tool and make sure you have the spelling and grammar checking tools activated to assist you in the composition process. You will also need to become comfortable with the publication style required by your school or instructor. One popular style is by the American Psychological Association (2010), and you may be required to use this resource. These basic tools and your development of skill in these areas will facilitate your ease in making your case as you address the requirements of an assignment, whether a case study or a scholarly paper.

Another valuable resource is a professional librarian, especially one who can help you effectively search for materials, teach you how to access databases, and provide you with interlibrary loan materials. A librarian can show you how to access the library remotely over the Internet to help with your time management and cut down on travel to the library during certain hours. But be sure use all your time management skills when searching online to avoid getting distracted or lost in the sea of information.

Sooner or later in your program of study you will have a group assignment in which the group, not each individual, earns the grade. This type of activity can be accomplished in person or online and may be a wonderful team experience—or a disaster with an uncooperative member. Peer pressure is warranted; if that is not effective, consult your instructor. Remember, teams are an important part of collaborative practice and we need to continually refine our skills in this area.

Taking Examinations

The thought of taking tests is one of the most threatening to the adult learner. Stress management techniques such as deep breathing may help. Some of the most important considerations are adequate rest and being confident in your preparation and understanding of the content. Understanding the information is critical, especially since test questions in nursing focus on critical analysis and rarely involve the simple recall of isolated facts. Beyond simple memorization of facts such as the bones and muscles of the leg, more complexity is added for application of this information to a patient situation. And then grades are an issue, with the adult learner trying to do "the best" or else experience a personal sense of failure. Remember, a grading scale is just that: a scale that varies. There are certain acceptable numbers on your bathroom scale, just as there should be acceptable numbers or letters on a grading scale. There will be times when you excel and others when you succeed but do not achieve an A—and that is acceptable. Give yourself permission to be human and not always receive the top grade in the course. Understanding, retention, and application of knowledge are the more important considerations.

Thriving

One of the most important actions you can take as you pursue your nursing degree is to thrive on the acquisition of your new knowledge, skills, and abilities. Lifelong learning is a component of professional nursing. From your practice, armed with technical skills and experience in the practice setting, we advance to critical analysis and clinical judgment that embody professional practice. You have taken the first step in your ongoing learning. Now, what is your view of professional nursing?

YOUR PHILOSOPHY OF NURSING

Virginia Henderson (1897–1996) was an outstanding leader in nursing. Her classic definition of nursing embodied her view of the unique role of the professional nurse as:

[a]ssisting the individual, sick or well, in the performance of those activities contributing to health or its recovery (or to a peaceful death) that he would perform unaided if he had the necessary strength, will, or knowledge. And to do this in such a way as to help him gain independence as rapidly as possible. (Henderson, 1966, p. 15)

This concrete definition was expanded and applied to nursing practice, education, and research. Henderson's philosophy of nursing was one of caring, assisting, and supporting the person. In her writings, she encouraged every nurse to develop a personal concept of nursing—in essence, a philosophy of nursing.

A **philosophy** of nursing presents a particular professional nurse's belief system or worldview of nursing—the nurse's personal definition of nursing. Recall that the first component on the structural hierarchy of contemporary nursing knowledge was the metaparadigm, followed by the influence of the belief system or philosophy. Fawcett and DeSanto-Madeya (2013) describe the function of a philosophy as communication of what the members of a discipline believe to be true relative to the phenomena of interest, how knowledge is developed, and the values with regard to actions and practices (p. 8).

As discussed previously, the metaparadigm concept of human beings relates to the people of concern for nursing. Nurses in different settings define patients uniquely within their practice—for example, as individuals versus families. The nurse's practice area and patient populations also influence the environment—for example, an intensive care unit in an acute care setting or a rural healthcare clinic located in a community school or modular building. The concept of health also varies, being different for the professional who provides care for trauma victims and the nurse involved with health initiatives in an employee group. Specific nursing roles, and the services provided, influence the concept of nursing. In addition to the metaparadigm concepts in a personal philosophy of nursing, certain other values and beliefs are generally apparent as one's beliefs about nursing are illustrated.

Consider the following essential features of professional nursing definitions identified in the ANA's *Nursing's Policy Statement: The Essence of the Profession* (2010a):

- Provision of a caring relationship that facilitates health and healing
- Attention to the range of human experiences and responses to health and illness within the physical and social environments
- Integration of objective data with knowledge gained from an appreciation of the patient or the group
- Application of scientific knowledge to the processes of diagnosis and treatment through the use of judgment and critical thinking
- Advancement of professional nursing knowledge through scholarly inquiry
- Influence on social and public policy to promote social justice
- Assurance of safe, quality, and evidence-based practice (p. 9)

Along with these criteria are interwoven ethical principles, standards of practice, and professional performance expectations. These are your values and beliefs.

At this point, you should critically analyze your belief system and express your views of nursing. We all have prior experiences that influence our thinking and actions. Try to place those aside and begin to craft your philosophy of nursing. Using these definitions and criteria, develop your views into a personal philosophy of nursing. Periodically reflect on your philosophy to analyze how your professional practice is enhanced in your ongoing quest for knowledge and expertise in your profession. This is your unique professional identity.

KEY POINTS

- The following are characteristics of a profession: (1) systematic theory and knowledge base, (2) authority, (3) community sanction, (4) an ethical code, and (5) a professional culture.

- Kerlinger and Lee (2000) define a theory as "a set of interrelated constructs (concepts), definitions, and propositions that present a systematic view of phenomena by specifying relations among variables, with the purpose of explaining and predicting the phenomena" (p. 11).

- A paradigm used by professionals in a scientific community consists of the beliefs and the belief system shared by members of that particular community to explain phenomena, practice the profession, and conduct research.

- The metaparadigm of nursing is the overall concern of nursing common to each nursing model, whether a conceptual model/paradigm or formal theory, and it includes the concepts of human beings, environment, health, and nursing.

- The *Code of Ethics for Nurses* (ANA, 2015) is the ethical standard for professional nursing practice. It identifies expected professional practice behaviors with patients, colleagues, and other professionals within nine provisions with interpretative statements.

- Autonomy involves judgment and self-governing within one's scope of practice. This self-governing requires ongoing evaluation of both responsibility and accountability in professional practice. In the ANA's *Code of Ethics for Nurses*, responsibility is defined as "an obligation to perform required professional activities at a level commensurate with one's education and in compliance with applicable laws and standards . . ." (ANA, 2015, p. 45) whereas, accountability is being answerable to self and others for one's own choices, decisions and actions as measured against a standard . . ." such as the Code (ANA, 2015, p. 41).

- The ANA (2010b) *Standards of Professional Performance* are ethics, education, evidence-based practice and research, quality of practice, communication, leadership, collaboration, professional practice evaluation, resource utilization, and environmental health.

- The five competencies for health professionals are providing patient-centered care, working in interdisciplinary teams, employing evidence-based practice, applying quality improvement, and using informatics (Greiner & Knebel, 2003).

- Roles are organized behavioral patterns and expectations.

- Learning is the perception and assimilation of the information presented to us in a variety of ways.

- Knowledge is the accumulation of the appropriate information through learning and experience. Skill is the ability to retrieve this knowledge through mental and psychomotor activities and apply it appropriately to the situation. Ability is your competence and proficiency in the demonstration of the knowledge and skill.

- Learning style or preference is simply the ways you best perceive, think, organize, use, and retain knowledge.

- Resources are tools or means of support.

- A personal philosophy of nursing presents the belief system or worldview of nursing for a particular professional nurse. Incorporated into such a philosophy are definitions, values, and assumptions about the metaparadigm concepts of human beings, environment, health, and nursing

Thought and Discussion Questions

1. Be prepared to participate in a discussion to be scheduled by your instructor on how you demonstrate the five core competencies of health professionals.

2. Explain your views on professional responsibility and accountability.

3. Describe how you demonstrate and document your continued competency.

4. Reflect carefully and identify your reasons for continuing your nursing education.

5. Consider your responsibilities.
   • Identify all your current roles. Which ones can be streamlined?
   • What resources can you classify as readily available, sometimes available, or in need of locating?
   • What strategies can you identify for improved time management for your new role as a student?

6. Review the Chapter Thought located on the first page of the chapter, and discuss it in the context of the contents of the chapter.

Interactive Exercises

Go to the Intranet site and complete the interactive exercises provided for this chapter.

REFERENCES

American Association of Colleges of Nursing. (2008). *The essentials of baccalaureate education for professional nursing practice*. Washington, DC: Author.

American Association of Colleges of Nursing. (2011). The *essentials of master's education in nursing*. Washington, DC: Author.

American Association of Colleges of Nursing. (2013). *Competencies and curricular expectations for clinical nurse leader education and practice*. Retrieved from http://www.aacn.nche.edu/publications/white-papers/cnl

American Association of Colleges of Nursing. (2014). *Mission*. Retrieved from http://www.aacn.nche.edu/about-aacn/mission-values

American Association of Critical-Care Nurses. (2014). *Mission*. Retrieved from http://www.aacn.org/wd/memberships/content/mission_vision_values_ethics.pcms?menu=aboutus

American Nurses Association. (2010a). *Nursing's policy statement: The essence of the profession* (2010 ed.). Silver Spring, MD: Nursesbooks.org.

American Nurses Association. (2010b). *Nursing: Scope and standards of practice* (2nd ed.). Silver Spring, MD: Nursesbooks.org.

American Nurses Association. (2014). *About the ANA*. Retrieved from http://nursingworld.org/FunctionalMenu Categories/AboutANA

American Nurses Association. (2015). *Code of ethics for nurses with interpretative statements*. Silver Spring, MD: Nursesbooks.org.

Benner, P. (1984). *From novice to expert: Excellence and power in clinical nursing practice*. Menlo Park, CA: Addison-Wesley.

Corrigan, M. S., Donaldson, M. S., Kohn, L. T., Maguire, S. K., & Pike, K. C. (2001). *Crossing the quality chasm: A new health system for the 21st century*. Washington, DC: National Academy Press.

Fawcett, J. (1995). *Analysis and evaluation of conceptual models of nursing* (3rd ed.). Philadelphia: F. A. Davis.

Fawcett, J. (2000). *Analysis and evaluation of contemporary nursing knowledge: Nursing models and theories*. Philadelphia: F. A. Davis.

Fawcett, J. (2005). *Contemporary nursing knowledge: Analysis and evaluation of nursing models and theories* (2nd ed.). Philadelphia: F. A. Davis.

Fawcett, J., & DeSanto-Madeya, S. (2013). *Contemporary nursing knowledge: Analysis and evaluation of nursing models and theories* (3rd ed.). Philadelphia: F.A. Davis.

Greenwood, E. (1957). Attributes of a profession. *Social Work, 2*(3), 45–55.

Greiner, A. C., & Knebel, E. (Eds.). (2003). *Health professions education: A bridge to quality*. Washington, DC: Institute of Medicine.

Henderson, V. (1966). *The nature of nursing: A definition and its implications for practice, education, and research*. New York: Macmillan.

Institute of Medicine (IOM). (2011). *The future of nursing: Advancing health, leading change*. Washington, DC: National Academies Press. Retrieved from http://www.iom.edu/Reports/2010/The-Future-of-Nursing-Leading-Change-Advancing-Health.aspx

International Council of Nurses (2012). *The ICN code of ethics for nurses*. Retrieved from http://www.icn.ch/images/stories/documents/about/icncode_english.pdf

International Council of Nurses. (2013). *About ICN*. Retrieved from http://www.icn.ch/about-icn/icns-mission/

Kerlinger, F. N., & Lee, H. B. (2000). *Foundations of behavioral research* (4th ed.). Belmont, CA: Wadsworth Thompson Learning.

Kuhn, T. S. (1970). *The structure of scientific revolutions* (2nd ed.). Chicago: University of Chicago Press.

Mezirow, J. (1991). *Transformative dimensions of adult learning*. San Francisco: Jossey-Bass.

Mezirow, J. (2000). Learning to think like an adult: Core concepts of transformation theory. In J. Mezirow and Associates, *Learning as transformation: Critical perspectives on a theory in progress* (pp. 3–33). San Francisco: Jossey-Bass.

Miller, B. K., Adams, D., & Beck, L. (1993). A behavioral inventory for professionalism in nursing. *Journal of Professional Nursing, 9,* 290–295.

Myers & Briggs Foundation. (2014). MBTI basics. Retrieved from http://www.myersbriggs.org/my-mbti-personality-type/mbti-basics/

National Council of State Boards of Nursing. (2014). *About NCSBN: Mission and values.* Retrieved from https://www.ncsbn.org/182.htm

National League for Nursing. (2013). *Mission/goals/core values.* Retrieved from http://www.nln.org/aboutnln/ourmission.htm

Sigma Theta Tau. (2014). *STTI organizational fact sheet.* Retrieved from http://www.nursingsociety.org/aboutus/mission/Pages/factsheet.aspx

VandenBos, G. R. (ed). (2013). *APA dictionary of clinical psychology.* Washington, DC: American Psychological Association.

BIBLIOGRAPHY

American Nurses Association. (2009). *Forensic nursing: Scope and standards of practice.* Silver Spring, MD: Nursebooks.org.

American Nurses Association. (2009). *Nursing administration: Scope and standards of practice.* Silver Spring, MD: Nursebooks.org.

American Nurses Association. (2009). *Transplant nursing: Scope and standards of practice.* Silver Spring, MD: Nursebooks.org.

American Nurses Association. (2010). *Gerontological Nursing: Scope and standards practice.* Silver Spring, MD: Nursebooks.org.

American Nurses Association. (2010). *Nursing professional development: Scope and standards of practice.* Silver Spring, MD: Nursebooks.org.

American Nurses Association. (2010). *Position statement: The nurse's role in ethics and human rights: Protecting and promoting individual worth, dignity, and human rights in practice settings.* Retrieved from http://www.nursingworld.org/ethicsrole

American Nurses Association. (2011). *School nursing: Scope and standards of practice* (2nd ed.). Silver Spring, MD: Nursebooks.org.

American Nurses Association. (2012). *Faith community nursing: Scope and standards of practice.* (2nd ed.). Silver Spring, MD: Nursebooks.org.

American Nurses Association. (2013). *Addictions nursing: Scope and standards of practice.* Silver Spring, MD: Nursebooks.org.

American Nurses Association. (2013). *Corrections nursing: Scope and standards of practice* (2nd ed.). Silver Spring, MD: Nursebooks.org.

American Nurses Association. (2013). *Holistic nursing: Scope and standards of practice* (2nd ed). Silver Spring, MD: Nursebooks.org.

American Nurses Association. (2013). *Intellectual and developmental disabilities nursing: Scope and standards of practice* (2nd ed.). Silver Spring, MD: Nursebooks.org.

American Nurses Association. (2013). *Neonatal nursing: Scope and standards of practice* (2nd ed.). Silver Spring, MD: Nursebooks.org.

American Nurses Association. (2013). *Neuroscience nursing: Scope and standards of practice.* Silver Spring, MD: Nursebooks.org.

American Nurses Association. (2013). *Plastic surgery nursing: Scope and standards of practice* (2nd ed.). Silver Spring, MD: Nursebooks.org.

American Nurses Association. (2013). *Public health nursing: Scope and standards of practice* (2nd ed.). Silver Spring, MD: Nursebooks.org.

American Nurses Association. (2013). *Radiology and imaging nursing: Scope and standards of practice.* Silver Spring, MD: Nursebooks.org.

American Nurses Association. (2013). *Rheumatology nursing: Scope and standards of practice.* Silver Spring, MD: Nursebooks.org.

American Nurses Association. (2014). *Palliative nursing: Scope and standards of practice.* Silver Spring, MD: Nursebooks.org.

American Nurses Association. (2014). *Psychiatric-mental health nursing: Scope and standards of practice* (2nd ed.). Silver Spring, MD: Nursebooks.org.

Kohn, L. T., Corrigan, M. S., & Donaldson, M. S. (1999). *To err is human: Building a safer health system.* Washington, DC: National Academy Press.

O'Neil, E. H. (1998). *Recreating health professional practice for a new century.* San Francisco: Pew Health Professions Commission.

Pew Health Professions Commission. (1995). *Critical challenges: Revitalizing the health professions for the twenty-first century.* San Francisco: USCF Center for the Health Professions.

ONLINE RESOURCES

American Association of Colleges of Nursing
http://www.aacn.nche.edu/

American Nurses Association
http://www.nursingworld.org

ANA Code of Ethics for Nurses
http://www.nursingworld.org/codeofethics

ICN Code of Ethics for Nurses
http://www.icn.ch/icncode.pdf

● Rose Kearney-Nunnery

Theory as the Basis for Practice

"Theory and research are not solely the province of the academic, just as practice is not solely the field of the practitioner."

(Glanz, Rimer, and Lewis 2002)

Chapter Objectives

On completion of this chapter, the reader will be able to:

1. Define key terms in theory development and utilization.
2. Discuss Maslow's theory of motivation with the hierarchy of basic needs.
3. Describe the components of developmental theories and their application to individuals across the life span.
4. Describe the components and application of systems theory.
5. Discuss the impact of theory on practice.

Key Terms

Theory
Model
Framework
Conceptual Model or Framework
Concept

Construct
Variable
Proposition
Theory Description and Evaluation
Hierarchy of Needs

Developmental Theories
General System Theory
Quantum Theory

One characteristic of a profession is that it is built on a theoretical base. This base includes theoretical foundations unique to the profession, as well as those borrowed or adapted from other scientific disciplines. Chapter 1 discussed paradigms and the metaparadigm concepts of nursing. Recall that Kuhn (1970) described a paradigm as "universally recognized scientific achievements that for a time provide model problems and solutions to a community of practitioners" (p. vii). When the paradigm is no longer useful in explaining phenomena, practice, and research in that particular scientific community, a paradigm shift occurs, and a new structure evolves.

In 1957, Merton used a paradigm to analyze sociological theory. He viewed the paradigm as a "field glass" to illuminate and view concepts and interrelationships and to make assumptions clear on the body of knowledge for analysis and testing. Merton (1957) identified the purposes of a paradigm as providing for the following:

1. Parsimonious arrangement of concepts and propositions showing interrelationships
2. A logical guide showing derivations and avoiding hidden assumptions and concepts
3. Culmination in theory development as a building process
4. Systematic arrangement and cross-tabulation of concepts for analysis
5. Codification of qualitative research methods (pp. 13–16)

From a cultural perspective, Leininger (2006) defined *worldview* as "the way an individual or group looks out on and understands their world about them as a value, stance, picture, or perspective about life or the world" (p. 83). In the professional culture of nursing, these are the values, attitudes, beliefs, and practices unique to the profession. Thus, a scientific community has the tools to create and test a theory for knowledge development and the use of this knowledge in practice. The worldview furnishes the philosophical assumptions that are considered "givens" by the theorist or the scientific community. In nursing, this provides us with the process: the metaparadigm concepts to various paradigms, and the development of theories on which to base research, practice, administration, and education.

TERMINOLOGY IN THEORY AND DEVELOPMENT ANALYSIS

Professions such as nursing are based on unique theory. Kerlinger and Lee (2000) defined a **theory** as "a set of interrelated constructs (concepts), definitions, and propositions that present a systematic view of phenomena by specifying relations among variables, with the purpose of explaining and predicting the phenomena" (p. 11). This definition provides us with the components and aims of a theory, which must initially be described and then evaluated for potential use in practice, education, and research in a discipline. Some theorists, however, believe this definition is too narrow and excludes descriptive theories; descriptive theories, which focus on factor naming, are abundant in professional nursing and are often a first step for further research and development.

Before moving to the components of a theory, we need to address three similar terms frequently associated with theory: model, framework, and conceptual model (or conceptual framework). A **model** is a graphic representation of some phenomenon. It may be a mathematical model (such as A + B = C) or a diagrammatic model that links words with symbols and lines. A theoretical model provides a visual description of a theory using limited narrative and displaying components and relationships symbolically. A **framework** is another means of providing a structural view of the concepts and relationships proposed in a theory. Again, use of words and narrative is limited, but the structure of the theory is presented as the framework and allows translation, interpretation, and illumination of the narrative or text.

A **conceptual model or framework** is similar to a theory in that it represents some phenomenon of interest and contains concepts and propositions. However, with a conceptual model or framework, the concepts and especially the propositions are broader in scope, less defined, and less specific to the phenomenon of concern. As Fawcett and DeSanto-Madeya (2013) note, "the concepts of a conceptual model are so abstract and general that they are not directly observed in the real world, nor are they limited to any particular individual, group, situation, or event" (p. 13).

A theory can evolve from a conceptual model or framework as concepts are further defined, specified, tested, and interrelated to represent some aspect of reality. Fawcett (1995, 2000, 2005) and, subsequently, Fawcett and DeSanto-Madeya (2013) have described the structural hierarchy of contemporary nursing knowledge (Fig. 2.1) with its components, from the most abstract metaparadigm, influenced by different philosophies, to conceptual models that further evolve into theories and specific empirical indicators for testing. They

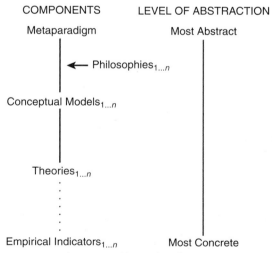

Figure 2.1 The structural hierarchy of contemporary nursing knowledge: Components and levels of abstraction. (*From Fawcett, J., and DeSanto-Madeya, S. (2013). Contemporary nursing knowledge: Analysis and evaluation of nursing models and theories [3rd ed., p. 4]. Philadelphia: F. A. Davis, with permission.*)

further define the function of conceptual models "to provide a framework to organize and visualize abstract and general phenomena and relations between various phenomena encompassed by the model" (Fawcett and DeSanto-Madeya, 2013, p. 13). Then, the function of a theory is "to narrow and more fully specify the phenomena contained in a conceptual model" (Fawcett and DeSanto-Madeya, 2013, p. 16). Concepts become less abstract, and the population of interest is identified. This increase in specificity is evident in the examples proposed by Alligood (2014c), who, on the basis of Fawcett's structural hierarchy of nursing knowledge, correlated examples in theoretical structures by different nursing theorists as follows:

- Metaparadigm: Person, environment, health, and nursing
- Philosophies: Nightingale, Watson, Benner
- Conceptual Models: King, Levine, Neuman, Orem, Rogers, Roy, Johnson
- Theories: Leininger, Newman, Parse, Pender, Meleis, Husted and Husted, Boykin and Schoenhofer
- Middle-Range Theories: Mercer, Mishel, Wiener and Dodd, Kolcaba, Swanson, Beck, Rutland and Moore

As more is known about the phenomenon, this knowledge can be used in specific, meaningful patient applications.

As knowledge about some phenomena increases, a theory is proposed to address the phenomena or reality within the discipline. The components of a theory are the constructs (concepts), with their specific definitions, and the propositions that describe or link those constructs (concepts). At the simplest level, a **concept** is a view or idea that we hold about something. It can be something highly concrete, such as a pencil, or something highly abstract, such as quality. The more concrete the concept, the easier it is understood and consistently used. For instance, we are comfortable envisioning a pencil and can easily describe it to others. This ability to describe something directly in the concrete world shares the "concept." But the concept of quality is more abstract, and ensuring that all individual definitions are the same is difficult, often requiring indirect measures.

We strive to define a concept in operational terms—that is, how we view a specific entity and how it can be measured so that others know exactly what we mean. To meet the criteria of a theory, we need to define the concepts. Consider the concept of a pencil. We think of a pencil as a writing implement. This is the theoretical or conceptual definition of a pencil we read in a dictionary. But what do we truly mean by *pencil*? It is a yellow-painted, wooden-covered graphite instrument that we use to make marks on a paper. Does it have an eraser? Does a mechanical pencil fit into this definition? An operational definition narrows the definition to precisely what we view and how it can be measured for use in practice or research as a measurable, empirical indicator. In addition, concepts are broadened to constructs, such as with quality or identity, which can be multidimensional and difficult—if not impossible—to break down into component parts.

A **construct** is a more complex idea package of some phenomenon that contains many factors but cannot be truly isolated or confined to a more concrete concept. The construct of *identity*, for example, contains many pieces, such as personal perception, role expectations, and status. However, we must still provide an operational definition of a construct by specifying certain elements it contains (as indirect measures), such as self-image, ideal image, group image, role expectations, and status. The same multidimensionality occurs when we assess the quality of healthcare.

In research, we often see the term *variables*, referring to some concept in the theory under study. A **variable** is a concept that can change and that contains a set of values that can be measured in a practice or research situation. For example, a client's cholesterol reading is a variable. The concept of blood cholesterol has been operationally defined within certain parameters, and the level of the reading is the value for the variable.

Whether concepts, constructs, or a combination of the two are included in a specific theory, they are the building blocks of the theory. Definitions are provided to help us understand the nature and characteristics of each block in the construction. We then need to relate these building blocks to each other. Describing and stating the relationships between or among the constructs (or concepts) provides the propositions of a theory. Also called relational statements, **propositions** show how the concepts are linked in the theory and how they relate to one another and to the total theoretical structure. They define how the structure is held together. In nursing theory, propositions refer to how the individual is characterized with specific abilities, knowledge, values, and traits and how these factors interrelate with the characteristics of health, the environment, and nursing.

Research is a means of supporting the concepts and relationships proposed in a theory. It provides supportive evidence and suggests further study and possible gaps or revisions needed in the theoretical structure. We can see this in the next chapters, which cover refinement of nursing and other health models, such as the health-belief model revision. Research can be qualitative and inductive, for generating theory, or more quantitative, for deductively testing hypotheses as theoretical propositions.

As stated previously, Kerlinger and Lee (2000) defined the aims or purpose of theory as describing or explaining some phenomena of interest. In nursing, theory is further differentiated into levels that describe, explain, predict, and control. Dickoff and James (1968) developed a classic position paper proposing four levels of nursing theory (Box 2.1). All levels may be present as a practice theory

---

BOX 2.1 **Dickoff and James (1968): Four Levels of Nursing Theory**

1. Factor-isolating (naming) theories
2. Factor-relating (situation-depicting) theories
3. Situation-relating (predictive or promoting/inhibiting theories)
4. Situation-producing (prescriptive) theories

Dickoff, J., & James, P. (1968). A theory of theories: A position paper. *Nursing Research, 17*, 197–203.

evolves (factor-isolating and then factor-relating), is subjected to further research, and is refined, becoming predictive and prescriptive. In application, testing, and refinement, a theory is a continuum as long as the content meets the intent of the discipline and metaparadigm.

In addition, theories are classified according to their scope as grand, middle-range, or limited in scope or practice. This is the breadth of coverage of some phenomena. General system theory is an example of a grand theory, or one with a broad scope. This theory, discussed later in the chapter, has been used in development, testing, and application in many scientific disciplines.

Merton (1957) was the first theorist to suggest "theories of the middle range: theories intermediate to the minor working hypotheses evolved in abundance during the day-by-day routines of research, and the all inclusive speculations comprising a master conceptual scheme from which it is hoped to derive a very large number of empirically observed uniformities of . . . behavior" (pp. 5–6). As you will see in the next chapter, middle-range theories are narrower in scope, with a limited view of a phenomenon, and contain concepts and propositions that are measurable and can be empirically tested. Some of our traditional nursing theories meet the characteristics of a middle-range theory, as described in Chapter 3. Other middle-range theories include the developmental theories reviewed later in this chapter. Although these theories address psychosocial, cognitive, and moral development, they apply across disciplines as continual, incremental knowledge and skills developed by individuals. More limited nursing practice theories are evolving as hypotheses derived from middle-range theories are tested, clarified, and made specific to certain practice areas or types of patients. Chapter 4 shows examples of limited nursing practice models that are being tested and refined into theoretical frameworks, including Pender's health promotion model. Even more narrow in scope are practice theories, which focus on measurable variables and propositions that are based on empirical research and now may be refined further, perhaps to a specific population or group of individuals with a common characteristic.

You can also enter "middle-range nursing theory" in your Internet search engine to locate additional sources of information from a variety of nursing programs.

THEORY DESCRIPTION AND EVALUATION

To understand theories for use and application in practice, we use certain criteria to describe and evaluate them. Theory development is both an inductive and a deductive process. An inductive process is used to generate concepts and make inferences by stating interrelationships (propositions) within a framework to view phenomena. From observations of phenomena, we can name concepts and enumerate proposed relationships. Once the theory is generated, it is applied, in whole or in part, for testing as a deductive process. For nursing **theory description and evaluation**, we consider the following three sets of criteria proposed by nursing scholars Chinn and Kramer, Barnum, and Fawcett.

Chinn and Kramer (2011) differentiate between theory description and critical reflection of empiric theory. The theory is described by answering questions in the following areas: purpose, concepts, definitions, relationships and structure, and assumptions. This process provides an understanding of the components and aims of the theory. Once the theory has been described, five issues are addressed in critical reflection:

• Clarity and consistency in presentation
• Simplicity and meaningfulness of relationships
• Generality or scope
• Accessibility as potential for use with empirically identifiable phenomena
• Significance as leading to the values in practice, education, and research (Chinn & Kramer, 2011, p. 205).

This differentiation allows us to discriminate between understanding the theoretical structure and evaluating the theory's soundness and usefulness in practice, education, or research. Alligood (2014c) refers to these five areas for theory analysis as clarity, simplicity, generality, accessibility, and importance (p. 9).

Barnum (1998) proposes two categories of theory: descriptive theory and explanatory theory. *Descriptive theory* is a factor-naming and factor-relating theory developed initially to characterize some phenomena. *Explanatory theory* brings us to the situation-relating and situation-producing levels of theory, looking at the "how," the "why," and the interrelationships in the theory (Barnum, 1998). Theory description is delineated as theory interpretation, with questions addressing the following areas:

• Major elements of the theory and their definitions
• Relationships among the elements
• Differentiation between descriptive and explanatory theory
• How the theory addresses, defines, and differentiates nursing
• The focus on the patient, nurse, action, or relationship
• Unique language used and defined by the theorist (Barnum, 1990, 1994, 1998)

For critical analysis, internal criticism and external criticism are differentiated. *Internal criticism* is used to evaluate how the theory components fit together: the clarity, consistency, adequacy, logical development, and, sometimes, level of theory development (Barnum, 1998). *External criticism* deals with real-world issues such as reality convergence, usefulness, significance, and discrimination from other healthcare disciplines (Barnum, 1998). This process allows us to discriminate between understanding the theoretical structure (internal criticism) and evaluating the soundness and usefulness of the theory for application in practice, education, or research (external criticism).

Fawcett and DeSanto-Madeya (2013) have proposed criteria for theory analysis and evaluation that have undergone several revisions. They further differentiate between

ONLINE CONSULT

Nursing Theories at
http://nursingtheories.info/

analysis and evaluation of nursing conceptual models and theories. Recall that conceptual models are more abstract than theories. As described by Fawcett and DeSanto-Madeya (2013) a theory is more concrete and more specific, and is restricted to a more limited range of phenomena, than a conceptual model, with the purpose of middle-range theories to describe, explain, or predict concrete and specific phenomena (p. 20).

Analysis refers to the description of the theory. Fawcett and DeSanto-Madeya (2013) have described an analysis as "a nonjudgmental examination" of the nursing model, while an evaluation requires judgments to be made about the extent to which a nursing model satisfies certain criteria (p. 442). Theory analysis is followed by theory evaluation, which requires thoughtful interpretation of the theory. Fawcett and DeSanto-Madeya (2013) have identified a series of questions for analysis and evaluation of nursing theories appropriate to their level of abstraction as compared with conceptual models. In this revision, Fawcett and DeSanto-Madeya (2013) have proposed steps in a framework for the analysis and the evaluation of the theory, as follows:

Theory Analysis	Theory Evaluation
Step 1: Model Origins	*Step 1:* Explication of origins
Step 2: Unique Focus	*Step 2:* Comprehensiveness of content
Step 3: Content	*Step 3:* Logical congruence
	Step 4: Generation of theory
	Step 5: Legitimacy (social utility, congruence, and significance)
	Step 6: Contributions to nursing knowledge and the discipline

Application of this framework for theory analysis and evaluation will be evident in Chapter 3, which deals with specific grand and middle-range nursing theories. Each of these sets of criteria involves a careful identification of the components and evaluation components for determination of applicability to nursing practice.

THEORIES FROM OUTSIDE OF NURSING

Nursing and other healthcare disciplines have long used a variety of theories to guide practice. Some are discipline-specific, such as the nursing theories reviewed in Chapter 3. For example, Fawcett and DeSanto-Madeya (2013) differentiate between theories developed unique to nursing (Newman, Orlando, Parse, Peplau, and Watson) and models borrowed from other disciplines (stress, coping, and self-efficacy) (p. 17). Early nursing theories were described by Barnum (1990) as follows:

> As an applied science, much of nursing's theory is "borrowed" from other disciplines. Every discipline has similar boundary ambiguities, where the inquiry and answers in one field overlap those in another. . . . Nursing's uniqueness in this respect does not lie in boundary overlap but in the number of boundary overlaps with which it must contend. A high number of overlaps occur in the discipline of nursing because it often attempts to deal holistically with a phenomenon (man) that has previously been dealt with in compartmentalized ways by other disciplines. (p. 218)

But, nursing theory has come a long way since that time. In her description of the development of nursing theory from the Curriculum Era in the early 20th century, through the Research and Graduate Education Eras in the middle 20th century, and the Theory Era in the latter part of the 20th century, into the 21st century and the Era of Theory Utilization, Alligood (2014a)—described the process resulting in theory is not just to know but to use (p. 8) with the growth of the discipline (p. 9). As proposed by Fawcett (2014), nurses must embrace nursing knowledge in the form of explicit nursing conceptual models and theories; indeed, "the use of discipline-specific nursing knowlege to guide nursing practice is the hallmark of professional nursing" (p. 427). Recall the metaparadigm concepts. Borrowed theories may address human beings, health, and the environment, but what of nursing? With collaborative practice, however, these theories provide a common ground and the opportunity for the application and sharing of middle-range theories. They also enable us to understand human nature, motivation, and development. But, as noted by Chinn and Kramer (2011), always consider specific factors that influence a nursing situation (p. 40).

Several classic theories have been applied in nursing to view the person, family, community, and group. We use Maslow's hierarchy of needs to view human beings and basic human needs. Developmental theories have been applied across the human life span as we seek to understand the complexity of human behavior. In looking at the person or group, we have applied systems theory to understand the interaction of human beings with their environment. The following section briefly describes selected theories that are applied in certain areas and have been used in the evolution of nursing models more specific to our metaparadigm concepts.

Maslow's Theory of Human Motivation and Hierarchy of Basic Needs

A theory widely used in many disciplines is Maslow's theory of human motivation. In his original 1954 book, *Motivation and Personality*, Maslow described how his work emerged. The book begins by presenting Maslow's philosophy as an approach to science. Human values are prevalent in the philosophy, and Maslow's worldview is described as holistic, functional, dynamic, and purposive. In his 1970 revised edition, Maslow reinforced his worldviews and described his theory as holistic-dynamic. He supported his original 16 propositions on motivation, on which his theory was based (see Chapter 9, on motivation in the teaching-learning process). This is a grand theory that views the complexity of human behavior, especially in relation to motivation of behavior. The theory of motivation is based on clinical and experimental data from psychology, psychiatry, education, and philosophy. It does not address specific nursing concerns except as they relate to human behavior with environmental influences.

Maslow's theory includes a hierarchical structure for human needs. This **hierarchy of needs** can be visualized as a pyramid (Fig. 2.2). At the base of the pyramid are the physiologic drives. Higher needs progress upward as safety, love and belonging, esteem, and self-actualization needs. Maslow (1954, 1970) described this as a "hierarchy of pre-potency" to explain that the individual concentrates on the physiologic drives. The physiologic drives are considered the most powerful, but as physiologic needs are satisfied, the individual focuses on emerging higher needs. This is the general structure for the hierarchy.

Individual differences are provided for in this theory. Some individuals have altered placement of needs in the hierarchy. Maslow (1970) described differences among individuals in placement of some of the higher needs such as a reversal of esteem and love/belonging needs. In addition, individuals may have different levels of need satisfaction. For example, one person might meet the physiologic drives at a 75 percent level, whereas another person's level for satisfaction is 85 percent. Individual differences also apply to the emergence of higher needs. Maslow (1970) regarded this as a gradual process; one person's safety needs may begin to emerge when his or her physiologic needs are being met at 25 percent, whereas another person may not begin to satisfy his or her safety needs until 30 percent of his or her physiologic needs are met. Levels of satisfaction and emergence of higher needs therefore occur at different points in different people, as do pain thresholds in different people.

Looking again at the theoretical hierarchy, we see at the bottom level of the pyramid the physiologic drives, including the need to maintain homeostasis and the needs of satisfying hunger and thirst, sleep and rest, activity and exercise, sexual gratification and sensory pleasure, and maternal responses (Maslow, 1970). Meeting the physiologic hunger drive is very different from meeting one's nutritional requirements or treating anxiety or depression with a chocolate bar.

When the individual is truly hungry or thirsty, not merely satisfying an appetite for food or drink, all energies and thoughts are directed to satisfying that drive for food or water. Consider the physiologic need of an individual with a chemical dependency. The person will focus all efforts on attaining the drug or addictive substance at the required level of satisfaction—while ignoring other needs, including the physiologic need for food or the next level of safety needs. When the physiologic drives and needs are relatively satisfied, higher-level needs emerge.

Safety needs are the next level of the hierarchy. Safety, both physical and emotional, must be achieved. Threats to a person's safety can become all-consuming. Think of an isolated person in an inner-city apartment whose fear for his safety motivates him to place bars on his windows and multiple chains and dead-bolt locks on his door. This person fears for his physical safety from a threat, real or imagined, of bodily harm. This is the main concern, not whether access is impeded in the case of a fire or accident. He places all focus on the quest for freedom from perceived danger.

Perceived safety can also be related to health, as with the fear of the patient with chronic obstructive pulmonary disease (COPD) to be near anyone who is coughing or sneezing. This person's safety need is to avoid a respiratory infection that could lead to pneumonia or even diminished oxygenation in an already compromised respiratory system. Even if the other person in the room is experiencing symptoms of a seasonal allergy, the individual with COPD seeks immediate escape from that environment because of the perceived danger of infection. Maslow (1954, 1970) also viewed safety needs more broadly in the need for the familiar and spiritual, religious, or philosophical meaning in life. He describes the use of rituals and ceremonial behaviors in children and individuals with psychological disorders as examples of focusing on safety needs.

Once the person satisfies safety needs, the focus turns to the need for love and belonging. Inclusion and affection are important needs, as contrasted with the isolated sex

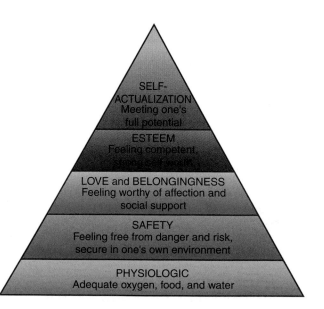

Figure 2.2 Maslow's hierarchy of human needs.

act, which is a physiologic drive. Maslow (1970) described the normal person as having a hunger and striving for affectionate relations and a place in a group, as opposed to the maladjusted person (pp. 43–44). Love and affection are manifested in many ways and are individually defined.

Satisfying the need for belonging and love brings us to the next level, esteem needs. Esteem needs involve a sense of dignity, worth, and usefulness in life. Maslow (1970) described two sets of esteem needs: (1) the sense of self-worth, including perceptions of strength, achievement, competence, and confidence, and (2) the esteem of others, including perceptions of deserved respect, status, recognition, importance, and dignity (p. 45). Satisfying the sense of self-worth and respect allows the next, and highest, level of basic needs to emerge.

The need for self-actualization, at the top of the pyramid, is the desire for self-fulfillment. This is the sense of being able to do all that a person can to answer the "why" of his or her existence. Maslow (1970) defined self-actualization as "the full use and exploitation of talents, capacities, potentialities, etc., such [that] people seem to be fulfilling themselves and . . . developing to the full stature of which they are capable" (p. 150). Originally, Maslow (1954) proposed that self-actualized people include both older people and college students and children. But when he further examined the concept of self-actualization, he separated psychological health from self-actualization, which he limited to older people whose human potentialities have been realized and actualized (Maslow, 1970).

Maslow then developed support for his theory of basic needs and human actions using case studies and other research. Through observation of people, he proposed specific phenomena that are determined by basic gratification of cognitive-affective, cognitive, character traits, interpersonal, and miscellaneous needs. He cited characteristics of people in relation to the hierarchy. For example, the following characteristics of self-actualized people emerged from Maslow's (1970) research and analysis of historical figures, public people, selected college students, and children:

1. More efficient and comfortable perceptions of reality
2. Acceptance of self, others, and nature
3. Spontaneity, simplicity, and naturalness in thoughts and behaviors
4. Problem-centered rather than ego-centered
5. Desire for detachment, solitude, and privacy
6. Autonomy with independence of culture and environment
7. Continued freshness of appreciation
8. Mystic and oceanic feelings with limitless horizons
9. Genuine desire to help people
10. Deeper and more profound interpersonal relationships
11. Democratic character structure
12. Strong ethical sense that discriminates means/ends and good/evil
13. Philosophical and unhostile sense of humor
14. Creativeness
15. Resistance to enculturation with an inner detachment (pp. 203–228).

Maslow created further hypotheses for testing. He described cases that diverged from his theory, such as the martyr who ignores survival needs for a principle. He called for further research, hypothesizing that satisfying basic needs earlier in life allows the individual to weather deprivation easier in later life (Maslow, 1954, p. 99). Maslow's work continued until his death in 1970. His hierarchy of needs has endured, and its applications have been extended in healthcare, education, industry, and marketing to understand people and their motivators. Needs related to individual, environmental, and health concerns are applicable to the nursing discipline. However, this theory is still a grand theory and does not address the specific domain of nursing.

Developmental Theories

A group of theories widely used in healthcare and education are the **developmental theories**. Some of these middle-range theories address personality (Erikson), cognitive (Piaget), and moral (Kohlberg) development using a life-span perspective. This perspective is based on progression and complexity in motor, personal-social, cognitive, or moral behavior. A brief review of each of the theories demonstrates how the theorist moved from a philosophy or worldview to identify concepts, propositions, and a model or theory based on observations, existing research, or case study presentations. Common to the developmental theories are predictable steps or stages through which the individual progresses during the life cycle. This is a building process. These theories are based largely on research through observation or case studies. Subsequent applications and research have been guided by the use of these theories to explain more specific phenomena or to test hypotheses.

Personality Development

Erikson's (1963) eight ages of man represents a theory of psychosocial personality development in which the individual proceeds through critical periods in a step-by-step or epigenetic process (Fig. 2.3). This theory has been and continues to be used widely in healthcare and psychology. In offering the theory, Erikson presented his philosophy and case studies with Freudian and neo-Freudian applications. Each stage has positive and negative aspects that are defined and described. The basic goal is for the individual to develop a favorable ratio of the positive aspects for a healthy ego. Erikson (1963) further described basic virtues and essential strengths for each of his "ages" or stages of development. These strengths and basic virtues define the positive aspects of ego development required in each stage. Propositions are developed for each of the stages. This theory is supported mainly by case study, with suggestions and encouragement of further hypotheses for research and testing. Erikson's theory has been used widely in nursing to foster positive ego development and empowerment in individuals. Although this theory does not specifically address

ONLINE CONSULT

Learn more about Maslow and his work at
http://www.maslow.com

AGES	STRENGTHS & VIRTUES	DEVELOPMENTAL STAGE
8. Ego Integrity Vs. Despair	Renunciation & Wisdom	Older Adulthood
7. Generativity Vs. Stagnation	Production & Care	Middle Adulthood
6. Intimacy Vs. Isolation	Affiliation & Love	Young Adulthood
5. Identity Vs. Role Confusion	Devotion & Fidelity	Adolescence
4. Industry Vs. Inferiority	Method & Competence	School Age
3. Initiative Vs. Guilt	Direction & Purpose	Preschool
2. Autonomy Vs. Shame & Doubt	Self-control & Will Power	Toddler
1. Trust Vs. Mistrust	Drive & Hope	Infancy

Figure 2.3 Erikson's (1963) eight ages of man.

the domain of nursing, common concerns include human beings, the environment, and psychosocial health.

Havighurst was another theorist who focused on personality development as developmental tasks and education. His theory from the mid-20th century included principles of cognitive and moral development in which the individual proceeded through six stages, accomplishing critical tasks. Havighurst (1972) described his philosophy, including the origins of the concept, and proposed a method for analyzing individual developmental tasks based on his defining criteria as well as biological, psychological, and cultural bases. He also provided educational implications for each of the developmental periods. Although descriptions of the tasks represent some gender bias and cultural limitations in our current global society, the biological and psychological bases are applicable. The tasks represent major milestones in biological, psychological, emotional, and cognitive functioning or development that individuals must negotiate as they progress through life. As with Erikson's theory of personality development, concerns about the human being, the environment, and health promotion are apparent in Havighurst's life-span perspective. The age-specific tasks represent activities of daily living during specific life stages, along with cognitive development.

Cognitive Development

Piaget's theory of cognitive development focuses on the development of the intellect. Piaget was truly an example of a self-actualized person. He described himself as a naturalist and biologist by training, without formal training in psychology (Flavell, 1963, p. vii). Moving from the publication of his first monograph on birds at the age of 10, he detailed the development of the intellect in children through observations. His techniques were sometimes criticized by the scientific community, but his theory has since been accepted and used in practice and research by many students and professionals. Piaget's theory looks at innate and environmental influences on the development of the intellect. This theory has four major periods of cognitive development: sensorimotor, preoperational

ONLINE CONSULT

Learn more about psychosocial development and Erikson's Eight Ages (or Stages) at
http://www. childdevelopmentinfo.com/development/erickson.shtml

thought, concrete operations, and formal operations (Table 2.1).

Within his theory, Piaget provided us with the concepts of schema, object permanence, assimilation, and accommodation. *Schema* are patterns of thought or behavior that evolve into more complexity as more information is obtained through assimilation and accommodation. *Object permanence*, the knowledge that something still exists when it is out of sight, develops when the child is between 9 and 10 months of age. *Assimilation* is the acquisition and incorporation of new information into the individual's existing cognitive and behavioral structures. *Accommodation* is the change in the individual's cognitive and behavioral patterns based on the new information acquired. Piaget's theory has been translated and applied worldwide and across disciplines. His work continued until his death in 1980, and further research and theory is still evolving from his contributions.

Piaget's work concentrated on cognitive development in children, including views on moral development. As such, it is more limited but has provided major insight into working with children. Applications are seen in health teaching, especially in chronic or terminal illness situations. But with these limitations on cognitive development for some environmental influences, it can address only a portion of the domain of concern to nursing.

Moral Development

Kohlberg's theory of moral development was an outgrowth of Piaget's work on moral development in children. Kohlberg's extensive work on moral development (Kohlberg, 1984; Kohlberg et al., 1987) is based on research with children who were given scenarios to describe reactions and make judgments. He initially studied boys 10 to 16 years old from Chicago, later adding research with children of both genders and different backgrounds. Kohlberg's theory (Table 2.2) consists of six stages grouped into three major levels: preconventional, conventional, and postconventional (Kohlberg, 1984).

Kohlberg's theory confers major insight into moral development. He provided the theoretical structure, supportive research, and applications in educational practice. The individual progresses through the levels and stages, not as a natural process, but through intellectual stimulation with a central focus on moral justice. This requires thinking about moral problems and issues. Further research and practices have been based on this theory and are ongoing. Consider the usefulness of this theory when

TABLE 2.1

Piaget's Theory of Cognitive Development

Period of Cognitive Development	Age	Stage Description
Sensorimotor Stages		
Reflexive	Birth–1 month	Use of primitive reflexes, such as sucking and rooting
Primary circular reactions	1–4 months	Repeating an event for the result, such as thumb in mouth
Secondary circular reactions	4–10 months	Combining events for a result, such as kicking mobile over crib
Coordination of secondary schema	10–12 months	Creating a behavior for some result, such as standing in crib to reach mobile
Tertiary circular reactions	12–18 months	Looking for similar results from varying behaviors, such as shaking crib and jumping to observe movements of mobile
Representational thought begins	18–24 months	Symbolic representation in thought such as hanging objects to create mobile
Preoperational	2–7 years	Making overgeneralizations, such as all cats are named Tiger; egocentric Focuses only on one concrete attribute Magical thought and symbolic play present
Concrete operations	7–11 years	Logical and reversible thought appears; conservation of matter and numbers
Formal operations	After 11 years	Theoretical and hypothetical thinking now possible; higher-order mathematics and reasoning

TABLE 2.2

Kohlberg's Theory of Moral Development (Kohlberg, 1981; Kohlberg and Lickona, 1990)

Level	Stage	Stage Description
Level I: Preconventional morality	1. Heteronomous morality	Egocentric and applies a fixed set of rules from authorities, e.g., parents
	2. Individualism, purpose, and exchange	Sees that different individuals have different rules, e.g., parents and teachers
Level II: Conventional morality	3. Interpersonal expectations, relationships, and conformity	Motives of other person now emerge when considering right and wrong; use of the Golden Rule
	4. Social system and conscience	The good of society as a whole now emerges
Level III: Postconventional morality	5. Social contract and individual rights	Believes in upholding laws and legal contracts
	6. Universal ethical principles	Principles of justice and human rights as an ethical system

you are working with a child or adolescent whose parent was recently diagnosed with a terminal illness.

As with Piagetian theory, Kohlberg's theory is limited to a specific area of development. The focus is on human beings, such as the child, with ramifications for adult life. Environmental (e.g., social and cultural) factors provide insight for social and psychological health. The limitation

to moral development addresses only a portion of the domain of concern to nursing.

Many developmental models are used and applied in nursing. Examine the conceptual models and theories presented in Chapter 3 for their application of developmental concepts. Several nursing theories have a decidedly developmental focus, whether as a main component, as in Watson's theory, or with specific concepts included, defined, and built on, as in King's model.

A life span, developmental, or life processes focus has major relevance for nursing, because we view human beings in the context of environment and effects on health status. The interrelationships with health and nursing are complex and must be specified for their applicability to the domain of nursing.

Systems Theory

Perhaps the most widely used theory in multiple disciplines is systems theory. Systems have been in existence for ages, but in the late 1930s, Bertalanffy introduced systems theory to represent an aspect of reality. Thus, **general system theory** was incorporated in the paradigms of many scientific communities. This is a grand theory that is wide in scope, and that has generated numerous theories in many disciplines. Bertalanffy (1968) explained the wide applicability in many scientific communities as the various disciplines became concerned with "wholeness"— that is, not just focusing on isolated parts, but dealing with the interrelationships among them and between the parts and the whole. A system generally contains the following basic components: input, output, boundary, environment, and feedback. Figure 2.4 illustrates a basic view of a simple system.

The initial step in understanding and applying systems theory is to view the grand theory. Bertalanffy (1968) defined a *system* as a complex of interacting elements and proposed that every living organism is essentially an open system. The general system theory applies the following principles to human and organizational systems:

1. *Wholeness:* This indicates that the whole is more than merely the sum of its parts. To understand the whole, one must understand the components and their interactions with each other and the environment.
2. *Hierarchical order:* Some form of hierarchy exists in the system's components, structure, and functions.
3. *Exchange of information and matter (openness):* In an open system, there is an exchange and flow of information and matter with the environment through some boundary that surrounds the system. Inputs come through the boundary from the environment, are transformed through system processes (throughputs), and are sent as outputs through the boundary back into the environment. This exchange of information and matter is goal-oriented, whether to maintain the steady state or to fulfill the functions of the system. An important component of this process is feedback from the environment.

4. *Progressive differentiation:* Differentiation within the system leads to self-organization. Applying the laws of thermodynamics, entropy is a measure of order or organization in the system in the process of seeking equilibrium or some final goal. In an open system, entropy is decreased or negative, allowing for differentiation and self-organization.
5. *Equifinality:* In open systems, the final state can be reached from different initial conditions and in different ways. Initial conditions do not necessarily determine the final state or outcome of the system.
6. *Teleology:* Behavior in the system is directed toward some purpose or goal, as a human characteristic.

Environmental influences are a major consideration in health care. Systems theory provides a useful framework with which to visualize some phenomenon (the system), focusing on the components, structure, and functions as the internal environment (throughputs), and influenced by (inputs and feedback) and influencing (outputs) the environment. It is important to analyze the system carefully for all component parts, structures, and functions. Recall that the basis for general system theory is that "the whole is greater than the sum of the parts." This brings us to the need for a precise analysis of interrelationships among components and between the parts and the entire system. In addition, an open system has permeable boundaries receiving input and feedback from the environment. Problems occur when environmental factors are unknown, unclear, or ignored. Consider the broad health-service system. Since the Institute of Medicine began issuing a series of reports in 1998, we have been greatly concerned about safety in healthcare. Systems issues have been a major focus, but moving from a culture of blaming individual practitioners, the challenge became one of improving components in the system, input, feedback, and outputs. In addition, the broader healthcare environment and societal influences are included and visualized as crossing the system boundaries of an individual hospital setting.

In nursing, systems theory and various applications have been used to explain organizations, nursing and healthcare delivery, and groups of people. Several nursing models are based on systems theory. Johnson's Behavioral Systems conceptual model views the person as a behavioral system and nursing as an external force. It exemplifies how a grand theory (general system theory) from another scientific community provided a basis for developing the conceptual model of nursing (Johnson's Behavioral Systems). Specificity to the metaparadigm concepts and interrelationships unique to nursing have provided the basis for the nursing conceptual framework. Further delineation of concepts and propositions leads to more specific nursing theory. Neuman's

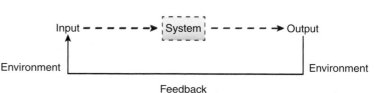

Figure 2.4 General systems model: A simple, open system.

Healthcare model, Roy's Adaptation model, and King's conceptual framework and Theory of Goal Attainment are examples of nursing conceptual models and theories based on systems models. Other nursing models use various components of general systems theory. Further applications of systems theory are evident in subsequent sections on management and leadership in organizations and change.

THEORETICAL CHALLENGES AND A PARADIGM SHIFT

Galbraith (1984) identified conventional wisdom as the structure of ideas that is based on acceptability, and to the people as their reality as they see and articulate it (p. 16). These ideas, which people generally consider as "truths," can be obstacles to new theories and to the development of new knowledge. Conventional wisdom may be that the current paradigm is on the brink of change. We must be open to new theories with new technology. Knowledge expansion can proceed at a much greater rate, as we have now seen with quantum physics or quantum mechanics.

For years, Newtonian physics provided the conventional wisdom of the three laws of motion: (1) inertia (objects in motion tend to stay in motion, and objects at rest tend to stay at rest unless there is interference from an outside force), (2) net force (the force on an object is mathematically equal to its mass times acceleration), and (3) reciprocal actions (for every action there is an equal and opposite reaction).

Based on the work of Galileo and others, Newton's theories from the 17th century prevailed until the 20th century with the addition of Einstein's theory of relativity and the discovery of **quantum theory**. As Nobel Laureate Robert Laughlin (2005) points out, although applicable to the macroscopic world, Newton's laws are incorrect at the atomic scale (p. 31). How we formerly pictured an atom, as a Newtonian-like solar system, is outdated and incorrect. Researchers and theorists have moved from classical physics to the era of the quantum.

We hear a good deal about the "quantum" nature of our world and universe. But it is all evolving as we develop new insight into the makeup of matter and how particles behave. A quantum is merely an energy bundle at the atomic and subatomic level—neutrons, protons, and electrons. The measurement of the quantum requires high-level mathematical computations looking at statistical probabilities of matter and waves. Hence, the discoveries from classic mechanics to quantum mechanics have occurred in areas of physics, chemistry, computers, and biology. This has provided the basis for certain transformations in healthcare, such as the introduction of the laser and magnetic resonance imaging (MRI). Biotechnology and advances in physical science will continue with our quest for discovery and knowledge. Laughlin (2005) notes, however, that we have experienced a paradigm shift, moving from a reductionist view of science to one of emergence, and that, "as in all other human activities, it is necessary in science to take stock now and then and reevaluate what one deeply understands and what one does not" (p. 13).

The language and concepts of quantum theory extend beyond the atom as we look at issues of holism, duality, uncertainty, causality, and probabilities in daily life and practice. Recognition and understanding of the paradigm shift are essential for the health sciences as we seek new knowledge and improvements in patient-care outcomes.

THE IMPACT OF THEORY ON PRACTICE

Alligood (2014a) proposes that professional nursing practice requires a systematic approach that is focused on the patient, and the theoretical works provide the perspectives of the patient (pp. 9–10). We use theory every day in our personal and professional lives, from learning the basic principles of asepsis in hygiene and standard precautions, to understanding the complex communication channels of the organizational system in which we practice.

Theory, practice, and research are interrelated and interdependent. We need theory to guide practice predictably and effectively. We need research to support the significance and usefulness of the theory, because the dynamic nature of our metaparadigm concepts of human beings, environment, health, and nursing makes theories tentative and subject to refinement and revision. Professional practice provides the questions for study based on problems and phenomena relevant to the discipline. Again, recall that nursing is a profession and a scientific community. We practice using principles provided by our metaparadigm and theoretical bases. This furnishes us with the tools for critical thinking, provision of care, education, administration, research, and interdisciplinary collaboration. We have a paradigm that provides the models for problems and solutions in our knowledge base and practice community in line with Kuhn's (1970) descriptions of a paradigm. Our paradigms and theories are designed to address problems and solutions in practice; otherwise we need to shift to a new structure with different theories and paradigms to explain our concerns for people, environments, health, and nursing.

The theory on which we base practice must be compatible with and must correspond to the phenomena of professional nursing practice. To ensure that the goals of theory and practice are consistent, Alligood (2014b) has recommended the following considerations for selecting a framework for practice:

1. Evaluate your values and beliefs held true about nursing.
2. Establish your philosophy statement of beliefs on the metaparadigm concepts.
3. Evaluate definitions of the metaparadigm concepts in selected models.
4. Select two to three frameworks that are consistent with your beliefs.
5. Look at the assumptions of the models.
6. Apply the models to your practice area to see if they work in the practice setting.

7. Compare the frameworks, looking at patient focus, nursing action, and outcomes.
8. Review the literature on applications of the selected models to practice.
9. Select the best framework appropriate to your practice and implement it. (p. 57)

But recall that conventional wisdom can be an obstacle to the discovery of new knowledge. Practice models are subject to change as new information is discovered and as patient needs change. The paradigm concepts must be in a constant state of evaluation to ensure that the model of practice is current and based on nursing science.

In the next chapter, conceptual models and theories unique to nursing are discussed. These models guide practice in our highly complex profession. Implementing models for practice, whether unique to nursing or adapted, is a necessary but arduous and time-consuming task. The process is worth the effort to ensure quality care for recipients, but it requires many of the skills addressed in subsequent chapters.

KEY POINTS

- Kerlinger and Lee (2000) define a theory as "a set of interrelated constructs (concepts), definitions, and propositions that present a systematic view of phenomena by specifying relations among variables, with the purpose of explaining and predicting the phenomena" (p. 11).

- A model is a graphic representation of some phenomena. A theoretical model provides a visual description of the theory using limited narrative and displaying components and relationships symbolically. A framework is another means of providing a structural view of the concepts and relationships proposed in a theory.

- A concept is a view or idea we hold about something, ranging from something highly concrete to something highly abstract. A construct is a more complex idea package of some phenomena. Definitions of concepts and constructs are theoretical or conceptual. An operational definition states precisely what we view as phenomena and how they can be measured as variables in a practice or research situation.

- Propositions in a theory are the descriptions and relationships among the constructs (or concepts) that propose how the concepts are linked and relate to each other and to the total theoretical structure.

- Dickoff and James (1968) developed a classic position paper proposing four levels of nursing theory: factor-isolating, factor-relating, situation-relating, and situation-producing theories.

- Theories are classified as grand, middle-range, or practice on the basis of their scope or breadth of coverage of phenomena.

- Theory description is a careful, nonjudgmental analysis of the component parts of a theory—its assumptions, concepts, definitions, propositions, context, and scope.

- Theory evaluation requires thoughtful interpretation relative to the clarity, significance, consistency, empirical support, and usefulness in explaining a phenomenon of concern.

- Maslow's theory of human motivation proposes a hierarchical structure for basic human needs.

- Developmental theories are widely used in nursing and other healthcare disciplines and include Erikson's (1963) eight ages of psychosocial development, Piaget's theory of cognitive development, and Kohlberg's theory of moral development.

- A system generally contains the following basic component parts: input, output, boundary, environment, and feedback. Bertalanffy's (1968) general system theory is a grand theory applied to many disciplines.

- Quantum theory, based on quantum physics, uses statistical probabilities for the actions of atomic and subatomic matter and waves and has provided some of the basis for advances in technology.

- Theory, practice, and research are interrelated and interdependent. When we are selecting a theory on which to base practice, the theory must be compatible with and correspond to the phenomena of professional nursing practice.

Thought and Discussion Questions

1. Consider the following statement by Barnum (1990) describing early nursing theories: "A high number of [boundary] overlaps occur in the discipline of nursing because it often attempts to deal holistically with a phenomenon (man) that has previously been dealt with in compartmentalized ways by other disciplines" (p. 218). What does she mean by "holistically"? How do you think other disciplines may deal with the human being in a compartmentalized way?

2. Identify individuals who you think are self-actualized, and explain why.

3. Identify a theory used in your practice setting. Identify the concepts (constructs), how the component concepts are defined, the propositions that link the concepts, and the aims of the theory.

4. Describe how theory is used in your practice setting, and propose how it could be used further.

5. Review the Chapter Thought located on the first page of the chapter, and discuss it in the context of the contents of the chapter.

Interactive Exercises

Go to the Intranet site and complete the interactive exercises provided for this chapter.

REFERENCES

Alligood, M. R. (2014a). The nature of knowledge needed for nursing practice. In M. R. Alligood, *Nursing theory: Utilization and application* (5th ed., pp. 1–12). St. Louis, MO: Elsevier Mosby.

Alligood, M. R. (2014b). Philosophies, models, and theories: Critical thinking structures. In M. R. Alligood (Ed.), *Nursing theory: Utilization and application* (5th ed., pp. 40–62). St. Louis, MO: Elsevier Mosby.

Alligood, M. R. (2014c). Introduction to nursing theory: Its history, significance, and analysis. In M. R. Alligood (Ed.), *Nursing theorists and their work* (8th ed., pp. 2–13). St. Louis, MO: Elsevier Mosby.

Barnum, B. J. S. (1990). *Nursing theory: Analysis, application, evaluation* (3rd ed.). Glenview, IL: Scott Foresman/Little, Brown Higher Education.

Barnum, B. J. S. (1994). *Nursing theory: Analysis, application, evaluation* (4th ed.). Philadelphia, PA: J. B. Lippincott.

Barnum, B. S. (1998). *Nursing theory: Analysis, application, evaluation* (5th ed.). Philadelphia, PA: Lippincott Williams & Wilkins.

Bertalanffy, L. V. (1968). *General system theory: Foundations, development, applications.* New York: George Braziller.

Chinn, P. L., & Kramer, M. K. (2011). *Integrated knowledge development in nursing* (8th ed.). St. Louis, MO: Elsevier Mosby.

Dickoff, J., & James, P. (1968). A theory of theories: A position paper. *Nursing Research, 17,* 197–203.

Erikson, E. H. (1963). *Childhood and society* (2nd ed.). New York: W. W. Norton.

Fawcett, J. (1995). *Analysis and evaluation of conceptual models of nursing* (3rd ed.). Philadelphia, PA: F. A. Davis.

Fawcett, J. (2000). *Analysis and evaluation of contemporary nursing knowledge: Nursing models and theories.* Philadelphia, PA: F. A. Davis.

Fawcett, J. (2005). *Contemporary nursing knowledge: Analysis and evaluation of nursing models and theories* (2nd ed.). Philadelphia, PA: F. A. Davis.

Fawcett, J. (2014). Nursing philosophies, models, and theories: A focus on the future. In A. M. Tomey & M. R. Alligood (Eds.), *Nursing theory: Utilization and application* (5th ed., pp. 425–441). St. Louis, MO: Mosby.

Fawcett, J., & DeSanto-Madeya, S. (2013). *Contemporary nursing knowledge: Analysis and evaluation of nursing models and theories* (3rd ed.). Philadelphia, PA: F. A. Davis.

Flavell, J. H. (1963). *The developmental psychology of Jean Piaget.* New York: Van Nostrand Reinhold.

Galbraith, J. K. (1984). *The affluent society.* Boston, MA: Houghton Mifflin.

Glanz, K., Rimer, B. K., & Lewis, F. M. (Eds.). (2002). *Health behavior and health education: Theory, research, and practice* (3rd ed.). San Francisco, CA: Jossey-Bass.

Havighurst, R. J. (1972). *Developmental tasks and education* (3rd ed.). New York: David McKay.

Kerlinger, F. N., & Lee, H. B. (2000). *Foundations of behavioral research* (4th ed.). Belmont, CA: Wadsworth Thompson Learning.

Kohlberg, L. (1984). *Essays in moral development: Vol. II. The psychology of moral development.* San Francisco, CA: Harper & Row.

Kohlberg, L., DeVries, R., Fein, G., Hart, D., Mayer, R., Noam, G., Snarey, J., & Wertsch, J. (1987). *Child psychology and childhood education: A cognitive-developmental view.* New York: Longman.

Kohlberg, L., & Lickona, T. (1990). Moral discussion and the class meeting. In R. DeVries & L. Kohlberg (Eds.), *Constructivist early education: Overview and comparison with other programs.* Washington, DC: National Association for the Education of Young Children.

Kuhn, T. S. (1970). *The structure of scientific revolutions* (2nd ed.). Chicago, IL: University of Chicago Press.

Laughlin, R. B. (2005). *A different universe: Reinventing physics from the bottom down*. New York: Basic Books.

Leininger, M. M. (2006). The culture care theory. In M. Leininger & M. R. McFarland (Eds.), *Culture care diversity and universality: A worldwide nursing theory* (2nd ed., pp. 1–41). Boston, MA: Jones and Bartlett.

Maslow, A. H. (1954). *Motivation and personality*. New York: Harper & Brothers.

Maslow, A. H. (1970). *Motivation and personality* (2nd ed.). New York: Harper & Row.

Merton, R. K. (1957). *Social theory and social structure* (Rev. ed.). Glencoe, IL: Free Press.

BIBLIOGRAPHY

Fawcett, J. (2011). Thoughts about nursing science and nursing sciencing on the event of the 25th anniversary of *Nursing Science Quarterly. Nursing Science Quarterly, 25,* 111–113.

Hardy, M. E. (1974). Theories: Components, development, evaluation. *Nursing Research, 23,* 100–107.

Power, F. C., Higgins, A., & Kohlberg, L. (1989). *Lawrence Kohlberg's approach to moral education*. New York: Columbia University.

Singer, D. G., & Revenson, T. A. (1998). *A Piaget primer: How a child thinks* (Rev. ed.). Madison, CT: International Universities Press.

ONLINE RESOURCES

Books by A. H. Maslow
http://www.maslow.com

Jean Piaget Society
http://www.piaget.org

Nursing Theories
http://www.nurses.info/nursing_theory.htm

● Jacqueline Fawcett

Evolution and Use of Formal Nursing Knowledge

3

The survival of the profession and discipline of nursing depends on nurses' understanding, acceptance, further development, and use of nursing discipline-specific knowledge, including nursing conceptual models and theories.

Chapter Objectives

On completion of this chapter, the reader will be able to:

1. Describe the meaning of formal nursing knowledge as the basis for professional nursing practice.

2. Identify the definitions and different functions of conceptual models and theories.

3. Discuss the advantages of using explicit conceptual models of nursing and nursing theories to guide professional nursing practice.

4. Apply a conceptual model of nursing or nursing theory to a particular practice situation.

Key Terms

Formal Nursing Knowledge
Nursing Knowledge
Conceptual Models of Nursing
Johnson's Behavioral System Model
King's Conceptual System
Levine's Conservation Model
Neuman's Systems Model
Orem's Self-Care Framework
Rogers' Science of Unitary Human
    Beings

Roy's Adaptation Model
Synergy Model
Grand Theories of Nursing
Leininger's Theory of Culture Care
    Diversity and Universality
Newman's Theory of Health as
    Expanding Consciousness
Parse's Theory of Humanbecoming

Middle-Range Nursing Theories
Peplau's Theory of Interpersonal
    Relations
Watson's Theory of Human Caring
Orlando's Theory of the
    Deliberative Nursing Process
Transitions Theory
Situation-Specific Nursing Theories

This chapter presents a discussion of the evolution of nursing knowledge—as it has been formalized—in conceptual models of nursing and nursing theories as well as a discussion of how that knowledge has influenced professional nursing practice.

FORMAL NURSING KNOWLEDGE

Conceptual models of nursing and nursing theories represent **formal nursing knowledge**. That knowledge was organized by several nurse scholars who devoted a great deal of time to observing people's experiences of wellness and illness, thinking about what is important to nurses and the profession of nursing in those experiences, and then testing their thoughts by conducting nursing research. **Nursing knowledge** continues to evolve as nurse researchers and practicing nurses use conceptual models and theories to guide their research and practice and then report the results at conferences and in publications. Consequently, all nurses can contribute to the evolution of nursing knowledge.

Nursing Defined

Nightingale's (1859) book, *Notes on Nursing: What It Is, and What It Is Not*, contains the first ideas that can be considered formal nursing knowledge. According to Nightingale, nursing ought to signify the proper use of fresh air, light, warmth, cleanliness, quiet, and the proper selection and administration of diet—all at the least expense of vital power to the patient; that is, she maintained that the purpose of nursing was to put the patient in the best condition for nature to act on him or her.

More than 100 years later, Henderson continued the evolution of formal nursing knowledge when she published a definition of nursing. "The unique function of the nurse," Henderson (1966) maintained, "is to assist the individual, sick or well, to perform those activities contributing to health or its recovery (or to peaceful death) that he [or she] would perform unaided if he [or she] had the necessary strength, will, or knowledge. And to do so in such a way as to help him [or her] gain independence as rapidly as possible" (p. 15). Although the intervening years were filled with many ideas about nursing, most of those ideas were, unfortunately, not presented as formal conceptual models and theories.

CONCEPTUAL MODELS

For our purposes, the terms *conceptual model, conceptual framework, conceptual system,* and *paradigm* have the same definition and functions and may be used interchangeably.

Definition

A **conceptual model** is defined as a set of relatively abstract and general concepts that address the phenomena of central interest to a discipline, the statements that broadly describe those concepts, and the statements that assert relatively abstract and general relations between two or more of the concepts (Fawcett & DeSanto-Madeya, 2013).

Each conceptual model presents a particular perspective about the phenomena of interest to a particular discipline, such as nursing. Conceptual models of nursing present diverse perspectives of human beings—including individuals, families and other groups, and communities—who are participants in nursing; the environment of the nursing participant and the environment in which nursing practice occurs; the health condition of the nursing participant; and the definition and goals of nursing as well as the practice methodology—typically referred to as the nursing process—used to assess, label, plan, intervene, and evaluate.

Functions

One function of any conceptual model is to provide a distinctive frame of reference, or "a horizon of expectations" (Popper, 1965, p. 47). Another function of each conceptual model is to identify a particular "philosophical and pragmatic orientation to the service nurses provide patients—a service which only nurses can provide—a service which provides a dimension to total care different from that provided by any other health professional" (Johnson, 1987, p. 195). Conceptual models of nursing provide explicit orientations not only for nurses but also for the general public. Johnson (1987) explained, "Conceptual models specify for nurses and society the mission and boundaries of the profession. They clarify the realm of nursing responsibility and accountability, and they allow the practitioner and/or the profession to document services and outcomes" (pp. 196–197).

Conceptual Models of Nursing

Currently, the works of several nurse scholars are recognized as broad **conceptual models of nursing** that can be used in many different practice situations. Among the best known of those conceptual models are Johnson's (1990) Behavioral System Model, King's (2006) Conceptual System, Levine's (1991) Conservation Model, Neuman's Systems Model (Neuman & Fawcett, 2011), Orem's (2001) Self-Care Framework, Rogers' (1990) Science of Unitary Human Beings, and Roy's (2009) Adaptation Model. An overview of each of these nursing models is presented in the following section, along with the implications of each one for professional nursing practice.

Dorothy Johnson's Behavioral System Model

Johnson's Behavioral System Model focuses on the person as a behavioral system, made up of all the patterned, repetitive, and purposeful elements of behavior that characterize life. Seven subsystems carry out specialized tasks or functions needed to maintain the integrity of the whole behavioral system and to manage its relationship to the environment. The subsystems and their functions are as follows:

1. *Attachment or affiliative*: The security—in terms of social inclusion, intimacy, and formation and maintenance of social bonds—that the individual needs for survival.

2. *Dependency*: The succoring behavior that calls for a response of nurturance as well as approval, attention or recognition, and physical assistance.
3. *Ingestive*: Appetite satisfaction—when, how, what, how much, and under what conditions the individual eats—all of which are governed by social and psychological considerations as well as biological requirements for food and fluids.
4. *Eliminative*: Elimination—when, how, and under what conditions the individual eliminates wastes.
5. *Sexual*: Procreation and gratification, with regard to behaviors dependent on the individual's biological sex and gender role identity, including but not limited to courting and mating.
6. *Aggressive*: Protection and preservation of self and society.
7. *Achievement*: Mastery or control of some aspect of self or environment, with regard to intellectual, physical, creative, mechanical, social, and caretaking (of children, partner, home) skills.

The structure of each subsystem involves four elements:

1. *Drive or goal*: The motivation for behavior.
2. *Set*: The individual's predisposition to act in certain ways to fulfill the function of the subsystem.
3. *Choice*: The individual's total behavioral repertoire for fulfilling subsystem functions, which encompasses the scope of action alternatives from which the person can choose.
4. *Action*: The individual's actual behavior in a situation. Action is the only structural element that can be observed directly; all other elements must be inferred from the individual's actual behavior and from the consequences of that behavior.

The three functional requirements listed below are needed by each subsystem to fulfill its functions:

1. *Protection* from noxious influences with which the system cannot cope
2. *Nurturance* through the input of appropriate supplies from the environment
3. *Stimulation* to enhance growth and prevent stagnation

Implications for Nursing Practice

Nursing practice is directed toward the restoration, maintenance, or attainment of behavioral system balance and dynamic stability at the highest possible level for the individual. Johnson's practice methodology, which is called the Nursing Diagnostic and Treatment Process, encompasses the four steps listed in Box 3.1. Each step is discussed in detail below.

Determination of the Existence of a Problem
The nurse obtains the following:

- Past and present family and individual behavioral system histories through interviews, structured and unstructured observations, and objective methodologies
- Data about the nature of behavioral system functioning in terms of the efficiency and effectiveness with which the patient's goals are obtained
- Information to determine the degree to which the behavior is purposeful, orderly, and predictable

---

BOX 3.1 **Johnson's Behavioral System Model: Diagnostic and Treatment Process**

- Determination of the Existence of a Problem
- Diagnostic Classification of a Problem
- Management of Nursing Problems
- Evaluation of Behavioral System Balance and Stability

- Information on the condition of the subsystem structural components to draw inferences about (1) drive strength, direction, and value; (2) the solidity and specificity of the set; (3) the range of behavior patterns available to the patient; and (4) the usual behavior in a given situation

The patient's behavior is compared with the following indices for behavioral system balance and stability, as well as the reorganization and integration of the subsystems:

- The behavior achieves the consequences sought.
- The behavior reveals the patient's effective use of motor, expressive, or social skills.
- The behavior is purposeful—actions are goal directed, reveal a plan, cease at an identifiable point, and are economical in sequence.
- The behavior is orderly—actions are methodical and systematic, build sequentially toward a goal, and form a recognizable pattern.
- The behavior is predictable—actions are repetitive under particular circumstances.
- The amount of energy expended to achieve desired goals is acceptable.
- The behavior reflects appropriate choices—actions are compatible with survival imperatives and the social situation.
- The behavior satisfies the patient sufficiently.

Diagnostic Classification of a Problem
A problem might occur in two areas:

- *Internal subsystem problems*: Functional requirements are not met, inconsistency or disharmony among the structural components of subsystems is evident, and/or the behavior is inappropriate in the ambient culture.
- *Intersystem problems*: The entire behavioral system is dominated by one or two subsystems, or a conflict exists between two or more subsystems.

Management of Nursing Problems
The general goals of action are to restore, maintain, or attain the patient's behavioral system balance and stability and to help the patient achieve an optimum level of balance and functioning when this goal is possible and desired. The nurse determines what nursing is to accomplish on behalf of the behavioral system by determining who makes the judgment regarding the acceptable level of behavioral system balance and stability. Nursing actions may occur in three areas:

- *Temporary external regulatory or control mechanisms*, by setting limits for behavior by either permissive or inhibitory means, inhibiting ineffective behavioral

responses, helping the patient acquire new responses, and reinforcing appropriate behaviors
- *Repair of damaged structural components*, by reducing drive strength by changing attitudes, redirecting goals by changing attitudes, altering the set by instruction or counseling, and adding choices by teaching new skills
- *Fulfillment of functional requirements* of subsystems, by protecting the patient from overwhelming noxious influences, supplying adequate nurturance, and providing stimulation to enhance growth and inhibit stagnation

The nurse negotiates the treatment modality with the patient by establishing a contract with the patient and helping him or her to understand the meaning of the nursing diagnosis and the proposed treatment.

Evaluation of Behavioral System Balance and Stability
The nurse compares the patient's behavior after treatment with indices of behavioral system balance and stability.

Imogene King's Conceptual System

King's Conceptual System focuses on the continuing ability of individuals to meet their basic needs so that they may function in their socially defined roles. This conceptual model also concentrates on individuals' interactions within three open, dynamic, interacting systems—the personal system, the interpersonal system, and the social system.

Personal Systems
Personal systems are individuals who are regarded as rational, sentient, social beings. Concepts related to the personal system are as follows:

- *Perception*: A process of organizing, interpreting, and transforming information from sense data and memory that gives meaning to one's experience, represents one's image of reality, and influences one's behavior
- *Self*: A composite of thoughts and feelings that constitute a person's awareness of individual existence, of who and what he or she is
- *Growth and development*: Cellular, molecular, and behavioral changes in human beings that are a function of genetic endowment, meaningful and satisfying experiences, and an environment conducive to helping individuals move toward maturity
- *Body image*: A person's perceptions of his or her body
- *Time*: The duration between the occurrence of one event and the occurrence of another event
- *Personal space*: The physical area, or territory, that exists in all directions as perceived by each individual
- *Learning*: Gaining knowledge

Interpersonal Systems
Interpersonal systems are defined as two or more individuals interacting in a given situation. The concepts associated with this system are as follows:

- *Interaction*: The act of two or more persons in mutual presence; a sequence of verbal and nonverbal behaviors that are goal directed
- *Communication*: The vehicle by which human relations are developed and maintained; encompasses intrapersonal, interpersonal, verbal, and nonverbal communications
- *Transaction*: A process of interaction in which human beings communicate with the environment to achieve goals that are valued
- *Role*: A set of behaviors expected of a person occupying a position in a social system
- *Stress*: A dynamic state whereby a human being interacts with the environment to maintain balance for growth, development, and performance, which involves an exchange of energy and information between the person and the environment for regulation and control of stressors
- *Coping*: A way of dealing with stress

Social Systems
Social systems are organized boundary systems of social roles, behaviors, and practices developed to maintain values, and the mechanisms to regulate these practices and rules. The concepts related to social systems are as follows:

- *Organization*: Composed of human beings with prescribed roles and positions who use resources to accomplish personal and organizational goals
- *Authority*: A transactional process characterized by active, reciprocal relations in which members' values, backgrounds, and perceptions play a role in defining, validating, and accepting the authority of individuals within an organization
- *Power*: The process whereby one or more persons influence other persons in a situation
- *Status*: The position of an individual in a group or a group in relation to other groups in an organization
- *Decision making*: A dynamic and systematic process by which a goal-directed choice of perceived alternatives is made and acted on by individuals or groups to answer a question and attain a goal
- *Control*: Being in charge

Implications for Nursing Practice
Nursing practice is directed toward helping individuals maintain their health so that they can function in their roles. King's practice methodology, which is the essence of her Theory of Goal Attainment, is called the Interaction-Transaction Process. The process encompasses the 10 steps listed in Box 3.2. Each step is discussed in detail below.

BOX 3.2 **King's Conceptual System Practice Methodology: Interaction-Transaction Process**

- Perception
- Judgment
- Action
- Reaction
- Disturbance
- Mutual Goal Setting
- Exploration of Means to Achieve Goals
- Agreement on Means to Achieve Goals
- Transaction
- Attainment of Goals

Perception

Perception is the first step in the assessment phase of the interaction-transaction process. The nurse and the patient meet in some nursing situation and perceive each other. The accuracy of the perception depends on verifying the nurse's inferences with the patient. The nurse can use the Goal-Oriented Nursing Record (GONR) to record both sets of perceptions.

Judgment

Judgment is the second step in the assessment phase of the interaction-transaction process. The nurse and the patient make mental judgments about the other, which the nurse can record on the GONR.

Action

Action is the third step in the assessment phase of the interaction-transaction process. Action is a sequence of behaviors of interacting persons, including recognition of the situation, activities related to the situation, and motivation to exert some control over the events to achieve goals. The nurse and the patient take some mental action, which the nurse can record on the GONR.

Reaction

Reaction is the fourth step in the assessment phase of the interaction-transaction process. The nurse and the patient mentally react to each one's perceptions of the other. The nurse can use the GONR to record these mental reactions.

Disturbance

Disturbance is the diagnosis phase of the interaction-transaction process. The nurse and the patient communicate and interact, and the nurse identifies the patient's concerns, problems, and disturbances in health. The nurse then conducts a nursing history to determine the patient's activities of daily living, using the Criterion-Referenced Measure of Goal Attainment Tool (CRMGAT); roles; environmental stressors; perceptions; and values, learning needs, and goals. The nurse records these data from the nursing history on the GONR.

The nurse also records the medical history and physical examination data, results of laboratory tests and x-ray examination, information gathered from other health professionals and the patient's family members, and any diagnoses on the GONR.

Mutual Goal Setting

Mutual goal setting is the first step in the planning phase of the interaction-transaction process. The nurse and the patient interact purposefully to set mutually agreed-on goals. If the patient cannot verbally participate in goal setting, the nurse interacts with family members instead.

Mutual goal setting is based on the nurse's assessment of the patient's concerns, problems, and disturbances in health; the nurse's and patient's perceptions of the interference; and the nurse's sharing of information with the patient and his or her family to help the patient attain the goals identified. Mutual goal setting includes consideration of the ethical aspects of the situation, including the following:

● Helping the patient and family to sort out the values inherent in the situation and encouraging them to think through their own value system and the consequences of action they decide to take in the situation

● Helping the patient and family to make decisions that take their value system into consideration by providing information that contributes to their decision, by emphasizing their reality as they have expressed it, and by not making decisions for them

● Becoming skillful in identifying options in every nursing situation and exploring those options with the patient and family

● Identifying those elements in the situation that can be changed and controlled and those that cannot, and concentrating energy and efforts on control and change

● Being especially sensitive to the ethical issues that may arise when considering the right to life, the right to die, and the right to information required for informed choice

The nurse records the mutually set goals on the GONR.

Exploration of Means to Achieve Goals

Exploration is the second step in the planning phase of the interaction-transaction process. The nurse and the patient interact purposefully to explore the means to achieve the mutually set goals.

Agreement on Means to Achieve Goals

Agreement is the third step in the planning phase of the interaction-transaction process. The nurse and the patient interact purposefully to agree on the means to achieve the mutually set goals. The nurse records the nursing orders with regard to the means to achieve goals on the GONR.

Transaction

Transaction is the implementation phase of the interaction-transaction process. Transaction refers to what is valued in the interaction. The nurse and the patient carry out the measures agreed on to achieve the mutually set goals. The nurse can use the GONR flow sheet and progress notes to record the implementation of measures used to achieve goals.

Attainment of Goals

Attainment of goals is the evaluation phase of the interaction-transaction process. The nurse and the patient identify the outcome of the interaction-transaction process. The outcome is expressed in terms of the patient's state of health or ability to function in social roles. The nurse and the patient make a decision with regard to whether the goal was attained and, if necessary, determine why the goal was not attained. The nurse can use the CRMGAT to record the outcome and the GONR to record the discharge summary.

Myra Levine's Conservation Model

Levine's Conservation Model focuses on conservation of the person's wholeness. Adaptation is the process by which people maintain their wholeness or integrity as they respond to environmental challenges and become congruent with the environment. There are three sources of environmental challenges:

1. *Perceptual environment*: That part of the environment to which individuals respond with their sense organs
2. *Operational environment*: Those aspects of the environment that are not directly perceived, such as radiation, odorless and colorless pollutants, and microorganisms

3. *Conceptual environment*: The environment of language, ideas, symbols, concepts, and invention

Individuals respond to the environment by means of four integrated processes that constitute the organismic response:

1. Flight-or-flight mechanism
2. Inflammatory-immune response
3. Stress response
4. Perceptual awareness, which includes the basic orienting, haptic, auditory, visual, and taste-smell systems

Implications for Nursing Practice

Nursing practice is directed toward promoting wholeness for all people, well or sick. Patients are partners or participants in nursing care and are temporarily dependent on the nurse. The nurse's goal is to end the dependence as quickly as possible. Levine's practice methodology is Nursing Process as Conservation, which is defined as "keeping together." The three steps of the process are listed in Box 3.3. Each step is discussed in detail below.

Trophicognosis

Trophicognosis is the formulation of a nursing care judgment arrived at by the scientific method. The nurse observes and collects data that will influence nursing practice, using appropriate assessment to establish an objective and scientific rationale for nursing practice. The nurse understands the basis for the prescribed medical regimen, including the medical diagnosis, the medical history, and the laboratory and x-ray examination reports, with specific reference to areas influencing the nursing care plan.

Assessment skills are directed at four conservation principles:

1. *Conservation of energy* determines the ability to perform necessary activities without producing excessive fatigue. Relevant observations include vital signs, the patient's general condition, the patient's behavior, the patient's tolerance of nursing activities required by his or her condition, and allowable activity for the patient based on his or her energy resources.
2. *Conservation of structural integrity* determines physical functioning. Relevant observations include status of any pathophysiological processes, status of healing processes, and effects of surgical procedures.
3. *Conservation of personal integrity* determines moral and ethical values and life experiences. Relevant observations include the patient's life story, interest in participating in decision making, and identifying sense of self.
4. *Conservation of social integrity* takes the patient's family members, friends, and conceptual environment into account. Relevant observations include identification of

the patient's significant others, participation in workplace and/or school activities, religion, and cultural and ethnic history.

The basis for implementation of the nursing care plan includes principles of nursing science and adaptation of nursing techniques to the unique cluster of needs demonstrated in the individual patient. The nurse identifies the provocative facts—that is, the data that provoke attention on the basis of knowledge of the situation—to provide the basis for a hypothesis, or trophicognosis. Observations are then recorded and transmitted.

Intervention/Action

Intervention/action is a test of the hypothesis. The nursing care plan is implemented and evaluated within the structure of administrative policy, availability of equipment, and established standards of nursing. The general types of nursing intervention required are therapeutic nursing intervention, which influences adaptation favorably, or toward renewed social well-being, and supportive nursing interventions, which cannot alter the course of the adaptation and can only maintain the status quo or fail to halt a downward course. Nursing interventions are structured according to the four conservation principles:

- *Conservation of energy* through an adequate deposit of energy resource and regulation of the expenditure of energy
- *Conservation of structural integrity* through maintenance or restoration of the structure of the body
- *Conservation of personal integrity* through maintenance or restoration of the patient's sense of identity, self-worth, and acknowledgment of uniqueness
- *Conservation of social integrity* through acknowledging the patient as a social being

Evaluation of Intervention/Action

The nurse's evaluation of the effects of the intervention/action is used to revise the trophicognosis as necessary. An indicator of the success of nursing interventions is the patient's organismic response.

Betty Neuman's Systems Model

Neuman's Systems Model focuses on the wellness of the patient system in relation to environmental stress and reactions to stress. The patient system, which can be an individual, a family or other group, or a community, is a composite of five interrelated variables:

1. *Physiological*: Bodily structure and function
2. *Psychological*: Mental processes and relationships
3. *Sociocultural*: Social and cultural functions
4. *Developmental*: Developmental processes of life
5. *Spiritual*: Aspects of spirituality on a continuum from complete unawareness or denial to a consciously developed, high level of spiritual understanding

The patient system is depicted as a central core, which is a basic structure of survival factors common to the species, surrounded by three types of metaphorical concentric rings:

1. *Flexible line of defense*: The outermost ring is a protective buffer for the patient's normal or stable state that

---

BOX 3.3 **Levine's Conservation Model Practice Methodology: Nursing Process as Conservation**

- Trophicognosis
- Intervention/Action
- Evaluation of Intervention/Action

prevents invasion of stressors and keeps the patient system free from stressor reactions or symptomatology.

2. *Normal line of defense*: This lies between the flexible line of defense and the lines of resistance and represents the patient system's normal or usual wellness state.

3. *Lines of resistance*: The innermost concentric rings are involuntarily activated when a stressor invades the normal line of defense. They attempt to stabilize the patient system and foster a return to the normal line of defense. If these rings are effective, the system can reconstitute; if they are ineffective, death may ensue.

The environment encompasses all internal and external factors or influences surrounding the patient system. The *internal environment* is all forces or interactive influences internal to or contained solely within the boundaries of the defined patient system; this is the source of intrapersonal stressors. The *external environment* is all forces or interaction influences external to or existing outside the defined patient system; this is the source of interpersonal and extrapersonal stressors. The *created environment* is subconsciously developed by the patient as a symbolic expression of system wholeness and supersedes and encompasses the internal and external environments; it functions as a subjective safety mechanism that may block the true reality of the environment and the health experience.

Implications for Nursing Practice

Nursing practice is directed toward facilitating optimal wellness through retention, attainment, or maintenance of client system stability. The nurse uses the Neuman Systems Model Assessment and Intervention Tool, the Systems Model Nursing Diagnosis Taxonomy, and any other relevant clinical tools to guide collection of data and facilitate documentation of nursing diagnoses, nursing goals, and nursing outcomes. The three steps of Neuman's practice methodology, which is called the Nursing Process Format, are listed in Box 3.4. Each step is discussed in detail here.

Nursing Diagnosis

The nurse establishes the database, which involves simultaneous consideration of the dynamic interactions of physiological, psychological, sociocultural, developmental, and spiritual variables. The nurse identifies the patient/patient system's perceptions and his or her own perceptions, including basic structure factors and energy resources; flexible and normal lines of defense, lines of resistance, degree of potential or actual reaction, and potential for reconstitution following a reaction; and the internal and external environmental stressors that threaten the stability of the patient/patient system. The nurse then compares his or her own perceptions with the patient/patient system's perceptions. A comprehensive nursing diagnosis is presented that encompasses the patient/patient system's general condition

---

BOX 3.4	**Neuman's Systems Model Practice Methodology: Nursing Process Format**

- Nursing Diagnosis
- Nursing Goals
- Nursing Outcomes

---

or circumstances, including identification of actual or potential variances from wellness and available resources.

Nursing Goals

The nurse prioritizes goals by considering the patient/patient system's wellness level, the meaning of the experience to the patient/patient system, system stability needs, and total available resources. Outcome goals and interventions are proposed that will facilitate the highest possible level of patient/patient system stability or wellness, maintain the normal line of defense, and retain the flexible line of defense. Desired prescriptive change or outcome goals are developed to correct variances from wellness with the patient/patient system, taking patient/patient system needs and resources into account. Specific preventions, presented as intervention modalities, are negotiated with the patient/patient system.

Nursing Outcomes

The nurse implements nursing interventions through the use of one or more of the three "prevention as intervention" modalities:

1. *Primary prevention*: Nursing actions to retain system stability are implemented through such measures as preventing stressor invasion, providing resources to retain or strengthen existing patient/patient system strengths, and supporting positive coping and functioning.

2. *Secondary prevention*: Nursing actions to attain system stability are implemented through such measures as protecting the patient/patient system's basic structure, mobilizing and optimizing the patient/patient system's internal and external resources to attain stability and energy conservation, and facilitating purposeful manipulation of stressors and reactions to stressors.

3. *Tertiary prevention*: Nursing actions to maintain system stability are implemented through such measures as attaining and maintaining the highest possible level of patient/patient system wellness and stability during reconstitution; educating, reeducating, and/or reorienting the patient/patient system as needed; and supporting the patient/patient system toward appropriate goals.

The nurse evaluates the outcome goals by confirming (with the patient/patient system) their attainment and reformulating goals as necessary. The nurse and patient/patient system set intermediate and long-range goals for subsequent nursing action.

Dorothea Orem's Self-Care Framework

Orem's Self-Care Framework focuses on patients' deliberate actions to meet their own and dependent others' therapeutic self-care demands. The model also focuses on nurses' deliberate actions to implement nursing systems designed to assist individuals and multiperson units who have limitations in their abilities to provide continuing and therapeutic self-care or care of dependent others. The concepts of Orem's conceptual model are as follows:

Self-Care

Self-care is behavior directed by individuals to themselves or their environments to regulate factors that affect their own development and functioning in the interests of life, health, or well-being.

Self-Care Agency

A self-care agency is the complex capability of maturing and mature individuals to determine the presence and characteristics of specific requirements for regulating their own functioning and development, make judgments and decisions about what to do, and perform care measures to meet specific self-care requisites.

Power Components

A person's ability to perform self-care is influenced by 10 power components:

1. Ability to maintain attention and exercise requisite vigilance with respect to self as self-care agent and internal and external conditions and factors significant for self-care
2. Controlled use of available physical energy that is sufficient for the initiation and continuation of self-care operations
3. Ability to control the position of the body and its parts in the execution of the movements required for the initiation and completion of self-care operations
4. Ability to reason within a self-care frame of reference
5. Motivation (i.e., goal orientations for self-care that are in accord with its characteristics and its meaning for life, health, and well-being)
6. Ability to make decisions about self-care and to operationalize these decisions
7. Ability to acquire technical knowledge about self-care from authoritative sources, to retain it, and to operationalize it
8. A repertoire of cognitive, perceptual, manipulative, communication, and interpersonal skills adapted to the performance of self-care operations
9. Ability to order discrete self-care actions or action systems into relationships with prior and subsequent actions toward the final achievement of regulatory goals of self-care
10. Ability to consistently perform self-care operations, integrating them with relevant aspects of personal, family, and community living

Basic Conditioning Factors

The person's ability to perform self-care also is influenced by 10 internal and external factors called basic conditioning factors:

1. Age
2. Gender
3. Developmental state
4. Health state
5. Sociocultural orientation
6. Healthcare system factors, such as medical diagnostic and treatment modalities
7. Family system factors
8. Patterns of living, including regular activities
9. Environmental factors
10. Resource availability and adequacy

Therapeutic Self-Care Demand

Therapeutic self-care demand is the action demand on individuals to meet three types of self-care requisites:

1. *Universal self-care requisites*: Actions that need to be performed to maintain life processes, the integrity of human structure and function, and general well-being
2. *Developmental self-care requisites*: Actions that need to be performed in relation to human developmental processes, conditions, and events and in relation to events that may adversely affect development
3. *Health deviation self-care requisites*: Actions that need to be performed in relation to genetic and constitutional defects, human structural and functional deviations and their effects, and medical diagnostic and treatment measures prescribed or performed by physicians

Self-Care Deficit

The self-care deficit is the relationship of inadequacy between self-care agency and the therapeutic self-care demand. A self-care deficit occurs when the therapeutic self-care demand exceeds self-care agency.

Nursing Agency

Nursing agency is a complex property or attribute that enables nurses to know and help others to know their therapeutic self-care demands, to meet their therapeutic self-care demands, and to regulate the exercise or development of their self-care agency. A nursing system is a series of coordinated deliberate practical actions performed by nurses and patients directed toward meeting the patient's therapeutic self-care demand and protecting and regulating the exercise or development of the patient's self-care agency.

Implications for Nursing Practice

Nursing practice is directed toward helping people meet their own and their dependent others' therapeutic self-care demands. Orem's practice methodology, which is called Professional-Technological Operations of Nursing Practice, involves the seven steps listed in Box 3.5. A detailed discussion of the operations is given below.

Case Management Operations

The nurse uses a case management approach to direct each of the nursing diagnostic, prescriptive, regulatory, and control operations. The nurse also maintains an overview of the interrelationships between the social, interpersonal, and professional-technological systems of nursing. Finally, the nurse uses the nursing history and other appropriate tools for collection of information,

---

BOX 3.5 **Orem's Practice Methodology: Professional-Technological Operations of Nursing Practice**

- Case Management Operations
- Diagnostic Operations
- Prescriptive Operations
- Regulatory Operations: Design of Nursing Systems for Performance of Regulatory Operations
- Regulatory Operations: Planning for Regulatory Operations
- Regulatory Operations: Production of Regulatory Care
- Control Operations

documentation of information, and measurement of the quality of nursing.

Diagnostic Operations

The nurse identifies the unit of service for nursing practice as an individual, an individual member of a multiperson unit, or a multiperson unit. The nurse determines why the individual needs nursing and collects demographic data about the patient and information about the nature and boundaries of the patient's healthcare situation and nursing's jurisdiction within those boundaries.

Prescriptive Operations

In collaboration with the patient or family, the nurse identifies all care measures needed to meet the entire therapeutic self-care demand. In addition, the nurse specifies the roles to be played by the nurse(s), patient, and dependent-care agent(s) in meeting the therapeutic self-care demand and in regulating the patient's exercise or development or self-care agency or dependent-care agency.

Regulatory Operations: Design of Nursing Systems for Performance of Regulatory Operations

The nurse designs a nursing system, a series of coordinated deliberate practical actions performed by the nurse and the patient. The actions are directed toward meeting the patient's therapeutic self-care demand and protecting and regulating the exercise or development of the patient's self-care agency or dependent-care agency. The selection of the appropriate nursing system depends on who can or should perform self-care actions:

- The *wholly compensatory nursing system* is selected when the patient cannot or should not perform any self-care actions, and thus the nurse must perform them.
- The *partly compensatory nursing system* is selected when the patient can perform some, but not all, self-care actions.
- The *supportive-educative nursing system* is selected when the patient can and should perform all self-care actions.

Each nursing system is implemented using one or more of the following *methods of helping*:

- Acting for or doing for the patient
- Providing a developmental environment
- Supporting the patient psychologically
- Guiding the patient
- Teaching the patient

Regulatory Operations: Planning for Regulatory Operations

The nurse specifies what is needed to produce the nursing system(s) selected for the patient, including the following elements:

- The time during which the nursing system will be produced
- The place where the nursing system will be produced
- The environmental conditions necessary for the production of the nursing system, as well as the equipment and supplies required
- The number and qualifications of nurses and other healthcare providers necessary to produce the nursing system and to evaluate its effects

- The organization and timing of tasks to be performed
- The designation of who (nurse or patient) is to perform the tasks

Regulatory Operations: Production of Regulatory Care

Nursing systems are produced by means of the actions of nurses and patients during nurse-patient encounters; the nurse produces and manages the designated nursing system(s) and method(s) of helping for as long as the patient's self-care deficit or dependent-care deficit exists.

- The nurse performs and regulates the self-care or dependent-care tasks for patients or assists patients with their performance of self-care or dependent-care tasks.
- The nurse coordinates self-care or dependent-care task performance so that a unified system of care is produced and coordinated with other components of healthcare.
- The nurse helps patients, their families, and others bring about systems of daily living for patients that support the accomplishment of self-care or dependent care and are, at the same time, satisfying in relation to patients' interests, talents, and goals.
- The nurse guides, directs, and supports patients in their exercise of, or in the withholding of the exercise of, their self-care agency or dependent-care agency.
- The nurse stimulates patients' interests in self-care or dependent care by raising questions and promoting discussions of care problems and issues when conditions permit.
- The nurse is available to patients at times when questions are likely to arise.
- The nurse supports and guides patients in learning activities and provides cues for learning as well as instructional sessions.
- The nurse supports and guides patients as they experience illness or disability and the effects of medical care measures and as they experience the need to engage in new measures of self-care or change their ways of meeting ongoing self-care requisites.

Control Operations

The nurse performs control operations concurrently or separately from the production of regulatory care. The nurse makes observations and evaluates the nursing system to determine whether the following goals are being met:

- The nursing system that was designed is actually produced.
- There is a fit between the current prescription for nursing and the nursing system that is being produced.
- Regulation of the patient's functioning is being achieved through performance of care measures to meet the patient's therapeutic self-care demand.
- Exercise of the patient's self-care agency or dependent-care agency is being properly regulated.
- Developmental change is in process and is adequate.
- The patient is adjusting to any decline in powers to engage in self-care or dependent care.

Martha Rogers' Science of Unitary Human Beings

Rogers' Science of Unitary Human Beings focuses on unitary, irreducible human beings and their environments. The four basic concepts are as follows:

1. *Energy fields* are irreducible, indivisible, pandimensional unitary human beings and environments that are identified by pattern and manifesting characteristics that are specific to the whole and that cannot be predicted from knowledge of the parts. Human and environmental energy fields are integral with each other.
2. *Openness* is a characteristic of human and environmental energy fields; energy fields are continuously and completely open.
3. *Pattern* refers to the distinguishing characteristic of an energy field. Pattern is perceived as a single wave that gives identity to the field. Each human field pattern is unique and is integral with its own unique environmental field pattern. Pattern is an abstraction that cannot be seen; what is seen or experienced are manifestations of field patterns. Manifestations of pattern include perceptions, expressions, and experiences.
4. *Pandimensionality* is a nonlinear domain without spatial or temporal attributes.

The three principles of homeodynamics, which describe the nature of human and environmental energy fields, are as follows:

1. *Resonancy* asserts that human and environmental fields are identified by wave patterns that manifest continuous change from lower to higher frequencies.
2. *Helicy* asserts that human and environmental field patterns are continuous, innovative, and unpredictable and are characterized by increasing diversity.
3. *Integrality* emphasizes the continuous mutual human field and environmental field process.

Implications for Nursing Practice

Nursing practice is directed toward promoting the health and well-being of all persons, wherever they are. The three steps of Rogers' practice methodology, which is called the Health Patterning Practice Method, are listed in Box 3.6. Each step is discussed in detail below.

Pattern Manifestation Knowing and Appreciation— Assessment

- Assessment refers to the continuous process of apprehending and identifying manifestations of the human energy field and environmental energy field patterns

---

BOX 3.6 **Rogers' Science of Unitary Human Beings Practice Methodology: The Health Patterning Practice Method**

- Pattern Manifestation Knowing and Appreciation— Assessment
- Voluntary Mutual Patterning
- Pattern Manifestation Knowing and Appreciation— Evaluation

---

that relate to current health events, including perceptions, expressions, and experiences.

- The nurse uses one or more research instruments or clinical tools based on the Science of Unitary Human Beings to guide application and documentation of the practice methodology.
- The nurse acts with pandimensional authenticity— that is, with a demeanor of genuineness, trustworthiness, and knowledgeable caring.
- The nurse focuses on the patient as a unified whole, a unitary human being.

Voluntary Mutual Patterning

- Voluntary mutual patterning is the continuous process whereby the nurse, with the patient, patterns the environmental energy field to promote harmony related to the health events.
- The nurse facilitates the patient's actualization of potentials for health and well-being. The nurse has no investment in the patient's changing in a particular way.
- The nurse does not attempt to change anyone to conform to arbitrary health ideals. Rather, the nurse enhances the patient's efforts to actualize health potentials from the patient's point of view.

Pattern Manifestation Knowing and Appreciation— Evaluation

- The nurse evaluates voluntary mutual patterning by means of pattern manifestation knowing.
- Additional pattern information is monitored and collected as it unfolds during voluntary mutual patterning.
- The nurse considers the pattern information within the context of continually emerging health patterning goals affirmed by the patient.

Callista Roy's Adaptation Model

Roy's Adaptation Model focuses on the responses of the human adaptive system, which can be an individual or a group, to a constantly changing environment. Adaptation is the central feature of the model. Problems in adaptation arise when the adaptive system is unable to cope with or respond to constantly changing stimuli from the internal and external environments in a manner that maintains the integrity of the system.

Environmental stimuli are categorized as follows:

- *Focal*: The stimuli most immediately confronting the person.
- *Contextual*: The contributing factors in the situation.
- *Residual*: Other unknown factors that may influence the situation. When the factors making up residual stimuli become known, they are considered focal or contextual stimuli.

Adaptation occurs through innate or acquired coping mechanisms used to respond to changing environmental stimuli:

- The *regulator coping subsystem* (*for individuals*) receives input from the external environment and from changes in the individual's internal state and processes the changes through neural-chemical-endocrine channels to produce responses.

- The *cognator coping subsystem* (*for individuals*) also receives input from external and internal stimuli that involve psychological, social, physical, and physiological factors, including regulator subsystem outputs. These stimuli are then processed through cognitive/emotive pathways, including perceptual/information processing, learning, judgment, and emotion.
- The *stabilizer subsystem control process* (*for groups*) involves the established structures, values, and daily activities used by a group to accomplish its primary purpose and contribute to common purposes of society.
- The *innovator subsystem control process* (*for humans in groups*) involves the structures and processes necessary for change and growth in human social systems.

Responses take place in four modes of adaptation for individuals and groups:

1. *Physiological/physical mode*
   - *Physiological mode* (*for individuals*) is concerned with basic needs requisite to maintaining the physical and physiologic integrity of the individual human system. It encompasses oxygenation; nutrition; elimination; activity and rest; protection; senses; fluid, electrolyte, and acid-base balance; neurologic function; and endocrine function. The basic underlying need is physiologic integrity.
   - *Physical mode* (*for groups*) pertains to the manner in which the collective human adaptive system manifests adaptation relative to basic operating resources, including participants, physical facilities, and fiscal resources. The basic underlying need is resource adequacy, or wholeness achieved by adapting to change in physical resource needs.
2. *Self-concept/group identity mode*
   - *Self-concept mode* (*for individuals*) addresses the composite of beliefs and feelings that a person holds about himself or herself at a given time. The basic underlying need is psychic and spiritual integrity, the need to know who one is so that one can be or exist with a sense of unity, meaning, and purposefulness in the universe. The *physical self* refers to the individual's appraisal of his or her own physical being, including physical attributes, functioning, sexuality, health and illness states, and appearance. It includes the components of body sensation and body image. The *personal self* refers to the individual's appraisal of his or her own characteristics, expectations, values, and worth, including self-consistency, self-ideal, and the moral-ethical-spiritual self.
   - *Group identity mode* (*for groups*) addresses shared relations, goals, and values, which create a social milieu and culture, a group self-image, and co-responsibility for goal achievement. Identity integrity is the underlying need, which implies the honesty, soundness, and completeness of the group members' identification with the group and involves the process of sharing identity and goals. This mode encompasses interpersonal relationships, group self-image, social milieu, and group culture.
3. *Role function mode* (*for individuals and groups*) focuses on the roles that the individual occupies in society. The basic underlying need is social integrity—the need to know who one is in relation to others so that one can act. For the group, this mode focuses on the action components associated with group infrastructure that are designed to contribute to the accomplishment of the group's mission or the tasks or functions associated with the group. The basic underlying need is role clarity—the need to understand and commit to fulfill expected tasks—so that the group can achieve common goals.
4. *Interdependence mode* (*for individuals and groups*) focuses on the basic underlying need of relational integrity, defined as the feeling of security in nurturing relationships. For the individual, the mode focuses on interactions related to the giving and receiving of love, respect, and value and encompasses affectional adequacy, developmental adequacy, resource adequacy, significant others, and support systems. For the group, it pertains to the social context in which the group operates, including both private and public contacts within the group and with those outside the group, and encompasses affectional adequacy, developmental adequacy, resource adequacy, context, infrastructure, and resources.

The four modes are interrelated. Responses in any one mode may have an effect on or act as a stimulus in one or all of the other modes. Responses in each mode are judged as either adaptive or ineffective. A judgment of "adaptive responses" indicates promotion of the goals of the human adaptive system, including survival, growth, reproduction, mastery, and person-environment transformation. A judgment of "ineffective responses" does not contribute to the goals of the human adaptive system.

Adaptation level is determined by the total effect of focal, contextual, and residual stimuli on the modes of adaptation. The three levels of adaptation are as follows:

1. *Integrated life process*: Level of adaptation at which the structures and functions of a life process are working as a whole to meet human needs
2. *Compensatory life process*: Level of adaptation at which the cognator and regulator [or stabilizer and innovator] have been activated by a challenge to the integrated life processes
3. *Compromised life process*: Level of adaptation resulting from inadequate integrated and compensatory life processes; an adaptation problem

Implications for Nursing Practice

Nursing practice is directed toward promoting adaptation in each of the four response modes, thereby contributing to the person's health, quality of life, and dying with dignity. Roy's practice methodology is the Adaptation Model Nursing Process, which encompasses the six steps listed in Box 3.7. Each step is discussed in detail below.

Assessment of Behavior

The nurse systematically gathers data about the behavior of the human adaptive system and judges the current state of adaptation in each adaptive mode. The nurse uses one or more of Roy's Adaptation Model–based research instruments or clinical tools to guide application and documentation of the practice methodology.

BOX 3.7 **Roy's Adaptation Model Practice Methodology: The Nursing Process**

- Assessment of Behavior
- Assessment of Stimuli
- Nursing Diagnosis
- Goal Setting
- Intervention
- Evaluation

Assessment of Stimuli

The nurse recognizes that stimuli must be amenable to independent nurse functions. Consequently, factors such as medical diagnoses and medical treatments are not considered stimuli because those factors cannot be independently managed by nurses. The nurse identifies the internal and external focal and contextual stimuli that are influencing the behaviors of particular interest, in the order of priority established at the end of the Assessment of Behavior component of Roy's Adaptation Model Nursing Process.

Nursing Diagnosis

The nurse uses a process of judgment to make a statement conveying the adaptation status of the human adaptive system of interest. The nursing diagnosis is a statement that identifies the behaviors of interest together with the most relevant influencing stimuli. The nurse uses one of the following three approaches to state the nursing diagnosis:

1. The nurse states the behaviors within each adaptive mode and with their most relevant influencing stimuli.
2. The nurse uses a summary label for behaviors in each adaptive mode with relevant stimuli.
3. The nurse uses a label that summarizes a behavioral pattern across adaptive modes that is affected by the same stimuli.

The nurse may link Roy's Adaptation Model–based nursing diagnosis with a relevant diagnosis from the taxonomy of the North American Nursing Diagnosis Association (NANDA).

Goal Setting

The nurse articulates a clear goal statement, identifying the specific short-term and long-term behavioral outcomes in response to nursing provided to the human adaptive system. The goal statement designates each behavior of interest, the way in which the behavior will change, and the time frame for attainment of the goal. Goals may be stated for ineffective behaviors that are to be changed to adaptive behaviors and also for adaptive behaviors that should be maintained or enhanced.

Intervention

Nursing intervention is the management of stimuli. The nurse selects and implements nursing approaches that have

a high probability of changing stimuli or strengthening adaptive processes. The nurse may alter, increase, decrease, remove, or maintain stimuli.

Evaluation

The nurse judges the effectiveness of nursing interventions in relation to the behaviors of the human adaptive system. The nurse systematically reassesses observable and nonobservable behaviors for each aspect of the four adaptive modes.

Other Nursing Conceptual Models

Most conceptual models are applicable to many, if not all, nursing specialities. However, some nurses prefer to use conceptual models that were developed for a particular area of nursing specialty practice. For example, the **Synergy Model** (Hardin & Kaplow, 2005) was developed by members of the American Association of Critical-Care Nurses to guide practice with hospitalized critically ill patients. Noteworthy is that this conceptual model is now used in several other clinical settings with several other patient populations. Practice guided by the Synergy Model focuses attention on the match between eight characteristics of patients and eight competencies of nurses. According to the model, when nurse competencies are a good match with patient characteristics, the likelihood of attaining optimal outcomes is increased. Each patient characteristic and each nurse competency may be rated on a scale of 1 to 5, with 1 = lowest level and 5 = highest level (http://www.aacn.org/wd/certifications/content/synmodel.pcms?menu=certification). (http://www.aacn.org/wd/certifications/content/synmodel.pcms?pid=1&&menu=).

The eight patient characteristics are as follows:

1. *Resiliency*
2. *Vulnerability*
3. *Stability*
4. *Complexity*
5. *Resource availability*
6. *Participation in care*
7. *Participation in decision making*
8. *Predictability*

The eight nurse competencies are as follows:

1. *Clinical judgment*
2. *Advocacy*
3. *Caring practices*
4. *Collaboration*
5. *Systems thinking*
6. *Response to diversity*
7. *Clinical inquiry*
8. *Facilitation of learning*

Three categories of outcomes are relevant: those experienced by patients and families, those that occur as the result of nursing care, and those that occur within the healthcare system.

1. *Patient and family outcomes*: Functional and behavioral changes, trust, satisfaction, comfort, and quality of life.
2. *Nursing care outcomes*: Physiological changes, presence or absence of complications, and extent to which care or treatment objectives were attained.
3. *System outcomes*: Readmission rate, length of stay, and cost utilization per case.

ONLINE CONSULT

North American Nursing Diagnosis Association (NANDA) at
http://www.nanda.org

NURSING THEORIES

For our purposes, the terms *theory*, *theoretical framework*, *theoretical model*, and *theoretical rationale* have the same definition and may be used interchangeably.

Definition

A nursing theory is defined as one or more relatively concrete and specific concepts that are derived from a conceptual model, the statements that describe those concepts, and the statements that assert relatively concrete and specific relations between two or more concepts (Fawcett & DeSanto-Madeya, 2013). Each theory presents a unique perspective about a particular phenomenon, such as a nursing participant, the environment, health, or a step of the nursing process or practice methodology.

Function

The function of a nursing theory is to provide considerable specificity in the description, explanation, or prediction of some phenomenon.

Nursing Grand Theories

Theories vary in scope—that is, they vary in the relative level of concreteness and specificity of their concepts and statements. Theories that are broadest in scope are called grand theories. These theories are made up of rather abstract and general concepts and statements that cannot be generated or tested empirically. Indeed, grand theories are developed through thoughtful and insightful appraisal of existing ideas or creative intellectual leaps beyond existing knowledge. Examples of **grand theories of nursing** are Leininger's Theory of Culture Care Diversity and Universality (Leininger & McFarland, 2006), Newman's (1994) Theory of Health as Expanding Consciousness, and Parse's (1998) Theory of Humanbecoming. Some nurses prefer to use a nursing grand theory rather than a conceptual model to guide their practice. An overview of each grand theory, along with implications for practice, is presented below. The less abstract nature of grand theories compared with conceptual models is illustrated by Parse's (1998) theory, which was derived in part from Rogers' (1970, 1990) conceptual model. Rogers' conceptual model is a frame of reference for all of nursing, whereas Parse's theory limits the domain of interest to the unitary human's experience of becoming.

Madeleine Leininger's Theory of Culture Care Diversity and Universality

Leininger's Theory of Culture Care Diversity and Universality focuses on the discovery of human care diversities and universalities and ways to provide culturally congruent care to people. The concepts of this grand theory are as follows:

- *Care*: Abstract and concrete phenomena related to assisting, supporting, or enabling experiences or behaviors toward or for others with evident or anticipated needs to ameliorate or improve a human condition or lifeway

- *Caring*: The actions and activities directed toward assisting, supporting, or enabling another individual or group with evident or anticipated needs to ameliorate or improve a human condition or lifeway or to face death

- *Culture*: The learned, shared, and transmitted values, beliefs, norms, and lifeways of a particular group that guide thinking, decisions, and actions in patterned ways; encompasses several cultural and social structure dimensions: technological factors, religious and philosophical factors, kinship and social factors, political and legal factors, economic factors, educational and cultural values, and lifeways

- *Language*: Word usages, symbols, and meanings about care

- *Ethnohistory*: Past facts, events, instances, and experiences of individuals, groups, cultures, and institutions that are primarily people centered (ethno) and that describe, explain, and interpret human lifeways within particular cultural contexts and over short or long periods of time

- *Environmental context*: The totality of an event, situation, or particular experience that gives meaning to human expressions, interpretations, and social interactions in particular physical, ecological, sociopolitical, and/or cultural settings

- *Health*: A state of well-being that is culturally defined, valued, and practiced and that reflects the ability of individuals (or groups) to perform their daily role activities in culturally expressed, beneficial, and patterned lifeways

- *Worldview*: The way people tend to look out on the world or their universe to form a picture of or a value stance about their life or the world around them

- *Cultural care*: The subjectively and objectively transmitted values, beliefs, and patterned lifeways that assist, support, or enable another individual or group to maintain their well-being and health, to improve their human condition and lifeway, and to deal with illness, handicaps, or death; the two dimensions of cultural care are:
  1. *Cultural care diversity*: The variabilities and/or differences in meanings, patterns, values, lifeways, or symbols of care within or between collectivities that are related to assistive, supportive, or enabling human care expressions
  2. *Cultural care universality*: The common, similar, or dominant uniform care meanings, patterns, values, lifeways, or symbols that are manifest among many cultures and reflect assistive, supportive, facilitative, or enabling ways to help people

- *Care systems*: The values, norms, and structural features of an organization designed for serving people's health needs, concerns, or conditions; the two types of care systems are as follows:
  1. *Generic lay care systems*: Traditional or local indigenous healthcare or cure practices that have special meanings and uses to heal or assist people, which are generally offered in familiar home or community environmental contexts with their local practitioners
  2. *Professional healthcare systems*: Professional care or cure services offered by diverse health personnel who

have been prepared through formal professional programs of study in special educational institutions

- *Cultural-congruent nursing care*: Cognitively based assistive, supportive, facilitative, or enabling acts or decisions that are tailor-made to fit with individual, group, or institutional cultural values, beliefs, and lifeways in order to provide or support meaningful, beneficial, and satisfying healthcare or well-being services; the three modes of cultural-congruent nursing care are as follows:
    1. *Cultural care preservation or maintenance*: Assistive, supportive, facilitative, or enabling professional actions and decisions that help people of a particular culture retain and/or preserve relevant care values so that they can maintain their well-being, recover from illness, or face handicaps and/or death
    2. *Cultural care accommodation or negotiation*: Assistive, supportive, facilitative, or enabling creative professional actions and decisions that help people of a designated culture adapt to, or negotiate with, others for a beneficial or satisfying health outcome with professional care providers
    3. *Cultural care repatterning or restructuring*: Assistive, supportive, facilitative, or enabling professional actions and decisions that help patients reorder, change, or greatly modify their lifeways for a new, different, and beneficial healthcare pattern while respecting the patients' cultural values and beliefs and still providing a beneficial or healthier lifeway than before the changes were coestablished with the patients.

Implications for Nursing Practice

Nursing practice is directed toward improving and providing culturally congruent care to people. The components of the practice methodology for the Theory of Culture Care Diversity and Universality are shown in Box 3.8. Each component is discussed in detail here.

Goals of Nursing Practice

The goals of nursing practice are to provide culturally congruent care that will be beneficial to, fit with, and be useful to the patient, family, or culture group healthy lifeways, and to offer a different kind of nursing care service to people of diverse or similar cultures.

Patients

- Individuals
- Families
- Subcultures
- Groups
- Communities
- Institutions

BOX 3.8 **Leininger's Theory of Culture Care Diversity and Universality Practice Methodology**

- Goals of Nursing Practice
- Patients
- Culturalogical Assessment
- Nursing Judgments, Decisions, and Actions
- Clinical Protocols

Culturalogical Assessment

The nurse maintains a holistic or total view of the patient's world by using the Sunrise Enabler to guide assessment of cultural beliefs, values, and lifeways, which are identified by assessing the seven cultural and social structure dimensions that make up the patient's worldview: *technological; religious and philosophical; kinship and social; cultural values, beliefs, and lifeways; political and legal;, economic;* and *educational factors.* In most cases, more than one session with the patient is required to cover all components of the Sunrise Enabler. The first session in a hospital or clinic lasts approximately 20 minutes; subsequent sessions may be longer. The nurse begins by clarifying and explaining the focus of the assessment to the patient, which is the patient's internal (emic) world, not the nurse's outsider (etic) world.

The nurse knows his or her own culture and subculture and particular variabilities, strengths, and assets. The nurse must also discover and remain aware of his or her own cultural beliefs, values, lifeways, biases, attitudes, and prejudices to avoid cultural blindness. The nurse must be aware that the patient may belong to a subculture or special group that maintains its own values and beliefs that differ from the values and beliefs of the dominant culture. The nurse gives attention to patient gender differences, communication modes, special language terms, interpersonal relationships, and use of space and foods.

The nurse shows a genuine interest in the patient and learns from and maintains respect for the patient. The nurse asks open-ended questions and maintains the role of an active listener, learner, and reflector. The nurse shares professional knowledge only if the patient asks about such knowledge.

The nurse begins the assessment with questions such as the following:

- "What would you like to share with me today about your experiences or beliefs to help you keep well?" or "Please tell me what is important to you and about your lifestyle."
- "Are there some special ideas or ways you would like nurses to care for you?"
- "From whom do you usually receive care?"
- "What aspects of your care do you want to change?"

Nursing Judgments, Decisions, and Actions

Nursing practice requires the co-participation of nurses and patients working together to identify, plan, implement, and evaluate the appropriate mode(s) of cultural-congruent nursing care. Nursing decisions and actions encompass the following:

- Assisting
- Supporting
- Facilitating
- Enabling

Together, the nurse and the patient select one or more modes of cultural-congruent nursing care:

- *Cultural care preservation or maintenance*
- *Cultural care accommodation or negotiation*
- *Cultural care repatterning or restructuring*

Clinical Protocols

Specific nursing practices or clinical protocols are derived from the findings of research guided by the Theory of

Culture Care Diversity and Universality. The research findings are used to develop protocols for cultural-congruent care that blends with the particular cultural values, beliefs, and lifeways of the patient and is assessed to be beneficial, satisfying, and meaningful to the patient.

Margaret Newman's Theory of Health as Expanding Consciousness

Newman's Theory of Health as Expanding Conscious-ness emphasizes the idea that every person in every situation, no matter how disordered and hopeless the situation may seem, is part of the universal process of expanding consciousness. The concepts of the theory are consciousness and pattern.

Consciousness

Consciousness is the informational capacity of human beings—that is, the ability of humans to interact with their environments. Consciousness encompasses interconnected cognitive and affective awareness; physiochemical maintenance, including the nervous and endocrine systems; growth processes; the immune system; and the genetic code. Consciousness can be seen in the quantity and quality of the interaction between human beings and their environments. The process of life moves toward higher levels of consciousness. Sometimes this process is smooth, pleasant, and harmonious; other times it is difficult and disharmonious, as in disease.

Pattern

Pattern is information that depicts the whole; it is relatedness. People are identified by their pattern. The evolution of expanding consciousness is seen in the pattern of movement-space-time. Pattern is manifested as exchanging, communicating, relating, valuing, choosing, moving, perceiving, feeling, and knowing. Pattern encompasses three dimensions:

1. *Movement-space-time*: Movement is an essential property of matter, a means of communicating, the means whereby one perceives reality and becomes aware of self, and the natural condition of life. Space encompasses personal space, inner space, and life space as dimensions of space relevant to the individual; and territoriality, shared space, and distancing as dimensions relevant to the family. Time can be both subjective (the amount of time perceived to be passing) and objective (clock time).
2. *Rhythm*: Basic to movement, rhythm is an integrating experience.
3. *Diversity*: Seen in the parts

Implications for Nursing Practice

Nursing practice is directed toward facilitating pattern recognition by connecting with the patient in an authentic way and assisting him or her to discover new rules for a higher level of organization or consciousness. The components of Newman's research/practice methodology, which is called the Research as Praxis Protocol, are listed in Box 3.9. Each component is discussed in detail here.

BOX 3.9 **Newman's Health as Expanding Consciousness Practice Methodology: Research as Praxis Protocol**

- Phenomenon of Interest
- The Interview
- Transcription
- Development of the Narrative: Pattern Recognition
- Diagram: Pattern Recognition
- Follow-up: Pattern Recognition
- Application of the Theory of Health as Expanding Consciousness

---

Phenomenon of Interest

The phenomenon of interest is the process of expanding consciousness.

The Interview

The meeting of the nurse and the study participant/patient occurs when there is a mutual attraction through congruent patterns—that is, an interpenetration of the two fields. The nurse and the study participant/patient enter into a partnership with the mutual goal of participating in an authentic relationship, trusting that in the process of its unfolding, both will emerge at a higher level of consciousness.

First, the nurse explains the study. The study participant/patient agrees to continue with the study and agrees to have the interview recorded. The initial interview lasts 45 to 60 minutes. The nurse begins with a simple, open-ended statement, such as, "Tell me about the most meaningful people and events in your life." This question may be modified to fit the focus of the study. The nurse continues the interview in a nondirectional manner, although direct questions may be used occasionally. Examples of additional questions are, "Tell me what it has been like living with [a particular medical diagnosis, clinical condition, or life circumstance]," "What is meaningful to you?" and "What do you think about what we have been talking about?" The nurse may prompt the study participant/patient to bring to mind something from childhood that stands out in memory, if he or she needs help in thinking of something considered important.

The nurse acts as an active listener and clarifies and reflects as necessary. The nurse is fully present in the moment, is sensitive to intuitive hunches about what to say or ask, and waits for insight into the meaning of the pattern. The nurse is free to disclose aspects of himself or herself that are deemed appropriate.

Transcription

The nurse listens carefully to and transcribes the audio recording of the interview soon after the interview is completed. The nurse is sensitive to the relevance of the data and may omit comments made by the study participant/patient that do not directly relate to his or her life pattern, with a reference to the time during the interview that such comments occurred, in case those comments seem important later.

Development of the Narrative: Pattern Recognition

The nurse selects the statements deemed most important to the study participant/patient and rearranges the key segments of the data in chronological order to highlight the most significant events and persons. Natural breaks where a pattern shift occurs are noted and form the basis of the sequential patterns. The nurse will recognize the pattern of the whole, made up of segments of the study participant/patient's relationships over time.

Diagram: Pattern Recognition
The nurse then transmutes the narrative into a simple diagram of the sequential pattern configurations.

Follow-up: Pattern Recognition
The nurse conducts a second interview with the study participant/patient to share the diagram or other visual portrayal of the pattern. The nurse does not interpret the diagram but rather uses it simply to illustrate the study participant/patient's story in graphic form, which tends to accentuate the contrasts and repetitions in relationships over time.

The mutual viewing of the graphic form is an opportunity for the study participant/patient to confirm and clarify or revise the story being portrayed. It is also an opportunity for the nurse to clarify any aspect of the story about which he or she has any doubt.

The nature of the pattern of person-environment interaction will begin to emerge in terms of energy flow—for example, blocked, diffuse, disorganized, repetitive, or whatever descriptors and metaphors come to mind to describe the pattern. The study participant/patient may express signs that pattern recognition is occurring (or has already occurred in the interval following the first interview) as the nurse and study participant/patient reflect together on the study participant/patient's life pattern.

If no signs of pattern recognition occur, the nurse and study participant/patient may want to proceed with additional reflections in subsequent interviews until no further insight is reached. Sometimes, no signs of pattern recognition emerge, and if so, that characterizes the pattern for that person. It is not to be forced.

Application of the Theory of Health as Expanding Consciousness
After the interviews are completed, the nurse undertakes more intense analysis of the data in light of the Theory of Health as Expanding Consciousness. The nurse evaluates the nature of the sequential patterns of interaction in terms of quality and complexity and interprets the patterns according to the study participant/patient's position on Young's spectrum of consciousness. The sequential patterns represent presentational construing or relationships. Any similarities of pattern among a group of study participants/patients having a similar experience may be designated by themes and stated in propositional form.

Rosemarie Parse's Theory of Humanbecoming

Parse's Theory of Humanbecoming focuses on human experiences of participation with the universe in the co-creation of health. The concepts of the theory are as follows:

- *Humanbecoming*: A unitary construct referring to the human being's living health

- *Meaning*: The linguistic and imagined content of something and the interpretation that one gives to something
  - *Imaging*: Reflective-prereflective coming to know the explicit-tacit-all-at-once
  - *Valuing*: Confirming-not confirming cherished beliefs in light of a personal worldview
  - *Languaging*: Signifying valued images through speaking-being silent and moving-being still
- *Rhythmicity*: The cadent, paradoxical patterning of the human-universe mutual process
  - *Revealing-concealing*: Disclosing-not disclosing all-at-once
  - *Enabling-limiting*: Living the opportunities-restrictions present in all choosings all-at-once
  - *Connecting-separating*: Being with and apart from others, ideas, objects, and situations all at once
- *Transcendence*: Reaching beyond with possibles—the hopes and dreams envisioned in multidimensional experiences and powering the originating of transforming
  - *Powering*: The pushing-resisting process of affirming-not affirming being in light of nonbeing
  - *Originating*: Inventing new ways of conforming-nonconforming in the certainty/uncertainty of living
  - *Transforming*: Shifting the view of the familiar-unfamiliar, the changing of change in co-constituting anew in a deliberate way

The three major principles of the theory of humanbecoming are as follows:

1. *Structuring meaning* is the imaging and valuing of languaging and means that humans construct what is real for them from choices made at many realms of the universe.
2. *Configuring rhythmical patterns of relating* is the revealing-concealing and enabling-limiting of connecting-separating and means that humans live in rhythm with the universe co-constituting patterns of relating.
3. *Co-transcending with possibles* is the powering and originating of transforming and means that humans forge unique paths with shifting perspectives as a different light is cast on the familiar.

Implications for Nursing Practice
Nursing practice is directed toward respecting quality of life as perceived by the person and the family. Part I of Parse's Practice Methodology is summarized in Box 3.10. Each aspect of Part II of Parse's Practice Methodology is outlined below.

Part II of Parse's Practice Methodology
Contexts for Nursing
- Nurse-person situations
- Nurse-group situations
- Participants: Children, adults
- Locations: Homes, shelters, healthcare centers, parish halls, all departments of hospitals and clinics, rehabilitation centers, offices, other milieus where nurses interact with people

BOX 3.10 Parse's Practice Methodology: Part I		
Theory of Humanbecoming	Practice Methodology Dimension	Practice Methodology Principle Process (Empirical Activity)
1. Structuring meaning	*Illuminating meaning*: Explicating what was, is, and will be	*Explicating*: Making clear what is appearing now through languaging
2. Configuring rhythmical patterns of relating	*Synchronizing rhythms*: Dwelling with the pitch, yaw, and roll of the human universe process	*Dwelling with*: Immersing with the flow of connecting-separating
3. Co-transcending with possibles	*Mobilizing transcendence*: Moving beyond the meaning moment with what is not-yet	*Moving beyond*: Propelling with envisioned possibles of transforming

Goal of the Discipline of Nursing

The goal of nursing is to enhance the quality of life from the person's, family's, and community's perspectives.

Goal of the Humanbecoming Nurse

The goal of the humanbecoming nurse is to be truly present with people as they enhance the quality of their lives.

True Presence

True presence refers to a special way of "being with" in which the nurse is attentive to moment-to-moment changes in meaning as he or she bears witness to the person's or group's own living of value priorities.

- *Coming-to-be-present*: True presence begins in the coming-to-be-present moments of preparation and attention—an all-at-once gentling down and lifting up. True presence begins in the coming-to-be-present moments of preparation and attention. Preparation involves an emptying to be available to bear witness to the other or others and being flexible, not fixed but gracefully present from one's center, as well as dwelling with the universe at the moment, considering the attentive presence about to be. Attention involves focusing on the moment at hand for immersion.
- *Face-to-face discussions*: The nurse and the person engage in dialogue, and the nurse tries to understand the person's perspective by initiating discussions. Conversation may be through discussion in general or through interpretations of stories, films, drawings, photographs, music, metaphors, poetry, rhythmical movements, and other expressions. The nurse really listens to the person, without interrupting. The nurse may seek clarification of the person's comments. The nurse tries to understand the person's perspective by initiating discussions using questions such as: How are you doing? How are things going? How was your day (or night)? What is life like for you? What is most important to you at this time? What do you need most right now? The nurse may seek clarification through such statements as: Tell me more about that. What does . . . mean for you? What is it like for you to live with . . . ? What do you see yourself doing? What can you do to get help? What might help you to go on? What do you hope happens?
- *Silent immersion*: Silent immersion is a process of the quiet that does not refrain from sending and receiving messages, a chosen way of becoming in the human-universe process lived in the rhythm of speaking-being

silent, moving-being still as valued images incarnate meaning. Silent immersion is true presence without words.
- *Lingering presence*: Lingering presence refers to recalling a moment after an immediate engagement—a reflective-prereflective "abiding with" attended to through glimpses of the other person, idea, object, or situation.

Ways of Changing Health Patterns in True Presence

- *Creative imagining*: Picturing—by seeing, hearing, and feeling—what a situation might be like if lived in a different way
- *Affirming personal becoming*: Uncovering preferred personal health patterns by critically thinking about how or who one is
- *Glimpsing the paradoxical*: Changing one's view of a situation by recognizing incongruities in that situation

Middle-Range Theories

Middle-range theories are narrower in scope than grand theories, encompassing a smaller number of concepts and a limited aspect of the real world. Middle-range theories are, therefore, made up of concepts that are empirically measurable and statements that are empirically testable. Indeed, the product of any nursing study can be considered a middle-range theory that constitutes the evidence for nursing practice (Fawcett & Garity, 2009). Middle-range theories may describe a concept, explain the relation between two or more concepts, or predict the effects of one or more concepts that are interventions on one or more other concepts that are outcomes.

Examples of widely used middle-range nursing theories are **Peplau's (1952, 1992) Theory of Interpersonal Relations, Watson's (2006) Theory of Human Caring,** and **Orlando's (1961) Theory of the Deliberative Nursing Process.** Peplau's middle-range descriptive nursing theory focuses on the phases of the interpersonal process that occur when an ill person and a nurse come together to resolve a health difficulty. Watson's middle-range explanatory nursing theory focuses on the human component of caring and the moment-to-moment encounters between the one who is caring and the one who is being cared for, especially the caring activities performed by nurses as they interact with others. Her theory asserts a relation between clinical caritas processes (nursing interventions) and a transpersonal caring relationship between nurse and patient. Orlando's middle-range predictive nursing theory focuses on an interpersonal process between people. Her theory asserts that the outcome of use of the deliberative nursing process is identification of the patient's immediate need for help.

More than 80 middle-range theories have been directly derived from the seven nursing conceptual models discussed earlier in this chapter (Table 3.1). Many other middle-range nursing theories and middle-range theories from other disciplines are used by nurses (see, for example, Alligood & Tomey, 2010; Peterson & Bredow, 2004; Smith & Liehr, 2014; Ziegler, 2005) but are not explicitly derived from any nursing conceptual model or a conceptual model from any other discipline.

TABLE 3.1

Explicit Middle-Range Theories Derived from Selected Conceptual Models of Nursing

Conceptual Model	Middle-Range Theory
Johnson's Behavioral System Model	Theory of a Restorative Subsystem
	Theory of Sustenal Imperatives
King's Conceptual System	Theory of Asynchronous Development
	Theory of Basic Empathy, Self-Awareness, and Learning Styles
	Theory of Decision Making
	Theory of Departmental Power [retitled Theory of Group Power]
	Theory of Families, Children, and Chronic Illness
	Theory of Family Health [retitled Family Health Theory]
	Theory of Goal Attainment
	Theory of Health and Social Support
	Theory of Social Support and Health of Older Adults
	Theory of Intrapersonal Perceptual Awareness
	Theory of Health Perception
	Theory of Interaction Enhancement
	Theory of Nursing Administration
	Theory of Nursing Empathy
	Theory of Organizational Health
	Theory of Personal System Empathy
	Theory of Transaction Process
	Theory of Integration
	Theory of Quality of Life of Stroke Survivors
	Theory of Patient Satisfaction with Nursing Care
	Theory of Social and Interpersonal Influences on Health
Levine's Conservation Model	Theory of Health Promotion for Preterm Infants
	Theory of Redundancy
	Theory of Therapeutic Intention
Neuman's Systems Model	Codependency-Overeating Model
	Theory of Adolescent Vulnerability
	Theory of Caregiver Role Strain
	Theory of Infant Exposure to Environmental Tobacco Smoke
	Theory of Maternal Student Role Stress
	Theory of Moderation of Stress Levels in Women in Multiple Roles
	Theory of Optimal Patient System Stability
	Theory of Prevention as Intervention

TABLE 3.1

Explicit Middle-Range Theories Derived from Selected Conceptual Models of Nursing—cont'd

Conceptual Model	Middle-Range Theory
Orem's Self-Care Framework	Theory of Well-Being
	Theory of Well-Being for Fatigue in Diabetics
	A Theory of Palliative Care Nursing Self-Competence
	Theory of Dependent Care
	Theory of Diabetes Self-Care Management
	Theory of Taking Care of Oneself in a High-Risk Environment
	Theory of Testicular Self-Examination
	White's Theory of Spirituality and Spiritual Self-Care
Rogers' Science of Unitary Human Beings	Theory of Aging
	Theory of Aging as Emerging Brilliance
	Theory of the Art of Professional Nursing
	Theory of Creativity, Actualization, and Empathy
	Theory of Energetic Patterning
	Theory of Diversity of Human Field Pattern
	Theory of Enfolding Health as Wholeness and Harmony
	Theory of Enlightenment
	Theory of Healthiness
	Theory of Human Field Motion
	Theory of Intentionality
	Theory of Kaleidoscoping in Life's Turbulence
	Theory of Participation
	Theory of Pattern
	Theory of Perceived Dissonance
	Theory of Power as Knowing Participation in Change
	Theory of Self-Transcendence
	Theory of Sentience Evolution
	Theories of Spirituality
Roy's Adaptation Model	Parrett and Biley Negotiating Uncertainty Theory
	Theory of Adaptation during Childbearing
	Theory of Adaptation to Chronic Pain
	Theory of Adapting to Diabetes
	Theory of Adapting to Chronic Health Conditions
	Theory of the Adapting Family
	Theory of Adapting to Life Events
	Theory of Adapting to Loss
	Theory of Caregiver Stress
	Theory of Chronic Pain
	Theory of Coping
	Theory of Holistic Clinical Education
	Theory of Psychosocial Adaptation to Termination of Pregnancy for Fetal Anomaly
	Theory of Sexuality Adaptation

Continued

Explicit Middle-Range Theories Derived from Selected Conceptual Models of Nursing—cont'd

Conceptual Model	Middle-Range Theory
	Theory of Successful Aging
	Theory of Urine Control
	Theory of the Physiological Mode
	Theory of Self-Concept Mode
	Theory of Role Function Mode
	Theory of Interdependence Mode
	Nursing Model of Cognitive Processing
	Theory of Facilitated Sensemaking

Source: Adapted from Fawcett, J., (2009). *Evaluating research for evidence-based nursing practice.* Philadelphia: F. A. Davis. Adapted from Fawcett, J., & Garity, J. (2009). *Evaluating research for evidence-based nursing practice.* Philadelphia, PA: F. A. Davis.

Transitions Theory has become more widely known during the past few years (Meleis, 2010). This middle-range theory focuses people's experiences during developmental, wellness-illness, situational, and organizations transitions.

Situation-Specific Theories

Situation-specific theories are even more specific and concrete than middle-range theories. As Meleis (2012) explained, situation-specific theories "are closer [than conceptual models, grand theories, and middle-range theories] to the clinical realities of caring for patients, as well as reflective of variations in the contexts and situations of populations" (p. 419). More specifically, situation-specific theories focus on a particular population of people who are experiencing a specific health condition.

Situation-Specific Nursing Theories

Development of **situation-specific nursing theories** may be guided by a conceptual model of nursing. For example, the situation-specific theory of Men's Healing from Childhood Maltreatment was constructed by viewing findings of a study of men's perceptions of their experiences of abuse and neglect during childhood within the context of Rogers' Science of Unitary Human Beings (Willis, DeSanto-Madeya, & Fawcett, 2015).

Development of nursing situation-specific theories also may be guided by a middle-range theory. For example, Im (2014) used Transitions Theory (Meleis, 2010) to guide development of her situation-specific theories of Caucasian Cancer Patients' Pain Experience, Asian American Cancer Patients' Pain Experience, and Asian Immigrant Women's Menopausal Symptom Experience in the United States. Hanna (2012) used Transitions Theory to guide development of her situation-specific theory of Emerging Adults' Experience of Type 1 Diabetes.

ADVANTAGES OF USING FORMAL NURSING KNOWLEDGE

Recognition of nursing as a profession bestows a certain status on nurses. The status conferred by being a member of a profession, rather than having an occupation or a trade, carries with it the responsibility to use formal nursing knowledge. Anderson (1995) explained that, as members of a profession, nurses "must ensure that we have a solid scholarly and scientific foundation upon which to base our practice" (p. 247). Conceptual models of nursing and nursing theories are that foundation; they provide explicit frames of reference for professional nursing practice by delineating the scope of nursing practice. Furthermore, conceptual models of nursing and nursing theories (1) specify innovative goals for nursing practice, (2) introduce ideas that are designed to improve practice (Lindsay, 1990), and (3) enhance the quality of people's lives by facilitating the identification of relevant information, reducing the fragmentation of healthcare, and improving the coordination of all aspects of healthcare (Chalmers, as cited in Chalmers et al., 1990).

More specifically, the use of formal nursing knowledge to guide nursing practice "represents nursing's unique contribution to the health-care system" (Parse, 1995, p. 128). It is the hallmark of professional nursing practice. As Chalmers pointed out, "Nursing models [and theories] have provided what many would argue is a much needed alternative knowledge base from which nurses can practice in an informed way. An alternative, that is, to the medical model which for so many years has dominated many aspects of health care" (Chalmers et al., 1990, p. 34).

Formal nursing knowledge also provides an alternative to the institutional model of practice, in which "the most salient values [are] efficiency, standardized care, rules, and regulations" (Rogers, 1989, p. 113). The institutional model, moreover, typically upholds, reinforces, and supports the medical model (Grossman & Hooton, 1993). Thus, the use of conceptual models of nursing and nursing theories moves the practice of nursing away from that driven by a medical or institutional model and, therefore, fosters autonomy from medicine and a coherent purpose of practice (Bélanger, 1991; Bridges, 1991; Ingram, 1991; Parse, 1995).

The major practical advantage of using a conceptual model of nursing is the identification of a comprehensive nursing process format or practice methodology that encompasses particular parameters for assessment, labels for problems, a strategy for planning nursing interventions, a typology of nursing interventions, and criteria for evaluation of the outcomes of nursing practice. The major practical advantage a nursing theory provides is greater specificity in one or more phases of the nursing process. Middle-range theories may be linked with conceptual models or grand theories, with the proviso that logical congruence is evident. For example, Orlando's (1961) Theory of the Deliberative Nursing Process tells the nurse exactly how to identify the patient's immediate need for help. Orlando's theory can be used very effectively in combination with Roy's (2009) Adaptation Model and other conceptual models of nursing.

It should be obvious by now that formal nursing knowledge identifies the distinctive nursing territory within the vast arena of multidisciplinary healthcare (Feeg, 1989). In addition, the use of formal nursing knowledge "help[s] nurses better communicate what they do" (Neff, 1991, p. 534) and why they do it. The importance of communicating what nursing is and what nurses do was underscored by Feeg (1989), who identified three reasons for implementing conceptual model-based or theory-based nursing practice that are as relevant today as they were in the 1980s. The three reasons are as follows:

1. In this time of information saturation and rapid change, we know it is not valuable to focus on every detail and, therefore, we need [conceptual models and theories] to help guide our judgments in new situations.
2. In this time of technologic overdrive, we need a holistic orientation to remind us of our caring perspective.
3. In this time of professional territoriality, it has become even more important to understand our identity in nursing and operationalize our practice from a [formal nursing] knowledge base. (p. 450)

The number of nurses throughout the world who recognize the advantages of using formal nursing knowledge is rapidly increasing, which is very important as the healthcare reforms that are occurring in many countries emphasize the expanded role of nursing in providing primary and specialized care. Use of formal nursing knowledge enables nurses to engage in "thinking nursing" (Allison & Renpenning, 1999), rather than just doing tasks and carrying out physicians' orders (Le Storti et al., 1999). Nurses are able to think nursing and talk nursing because the conceptual models and theories that constitute formal nursing knowledge provide a distinctive nursing language. The lack of a nursing language in the past—and in the present when conceptual models of nursing and nursing theories are not used—"has been a handicap in nurses' communications about nursing to

the public as well as to persons with whom they work in the health field" (Orem, 1997, p. 29). Thus, the content of each conceptual model of nursing and nursing theory, which is stated in a distinctive vocabulary, should not be considered jargon. Rather, the terminology used by the author of each conceptual model or theory should be recognized as the result of considerable thought about how to convey the meaning of that particular perspective to others (Biley, 1990). "The attention to language," Watson (1997) maintained, "is especially critical to an evolving [profession], in that during this postmodern era, one's survival depends on having language; writers in this area remind us 'if you do not have your own language you don't exist'" (p. 50). Elaborating, Akinsanya (1989) explained, "Every science has its own peculiar terms, concepts, and principles which are essential for the development of its knowledge base. In nursing, as in other sciences, an understanding of these is a prerequisite to a critical examination of their contribution to the development of knowledge and its application to practice" (p. ii). Indeed, the differences in the vocabularies of the various conceptual models and theories are the same as the differences in the vocabularies of diverse medical specialties, such as obstetrics, gynecology, cardiology, neurology, psychiatry, and geriatrics.

Thinking nursing within the context of formal nursing knowledge helps nurses to "clarify their thinking on their role, especially at a time when the roles of many health professionals are becoming blurred" (Nightingale, 1993, p. 2).

Risks and Rewards of Using Formal Nursing Knowledge

Johnson (1990) noted that although individual nurses and nursing departments take risks when the decision is made to implement conceptual model- or theory-based nursing practice, the rewards far outweigh the risks. She stated:

To openly use a nursing model [or theory] is risk-taking behavior for the individual nurse. For a nursing department to adopt one of these models [or theories] for unit or institution use is risk-taking behavior of an even higher order. The reward for such risk-taking for the individual practitioner lies in the great satisfaction gained from being able to specify explicit concrete nursing goals in the care of patients and from documenting the actual achievement of the desired outcomes. The reward for the nursing department is having a rational, cohesive, and comprehensive basis for the development of standards of nursing practice, for the evaluation of practitioners, and for the documentation of the contribution of nursing to patient welfare. (Johnson, 1990, p. 32)

Accumulating anecdotal and empirical evidence indicates that additional rewards of using formal nursing knowledge to guide nursing practice include reduced staff nurse turnover, more rapid movement from novice to expert nurse, greater patient and family satisfaction with nursing, increased nurse job satisfaction, and considerable cost savings (Fawcett & DeSanto-Madeya, 2013). Furthermore, as the use of formal nursing knowledge grows, both nurses and participants in nursing are empowered.

SELECTING A CONCEPTUAL MODEL OR NURSING GRAND THEORY FOR PROFESSIONAL NURSING PRACTICE

Although formal nursing knowledge is made up of many conceptual models and theories, using more than one conceptual model or grand theory at the same time will create much confusion. Therefore, each nurse should select just one as a guide for professional practice. The following six steps can help you select an appropriate conceptual model of nursing or nursing grand theory:

1. Identify your own beliefs and values related to the phenomena of interest to all nurses. State your beliefs about the participants in nursing, the relevant environment, health, and the goals of professional nursing practice.
2. Identify the patient population with which you would like to work. The population may be based on a specific medical diagnosis, such as cancer or renal failure; an age group, such as children or the older adults; a type of illness, such as an acute crisis or chronic illness; or a particular symptom, such as chest pain or an elevated temperature.
3. Systematically analyze and evaluate the content of several conceptual models of nursing and nursing grand theories. Review the summaries of the conceptual models and grand theories presented in the chapter as well as the primary-source material for each conceptual model and grand theory. This review will provide a firm foundation for your selection of the conceptual model or grand theory.
4. Compare your own beliefs and values with the philosophical claims undergirding the selected conceptual model or grand theory.
5. Identify the conceptual models and nursing grand theories that are appropriate guides for nursing with the patient population in which you are interested.
6. Choose the conceptual model or grand theory that most closely matches your beliefs and values and the patient population with which you want to work. Then use the model or theory to guide your practice with several nursing participants so that you can determine its utility. If you find that the conceptual model or grand theory you have chosen is not useful, select another model or theory and test its utility.

USING CONCEPTUAL MODELS OR GRAND THEORIES TO GUIDE PROFESSIONAL NURSING PRACTICE

Research findings indicate that nurses feel vulnerable and experience a great deal of stress when they attempt to achieve professional aspirations within a rapidly changing, medically dominated, bureaucratic healthcare delivery system (Graham, 1994). As a structure for critical thinking within a distinctively nursing context, formal nursing knowledge provides the intellectual skills and points to the practical skills that nurses need to survive at a time when cost containment through reduction of professional nursing staff is the modus operandi of managed care and the administrators of healthcare delivery systems, including hospitals, home healthcare agencies, and health maintenance organizations.

As a novice user of a conceptual model of nursing or nursing grand theory, you should not become discouraged if your initial experiences with the model or theory seem forced or awkward. Adopting an explicit nursing model or theory does require using a new vocabulary and a new way of thinking about nursing situations. Repeatedly using the conceptual model or grand theory should, however, lead to more systematic and organized applications. Broncatello's (1980) words, written more than 30 years ago, continue to provide the encouragement needed to start using a conceptual model of nursing or nursing theory to guide professional nursing practice:

The nurse's consistent use of any model [or theory] for the interpretation of observable [patient] data is most definitely not an easy task. Much like the development of any habitual behavior, it initially requires thought, discipline, and the gradual evolvement of a mind-set of what is important to observe within the guidelines of the model [or theory]. As is true of most habits, however, it makes decision making less complicated. (p. 23)

Using formal nursing knowledge allows the nursing profession to be clear about its mission in the constantly changing healthcare arena. Now, perhaps more than ever before, it is crucial that nurses explicate what they know and why they do what they do. In other words, it is crucial that all nurses communicate distinctive nursing knowledge and explain how that knowledge governs the actions performed on behalf of or in conjunction with people who require nursing. Thus, it is incumbent on all nurses to use formal nursing knowledge. Only if they do so can nurses continue to claim a place on the multidisciplinary healthcare team.

KEY POINTS

● Conceptual models of nursing present diverse perspectives of the participant in nursing, who can be an individual, a family, or a community; the environment of the nursing participant and the environment in which professional nursing practice occurs; the participant's health state; and the definition and goals of nursing as well as nursing actions or interventions.

KEY POINTS—cont'd

● The most practical function of a conceptual model is its delineation of goals for nursing practice and a practice methodology (that is, a nursing process) that encompasses parameters for assessment, labels for problems, a strategy for planning nursing interventions, a typology of nursing interventions, and criteria for evaluation of the outcomes of nursing practice. A conceptual model of nursing provides a structure for documentation of all aspects of the nursing process, from patient assessment to evaluation of outcomes. A conceptual model also helps identify standards of nursing practice and criteria for quality assurance reviews. Nursing grand theories can be used in place of conceptual models and, therefore, have the same functions.

● The function of nursing middle-range theories and situation-specific theories is to provide considerable specificity in the description, explanation, or prediction of some phenomenon. Theories are more concrete and specific than conceptual models. A conceptual model is an abstract and general system of concepts and statements, whereas a theory deals with one or more relatively concrete and specific concepts and statements. In addition, conceptual models are general guides that must be specified further by relevant and logically congruent theories before action can occur.

● Conceptual models of nursing and nursing grand theories, middle-range theories, and situation-specific theories move the professional practice of nursing away from that driven by a medical or institutional model and, therefore, foster autonomy from medicine and a coherent purpose for professional nursing practice.

● Six steps are used to select a conceptual model or nursing grand theory to guide professional nursing practice: (1) state your philosophy of nursing, in the form of beliefs and values about human beings who are nursing participants, the environment, health (including wellness and illness), and nursing goals; (2) identify the particular patient population with which you wish to practice; (3) thoroughly analyze and evaluate several conceptual models of nursing and nursing grand theories; (4) compare the philosophical claims on which each conceptual model and nursing grand theory is based with your own philosophy of nursing; (5) determine which conceptual models or nursing grand theories are appropriate for use with the patient population you are interested in; and (6) select the one conceptual model or nursing grand theory that most closely matches your philosophy of nursing and the patient population of interest.

Thought and Discussion Questions

1. List two ways in which a conceptual model differs from a grand theory, a middle-range theory, and a situation-specific theory.

2. Many people select nursing as a career because they enjoy "taking care of" other people. Orem's conceptual model of nursing focuses on individuals with limited abilities to provide continuing self-care or care of dependent others. Describe the difference between "taking care of people" as a general term and professional nursing practice directed toward helping people meet their own and their dependent others' therapeutic self-care demands.

3. Describe the focus of Neuman's systems model in relation to chronically ill patients and their families as they struggle to respond to stressors associated with periodic changes in the patients' health status. For example, what level(s) of prevention interventions are needed as chronically ill patients' health status changes?

4. Some nurses at a nursing home describe a particular resident as a "difficult patient." How does use of Orlando's theory of the deliberative nursing practice influence the way you think about and interact with patients who are regarded as "difficult"?

5. Explain how Roy's adaptation model provides guidelines for patient-centered and family-centered nursing care.

6. Patient-centered care requires that nurses understand and acknowledge culturally diverse patients' health-related beliefs, values, and lifeways. What types of health-related beliefs, values, and lifeways can be identified by applying the practice methodology of Leininger's Theory of Culture Care Diversity and Universality?

Interactive Exercises

Go to the Intranet site and complete the interactive exercises provided for this chapter.

REFERENCES

Portions of this chapter were adapted from Fawcett, J., & DeSanto-Madeya, S. (2013). Contemporary nursing knowledge: Analysis and evaluation of nursing models and theories (3rd ed.). Philadelphia: F. A. Davis; and Fawcett, J. (2013). Appendix N-1: Conceptual models and theories of nursing. In D. Venes (Ed.), Taber's cyclopedic medical dictionary (22nd ed., pp. 2629–2660). Philadelphia: F. A. Davis, with permission.

Akinsanya, J. A. (1989). Introduction. *Recent Advances in Nursing, 24*, i–ii.

Alligood, M. R., & Tomey, A. M. (2010). *Nursing theorists and their work* (7th ed.). St. Louis, MO: Mosby Elsevier.

Allison, S. E., & Renpenning, K. (1999). *Nursing administration in the 21st century*. Thousand Oaks, CA: Sage.

Anderson, C. A. (1995). Scholarship: How important is it? *Nursing Outlook, 43*, 247–248.

Bélanger, P. (1991). Nursing models: A major step towards professional autonomy. *AARN Newsletter, 48*(8), 13.

Biley, F. (1990). Wordly wise. *Nursing (London), 4*(24), 37.

Bridges, J. (1991). Working with doctors: Distinct from medicine. *Nursing Times, 87*(27), 42–43.

Broncatello, K. F. (1980). Auger in action: Application of the model. *Advances in Nursing Science, 2*(2), 13–23.

Chalmers, H., Kershaw, B., Melia, K., & Kendrich, M. (1990). Nursing models: Enhancing or inhibiting practice? *Nursing Standard, 5*(11), 34–40.

Fawcett, J., & DeSanto-Madeya, S. (2013). *Contemporary nursing knowledge: Analysis and evaluation of nursing models and theories* (3rd ed.). Philadelphia, PA: F. A. Davis.

Fawcett, J., & Garity, J. (2009). *Evaluating research for evidence-based nursing practice*. Philadelphia, PA: F. A. Davis.

Feeg, V. (1989). From the editor: Is theory application merely an intellectual exercise? *Pediatric Nursing, 15*, 450.

Graham, I. (1994). How do registered nurses think and experience nursing? A phenomenological investigation. *Journal of Clinical Nursing, 3*, 235–242.

Grossman, M., & Hooton, M. (1993). The significance of the relationship between a discipline and its practice. *Journal of Advanced Nursing, 18*, 866–872.

Hanna, K. M. (2012). A framework for the youth with type 1 diabetes during the emerging adulthood transition. *Nursing Outlook, 60*, 401–410.

Hardin, S. R., & Kaplow, R. (2005). *Synergy for clinical excellence: The AACN synergy model for patient care*. Boston, MA: Jones and Bartlett.

Henderson, V. (1966). *The nature of nursing. A definition and its implications for practice, research, and education*. New York, NY: Macmillan.

Im, E.-O. (2014). Theory of transitions. In M. J. Smith & P. R. Liehr (Eds.), *Middle-range theory for nursing* (3rd ed., pp. 253–276. New York, NY: Springer.

Ingram, R. (1991). Why does nursing need theory? *Journal of Advanced Nursing, 16*, 350–353.

Johnson, D. E. (1987). Evaluating conceptual models for use in critical care nursing practice [Guest editorial]. *Dimensions of Critical Care Nursing, 6*, 195–197.

Johnson, D. E. (1990). The behavioral system model for nursing. In M. E. Parker (Ed.), *Nursing theories in practice* (pp. 23–32). New York, NY: National League for Nursing.

King, I. M. (2006). Part One: Imogene M. King's theory of goal attainment. In M. E. Parker, *Nursing theories and nursing practice* (2nd ed., pp. 235–243). Philadelphia, PA: F. A. Davis.

Leininger, M. M., & McFarland, M. R. (2006). *Culture care diversity and universality: A worldwide nursing theory* (2nd ed.). Boston, MA: Jones and Bartlett.

Le Storti, L. J., Cullen, P. A., Hanzlik, E. M., Michiels, J. M., Piano, L. A., Ryan, P. L., & Johnson, W. (1999). Creative thinking in nursing education: Preparing for tomorrow's challenges. *Nursing Outlook, 47*, 62–66.

Levine, M. E. (1991). The conservation principles: A model for health. In K. M. Schaefer & J. B. Pond (Eds.), *Levine's conservation model: A framework for nursing practice* (pp. 1–11). Philadelphia, PA: F. A. Davis.

Lindsay, B. (1990). The gap between theory and practice. *Nursing Standard, 5*(4), 34–35.

Meleis, A. I. (2010). *Transitions theory: Middle-range and situation-specific theories in nursing research and practice*. New York, NY: Springer.

Meleis, A. I. (2012). *Theoretical nursing: Development and progress* (5th ed.). Philadelphia, PA: Wolters Kluwer Health/Lippincott Williams and Wilkins.

Neff, M. (1991). President's message: The future of our profession from the eyes of today. *American Nephrology Nurses Association Journal, 18*, 534.

Neuman, B., & Fawcett, J. (2011). *The Neuman systems model* (5th ed.). Upper Saddle River, NJ: Prentice Hall.

Newman, M. A. (1994). *Health as expanding consciousness* (2nd ed.). New York, NY: National League for Nursing Press.

Nightingale, F. (1859). *Notes on nursing: What it is, and what it is not*. London: Harrison and Sons. [Commemorative edition printed 1992, Philadelphia, PA: J. B. Lippincott]

Nightingale, K. (1993). Editorial. *British Journal of Theatre Nursing, 3*(5), 2.

Orem, D. E. (1997). Views of human beings specific to nursing. *Nursing Science Quarterly, 10*, 26–31.

Orem, D. E. (2001). *Nursing: Concepts of practice* (6th ed.). St. Louis, MO: Mosby.

Orlando, I. J. (1961). *The dynamic nurse-patient relationship: Function, process and principles*. New York: G. P. Putnam's Sons. [Reprinted 1990, New York: National League for Nursing]

Parse, R. R. (1995). Commentary. Parse's theory of humanbecoming: An alternative guide to nursing practice for pediatric oncology nurses. *Journal of Pediatric Oncology Nursing, 12*, 128.

Parse, R. R. (1998). *The humanbecoming school of thought: A perspective for nurses and other health professionals*. Thousand Oaks, CA: Sage.

Peplau, H. E. (1952). *Interpersonal relations in nursing*. New York: G. P. Putnam's Sons. [Reprinted 1991, New York, NY: Springer]

Peplau, H. E. (1992). Interpersonal relations: A theoretical framework for application in nursing practice. *Nursing Science Quarterly, 5*, 13–18.

Peterson, S. J., & Bredow, T. S. (2004). *Middle-range theories: Application to nursing research*. Philadelphia, PA: Lippincott Williams & Wilkins.

Popper, K. R. (1965). *Conjectures and refutations: The growth of scientific knowledge*. New York, NY: Harper & Row.

Rogers, M. E. (1970). *An introduction to the theoretical basis of nursing*. Philadelphia, PA: F. A. Davis.

Rogers, M. E. (1989). Creating a climate for the implementation of a nursing conceptual framework. *Journal of Continuing Education in Nursing, 20*, 112–116.

Rogers, M. E. (1990). Nursing: Science of unitary, irreducible, human beings: Update 1990. In E. A. M. Barrett (Ed.),

Visions of Rogers' science-based nursing (pp. 5–11). New York, NY: National League for Nursing.

Roy, C. (2009). *The Roy adaptation model* (3rd ed.). Upper Saddle River, NJ: Pearson.

Smith, M. J., & Liehr, P. R. (Eds.). (2014). *Middle range theory for nursing* (3rd ed.). New York, NY: Springer.

Watson, J. (1997). The theory of human caring: Retrospective and prospective. *Nursing Science Quarterly, 10,* 49–52.

Watson, J. (2006). Part One: Jean Watson's theory of human caring. In M. E. Parker, *Nursing theories and nursing practice* (2nd ed., pp. 295–302). Philadelphia, PA: F. A. Davis.

Willis, D. G., DeSanto-Madeya, S., & Fawcett, J. (2015). Moving beyond dwelling in suffering: A situation-specific theory of men's healing from childhood maltreatment. *Nursing Science Quarterly, 28,* 57–63.

Ziegler, S. M. (Ed.). (2005). *Theory-directed nursing practice* (2nd ed.). New York, NY: Springer.

● Rose Kearney-Nunnery

4

Health, Illness, and Holism

"I can enter your world, as one who invites your growth or as a strangler of your possibilities, a prophet of stasis."

Sidney M. Jourard (1971)

Chapter Objectives

On completion of this chapter, the reader will be able to:

1. Differentiate among the various health and illness models for applicability to professional nursing practice.

2. Discuss the advantages and disadvantages of the various models.

3. Apply a health belief or health promotion model to a given nursing care situation.

4. Examine the application of holism in professional practice.

5. Select a model for cultural competence and apply it to a patient population from a culture other than yours.

Key Terms

Health
Health Promotion
Health Protection
Preventive Services
Primary Prevention

Secondary Prevention
Tertiary Prevention
High-level Wellness
Health Belief Model
Health Promotion Model

Chronic Illness Trajectory
   Framework
Functional Health Patterns
Holistic Nursing
Cultural Competence

Health is a condition we seek, promote, and hope to maintain. Health is more than the absence of illness or infirmity. A multidimensional construct of health is determined by the individual's worldview and philosophical assumptions. Consider the four metaparadigm concepts of nursing and the fact that health is specified in the nursing theory that guides our practice. Health as a part of the metaparadigm is interrelated with the concepts of human beings, environment, and nursing. Considering your particular view of the world and your concept of health, we can now approach ways of promoting health using a sample of different models. However, consider that your patient population may have a different worldview. The selection of model is, again, determined by one's worldview and theoretical guide.

In Chapter 3, health is illustrated within individual theoretical structures. For example, compare the definitions of health provided by King, Roy, and Leininger. King (1981) defines health as "dynamic life experiences of a human being, which implies continuous adjustment to stressors in the internal and external environment through optimum use of one's resources to achieve maximum potential for daily living" (p. 5). Here we have the focus on human beings. Roy defines health as a state and process of being and becoming integrated and whole with a focus on the mutuality between human beings and the environmental (Andrews & Roy, 1991, p. 21). Leininger (2002b) defines health as "a state of well-being or restorative state that is culturally constituted, defined, valued, and practiced by individuals or groups that enables them to function in their daily lives" (p. 84). Care, rather than health, is considered the central concept. It refers to the secondary concepts of nursing—health, curing, and well-being, and especially culture care (Leininger & McFarland, 2006, p. 3).

In other nursing theories and models, the concept of health may not be well defined but is interpreted, as in Rogers's theory, as a "value term defined by the culture or individual" (Gunther, 2010, p. 246). Or, in Parse's (1981) theory, health is a process of becoming (p. 159). Still, health or well-being is represented in each framework on which practice is based. Before delving into the theories of health and illness—in the context of health promotion and illness prevention—and cultural perceptions of health, it is first important to understand the different levels and types of health promotion and illness prevention activities.

LEVELS OF PREVENTION

When considering health promotion activities, we frequently refer to illness and disability prevention. Over twenty years ago, national health promotion and disease prevention activities were developed under the auspices of the U.S. Department of Health and Human Services

ONLINE CONSULT

Nursing Theories at
http://www.nurses.info/nursing_theory.htm

(USDHHS) and published as *Healthy People 2000*. Interestingly, the publication distinguished between health promotion and health protection strategies, with an individual versus a community focus:

> **Health promotion** *strategies are those related to individual lifestyle—personal choices made in a social context—that can have a powerful influence over one's health prospects. These include physical activity and fitness, nutrition, tobacco, alcohol and other drugs, family planning, mental health and mental disorders and violent and abusive behavior. . . .* **Health protection** *strategies are those related to environmental or regulatory measures that confer protection on large population groups. These strategies address issues such as unintentional injuries, occupational safety and health, environmental health, food and drug safety, and oral health.* **Preventive services** *include counseling, screening, immunization, or chemoprophylactic interventions for individuals in clinical settings.* (USDHHS, PHS, 1992, pp. 6–7)

These preventive activities and services address the three levels of prevention: primary, secondary, and tertiary. Health promotion activities are both protective and preventive, but they require consumers actively involved in all levels of prevention. And this focus on health promotion and health protection strategies became an important component of *Healthy People 2020* (USDHHS, 2010) with the national goals for high quality and years of healthy life, health equity, healthy environments, and healthy development and behaviors across the lifespan. See Chapter 14 for more on population health.

Primary Prevention

Primary prevention refers to healthy actions taken to avoid illness or disease. Examples are healthy nutrition, smoking cessation, exercise programs, parenting classes, community awareness programs, and mental health programs and activities. The individual lifestyle health promotion strategies recommended in *Healthy People* are becoming more popular and prevalent as people take responsibility for their own health. Health columns appear frequently in publications. We have also seen a growing number of health food and holistic health stores, "healthy" fast food options, Web sites, and educational programs for the general public. But consumers can still have difficulty acquiring sufficient information on a selected topic before they become frustrated.

Secondary Prevention

Secondary prevention involves screening for early detection and treatment of health problems. With secondary prevention, the individual is seeking healthcare not for a specific problem but, rather, for early detection of a potential problem to mobilize resources and reduce its intensity or severity if the problem is identified. Secondary prevention usually involves use of some procedure or measurement tool in addition to the health history and physical assessment. Examples of secondary prevention are screening procedures used by healthcare consumers or healthcare professionals for physiological, developmental, or environmental problems. Physiological procedures include screening for hypertension or specific forms of cancer. Mental health screening procedures range from simple tests for orientation to more elaborate instruments such as mental status questionnaires for aging patients. In young children, examples of secondary prevention activities are use of growth charts to assess growth along established percentiles and developmental screening tests to detect problems in the areas of personal-social skills, motor activities, and language. Note the difference between using parenting classes as primary prevention for developmental stimulation and screening for developmental problems as secondary prevention. Environmental screening procedures include testing air and water quality and home safety assessments. If a problem is detected, a referral is made for a differential diagnosis and institution of early treatment.

Tertiary Prevention

Tertiary prevention occurs during the rehabilitative phase of an illness to prevent complications or further disability. The individual has already entered the healthcare system and is recovering from or learning to cope with a health deficit. Tertiary prevention builds on this care to prevent further deficits. Examples of tertiary prevention are counseling and teaching after recovery from a cardiovascular event, an accident or injury, an abusive situation, or any other physical, psychosocial, mental, or environmental disruption from usual health and functioning. Support from self-help groups is a large component of tertiary prevention. An example of tertiary prevention is family counseling after identification of a child in an abusive situation.

Professional nursing practice involves not only health promotion but also all three levels of preventive activities. Because the health of individuals, families, communities, and groups is a major concern in nursing, professional skill and expertise in the area of prevention activities are presumed in practice, education, research, and administrative functions.

THEORIES OF HEALTH AND ILLNESS

Aside from the conceptual or theoretical frameworks, different nursing models are available to guide assessment of health factors and promote and preserve health. Interestingly, Benner and Wrubel (1989) described five theories of health as (1) an ideal, (2) the ability to fulfill social roles, (3) a commodity, (4) a human potential, and (5) a sense of coherence. Health is more than an ideal. We strive for the person, family, community, or group to reach a positive state of well-being. Defining health as the ability to perform one's role is limiting and fails to meet our holistic concern for human beings. As Benner and Wrubel (1989) observe, "this view focuses on doing rather than being and ignores the person's sense of fulfillment and well-being" (p. 151). Health as a commodity implies that it can be bought, sold, traded, and withheld. This view fails to meet the intent of a caring professional practice discipline. Health as a commodity is described as

a "medicalized view," promising instant cures without personal involvement (Benner & Wrubel, 1989, pp. 151–153).

Health defined as a human potential is consistent with the beliefs of nursing and many other healthcare disciplines and is the basis of the first three health models presented here. Health as a human potential includes physical, mental, and spiritual health. Benner and Wrubel (1989) describe the limitation of this model in health promotion activities in that, although all people have the potential for health, they are continually pursuing increasing levels of health but not attaining health as a state or condition (pp. 156–157). This definition depends on whether health is viewed as a defined goal or a dynamic state that we continue to strive toward. Dunn's (1973) high-level wellness model, the health belief model, and Pender's (1996) health promotion model are consistent with health viewed as human potential.

The fifth view of health takes a phenomenological approach. *Phenomenology* is the lived experience of the individual, from his or her unique perspective. This view focuses on one's lived experience rather than on an opinion derived from another person's observations of the experience. Benner and Wrubel's (1989) approach to health as a mind-body-spirit integration in a state of becoming is an example of health as a sense of coherence. A focus on the person's belonging to a sociocultural group makes this integration unique. Benner and Wrubel define the term *well-being* as a better indication of health with challenges and involvement in the following definition: "Well-being is defined as congruence between one's possibilities and one's actual practices and lived meanings and is based on caring and feeling cared for" (Benner & Wrubel, 1989, p. 160).

In this view, a model must be based on a qualitative approach to address individuals' well-being, because it depends on the lived experience of those persons in their context. As Benner and Wrubel (1989) state, "health as well-being comes when one engages in sound self-care, cares, and feels cared for—when one trusts the self, the body, and others. Breakdown occurs when that trust is broken. Well-being can be restored" (p. 165). Newman's (2008) theory of health as the expansion of consciousness (p. 5) is applicable to this view. The chronic illness trajectory framework is also consistent with the view of health as coherence, as are holistic health practices focused on the interrelatedness of mind, body, and spirit.

Model of High-Level Wellness

Dunn developed his model of **high-level wellness** starting with the 1947 definition of health from the World Health Organization that emphasized physical, mental, and social well-being. He stressed that well-being includes the positive, dynamic, and unique integration of mind, body, and spirit of the individual within his or her environment, including work, family, community, and society. Dunn (1973) defined high-level wellness for an individual as "an integrated method of functioning which is oriented toward maximizing the potential of which the individual is capable [and] requires that the individual maintain a continuum of balance and purposeful direction within the environment where he is functioning" (pp. 4–5).

Dunn regarded high-level wellness as an ongoing challenge to the highest level possible—the individual's maximum potential. Meeting basic needs and striving for higher needs were components of his view of individual health and well-being. Dunn (1973) viewed high-level wellness as "an open-ended and ever-expanding tomorrow with its challenge to live at full potential" (p. 223). He also considered high-level wellness, with similar components, for the family, community, environment, and society.

Dunn's beliefs about high-level wellness evolved into a health grid (Fig. 4.1) that demonstrates a person or group at some point along a health continuum or horizontal axis, from death at the left side to peak wellness at the right. The person or group was further influenced by the environment (the vertical axis), from a very favorable environment at the top to a very unfavorable environment at the bottom. This grid illustrates the person or group in context, within one of the four quadrants ranging from poor health to protected poor health, high-level wellness, and emergent high-level wellness. The high-level wellness model provides an explanation of the person-environment relationship in health but gives no direction as to movement among quadrants, and it also compartmentalizes wellness.

The model could be used effectively to address health equity for the patient who is currently in an unfavorable environment (poorly accepted health services related to a language barrier) to a favorable environment where we strive to promote more culturally relevant, understandable, and acceptable services and healthcare.

Health Belief Model

The **health belief model** is a tool for looking at both health promotion and actions directed at maintaining or restoring health. Originally, the model was based on the following hypothesis:

Persons will not seek preventative care or health screening unless they possess minimal levels of relevant health motivation and knowledge, view themselves as potentially vulnerable and the condition as threatening, are convinced of the efficacy of intervention, and see few difficulties in undertaking the recommended action (Becker et al., 1977, p. 29).

The health belief model was designed as an organizing framework to advance health promotion activities

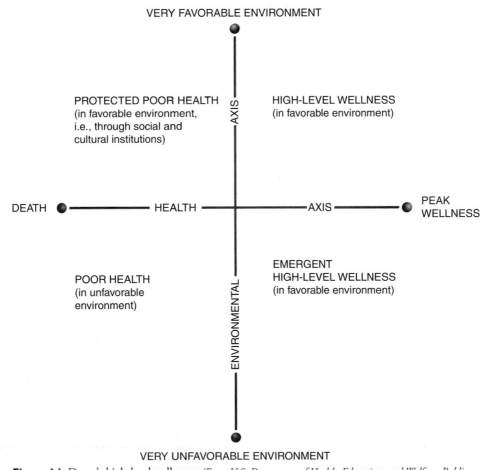

Figure 4.1 Dunn's high-level wellness. *(From U.S. Department of Health, Education, and Welfare. Public Health Service, National Office of Vital Statistics.)*

by targeting interventions on certain individual variables. The three major concepts in the model were individual perceptions, modifying factors, and likelihood of action. Individual perceptions involve how the person considers the risk of susceptibility or the severity of the illness—in other words, how likely he or she believes it is that the disease or condition could happen to him or her. Modifying factors are a set of demographic, sociopsychological cues to action from family, friends, professionals, or the media relative to the perceived threat of the disease. Sociopsychological variables include personality, interpersonal influences, and socioeconomic status. The modifying factors, along with individual perceptions, lead to the likelihood of action in the direction of health. The concept of motivation is central to this model (Becker et al., 1977, p. 31).

An extensive review of research on variables in the health belief model led to a subsequent revision. The model was expanded from a diagram of health belief concepts and their interrelationships to a full explanation of and prediction about health-related behaviors. The three major concepts were (1) readiness to undertake recommended compliance behavior, (2) modifying and enabling factors, and (3) compliant behaviors. On the basis of research, readiness to undertake recommended compliance behavior broadened individual perceptions from perception of susceptibility and severity to perceptions of motivations, values for threat reduction, and subjective risk/benefit considerations that the compliant behaviors would be safe and effective. Modifying factors were expanded to more inclusive modifying and enabling factors on the basis of research findings. A reciprocal relationship between readiness and modifying/enabling factors also became more apparent in the revised model. The outcome in the revised model was the likelihood of compliant behaviors with preventive recommendations or prescribed regimens.

The original version of the health belief model focused on health promotion or preventive behaviors. Since its inception, the model has been widely used in research and practice. In addition to use in understanding utilization of healthcare services and health promotion behaviors, the model has guided research in patient compliance to healthcare. An extensive body of research on patient compliance for the revised model demonstrated applicability in a wide range of healthcare situations. Insights for use of the model in practice and education were offered. Concerning patient education, Becker and associates (1977) recommended that healthcare providers understand the following principles:

1. Behavior is motivated.
2. Certain beliefs seem central to a person's decision to act.
3. Not all persons possess these beliefs and motives to equal degrees.
4. Intellectual information, although necessary, is often not sufficient to stimulate needed beliefs.
5. Health providers need to view the importance of patient education and accept substantial responsibility in this activity. (p. 42)

These principles are consistent with the discipline of professional nursing practice and are routinely incorporated into plans for care and health teaching. Consideration of the belief systems of the individual, family, or group is essential in assessing a patient and choosing interventions. The extent of detail and inclusion of this information is the challenge to the nurse, whose health-teaching role is an integral component of professional practice.

As a part of the health history, readiness, as a motivation in health behaviors, is easily included in the interview. The patient's "subjective estimates" of the potential to reduce the threat and care options are less commonly included in the assessment, depending on the professional's impressions of time restraints and knowledge of the patient or even on cultural or interpersonal differences between the professional and the patient. In a nursing health assessment, we frequently acquire demographic information and some structural information that provides insight into modifying and enabling factors. The challenge is to acquire the additional structural information, such as cost and accessibility, and to seek information from the patient about quality, satisfaction, and social pressures for additional knowledge of attitudinal, interaction, and enabling factors. This information can be used to increase compliant behaviors.

Nevertheless, the model has limitations. First, the language is directed to physician-patient relationships, quite possibly a product of the roles and functions of other healthcare providers in 1977. More recently, the health belief model has been used in further research consistent with views of nursing. Ongoing research and applications of health behavior have been demonstrated at the level of the individual, dyad, group, organization, and community (Glanz, Rimer, & Lewis, 2002). Second, as Pender (1987, 1996; Pender, Murdaugh, & Parsons, 2002, 2011) indicates, the health belief model is directed at preventive services or health protection behaviors in the context of a provider-consumer relationship rather than individual health promotion behaviors. To be empowered consumers in today's healthcare system, individuals must take personal responsibility for their own health long before they seek care from a health professional. This concept is now beginning to be addressed in the health belief model, especially in applications related to health education.

Health Promotion Model

Pender's **health promotion model**, an outgrowth of the health belief model, is based on research and information on health and health-protecting behaviors. It is primarily a nursing model and has been revised with evolving knowledge. In the health promotion model, health promotion is motivated by the desire to increase the level of wellness and actualization of an individual or an aggregate group (Pender, 1996, p. 7). Pender describes the health promotion model as a "competence- or approach-oriented model with applicability across the life span for motivating overall healthy lifestyles" (Pender et al., 2006, p. 48). A further holistic focus is apparent in the revisions of the health promotion model; to include considerations of the family, the community, the nation, and the world (Pender et al., 2011, p. 31). Health is defined as "the realization of human potential through goal-directed behavior, competent self-care, and satisfying relationships with others, while adapting to maintain structural integrity and harmony with the social and physical environments" (Pender et al., 2011, p. 22). She points out that unlike the health belief model "the health promotion model does not include ,'fear' or 'threat' as a source of motivation for the health behavior" (Pender et al., 2011, p. 44).

Structurally, the model had been designed as a schematic representation similar to the original health belief model. After extensive research, however, the model was revised, and significant variables were reorganized (Fig. 4.2). The knowledge obtained through research led to the later addition of three new variables in the health promotion model: activity-related affect, commitment to a plan of action, and immediate competing demands and preferences.

The revised health promotion model contains two principal components that interact for participation in health-promoting behaviors: (1) individual characteristics and experiences and (2) behavior-specific cognitions and affect. Individual characteristics and experiences are similar to the individual perceptions in the health belief model, in that they involve looking at health through past experiences (prior related behavior) and personal factors. Pender points out that "research indicates that often the best predictor of behavior is the frequency of the same or a similar behavior in the past" (Pender et al., 2011, p. 45). Personal factors include biologic variables (age, gender, body mass, etc.), psychological variables (such as self-esteem, self-motivation, perceived health status), and sociocultural variables (race, ethnicity, acculturation, education, socioeconomic status) (Pender et al., 2011, p. 46).

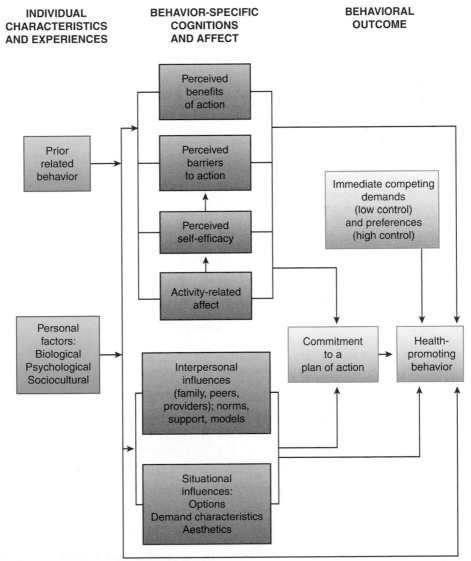

Figure 4.2 Pender's health belief model. (Pender, N. J., Murdaugh, C. L., and Parsons, M. A. [2011]. *Health promotion in nursing practice* [6th ed.]. Upper Saddle River, NJ: Pearson Education, Inc., p. 45. Reprinted by permission of Pearson Education, Inc.)

On the basis of research evidence, these biological, psychological, and sociocultural personal factors were included in the model as further predictors of individual health perceptions and behaviors. For example, consider the health-seeking behaviors demonstrated by patients of different socioeconomic groups, family backgrounds, and experiences in the healthcare system. A later section of this chapter addresses cultural differences in health beliefs that also influence health-seeking behaviors.

The behavior-specific cognitions and affect are similar to the health belief model's modifying or enabling factors but relate more to the nomenclature of nursing. As Pender has indicated, this category of variables is of "major motivational significance" and provides the critical "core," because they are subject to modification based on interventions (Pender et al., 2011, p. 46). These behavior-specific cognitions and affects include perceived benefits, perceived barriers, perceived self-efficacy, activity-related affect (subjective feelings), interpersonal influences, and situational influences. Interpersonal and situational influences are identified as having both direct and indirect effects on health promotion behaviors. Consider the older adult walking through a shopping mall and noticing a free hypertension screening clinic. Indirect situational influences to obtain a screening test may include the perceived camaraderie of people in the clinic compared with a tedious wait for an office appointment. The direct influence is the availability of the screening during this older adult's routine exercise program at the mall.

The variables of perceived benefits, perceived barriers, self-efficacy, interpersonal influences, and situational influences have been supported in research studies as predictors of health promotion behaviors (Pender, 1996; Pender et al., 2002, 2006, 2011). Activity-related affect, a variable added in the revised health promotion model, addresses the individual's subjective feelings related to the health promotion behavior. Although research studies have supported constructs in the model, Pender et al. (2011) have observed that inadequate testing of the entire model is possibly related to the complexity and the large number of concepts (p. 50).

Behavioral outcome, the third component of the model, includes actions toward the healthy behavior. These actions lead to the attainment of a positive health outcome. Two variables (immediate competing demands and preferences, and commitment to a plan of action) were added to the revised health promotion model to explain further the behavioral outcome of the health-promoting behavior. Pender describes the commitment to the plan of action with two distinct cognitive processes: "[a] commitment to carry out a specific action at a given time and place and with specified persons or alone, irrespective of competing preferences . . . and (2) identification of definitive strategies for eliciting, carrying out, and reinforcing the behavior" (Pender et al., 2011, p. 49).

The health-promoting behavior can be affected by the immediate competing demands and preferences the individual perceives. These are viewed as alternate behaviors. Competing demands are behaviors over which the person has little control because of environmental factors, like family commitments. Competing preferences are behaviors

with powerful reinforcing properties—such as a sudden urge for a particular food—over which the person has a high level of control (Pender et al., 2011, p. 50). This component is greatly influenced by nursing interventions related to values clarification, encouragement, and reinforcement of healthy behaviors.

In the earlier version of the health promotion model, Pender (1987) described the model as a flexible organizing framework, subject to revision after further testing. This was followed by the identification of theoretical basis from both the Expectancy-Value Theory and the Social Cognitive Theory with the specification of first seven assumptions (Pender, 1996) and then 15 theoretical propositions (Pender et. al., 2002). Research has been ongoing for testing of the model. With the empirical support of variables, the revised model has greater potential to predict and intervene for health promotion activities. Health promotion settings are the social environment in which we live, work, and play, such as family, school, workplace, healthcare agencies, and the community at large. Ongoing research studies have focused on a variety of populations to target health promotion activities.

Comparison of the Two Models

Table 4.1 compares the health belief model and the health promotion model. Both models propose that the health professional must understand how the person perceives the world and that the person makes personal decisions through identified readiness or individual characteristics and experiences. The modifying factors or behavior-specific cognitions and affect are the social, situational, and environmental influences related to the person's conception of healthy behavior. Both models include demographic variables, because research supports the importance of differences. For example, the choice between surgery and irradiation is very different for a 28-year-old patient and an 88-year-old patient, in terms not only of physiological differences but also of past experiences. Attention to these differences turns the focus of healthcare consumers to their specific outcomes and increases chances of success in the health promotion activity.

Chronic Illness Model

Although the health belief model has been used in research and practice settings with patients who have chronic illnesses, Corbin and Strauss's chronic illness model is specific to chronicity. Despite its focus on chronic illness, it is still a health promotion model. As Corbin and Strauss (1992a) have stated:

The focus of care in chronicity is not on cure but first of all on the prevention of chronic conditions, then on finding ways to help the ill manage and live with their illness should these occur. Interventions are aimed at fostering the prevention of, living with, and shaping the course of chronic illnesses, especially those requiring technologically complex management, while promoting and maintaining quality of life. (p. 20)

The **chronic illness trajectory framework** (Corbin & Strauss, 1992a) was developed as a substantive theory for

TABLE 4.1

Comparing the Health Belief Model and the Health Promotion Model

Model	Individual Characteristics	Mediating Factors	Outcomes
Health Belief Model (Becker et al., 1977)	Readiness for recommended behavior: Motivations, including general health concerns, willingness and compliance behaviors, positive health attitudes Value of illness threat reduction, including subjective estimates and past experiences Probability that compliant behavior will reduce threat (subjectively)	Modifying/enabling factors: Demographic Structural Attitudes Interaction Enabling	Compliant behaviors: Likelihood of compliance with preventive health recommendations and prescribed regimens
Pender's Health Promotion Model (Pender, Murdaugh, & Parsons, 2011)	Individual characteristics and experiences: Prior related behavior Personal factors Biological Psychological Sociocultural	Behavior-specific cognitions and affect: Perceived benefits Perceived barriers Perceived self-efficacy Activity-related affect Interpersonal influences Situational influences	Behavioral outcomes: Commitment to a plan of action Immediate competing demands and preferences Health promoting behaviors

application to individuals with a broad range of chronic conditions. Benner and Wrubel's (1989) concept of health as coherence applies to this model. Corbin and Strauss (1992a) describe the development of the framework as based on 30 years of qualitative, grounded theory research. The original framework was developed with the following concepts: key problems, basic strategies, organizational or family arrangements, and consequences (Strauss & Glaser, 1975; Strauss et al., 1984). It evolved into a nursing theory through its use and research base, but the developers maintain that it potentially applies to all healthcare disciplines. The framework was based on the following assumptions:

1. The course of chronic conditions varies and changes over time.
2. The course of a chronic condition can be shaped and managed.
3. The technology involved is complex and can potentially create side effects.
4. The illness and technology pose potential consequences for the individual's physical well-being, biographical fulfillment (identify over time), and performance of daily activities.
5. Biographical needs and performance of daily activities can affect illness management choices and the course of the illness.
6. The course of illness is not inevitably downward.
7. Chronic illnesses do not necessarily end in death. (Corbin & Strauss, 1992a, p. 10; 1992b, p. 97)

Corbin and Strauss (1992a) described the framework as a conceptual model organized under the central concept of trajectory. This central concept was proposed to indicate the management of the evolving course of the chronic condition, as "shaped" by the person, family members, and healthcare providers. Corbin (1998) subsequently updated the model with "a greater emphasis on health promotion and illness prevention," along with simplified language, greater emphasis on the role of nurses, and global health considerations (p. 33). Refer to Table 4.2. The revision provided nine, rather than eight, phases for a trajectory with a focus on quality of life. In the acute phase, the illness is treated with a goal of returning to normal activities. However, in a life-threatening situation, the goal of management is to remove the threat, with everyday activities suspended until the crisis has past, but the downward phase is focused on adaptation to disability (Corbin, 1998, p. 36). However, if the patient returns to the stable phase, normal activities of daily living will take place in the home and community environment. Corbin (1998) describes the implementation of the model as the problem-solving approach, similar to the steps of the nursing process, as data gathering, problem prioritizing and goal setting, developing the plan of action, implementing the plan, and following up with any needed changes in the plan.

This model focuses on the person to illustrate the management of an evolving course of a chronic condition and the individual experiences that are influenced by that individual, the family, and healthcare providers. The ultimate goals are health promotion and disability prevention, but with the recognition of the incidence of increasing chronic illness. It takes us a step farther than the health belief model because this model is more grounded in the individual's unique, personal history and patterns of life. Individuals with various chronic illnesses have been studied in many countries around the world using grounded theory and the Chronic Illness Trajectory Framework. The framework has also been used in research on dementia in family members and considerations on placement that was funded by the National Institute of Nursing Research

TABLE 4.2	

The Chronic Illness Trajectory Framework (Corbin, 1998)

Trajectory phases	Pretrajectory Trajectory onset Stable Unstable Acute Crisis Comeback Downward Dying
Trajectory, defined	The illness/condition course and actions taken to shape or control the course (Corbin, 1998, p. 35)
Trajectory, overall goal	"To keep populations free of chronic conditions, and when chronic conditions strike, to assist those affected to control symptoms, prevent complications, and maintain stability . . . [for] quality and quantity to life" (Corbin, 1998, p. 37)
Management strategies	Technology used, resources, past experience, motivation, setting of care, lifestyle/beliefs, interactions/relationships, service providers, chronic condition and physiological involvement, symptoms, political and economic trends
Approach to care	Holistic, individualized, flexible with consideration of the cultural setting and changes in trajectory phases, and applicable to the care setting

(NINR). This model has also been used to study adherence to treatment over time in patients with congestive heart failure (Granger, Moser, Harrell, Sandelowski, & Ekman, 2007). Additional chronic illness models have evolved (Curry, Walker, Moore, & Hogstel, 2010; McEvoy & Barnes, 2007; Weinert, Cudney, & Spring, 2008) as we focus on the growing population of patients with chronic illnesses. The model has also been adapted for application to cancer survivorship patients (Klimmek & Wenzel, 2012). The use of grounded theory as an inductive approach to understanding the individual's experience with chronic illness and all the associated contextual factors is predominant in these research studies. For example, the chronic illness experience is distinctively different for an elderly, frail Anglo-American woman living alone in an urban high-rise apartment than for the African American elder with a physical disability living with her grandson in a rural farm area or for the Asian American elder in a multigenerational environment. The difference involves more than the issue of compliance; it focuses on quality. This model is extremely relevant to nursing care as we experience the rising numbers of chronic illnesses managed in contemporary practice and the growing population of aging adults who are living longer while dealing with a chronic illness. In addition, the importance of cultural relevance, the beliefs and values of individuals, families, communities, and groups, and environmental factors are major considerations in holistic healthcare.

All of these models require a thoughtful and thorough nursing assessment. Valid data are needed for their application. As part of the nursing assessment, the application of Gordon's (2008) **functional health patterns** could assist in this application (Box 4.1). Nursing assessment

BOX 4.1	**Functional Health Patterns**

Gordon (2008) has identified 11 functional health patterns for inclusion in the nursing assessment and diagnosis process:
● Health perception and health management
● Nutrition and metabolic
● Elimination
● Activity and exercise
● Sleep and rest
● Cognitive and perceptual
● Self-perception and self-concept
● Role and relationship
● Sexuality and reproductive
● Coping and stress tolerance
● Values and beliefs

of each of these areas provides valuable data for application of a health or illness model to address health and illness focused on human potential or a sense of coherence and holism. In addition, this assessment data and identification of functional health patterns provide the basis of the nursing process and identification of nursing diagnoses.

Holism

Holism is a term frequently used in nursing and other health professions as we focus on human beings in their environment. As simply stated by Antigoni and Dimitrios (2009), **holistic nursing** is "healing the whole person"

(p. 150). In her review of the philosophy and theory of holism, Erickson (2007) points out that although the concept of holism has been present for many centuries, the word *holism* is a product of the 20th century application in nursing in the 1970s when "central to each holistic nurse's philosophy were the beliefs that the whole is greater than the sum of the parts, the patient's world view guides practitioners in understanding the whole, and the nurse is instrumental in helping people to heal and grow"(p. 145). Recall that "wholeness" is one of the principles in systems theory and also included in many nursing models. More recently, Zborowsky and Kreitzer (2009) applied systems theory to their model designed at three overlapping circles for people, process, and place, with the common center that was created and entitled the optimum healing environment (OHE). In fact, they propose that the OHE is "created when people, place, and care processes converge at a particular time and within a particular culture" (Zborowsky & Kreitzer, 2009, p. 187). And, as Ray (2010) points out, "the holistic science of nursing has provided nursing with understanding of the complexity of human relationships and the complexity of the meaning of the integral relationship of the human and environment" (p. 138).

The American Holistic Nurses Association (AHNA) and the American Nurses Association (ANA) (2013) have identified the *Holistic Nursing: Scope and Standards of Practice* guided by principles for the concepts of person, health/healing, practice, nursing roles, self-reflection, and self-care. As with the general *Scope and Standards of Practice* (ANA, 2010), holistic nursing is described with six standards of practice in line with the steps of the nursing process and standards of professional performance focused on quality, education, practice evaluation, collegiality, collaboration, ethics, research, resource utilization, and leadership. Holistic nursing is described as "focus[ing] on protecting, promoting, and optimizing health and wellness; assisting healing; preventing illness and injury; alleviating suffering; supporting people to find peace, comfort, harmony, and balance through the diagnosis and treatment of human response; and advocacy in the care of individuals, families, communities, populations, and the planet" (AHNA & ANA, 2013, p. 1). The focus is on the whole person in their unique context. Andrews (2008b) describes the holistic paradigm as seeking "to maintain a sense of balance or harmony between humans and the larger universe [with] explanations for health and disease based not so much on external agents as on imbalance or disharmony among the human, geophysical, and metaphysical forces of the universe" (p. 69). As illustrated in Chapter 3, several nursing models are consistent with this model of practice. The patient is the focus, with the goal of returning to a state of harmony or balance, and care may include both conventional treatment as well as a traditional and complementary and alternative therapies (CAM).

While holistic nursing practice is a specialty practice with its unique scope and standards identified by the profession, components of holism are evident in all nursing practice areas. The American Association of Colleges of Nursing (AACN, 2006, 2008b) in its *Essentials* documents for both baccalaureate and graduate education, includes the expectation for holistic practice. At the undergraduate level, the first assumption is that "the baccalaureate generalist graduate is prepared to practice from a holistic, caring framework" (AACN, 2008b, p. 8), and the direct practice of the advanced practice nurse is characterized by the use of a holistic perspective (AACN, 2006, p. 18).

As stated in the *Holistic Nursing: Scope and Standards of Practice* (AHNA & ANA, 2013), "holistic nursing is a world view—a way of 'being' in the world and not just a modality—holistic nurses can practice in any setting, anywhere, and with individuals throughout the life span" (p. 22). The holistic caring process is aligned with the steps of the nursing process but, as with any specialty practice, requires specialty knowledge, skills, and abilities. In addition, as in the ANA (2010) *Nursing: Scope and Standards of Practice,* holistic practice competencies are delineated for the RN and the nurse with graduate-level preparation. All professional nursing practice requires a holistic perspective. As stated in the ANA (2010) *Nursing: Scope and Standards of Practice*, "the nursing needs of human beings are identified from a holistic perspective and are met within the context of a culturally sensitive, caring interpersonal environment" (p. 18). This holistic perspective includes the physical, emotional, social, and spiritual needs of the individual and the family. And the spiritual dimension includes feelings, thoughts, experiences, and behaviors in a search for meaning, not necessarily synonymous with religion (AHNA & ANA, 2013, p. 91). The need for holistic nursing practice is important for the patient, family, and nurse whether the situation involves routine, emergency, or palliative care, the care is applicable to individual preferences and culture.

CULTURAL INFLUENCE ON HEALTH PERCEPTIONS

Over the past 30 years, national initiatives in *Healthy People 2000, 2010,* and *2020,* have targeted selected groups of at-risk populations requiring special health promotion strategies. These reports illustrated significant health problems in some minority groups, but more importantly, they emphasized individuals within subgroups. As originally reported in *Healthy People 2000,* individual differences, beyond racial group, socioeconomic status, and educational level, affect health status and access to healthcare. These reports pointed out that "our healthcare programs are characterized by unacceptable disparities linked to membership in certain racial and ethnic groups" (USDHHS, PHS, 1992, p. 31). Since that time, studies and outreach efforts have investigated racial, cultural, environmental, social, and linguistic issues. As an example, the Commonwealth Foundation conducted a field study, reporting that "minorities have difficulty getting appropriate, timely, high-quality care because of language barriers and that they may have different perspectives on health, medical care, and expectations about diagnosis and treatment" (Betancourt et al., 2002, p. 3). Further research into managed care, education, and government illustrated "a clear link between cultural competence, improving quality, and eliminating racial and ethnic disparities in health care" (Betancourt et al., 2005, p. 1). Pender et al. (2011) describe designing culturally competent health promotion programs and identify specific demographic, cultural, and health system factors to assess in vulnerable populations (p. 293). The issue then goes beyond access to the need for the provision of acceptable healthcare to address the issue of health equity.

These reports began to highlight the need for a concerted effort to understand and embrace diversity in our daily personal and professional lives. But much is implied within the construct of "diversity." When people speak of ethnicity and race, they generally refer to a group, tribe, or nation of people united by some common characteristics, whether biological, environmental, or social. In the United States, we tend to classify people into five ethnic groups: African Americans, Asian Americans and Pacific Islanders, Hispanic Americans, Native Americans, and white Americans. But this tendency does little to help us understand the health beliefs, practices, needs, or diversity represented within each of these population classifications. It may, in fact, encourage us to impose stereotypical judgments on persons within these groups.

This point leads us to the concept of culture as a way of life and the increasing focus on **cultural competence**. Purnell (2013) describes competence in healthcare as "having the knowledge, skills, and abilities to deliver care congruent with the patient's cultural beliefs and practices" (p. 7). Purnell (2013) further states that increasing one's consciousness of cultural diversity improves the possibilities for healthcare practitioners to provide culturally competent care (p. 7).

Our cultural inheritance has a powerful influence on our health beliefs, both conscious and unconscious. We bring into our personal and professional lives the influences from our ancestors, family, peers, and colleagues. We are affected by history, genetics, social customs, religion, language, politics, law, economics, education, and many other factors. We mutually influence and are influenced by others because of these endowments. When we talk about cultural diversity, we mean more than an inherited background. "Culture" implies social, familial, religious, national, and professional characteristics that affect the way we think and act; it is a combination of all these things.

Research demonstrating individual differences and perceptions provided valuable data for the revision of the health belief model. Educational, ethnic, and social class differences were identified for careful assessment of patient beliefs and perceptions (Becker et al., 1977). These data

ONLINE CONSULT

Agency for Healthcare Research and Quality at
http://www.ahrq.gov

The Commonwealth Fund at
http://www.cmwf.org

Healthy People at
http://www.healthypeople.gov

U.S. Department of Health & Human Services at
http://www.hhs.gov

are significant whether one is dealing with individual patients or families with a specific healthcare deficit or a larger population group with informational needs for health promotion activities.

But it is important to consider the characteristics of both the patient and the health professional. The values for cultural diversity and culturally sensitive care are clearly illustrated in position statements of our nursing organizations. In addition, AACN (2008a, 2009) has identified core cultural competences for nurses prepared at both the baccalaureate and graduate levels (see Table 4.3). As Andrews (2008b) indicates, however, healthcare professionals "must have positive experiences with members of other cultures and learn to value genuinely the contributions all cultures make to our multicultural society" (p. 9).

One's health beliefs are the result of cultural inheritance, education, reasoned opinions, and, often, unfounded impressions. The proportion of each of these factors is individually determined. Andrews (2008a) describes three worldviews for cultural influence on healthcare: (1) magico-religious, (2) scientific, and (3) holistic. The three different views show us how individuals differ in their beliefs in the supernatural, the scientific community, or the holistic mind-body-spirit interrelationship. It is worth noting that the traditional healthcare system operates from the scientific worldview, which diverges from that of many cultures and their subgroups.

The *magico-religious view* of health and healing focuses on the supernatural. It can include ancient rites and rituals, reliance on prayer and the will of a supreme being, pilgrimages, spiritual healing, and the like. The *scientific view* is the dominant one for the healthcare system, with reliance on allopathic medicine, biomedical treatments, and a focus on a cure for illness and disease. As noted by Spector (2013), the allopathic philosophy is predicated on a dualistic view of body and mind and adherence to scientific and technological norms of the system for acute care, chronic care, rehabilitation, psychiatric/mental health, and community/public health—and is a culture onto itself (pp. 108–109). The *holistic paradigm* sees health as a balance of the physical, mental, and spiritual whole and includes both alternative and complementary therapies (e.g., aromatherapy or massage) and ethnocultural practices (e.g., herbs or voodoo) used to treat the person rather than the disease (Spector, 2013). The holistic aim is for a sense of harmony and treatment to correct an imbalance. Significant differences can exist in health beliefs and roles between the patient with a healthcare need and the healthcare provider, considered the "expert."

In our healthcare system, we generally view the roles of healthcare providers and those of consumers in traditional ways. We consider the disease or illness, including all the pathophysiology and treatment modalities. We are aware of healthcare and health promotion services in both the hospital and community setting. We usually present them through our words and behaviors as norms to which patients must adhere. Otherwise, they are termed "bad patients," "noncompliant," or even "problem cases." For example, the healthcare community carefully conducts, evaluates, and uses research to identify biological, chemical, structural, and physical factors to treat, manage, or cure a disease. Faced with patients whose belief system

TABLE 4.3

AACN's (2008a, 2009) Identification of Cultural Care Competencies for Nurses by Educational Preparation

Baccalaureate Prepared Nurses	Master's and Doctorally Prepared Nurses
Apply knowledge of social and cultural factors that affect nursing and healthcare across multiple contexts.	Prioritize the social and cultural factors that affect health in designing and delivering care across multiple contexts.
Use relevant data sources and best evidence in providing culturally competent care.	Construct socially and empirically derived cultural knowledge of people and populations to guide practice and research.
Promote achievement of safe and quality outcomes of care for diverse populations.	Assume leadership in developing, implementing, and evaluating culturally competent nursing and other healthcare services.
Advocate for social justice, including commitment to the health of vulnerable populations and the elimination of health disparities.	Transform systems to address social justice and health disparities. Provide leadership to educators and members of the healthcare or research team in learning, applying, and evaluating continuous cultural competence development.
Participate in continuous cultural competence development.	Conduct culturally competent scholarship that can be utilized in practice.

Sources: American Association of Colleges of Nursing. (2008). *Cultural competency in baccalaureate nursing education.* Retrieved from http://www.aacn.nche.edu/education/pdf/competency.pdf; American Association of Colleges of Nursing. (2009). *Establishing a culturally competent master's and doctorally prepared nursing workforce.* Retrieved from http://www.aacn.nche.edu/Education/pdf/CulturalComp.pdf

includes the "hot/cold" theory of disease causation and treatment—which holds that imbalance of the four body humors of yellow and black bile, phlegm, and blood resulting in a "hot" infectious condition must be treated with appropriate foods or herbs—we may ignore or patronize the patient. Many scientific minds reject this theory, creating conflict and failure to provide healthcare. As Benner and Wrubel (1989) observe, "changes in lifestyles and health habits work best when they are integrated into the person's own cultural patterns and traditions [for] it is hard to sustain new patterns if they go against the grain of one's normal social patterns" (p. 155).

Models of Cultural Care and Competence in Practice

The movement for culturally competent care is an imperative for practice in the health professions. Although many models have been designed to assist practitioners, the following selected models are useful in nursing practice. To explore additional models of culturally competent care, see the Bibliography at the end of this chapter.

Culture Care Diversity and Universality

Madeleine Leininger proposed a transcultural nursing theory with the central focus on care, especially the concept of *culture care.* Leininger's (1970) early definition of *culture* referred to a way of "life belonging" to a designated group, through accumulated traditions, customs, and the

ways the group solves problems that are learned and transmitted systematically, largely through socialization practices that are reinforced through social and cultural institutions (pp. 48–49). Within her culture care theory, Leininger (2002c) defined culture as "patterned lifeways, values, beliefs, norms, symbols, and practices of individuals, groups, or institutions that are learned, shared, and usually transmitted intergenerationally over time" (p. 83). Taking this one step further as a health belief, Leininger (2002c) defined *cultural care* as "the synthesized and culturally constituted assistive, supportive, and facilitative caring acts toward self or others focused on evident or anticipated needs for the patient's health or well-being or to face disabilities, death or other human conditions" (p. 83). To this end, she states that "the purpose of theory of Culture Care was to discover, document, know and explain the interdependence of care and culture phenomena with differences and similarities between and among cultures" (Leininger & McFarland, 2006, p. 4).

On the basis of in-depth qualitative research, Leininger has identified dominant cultural values and culture care meanings and action modes for many different American subculture groups, showing differences with the Anglo-American healthcare value structure. She defines *subcultures* as "small or large groups living in a dominant culture that retain certain values and beliefs that are different from the dominant culture" (Leininger, 2002a, p. 122). The Anglo-American cultural values include individualism, independence and freedom, competition and achievement, materialism, technology, instant time and actions, youth and beauty, equal rights (gender), leisure time, scientific facts and numbers, and a sense of generosity in time of crisis; action modes include stress alleviation, personalized acts, self-reliance, and health instruction. These characteristics are consistent with the prevailing culture of the practitioners and organizations that make up the healthcare system. In her book *Culture Care Diversity and Universality: A Theory of Nursing*, Leininger lists information on a sample of some American subgroups (Leininger, 1991a, p. 355). She has identified further special groups as subgroups, such as the homeless, drug users, homosexual individuals, the deaf, those infected with HIV, and nurses. Valencia-Go (2006) supports the identification of these subgroups as *emerging populations* in healthcare to include ethnic minorities, the homeless, and those afflicted with AIDS (p. 24).

Difficulties arise when significant values are unknown, in conflict, or poorly understood. The patient's cultural values can be quite different from those of the healthcare provider. As Leininger (1991a) details in her book, of the 15 sample subgroups presented, 10 share none of the dominant characteristics of healthcare systems and Anglo-American patients, and few characteristics are shared by the remaining subgroups. In addition, consider the importance of religious or dominant spiritual influence in all but three of the cultural subgroups she described. Knowledge of the dominant values can assist in providing health promotion or health maintenance information, activities, and programs. An example can be seen with the increasing importance of the use of faith communities in health promotion activities. Leininger (1994) stresses that nurses as primary, secondary, and tertiary care providers, through their close and continuous contact with culturally diverse patients, must move from unicultural personal and professional knowledge to provide meaningful culturally based nursing care (p. 255). Time, openness, and a growing understanding are critical components of a clinician's development of higher levels of cultural competence.

The Giger and Davidhizar Transcultural Assessment Model

Another nursing model directed at the importance of culture and care focuses on the assessment process. Giger and Davidhizar have identified a variety of cultural behavior patterns relevant to health assessment that have an influence on the delivery of care. They define culture as "a patterned behavioral response that develops over time as a result of imprinting the mind through social and religious structures and intellectual and artistic manifestations" (Giger & Davidhizar, 2008, p. 2). Their assessment model has been used in a variety of research and clinical practice settings and includes the concepts listed in Box 4.2. Cultures of origin, subcultures, and acculturalization are important considerations in this assessment model.

Notice that in this assessment model, the focus is on the *culturally unique individual*. The initial area for assessment is on individual characteristics, including the individual's definition of culture. The next assessment areas

| BOX 4.2 | Patterns for Assessment in the Giger & Davidhizar (2008) Transcultural Assessment Model |

Culturally unique individual factors
● Communication
● Space
● Social orientation
● Time
● Environmental control
● Biologic variations
● Nursing assessment

Source: J. N. Giger & R. E. Davidhizar (2008). *Transcultural Nursing: Assessment and Intervention* (5th ed.). Philadelphia: Mosby.

include specifics on communication patterns and use of space, which reveal cultural differences but also have a profound influence on interactions and acceptability of information sharing. Social organization is designed to obtain information on current health status as well as family, work, social, political and religious affiliations, practices, and preferences. Assessment of time consideration also looks at cultural patterns, practices, and preferences. Environmental control focuses on the individual's perception of locus of control (internal versus external as with the magico-religious paradigm), values and supernatural influences, and their description of their environment and their concept of health. The area of biological variations includes a complete physical examination with particular attention to cultural/sociocultural, physical, metabolic, and genetic variations. The nursing assessment focuses on clinical judgment of the individual and summarizes the assessment data for incorporation into the plan of care. Although identified in their assessment model as nursing assessment, applications have been extended to other health professions. As reported by Giger and Davidhizar (2008), application of the model in diverse settings is producing a means for clinical understanding and application of culturally competent care across disciplines (p. 16).

Spector's Health Traditions Model

Spector (2013) views a person as a unique cultural being, having personal health traditions and being affected by cultural phenomena. Her model for the individual is an oval with the outer band containing the concepts of communication, space, time, biological variations, environmental control and social organization, and with the middle band containing the concepts of culture, religion, and ethnicity. At the center of the model is the person as a unique being with personal health traditions. Using the concept of holistic health, health traditions are explored as a model for these unique individuals, as what people do in order to maintain, protect, and restore health from the perspective of their traditions (Spector, 2013, p. 92). This Health Traditions model is designed as a matrix with health maintenance, protection, and restoration on the vertical axis, which interrelate with three holistic concepts (physical, mental, and spiritual) on the horizontal axis.

Health maintenance concepts involve basic physical, mental, and spiritual needs. Health protection includes special foods, activities, customs, and religious practices or rituals. Restoration activities include holistic remedies for the body, mind, and spirit. Culture, heritage, and health traditions are important foci for this view of culture and the development of cultural awareness. Spector (2013) provides a heritage assessment tool to understand a person's traditional health and illness beliefs and practices, and to determine appropriate community care resources (pp. 376–378).

The Purnell Model for Cultural Competence

Purnell (2013) describes the need for self-awareness in cultural competence as a deliberative and emotional process of getting to know yourself (personality, values, beliefs, standards, ethics, etc.) and the impact of these factors when interacting with others different from yourself (p. 45). The Purnell model is an organizing framework, designed as a wheel with four rims representing the society, community, family, and the person, and spokes as 12 wedges representing interconnected cultural constructs or domains, to the unknown dark core at the center (Fig. 4.3). Purnell provides assessment questions for each of the 12 domains of culture, addressing the concepts under the various and interrelated domains. Purnell (2013) further describes the jagged line at the bottom of the model under the wheel representing "the concept of cultural consciousness," from left to right, as the unconsciously incompetent to the unconsciously competent practitioner (pp. 16–17). The development of cultural competence is implicit, as noted in one of 20 assumptions upon which the model is based: "to be effective, health care must reflect the unique understanding of the values, beliefs, attitudes, lifeways, and worldview of diverse populations and individual acculturation patterns" (Purnell, 2013, p. 15).

Purnell's model emphasizes human beings, health, and the environment; however, the model is not restricted to nursing and is applicable across disciplines. Information provided in the model is designed to understand holistically human beings with health issues within the various broad constructs.

What each of the models seems to have in common is a directive to actively seek to understand the uniqueness of human beings in their context, as cultural competence. And in doing this, care for individuals, families, and groups will result in more positive outcomes. They also point to the fact, however, that individuals within a selected culture are very different. As we seek to understand different cultures and heritages, we must still focus on human beings. Consider the results of a research study to validate an instrument used with hospitalized patients on advance directives. The researchers found that the instrument was valid, in both the English and Spanish versions. But differences were also found in the preferences, in that the Hispanic adult participants had less knowledge of advance directives and a higher preference for life-support interventions. Froman and Owen (2003) were able to support the validity of the instrument but did recommend

further study to address the "great diversity among Hispanic regions and culture" (p. 36).

Further, consider the following variables for culturally competent care:

- Time with patients to become accepted and gain an understanding of their belief system
- Differences in belief systems among generations and geographic origin
- Past experiences and current situation
- Religious influences
- Familial influences
- Understanding of advance directives
- Acceptance of the healthcare services, systems, and practitioners
- Linguistic issues

Other individual values may not be initially apparent or may grow more dominant. Complementary and alternative medicine (CAM) and healthcare practices, such as acupuncture, imagery, and herbal medicines, are being used as people become dissatisfied with the biomedical view and move to holistic care. These practices may differ from an individual's inherited cultural background but may be adopted or become more dominant. In addition, they may be used along with (complementary) or instead of (alternative) conventional medicine, and their use may or may not be reported by the patient to the healthcare provider. Spector (2013) reports the rapidly growing use of homeopathic healthcare choices as alternative or complementary (e.g., aromatherapy, biofeedback, hypnotherapy, massage) and ethnocultural or traditional (e.g., herbs and holistic healing practices and rituals). And the research and body of knowledge on many of these practices is growing. A review of current literature reveals a wide range of research studies reporting on the use of CAM in a variety of patient populations, from children, to normal childbearing families, to patients with medical diagnoses including breast and prostate cancer. The increase in use and acceptance of CAM points to the need for a comprehensive cultural assessment with the patient and may require of the clinician great openness, sensitivity, and time.

THE NURSE'S ROLE

Nurses have a primary responsibility in health promotion, health maintenance, and prevention activities; in fact, such activities represent the essence of professional nursing practice. The focus of nursing is on the health of the

---

ONLINE CONSULT

Office of Minority Health & Health Disparities (OMHD) at
http://www.cdc.gov/diversity/faqs/diversity.htm

National Center for Complementary and Alternative Medicine at
http://nccam.nih.gov

Transcultural Nursing at
http://www.culturediversity.org/ index.html

The Purnell Model for Cultural Competence

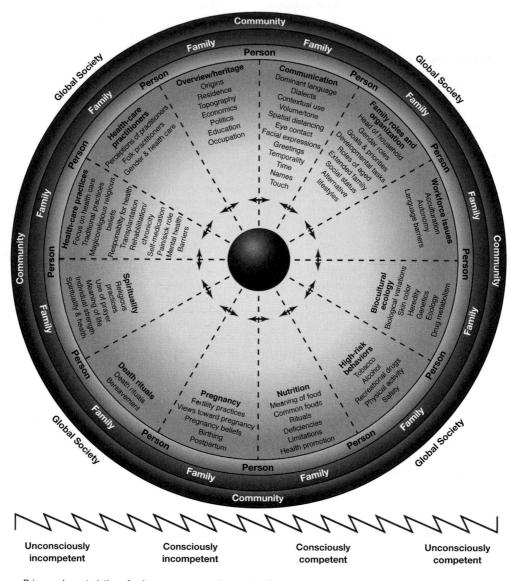

Primary characteristics of culture: age, generation, nationality, race, color, gender, religion

Secondary characteristics of culture: educational status, socioeconomic status, occupation, military status, political beliefs, urban versus rural residence, enclave identity, marital status, parental status, physical characteristics, sexual orientation, gender issues, and reason for migration (sojourner, immigrant, undocumented status)

Unconsciously incompetent: not being aware that one is lacking knowledge about another culture
Consciously incompetent: being aware that one is lacking knowledge about another culture
Consciously competent: learning about the client's culture, verifying generalizations about the client's culture, and providing culturally specific interventions
Unconsciously competent: automatically providing culturally congruent care to clients of diverse cultures

Figure 4.3 The Purnell Model for Cultural Competence. *Source: Purnell, L. (2013). Transcultural health care: A culturally competent approach (4th ed.). Philadelphia: F. A. Davis.*

individual, family, community, and societal group. Health promotion roles are guided within the theoretical framework on which nursing practice is based, including how you, as the professional, view the human beings, the concept of health, the environment, and the practice of nursing as well as your accord with a model's definitions and relationships. This is the purpose of the middle-range theories discussed in Chapter 3, from which you can move to a practice model that is applicable to your specific function or practice setting. Before you decide on the best framework to guide your own professional practice, consider the following two examples.

Example 1

Suppose your practice is guided by King's Theory of Goal Attainment. In this theory, nursing is defined as "a process of human interactions between nurse and patient whereby each perceives the other and the situation, and through communications, they set goals, explore the means to achieve them, agree to the means, [and] their actions indicate movement toward goal achievement" (King, 1987, p. 113). Health promotion, health maintenance, and prevention activities are all implied in this definition of *health* as adjustment to stressors in the system environments and use of resources. Health is viewed as a potential and the goal of the process.

Specific assessment and intervention activities must address the theory's theoretical concepts and propositions. Selected health and illness models can be used to guide practice. Personal perceptions of the patient are important components of the Health Belief Model, Pender's Health Promotion Model, and the Chronic Illness Trajectory Framework. If your practice setting is a clinic with a large population that needs health promotion strategies addressing individual lifestyles and the preventive services identified in *Healthy People 2020*, you may find the health belief model or Pender's Health Promotion Model quite useful

with your patients. These same models can address health maintenance as secondary and tertiary prevention. On the other hand, if your practice setting is a hospice or you work primarily with patients with cancer and their families, you may find the chronic illness trajectory framework more useful for guiding your practice and use of the nursing process.

Example 2

If your practice is guided by Leininger's Culture Care Diversity and Universality model, three modes of cultural care guide your nursing judgment, decisions, and actions: preservation and maintenance, accommodation and negotiation, and repatterning or restructuring (Leininger, 1991b, 2002c; Leininger & McFarland, 2006). In Leininger's concept of culturally congruent nursing care, these modes all focus on health promotion, health maintenance, and prevention activities within the context of the individual cultural belief system. Leininger defines culturally *congruent nursing care* as the specific use of "culturally based care, knowledge, acts and decisions in sensitive and knowledgeable ways to appropriately and meaningfully fit the cultural values, beliefs, and lifeways of human beings for their health and wellbeing, or to prevent illness, disabilities, or death" (Leininger & McFarland, 2006, p. 15). The practice models and assessment tools you select must be culturally sensitive and must include individual focus on each of the assessment factors in the Sunrise Enabler, which is used to depict the dimensions of her theory visually (Leininger, 1991b, 2002c; Leininger & McFarland, 2006).

Selecting a health model involves a deliberate and reflective process that takes into account your views, the theory that guides your professional practice, and the unique characteristics of the people and environment in which you work. You may practice under several similar models, depending on a changeable environment or consumer group interactions.

KEY POINTS

● Health promotion and health protection strategies relate to individual lifestyle and environmental influences on health status and health prospects. Preventive activities and services address three areas of prevention. Primary prevention consists of healthy actions taken to avoid illness or disease. Secondary prevention involves screening for early detection and treatment of health problems. Tertiary prevention during the rehabilitative phase of an illness prevents complications and further disability.

● Health is more than the absence of illness, disease, or infirmity. A concept of health is determined by one's worldview and philosophical assumptions.

● Benner and Wrubel (1989) describe five theories of health as (1) an ideal, (2) the ability to fulfill social roles, (3) a commodity, (4) a human potential, and (5) a sense of coherence.

● Dunn's (1973) high-level wellness emphasizes well-being, including the positive, dynamic, and unique integration of the mind, body, and spirit of the individual functioning within the environment and at the maximum potential.

● The health belief model (Becker et al., 1977) was designed as an organizing framework to advance health promotion activities by targeting interventions to certain individual variables. Three major concepts explain and predict health-related behaviors: (1) readiness to undertake recommended compliance behavior, (2) modifying and enabling factors, and (3) compliant behaviors.

Continued

KEY POINTS—cont'd

- Pender's health promotion model is a schematic representation with three components for health-promoting behaviors. Individual characteristics and experiences include prior related behavior and personal factors (biologic, psychological, and sociocultural factors). Behavior-specific cognitions and affect include perceived benefits, perceived barriers, perceived self-efficacy, activity-related affect interpersonal influences, and situational influences. The behavioral outcome is attainment of a positive health outcome through commitment to the plan of action and competing demands and preferences.

- The chronic illness trajectory framework (Corbin & Strauss, 1992a) is a conceptual model organized under the main concept of trajectory for managing an evolving course of a chronic condition.

- Gordon's (2008) 11 functional health patterns can be used as a valuable tool in the nursing assessment and diagnosis process and in the application of models to address health and illness focused on human potential or a sense of coherence.

- Holistic nursing is described as "focus[ing] on protecting, promoting, and optimizing health and wellness; assisting healing; preventing illness and injury; alleviating suffering; supporting people to find peace, comfort, harmony, and balance through the diagnosis and treatment of human response; and advocacy in the care of individuals, families, communities, populations, and the planet" (AHNA & ANA, 2013, p. 1).

- Culture involves a combination of social, familial, religious, national, and professional characteristics that affect the way we think, act, and interact with others. Differences among groups and subgroups produce diversity that can lead from uniculturalism to appreciation of a multicultural environment and healthcare behaviors.

- Leininger defines culturally congruent nursing care as "culturally based care, knowledge, acts and decisions in sensitive and knowledgeable ways to appropriately and meaningfully fit the cultural values, beliefs, and lifeways of human beings for their health and wellbeing, or to prevent illness, disabilities, or death" (Leininger & McFarland, 2006, p. 15).

- The Giger and Davidhizar Transcultural Assessment Model (2008), directed at the importance of culture and care focuses on the assessment process and patterns of culturally unique individual factors, communication, space, social orientation, time, environmental control, biological variations, and nursing assessment.

- Using the same concepts of communication, space, time, biological variations, and social orientation, Spector (2013) views a person as a unique cultural being with personal health traditions and considers how he or she is affected by cultural phenomena.

- The Purnell Model for Cultural Competence (2013) is an organizing framework, designed as a wheel with four rims representing the society, community, family, and the person, and spokes as 12 wedges representing cultural constructs, to the unknown dark core at the center.

- Complementary and alternative medicine (CAM) and healthcare practices are being tried as people become dissatisfied with the biomedical view and move to holistic care.

- Nursing focuses on the health of the individual, family, community, and societal group. Health promotion roles are guided by the theoretical framework on which practice is based.

Thought and Discussion Questions

1. Select a definition provided for health from the nursing theories presented in Chapter 3. Discuss which of the five models of health they fit into, and suggest health promotion models for each.

2. Use Pender's health promotion model to plan a health promotion campaign for one of the following situations:
   - Immunization program in an urban apartment complex with a high density of families with young children
   - Home safety program at a senior citizens' center
   - Wellness program for employees in a manufacturing company

3. Recall a patient with a chronic illness for whom you have provided nursing care in the past. Retrospectively apply the chronic illness trajectory framework to the patient experiences that you were able to observe.

4. Think of an example from your experience of a patient from a different culture with different perceptions of health, illness, or treatment from your own. How did you or could you alter your approach to the patient?

5. Review the Chapter Thought located on the first page of the chapter, and discuss it in the context of the contents of the chapter.

Interactive Exercises

Go to the Intranet site and complete the interactive exercises provided for this chapter.

REFERENCES

American Association of Colleges of Nursing (AACN). (2006). *The essentials of doctoral education for advanced nursing practice.* Retrieved from http://www.aacn.nche.edu/ DNP/pdf/Essentials.pdf

American Association of Colleges of Nursing (AACN). (2008a). *Cultural competency in baccalaureate nursing education.* Retrieved from http://www.aacn.nche.edu/ leading-initiatives/ education-resources/competency.pdf

American Association of Colleges of Nursing (AACN). (2008b). *The essentials of baccalaureate education for professional nursing practice.* Retrieved from http://www.aacn.nche.edu/ Education/pdf/BaccEssentials08.pdf

American Association of Colleges of Nursing (AACN). (2009). *Establishing a culturally competent master's and doctorally prepared nursing workforce.* Retrieved, from http://www.aacn .nche.edu/education-resources/CulturalComp.pdf

American Holistic Nurses Association (AHNA) & American Nurses Association (ANA). (2013). *Holistic nursing: Scope and standards of practice* (2nd ed.). Silver Springs, MD: Nursebooks.org.

American Nurses Association (ANA). (2010). *Nursing: Scope and standards of practice* (2nd ed.). Silver Springs, MD: Nursebooks.org.

Andrews, H., & Roy, C. (1991). *Essentials of the Roy Adaptation Model.* Norwalk, CT: Appleton-Century-Crofts.

Andrews, M. M. (2008a). The influence of cultural and health belief systems on health care practices. In M. M. Andrews & J. S. Boyle, *Transcultural Concepts in Nursing Care* (5th ed., pp. 66–81). Philadelphia, PA: Wolters Kluwer/Lippincott Williams & Wilkins.

Andrews, M. M. (2008b). Theoretical foundations of transcultural nursing. In M. M. Andrews & J. S. Boyle, *Transcultural Concepts in Nursing Care* (5th ed., pp. 3–14). Philadelphia, PA: Wolters Kluwer/Lippincott Williams & Wilkins.

Antigoni, F., & Dimitrios, T. (2009). Nurses' attitudes towards complementary therapies. *Health Science Journal, 3,* 149–157.

Becker, M. H., Haefner, D. P., Kasl, S. V., Kirscht, J. P., Maiman, L. A., & Rosenstock, I. M. (1977). Selected psychosocial models and correlates of individual health-related behaviors. *Medical Care, 15*(5, Supplement), 27–46.

Benner, P., & Wrubel, J. (1989). *The primacy of caring: Stress and coping in health and illness.* Menlo Park, CA: Addison-Wesley.

Betancourt, J. R., Green, A. R., & Carrillo, J. E. (2002). *Cultural competence in health care: Emerging frameworks and practical approaches* (Publication No. 576). New York: The Commonwealth Fund.

Betancourt, J. R., Green, A. R., Carrillo, J. E., & Park, E. R. (2005). Cultural competence and health care disparities: Key perspectives and trends. (Publication No. 821). New York: The Commonwealth Fund.

Bucher, D. (2008). Cultural competence: scholarly nature of clinical practice of nursing. *Clinical Scholars Review, 1*(2), 110–113.

Corbin, J. M. (1998). The Corbin and Strauss chronic illness trajectory model: An update. *Scholarly Inquiry for Nursing Practice: An International Journal, 12,* 33–41.

Corbin, J. M., & Strauss, A. (1992a). A nursing model for chronic illness management based upon the trajectory framework. In P. Woog (Ed.), *The chronic illness trajectory framework: The Corbin and Strauss nursing model* (pp. 9–28). New York: Springer.

Corbin, J. M., & Strauss, A. (1992b). Commentary. In P. Woog (Ed.), *The chronic illness trajectory framework: The Corbin and Strauss nursing model* (pp. 97–102). New York: Springer.

Curry, L. C., Walker, C., Moore, P., & Hogstel, M. (2010). Validating a model of chronic illness and family caregiving. *Journal of Theory Construction & Testing, 14*(1), 10–16.

Dunn, H. L. (1973). *High-level wellness.* Arlington, VA: Beatty.

Erickson, H. L. (2007). Philosophy and theory of holism. *Nursing Clinics of North America, 42,* 139–163.

Froman, R. D., & Owen, S. V. (2003). Validation of the Spanish life support preference questionnaire (LSPQ). *Journal of Nursing Scholarship, 35*(1), 33–36.

Giger, J. N., & Davidhizar, R. E. (2008). *Transcultural nursing: Assessment and intervention* (5th ed.). St. Louis, MO: Mosby Elsevier.

Glanz, K., Rimer, B. K., & Lewis, F. M. (Eds.) (2002). *Health behavior and health education: Theory, research, and practice* (3rd. ed.). San Francisco, CA: Jossey-Bass.

Gordon, M. (2008). *Assess notes: Assessment and diagnostic reasoning.* Philadelphia, PA: F. A. Davis.

Granger, B. B., Moser, D., Harrell, J., Sandelowski, M., & Ekman, I. (2007). *Progress in cardiovascular nursing, 22*(3), 152–158.

Gunther, M. E. (2010). Martha E. Rogers: Unitary human beings. In M. R. Alligood & A. M. Tomey (Eds.), *Nursing theorists and their work* (7th ed., pp. 242–264). St. Louis, MO: Mosby/Elsevier.

Jourard, S. M. (1971). *The transparent self.* New York: Litton Educational.

King, I. M. (1981). *A theory for nursing: Systems, concepts, process*. New York: John Wiley & Sons.

King, I. M. (1987). King's theory of goal attainment. In R. R. Parse (Ed.), *Nursing science: Major paradigms, theories, and critiques* (pp. 107–113). Philadelphia, PA: W. B. Saunders.

Klimmek, R., & Wenzel, J. (2012). Adaptation of the Illness Trajectory Framework to describe the work of transitional cancer survivorship. *Oncology Nursing Forum, 39*, E499–510.

Leininger, M. (1970). *Nursing and anthropology: Two worlds to blend*. New York: John Wiley & Sons.

Leininger, M. (2002a). Culture care assessments for congruent competency practices. In M. Leininger & M. R. McFarland, *Transcultural nursing: Concepts, theories, research, and practice* (3rd ed., pp. 117–143). New York: McGraw-Hill.

Leininger, M. (2002b). Cultures and tribes of nursing, hospitals, and the medical culture. In M. Leininger & M. R. McFarland, *Transcultural nursing: Concepts, theories, research, and practice* (3rd ed., pp. 181–204). New York: McGraw- Hill.

Leininger, M. (2002c). The theory of culture care and ethnonursing research method. In M. Leininger & M. R. McFarland, *Transcultural nursing: Concepts, theories, research, and practice* (3rd ed., pp. 71–98). New York: McGraw-Hill.

Leininger, M. M. (1991a). Selected culture care findings of diverse cultures using culture care theory and ethnomethods. In M. M. Leininger (Ed.), *Culture care diversity and universality: A theory of nursing* (Pub. No. 15–2402, pp. 345–371). New York: National League for Nursing.

Leininger, M. M. (1991b). The theory of culture care diversity and universality. In M. M. Leininger (Ed.), *Culture care diversity and universality: A theory of nursing* (Pub. No. 15–2402, pp. 5–68). New York: National League for Nursing.

Leininger, M. M. (1994). Transcultural nursing education: A worldwide imperative. *Nursing and Health Care, 15*, 254–257.

Leininger, M. M., & McFarland, M. R. (2006). *Culture care diversity and universality: A worldwide nursing theory* (2nd ed.). Boston, MA: Jones and Bartlett.

McEvoy, P., & Barnes, P. (2007). Using the chronic care model to tackle depression among older adults who have long-term physical conditions. *Journal of Psychiatric and Mental Health Nursing, 14*, 233–238.

Newman, M. A. (2008). *Transforming presence: The difference that nursing makes*. Philadelphia, PA: F.A. Davis.

Parse, R. R. (1981). *Man-living-health: A theory of nursing*. New York: John Wiley & Sons.

Pender, N. J. (1987). *Health promotion in nursing practice* (2nd ed.). Norwalk, CT: Appleton & Lange.

Pender, N. J. (1996). *Health promotion in nursing practice* (3rd ed.). Stamford, CT: Appleton & Lange.

Pender, N. J., Murdaugh, C. L., and Parsons, M. A. (2002). *Health promotion in nursing practice* (4th ed.). Upper Saddle River, NJ: Pearson Prentice Hall.

Pender, N. J., Murdaugh, C. L., and Parsons, M. A. (2006). *Health promotion in nursing practice* (5th ed.). Upper Saddle River, NJ: Pearson Prentice Hall.

Pender, N. J., Murdaugh, C. L., and Parsons, M. A. (2011). *Health promotion in nursing practice* (6th ed.). Upper Saddle River, NJ: Pearson Prentice Hall.

Purnell, L. (2013). *Transcultural health care: A culturally competent approach* (4th ed.). Philadelphia, PA: F.A. Davis.

Ray, M. A. (2010). *Transcultural caring dynamics in nursing and health care*. Philadelphia, PA: F. A. Davis.

Spector, R. E. (2013). *Cultural diversity in health and illness* (8th ed.). Upper Saddle River, NJ: Pearson.

Strauss, A. L., Corbin, J., Fagerhaugh, S., Glaser, B. G., Maines, D., Suczek, B., & Wiener, C. L. (1984). *Chronic illness and the quality of life* (2nd ed.). St. Louis, MO: C. V. Mosby.

Strauss, A. L., & Glaser, B. G. (1975). *Chronic illness and the quality of life*. St. Louis, MO: C. V. Mosby.

U.S. Department of Health and Human Services (USDHHS). (2010). *Healthy People 2020*. Retrieved from http://www.healthypeople.gov/2020/about/default.aspx

U.S. Department of Health and Human Services, Public Health Service (USDHHS, PHS). (1992). *Healthy People 2000: Summary Report*. Boston, MA: Jones & Bartlett.

Valencia-Go, G. (2006). Emerging populations and health. In C. L. Edlman & C. L. Mandle (Eds.), *Health promotion throughout the lifespan* (6th ed., pp. 23–49). St. Louis, MO: Mosby.

Weinert, C., Cudney, S., & Spring, A. (2008). Evolution of a conceptual model for adaptation to chronic illness. *Journal of Nursing Scholarship, 40*, 364–372.

Zborowsky, T, & Kreitzer, M. J. (2009). People, place, and process: The role of place in creating optimal healing environments. *Creative Nursing, 15*, 186–190.

BIBLIOGRAPHY

Burton, C. R. (2000). Rethinking stroke rehabilitation: The Corbin and Strauss chronic illness trajectory framework. *Journal of Advanced Nursing, 32*, 595–602.

Campinha-Bacote, J. (2003). *The process of cultural competence in the delivery of healthcare services: A culturally competent model of care* (4th. ed.). Cincinnati, OH: Transcultural C.A.R.E. Associates.

Erickson, H. L., Erickson, M. E., Campbell, J. A., Brekke, M. E., Sandor, M. K. (2012). Validation of holistic nursing competencies: Role-delineation study, 2012. *Journal of Holistic Nursing, 31*, 291–302.

Fontaine, K. L. (2011). *Complementary and alternative therapies for nursing practice* (3rd ed.). Upper Saddle River, NJ: Prentice Hall.

Halcomb, E., & Davidson, P. (2005). Using the illness trajectory framework to describe recovery from traumatic injury. *Contemporary Nurse: A Journal for the Australian Nursing Profession, 19*(1–2), 232–241.

Lubkin, I. M., & Larsen, P. D. (1998). *Chronic illness: Impact and interventions* (4th ed.). Sudbury, MA: Jones and Bartlett.

Purnell, L. (2005). The Purnell model for cultural competence. *Journal of Multicultural Nursing & Health, 11*(2), 7–15.

ONLINE RESOURCES

Agency for Healthcare Research and Quality
http://www.ahrq.gov

The Commonwealth Fund at
http://www.cmwf.org

Healthy People
http://www.healthypeople.gov

Office of Minority Health & Health Disparities
http://www.cdc.gov/minorityhealth/OMHHE.html

National Center for Complementary and Alternative Medicine
http://nccam.nih.gov

National Center for Cultural Competence
http://nccc.georgetown.edu/index.html

Office of Disease Prevention and Health Promotion
http://odphp.osophs.dhhs.gov

Transcultural C.A.R.E. Associates
http://www.transculturalcare.net

U.S. Department of Health & Human Services
http://www.hhs.gov

● Rose Kearney-Nunnery

5

Evidence-Based Practice

"We may search for information, but once gained how does it become wisdom?"

Rose Kearney-Nunnery

Chapter Objectives

On completion of this chapter, the reader will be able to:

1. Explain the importance of evidence-based practice for the profession of nursing.
2. Define basic terminology used in research for application of findings in practice.
3. Describe legal and ethical considerations applicable to research with human subjects.
4. Describe different ways to participate in nursing research.
5. Analyze barriers to evidence-based practice.
6. Prepare a basic critique of a published research study.
7. Plan for the inclusion of consistent evidence-based care in the practice setting.

Key Terms

Evidence-Based Practice	Knowledge Transformation	Operational Definition
Research	Translational Research	Variables
Ethical Codes	Critique	Sampling
Basic Human Rights	Research Problem	Data Collection Procedures
Minimal Risk	Literature Review	Instruments
Empirical Research	Hypotheses	Descriptive Statistics
Qualitative Research	Research Design	Inferential Statistics

Theory guides practice, but current knowledge and practice must be based on evidence of efficacy rather than intuition, tradition, or past practice. Out of a national concern for safety initiatives in 1999 and a focus on systems issues in 2001, the national call came for changes in the education and competencies of health professionals in all disciplines in 2003. The result was the identification of the five core competencies for health professionals identified in Chapter 1. The importance of employing evidence-based practice (EBP) was described as follows:

> *The committee feels that it is critical for interdisciplinary health teams and each of the disciplines to be able to tap this evidence base effectively at the point of patient care, determining whether an intervention, such as a preventive service, diagnostic test, or therapy, can be expected to produce better outcomes than alternatives—including the alternative of doing nothing. (Greiner & Knebel, 2003, p. 56)*

Sigma Theta Tau (2005), the International Honor Society of Nursing, defines the use of **evidence-based practice** as "an integration of the best evidence available, nursing expertise, and the values and preferences of the individuals, families, and communities who are selected" (p. 1). This does not sound unique to our view of nursing and quality healthcare. The question becomes Are we *consistently using* the best evidence available to guide care to patients? And the next questions are: Do we have the best evidence available? Where is the information? And, are we applying appropriate knowledge in clinical situations?

An actual paradigm shift has occurred with the call for evidence-based practice. Traditional practices are not appropriate unless supported by current evidence of efficacy and appropriateness for the patient. As will be discussed in subsequent chapters, Magnet Recognition also supports the use of evidence-based practice for enhanced outcomes for both patients and nurses (American Nurses Credentialing Center [ANCC], 2014):

> *A robust quality program with clinical decisions based on solid evidence translates into better patient outcomes. (p. 1)*

Research supports our knowledge base and answers questions of clinical concern. It provides sound information on which to base practice, as evidence-based nursing practice. Porter-O'Grady (2006) describes evidence-based practice as requiring "a degree of flexibility and fluidity based on firm scientific and clinical evidence validating appropriate and sustainable clinical practice" (p. 3). Evidence can come from a number of sources, but we need both seekers and users of the information in practice to develop and enhance knowledge. Clinicians in the practice setting have the questions. These questions must be refined and studied so that nurse researchers can find solutions to healthcare practice problems. And we need further validation from the consumer as to the appropriateness of the intervention. This is truly evidence-based practice.

THE EVOLUTION OF NURSING RESEARCH

Research has been defined as a "systematic, controlled, empirical, amoral, public, and critical investigation of natural phenomena guided by theory and hypotheses about the presumed relations among such phenomena" (Kerlinger & Lee, 2000, p. 14). Given this definition, research is still viewed by some as an academic exercise. But it is much more in nursing. The purposes of research are to describe, explain, predict, and control phenomena and to provide information for future use in practice or for expansion of the knowledge base. Specific to the discipline, the National Institute of Nursing Research (NINR, 2012) defines nursing research as the development of knowledge to (1) build the scientific foundation for clinical practice, (2) prevent disease and disability, (3) manage and eliminate symptoms caused by illness, and (4) enhance end-of-life and palliative care (p. 1).

Nursing research began with Florence Nightingale and her identification of environmental influences on health and illness. In her classic *Notes on Nursing: What It Is, and What It Is Not* (1859), Nightingale identified factors that influence health and wellness, supporting them with observational accounts, statistics, and deductive reasoning. Following her landmark efforts, non-nurse researchers performed limited research on nurses and nursing education. Then, in the mid-20th century, graduate nursing programs began to proliferate, as did nurses' involvement in research studies, often on nurses and delivery of nursing services. The introduction of the journal *Nursing Research* in 1952 provided a specific channel for disseminating research findings to other nurses.

During the second half of the 20th century, the number of graduate and baccalaureate nursing programs grew. Content on research became prevalent in baccalaureate nursing curricula during the 1970s and early 1980s. Graduate student enrollments increased with the growth in doctoral programs in the 1980s. Research findings were used to develop and refine conceptual and theoretical models. More nurses were now doing research, and the American Nurses Association (ANA) Cabinet on Nursing Research identified research expectations by level of education in 1981. The primary focus of research changed during this time from educational programs and methods to the focus of nursing: people as patients, consumers, and members of society. Support has grown for research as we see the needs to investigate the domain of nursing, test theories and interventions, and demonstrate efficacy and efficiency of nursing actions and patient outcomes. And now, with our emphasis on evidence-based practice, we need more than isolated studies. We depend on an evolving body of knowledge of efficacy for positive patient outcomes.

Nursing research was supported in a position statement of the American Association of Colleges of Nursing (AACN) that has gone through revisions as our body of knowledge has developed—as have our professionals with additional knowledge and education with the development of the generalist nurse prepared at master's level and the nurse with a practice doctorate. AACN has identified research expectations and competencies of graduates from baccalaureate through postdoctoral programs, moving from evaluation and utilization of research to generating new knowledge with advanced preparation (AACN, 2006a, p. 5). This progression has implications for the baccalaureate-prepared nurse in the identification of research problems, the support of ongoing research, the use of applicable findings in practice, and the expansion of the knowledge base following preparation at the graduate level. For example, at the baccalaureate level, AACN (2008) describes the scholarship needed for evidence-based practice as "grounded in the translation of current evidence into one's practice" (p. 4). Nursing programs are required to have content and practice in place in the baccalaureate curriculum with demonstration of these outcomes in students and graduates. And baccalaureate graduates are expected to demonstrate further evolution and skill in professional practice. In comparison, for the practice doctorate, AACN (2006b) illustrates additional skill where "the scholarship of application expands the realm of knowledge beyond mere discovery and . . . through its position where the sciences, human caring, and human needs meet and new understandings emerge" (p. 11).

The Growing Significance of Nursing Research

The establishment of the National Center for Nursing Research (NCNR) as part of the National Institutes of Health (NIH) in April 1986, under the Health Research Extension Act of 1985 (PL99–158), demonstrated the importance of research for and by the profession. In 1993, the National Institute of Nursing Research (NINR) was established, a change from the former divisional and center status, with fiscal year appropriations from Congress growing, thus further demonstrating the importance of generating knowledge in nursing. An important component of the mission of the NINR is to "promote and improve the health of individuals, families, communities, and populations [through] . . . clinical and basic research and research training on health and illness across the lifespan to build the scientific foundation for clinical practice, prevent disease and disability, manage and eliminate symptoms caused by illness, and improve palliative and end-of-life care" (NINR, 2013, p. 1). Extramural research programs for the NINR concern promoting health and preventing disease, improving quality of life, and addressing health disparities, end-of-life issues, and quality care. Research proposals are highly competitive at NINR, as with other areas of NIH. Research proposals are reviewed by a panel of experts and scored according to the consistency with the mission of NINR and the merit of the research project. During the initial phase of NINR initiatives, research priorities were specified for investigations. In 2004, the NINR issued research opportunities to focus on chronic illnesses or conditions, behavioral changes and interventions, and response to compelling health concerns. Important information is evolving with results presented to Congress and other audiences. Reports on these projects are available and are making a difference, as are the continued federal appropriations that are committed to the NINR. Scientific topics continue to be identified as areas of research emphasis and ongoing interests.

A vital issue is the need for reliable and valid research on questions of clinical concern for decision making and change in practice. In nursing, research must be directed at interventions over which nursing has control so that the knowledge developed can lead to needed change. This direction at nursing practice issues is also relevant in collaborative projects that address multiple disciplines. This focus on practice is the essence of evidence-based practice.

For some time, Sigma Theta Tau has recognized the importance of generating and using research. The purposes of this honor society include encouraging scholarly and creative work. This purpose is applicable to both the conduct and utilization of research for evidence-based practice. Scholarship involves discovery, integration, application, and teaching. Utilizing and communicating research in nursing practice projects and conferences have been foci of Sigma Theta Tau International. The organization also supports research investigations that generate nursing knowledge through competitive extramural grants for researchers, as does the American Nurses Foundation. Nurses have a major responsibility to identify research problems, support ongoing research, and use applicable findings in practice, along with continuing to learn in this area of scholarly nursing practice.

LEGAL AND ETHICAL CONSIDERATIONS IN RESEARCH

An essential responsibility in professional nursing practice is protecting the rights of research subjects. The rights of people in research have been of great concern to ethicists, legislators, and professionals, leading to ethical codes and guidelines for the protection of research subjects. History has provided much of the impetus for our professional codes and federal regulations. During World War II, experiments noted for the unethical treatment of subjects included the Nazi medical experiments and the Japanese concentration camp experiments on human subjects. As a result, international **ethical codes** evolved. In 1949, the Nuremberg Code set standards for involving human subjects in research, with guidelines for consent, protections, risks and benefits, and qualifications of researchers. For example, true informed and voluntary consent became an essential requirement. The Declaration of Helsinki (1990), formalized in 1964 and revised in 1975 and 1989, provided guidelines on therapeutic and nontherapeutic research, along with the requirements for

ONLINE CONSULT

American Nurses Foundation: Nursing Grant Scholars at
http://anfonline.org/Doc-Vault/Programs/NursingResearchGrant

Federal Opportunities for Research Funding at
http://www.grants.gov

National Institute of Nursing Research at
http://ninr.nih.gov

Sigma Theta Tau International: Research Grant Opportunities at
http://www.nursingsociety.org/Research/Pages/default.aspx

disclosing the risks and potential benefits of the research and obtaining written consent for participation from research subjects.

Safety, Health, and Welfare

In the United States, the Tuskegee syphilis study, the Jewish Chronic Disease Hospital study, and the Willowbrook hepatitis study are further examples of unethical treatment of research subjects (Box 5.1). In the quest for knowledge, researchers failed to consider the basic human rights of their subjects, especially the right of informed consent and considerations for vulnerable populations. Federal regulations evolved from the original guidelines of the former Department of Health, Education, and Welfare, culminating in the National Research Act in 1974. This law specified the composition and authority of institutional review boards (IRBs). IRBs are now mandated as oversight bodies to ensure protection of research subjects, especially for research projects seeking federal funding.

The Belmont Report was the outcome of a National Commission for the Protection of Human Subjects of Biomedical and Behavioral Research assembled by the National Research Act. This commission was charged with identifying principles and developing guidelines. The report specified boundaries between practice and research. Basic ethical principles were reinforced, highlighting respect for persons and defining the principles of beneficence (doing no harm, with maximum benefits and minimal risks) and justice (fairness relative to one's share, need, effort, contribution, and merit). Specific applications that resulted from the Belmont Report (1979) were (1) guidelines on informed consent, including provision of information and ensuring comprehension and voluntariness, (2) assessment of risks and benefits, and (3) selection of subjects. The Belmont Report provided the basis for federal laws.

All activities involving humans as subjects must provide for the safety, health, and welfare of every individual. Subjects do not abdicate rights with their participation in a research study. Four **basic human rights** must be ensured for research subjects. These principles speak to ethical considerations and human rights:

1. Beneficence ("Do no harm")
2. Full disclosure
3. Self-determination
4. Privacy and confidentiality

The "do no harm" concept includes careful consideration of the risk-benefit ratio with any research project. One must keep in mind that **minimal risk** requires that "the probability and magnitude of harm or discomfort anticipated in the research are not greater in and of themselves than those ordinarily encountered in daily life or during the performance of routine physical or psychological examinations or tests" (Protection of Human Subjects, 45 CFR 46, §46.102 [i], 2009). Full disclosure of information and self-determination by potential subjects are necessary conditions for informed consent. In addition, subjects' rights to privacy and confidentiality must be ensured throughout the process. As protections for these four rights, the guidelines must be considered by researchers and their respective IRBs (Box 5.2).

The issue of privacy of personal health information (PHI) was the focus of the Health Insurance Portability and Accountability Act (HIPAA) of 1996. PHI is "individually identifiable health information transmitted by electronic

---

| BOX 5.1 | Examples of Unethical Use of Vulnerable Populations in Research |

1932–1972 Tuskegee, Alabama
Longitudinal clinical study by the Public Health Service of untreated syphilis in sharecroppers, mostly African Americans, who did not receive full disclosure, did not give informed consent, and received deceptive and ineffective treatments.

1963 Brooklyn, New York
In a short-term study, debilitated patients at the Jewish Chronic Disease Hospital, who did not have cancer, were injected with live cancer cells to study their response. This study also had partial federal funding with subjects who were indigent and did not receive full disclosure or informed consent.

1963–1966 Staten Island, New York
At Willowbrook State School, a school for the mentally retarded (intellectually disabled), healthy children were intentionally injected with the hepatitis virus to study the disease and treatment process. Parents did not receive full disclosure, and needless to say, subjects were harmed.

| BOX 5.2 | General Principles/Ethical Guidelines for Research on Human Subjects |

- Risks to the subjects are minimized.
- Risks are reasonable in relation to anticipated benefits to subjects.
- Selection of subjects is equitable.
- Informed consent is sought from each prospective subject or the legally authorized representative.
- Informed consent is appropriately documented.
- The research plan makes adequate provision for monitoring the data collected to ensure the safety of subjects.
- Adequate provisions exist to protect the privacy of subjects and maintain the confidentiality of data.
- Additional safeguards are in place to protect the rights and welfare for subjects who are vulnerable—e.g., children, prisoners, pregnant women, mentally disabled persons, or economically or educationally disadvantaged persons—because these subjects are vulnerable to coercion or undue influence.

Source: Title 45 Code of Federal Regulations Part 46 (45 CFR 46), §46.111 at http://www.hhs.gov/ohrp/humansubjects/guidance/45cfr46.html

ONLINE CONSULT

National Institutes of Health: Regulations and Ethical Guidelines, including the Belmont Report (http://www.hhs.gov/ohrp/humansubjects/guidance/belmont.html), the Declaration of Helsinki (http://www.hhs.gov/ohrp/archive/irb/irb_appendices.htm#j6), and the Nuremberg Code at **http://www.hhs.gov/ohrp/archive/irb/irb_appendices.htm#j5**

Compensating for Research Injuries: The Ethical and Legal Implications of Programs to Redress Injured Subjects, Volume 1, a report by the President's Commission for the Study of Ethical Problems in Medicine and Biomedical and Behavioral Research, Washington, DC, June 1982, at **http://www.gwu.edu/~nsarchiv/radiation/dir/mstreet/commeet/meet16/brief16/tab_b/br16b1a.txt**

American Association of Critical-Care Nurses. (2013). Ethical foundations for critical care nursing research at **http://www.aacn.org/wd/practice/docs/research/ethical-foundations-critical-care-nursing-research.pdf**

media, maintained in electronic mediator transmitted or maintained in any other form or medium" (USDHHS, 2004, p. 6). The Act's Privacy Rule establishes:

[M]inimum federal standards for protecting the privacy of individually identifiable health information. The Rule confers certain rights on individuals, including rights to access and amend their health information and to obtain a record of when and why their PHI has been shared with others for certain purposes. (USDHHS, 2004, p. 6)

For researchers, informed consent is a necessary process. HIPAA's privacy provisions require further language in the consent process, with required elements for access to and use of PHI. A privacy authorization may be incorporated into the consent form or maintained as a separate document. De-identifying PHI before revealing it to others requires the removal of specific data identifiers that could link the individual to his or her PHI. The privacy rules do allow, however, for the use of selected categories of PHI, as a "limited data set" that may be used or disclosed for purposes of research, public health, or healthcare operations without obtaining either an individual's authorization or a waiver for its use and disclosure, with the removal of 16 data identifiers and a data use agreement (USDHHS, 2004, p. 19).

As with other areas of nursing practice, legal and ethical considerations are deliberated with any research activity. These issues occur in the planning, implementation, analysis, and reporting stages for a research endeavor. In the proposal or planning stage of any research study, the researcher must consider the rights of the subjects and the ethical nature of the study. When a researcher defines the problem and purpose of the research, the significance of the problem for the body of knowledge and the ethical issues associated with the proposed investigation are vital considerations.

ONLINE CONSULT

U.S. Department of Health & Human Services: Health Information Privacy at **http://www.hhs.gov/ocr/hipaa/**

The Institutional Review Board (IRB)

Once the basic research plan is developed, an IRB must review and approve the start of the study. Strict federal guidelines for review by an IRB must be adhered to, especially in agencies seeking funding for research. Human subjects' rights of full disclosure, self-determination (informed consent), privacy and confidentiality, and safety must be ensured. The research proposal, with statements of the problem and purpose or significance, literature support, theory and definitions, specific research questions or hypotheses, design, sampling plans, and data collection and analysis methods must be approved by the IRB for use with human subjects. The researcher submits a proposal to an IRB for approval to proceed to the next steps of subject selection and data collection. During this stage of implementing the research project, the investigator must adhere to the procedures specified for data collection and analysis. The IRB performs evaluations throughout the project to ensure that subjects are not placed at risk and that the integrity and confidentiality of the data are maintained during collection, analysis, and dissemination of the findings.

ANA Guidelines

In addition to basic ethical principles and federal, state, local, and institutional regulations, in 1985 the ANA specified human rights guidelines for nurses in research. Ten years later, and with the consideration of societal and professional practice changes that had occurred, new guidelines based on nine principles were published (Silva, 1995, p. 2). These principles addressed beneficence, full disclosure, self-determination, privacy and confidentiality, and the skills of the researcher.

Each of the nine principles charged the investigator with specific responsibilities. Explanatory commentary and specific research guidelines were presented for each of the nine principles. For example, with the protection of subjects against harm, vulnerable groups were discussed, such as pregnant women, children, persons with HIV or AIDS, and the elderly. All of the principles required that professionals in a practice setting be aware of any ongoing research and its associated risks to both subjects and participants. And nurses have both the right and the responsibility to participate in research. Participation of nurses should be evident; for example, they should function as members of research teams and IRBs. Nurses also can actively participate by giving support and assistance to others involved in research for the advancement of knowledge and enhancement of professional practice within the discipline and among the various healthcare disciplines. The process of research with human subjects must be diligent and must benefit subjects and participants through the acquisition and use of new knowledge. Consult the government and your institutional Web sites for information on protections for human subjects in research.

PROCESSES OF NURSING RESEARCH

The actual research process is generally thought of as the scientific method. This can be misleading, however, when one considers the different types of research. To understand the basics of nursing research, first think about the scientific method as a systematic process for answering a question or testing a hypothesis. One problem emerges: this is done more easily in a controlled laboratory setting, with variables such as chemicals, than in a natural setting in which the variables involve people, well or ill, who need nursing interventions. With this in mind, it is easier to begin with empirical research using quantitative methods.

The Empirical Method

First, consider the steps of research. **Empirical research** is based on the strict rules of the scientific method and on the philosophical perspective of positivism. With this perspective, the focus is on an observable, measurable, and predictable world. It is guided by a controlled set of steps that one goes through to make an observation or test a hypothesis. It is a deductive and linear method consisting of the following steps:

1. Identification of the problem
2. Statement of the purpose
3. Review of the literature
4. Description of the theoretical framework
5. Definition of terms
6. Statement of the hypothesis(es)
7. Selection of the research design, population, and sample
8. IRB approval
9. Data collection
10. Data analysis and interpretation
11. Presentation of findings and recommendations

Using this empirical approach, the researcher may return to a prior step in the planning stage—for example, to refine the problem after a review of the literature—but

---

ONLINE CONSULT

Agency for Healthcare Research and Quality (AHRQ) at
http://www.ahrq.gov/

National Institutes of Health at
http://www.nih.gov/

U.S. Department of Health & Human Services at
http://www.hhs.gov

Office for Human Research Protections (OHRP) at
http://www.hhs.gov/ohrp/

---

will still go through all successive steps in a systematic and controlled manner to maintain the integrity of the process. Once the plans for the study are finalized, strict research protocols are adhered to with quantitative methods to reduce threats to the validity of the study. Although some of the steps may be combined, nurse researchers using quantitative methods engage in the same process to describe, explain, predict, and control phenomena of concern to nursing. The following is a review of the empirical research process.

In the initial step of *problem* identification, the researchers specify what they are interested in studying. This is the "what" that will be done as the study progresses. For example, a specific nursing intervention is compared with a traditional nursing intervention for a selected group of patients. Next, researchers specify the reason they are interested in this problem, or the *purpose* of the research. At this time, the significance of the problem for the body of knowledge and ethical issues associated with the proposed investigation are considerations. This is "why" the researchers want to investigate the new intervention—for example, to effectively improve the health awareness or healthy behaviors of the patient group.

The researchers next search the *literature* to discover what is known on the topics: the interventions, the patient group, cultural factors, useful theoretical bases (e.g., self-care), and what problems have been studied in the area. This provides context and the current information known on the topic. This is a time-intensive process that requires absorbing a great deal of information for the planning stage of the project. Researchers perform literature searches, followed by careful critique and assimilation of the information. Next, researchers specify the *theoretical framework*, or philosophical orientation that will guide the research. For example, the study may be guided by one of the middle-range or practice theories discussed in Chapter 3. *Definitions of terms and variables* specific to the study emerge from the theoretical framework, as do specific research questions that will be addressed or the *hypotheses* (predictions) the study will test.

So far we have the basic idea for the investigation, but the researchers must select a design or plan for the study that is appropriate for the problem in light of the theoretical framework. For example, when studying the efficacy of an intervention with two groups of patients, the researcher may use an experimental control group design. However, true experiments require manipulation of the independent variable, control of other variables, and random assignment to study groups. Often we see quasi-experimental designs in nursing—for example, the use of a nonequivalent control group—because of the nature of the intervention.

Once the appropriate *design* has been selected, the researchers must define the *population*—those individuals or groups to whom the findings will be applicable or generalizable. Researchers know that not all of the people to whom the research applies can be studied, so they must study a select group of the population; this is known as a *sample*. The researchers' decision about the type and the size of the sample is based on the research design, theoretical framework, research purpose, and research problem. It all relates back in a linear manner, but the goals in sampling are to limit bias and statistical error and for the sample to be representative of the population.

The researchers now have the basic plan for their investigations, but no one has been studied yet. The rights of human subjects must be considered and protected. At this point the researcher submits a proposal to an IRB for *approval* or exemption to proceed to the next step of data collection. Once IRB approval has been secured, the researcher is ready to begin collecting *data*.

Plans for data collection and analysis have already been made in the research proposal and are strictly adhered to. Researchers must follow the proposed design when data are collected; for example, they cannot decide to replace interviews that were planned with a questionnaire. Data must be collected in an orderly and systematic manner and must be recorded before analysis and decision making begin.

Measurement issues are of prime concern. The type of data collected and the measurement instruments are, again, determined before the study is started, on the basis of the research problem, literature review, theoretical basis, research questions or hypotheses, research design, and sampling method. Issues of reliability (consistency of measurement) and validity (proper measurement of the variable of interest) are considered by the researcher from prior methodological studies, use in similar research, or a pilot study as a small-scale version or a formal trial designed to resolve any methodological issues. Measurements may be self-reported, in writing, by the subjects in the sample (via tests, questionnaires, diaries, etc.) or may require recording or note taking by researchers in personal or telephone interviews.

Measurements can also be observations of behavior (ability to perform a skill, such as a dressing change), responses by subjects on a scale (such as a Likert scale or a scale for pain perception from 0 to 10), physiological measures (such as blood pressure, electrocardiogram, electroencephalogram, or oxygen saturation), review of records, or other types of methods. Research protocols are strictly adhered to: the identical detailed process is used with each research subject. Scripts are used to read instructions to subjects to ensure that each subject has been given the same information for the data collection process.

Once all subjects have been investigated and all data collected, the researcher moves into the *analysis* stage. The analysis provides information to answer the research questions or support or refute the hypotheses. The analysis stage seems to be the most threatening to the research novice. Keep in mind that the research depends on a good analysis of the data so that reliable, valid information is made available on the topic. The most important decisions for this stage were made before the study was started, with the selection of the correct statistical tests. In addition, computers or statisticians can easily perform calculations. Try to see this stage as one of discovery and understanding how the data provide answers to the research questions or hypotheses. The findings are reported objectively for each research question or hypothesis.

The results of the descriptive statistics (such as frequencies, means, standard deviations, correlations) are reported to characterize the sample. Appropriate inferential statistics are used to generalize to the population (such as t-test, analysis of variance, correlations, and multivariate analysis), according to the type of measurement scale, the sample size, and the assumption of a normal distribution. From the point of reporting the statistics, the researcher then *interprets* the meaning and implications relative to the stated research questions or hypotheses. Recommendations for use of the findings and further research are then presented in the research report.

Presenting the *findings and recommendations* to others is the final responsibility of the researcher as part of the particular study. The findings can be disseminated locally, regionally, nationally, and/or globally through presentations or publications. It is vital that the information be shared with others. If the findings are important and point to a need for change, practicing nurses have the opportunity and responsibility to implement the information as appropriate to their practice settings. Additional research may also be needed. If the findings were not significant or were indifferent, then further research is needed, perhaps involving further specification of the problem, better measurement instruments, or a different environment or sample. If the research findings were negative, the new intervention was less effective than current ones. Still more research may be needed if there were problems with reliability and validity. For example, if a safety issue emerged during the research, a subject would have been withdrawn from the study or the study halted. Still, it is necessary for others to know about this in order to make use of the information or avoid problem areas.

Qualitative Research

The research process using qualitative research methods is somewhat different. **Qualitative research** is used to generate theory to explore, describe, and illuminate phenomena. The basis of qualitative research focuses on the meaning and interpretation of experiences to understand some phenomena. Types of research classified as qualitative include ethnography, field studies, grounded theory, historical research, analytic induction, and phenomenology.

Major data collection methods are naturalistic observation (hence the term *field studies*) and on-site interviewing. Some researchers describe the data that emerge from this research as "information rich," because the researcher begins a study with a need to understand from the perspective of people in the environment. The researcher is not limiting the data collection to a few variables. Rather, he or she is trying to have the people in their environment describe the phenomena; the researcher then classifies concepts, identifies themes, and generates theory. This is why some also see qualitative research as a "humanistic" form of research that investigates people and their unique experiences.

In qualitative research, the linear steps of the process are not the procedure. The researcher must still complete the initial process of developing the project, with identification of a *problem* or a little-understood area or phenomena, and the statement of *purpose* as an inquiry for "discovery" of the phenomena. The review of the *literature* looks at what is known, which is often tangential, because little may be known before the research uncovers the phenomena. The *theory* will evolve from this research, rather than be driven by it, as are the *terminology* and *future study hypotheses* that use quantitative methods for theory testing. The process of IRB approval is still required prior to data collection, for the protection of human subjects.

Qualitative methods have different inquiry forms and processes. *Data collection and analysis* are driven by the particular qualitative method, as with an ethnography to describe the phenomena from the perspective of the subjects. Reliability and validity issues can be difficult with this form of research, and investigators frequently use triangulation of data to provide valid results. *Triangulation* involves the use of multiple data sources, complementary investigations, or theoretical perspectives to improve the data's validity. Dissemination of the findings through presentations and publication is the final step in the process, along with identification of future areas for inquiry.

Choice of Research Method

Whether quantitative or qualitative research methods are selected depends on the phenomena of interest and the purpose of the research. For example, one researcher may use qualitative methods to investigate the health beliefs of a particular cultural group, while another researcher would use quantitative methods to test a new intervention designed to enhance the functional independence of older adults with a limitation in mobility. Comparisons of qualitative research to the empirical research process are illustrated in Table 5.1. Regardless of the methods selected to address the need for information on the problem, the

TABLE 5.1

Empirical and Qualitative Research Methods

	Empirical Research	Qualitative Research
Identification of the problem	Narrowly specify what is to be studied.	Identify little understood area or phenomena.
Statement of the purpose	Specify the reason the problem is of interest.	Specify the inquiry for discovery of the phenomena.
Review of the literature	Discover what is already known about the problem.	Using tangential subjects, demonstrate why little is known about the phenomena.
Description of the theoretical framework	Select and apply a theory or model.	Theory will evolve from the research.
Definition of terms	Define terms and variables to be studied, consistent with the theoretical model.	Terminology will emerge from the findings.
Statement of the hypothesis(es)	Specify questions or hypotheses to be tested, consistent with the theoretical model.	Develop broad questions to be asked that will lead to others during the research as discovery.
Selection of the research design, population, and sample	Select specific design and study instruments. Specify population of interest. Identify group and number of research subjects (sample).	Select a qualitative method and a group to seek their descriptions of their human experience. Propose methods to access the group.
Approval of institutional review board	Submit and obtain approval of research proposal.	Submit and obtain approval of research proposal.
Data collection	Strictly adhere to research protocol, controls, and steps specified with the study's measurement instruments; for example, the experimental group of subjects has one intervention while the control group received the usual treatment or intervention. Systematically record data.	Gain entry to the group, propose broad questions, receive information, and seek meaning. Further questions emerge as the study progresses and are pursued in search of meaning and understanding. For example, use grounded theory to see the data falling into differing categories.
Data analysis and interpretation	Apply the statistical tests on the study variables specified in the research proposal and draw conclusions from these tests.	Create meaning and themes from information in transcripts and documents that evolve into different areas and emerge into a theoretical framework.
Presentation of findings and recommendations	Report the statistics on the questions or hypotheses as findings. Draw conclusions based on the findings and propose applications and further investigation.	Propose a theoretical framework to pursue further investigation of the categories of meaning discovered, thus adding to our theoretical bases described in Chapter 3.

research must respect the individual or group in the quest for knowledge.

THE ROAD TO EVIDENCE-BASED PRACTICE

We have a responsibility to base nursing practice on current knowledge. This responsibility highlights an accountability issue for the profession and focuses the direction of nursing research on issues for improved patient outcomes and effective care in a time when resources are stretched beyond limits. We have evolved from the landmark work for research-based nursing practice that began in the 1970s. Between 1971 and 1975, the federally funded Western Interstate Commission for Higher Education (WICHE) project focused on both the conduct of research projects and the utilization of research findings, to support collaborative research endeavors followed by a focus on using research findings in practice (Lindeman & Krueger, 1977). Between 1975 and 1981, a second federally funded project, Conduct and Utilization of Research in Nursing (CURN), focused on use in the hospital setting of the knowledge from research already available. Finding the information and the applicability to the practice setting were the skills of concern. This led to the development of guidelines and specific protocols for research-based nursing interventions and educational media to help nurses base their practice and interventions with patients on research evidence. Since the 1970s, many professional journals are now dedicated to publishing research findings, and other journals include special columns or research features. Professional conferences, both general and specialty, provide research presentations as special and concurrent offerings. A focus on research and evidence-based practice has also emerged in certification examinations.

In 1981, the ANA Cabinet for Nursing Research developed guidelines for involvement in research based on level of nursing education, as mentioned earlier in the chapter. Subsequently, professional nursing organizations have delineated expectations for nurses' involvement in research according to level of educational preparation. In these guidelines, the graduate with doctoral or postdoctoral preparation is seen as providing leadership on investigating phenomena, applying theory, and developing methods to generate knowledge for the discipline. With an expertise in specialty practice, the nurse with graduate preparation in nursing is the facilitator for using research findings and conducting investigations. Baccalaureate nursing graduates are research consumers and are responsible for identifying researchable problems and findings from prior research on which to base practice.

Nevertheless, there have been problems with disseminating findings and applying them in practice. National practice guidelines have been available since the 1990s, but studies have shown they have not been incorporated consistently in practice. However, improvements are apparent with our current focus on evidence-based practice.

Evidence-based practice is fundamental to contemporary nursing, providing a firm foundation for nursing interventions and quality improvement in healthcare. EBP has been identified as one of the core competencies for health professionals in all disciplines.

To address this core competency, the Academic Center for Evidence-Based Practice (ACE) led the way with a project to establish a national consensus on essential competences for EBP for use in education and practice (Stevens, 2005, p. 1). Competencies by educational level (undergraduate, 20; masters, 32; and docoral, 31) were identified based on the five stages of the ACE Star Model of knowledge transformation (Fig. 5.1). In 2008, 10 additional competencies were identified to address Associate Degree Nursing preparation and the need for evidence-based practice at the different educational levels (Stevens, 2009). **Knowledge transformation** is defined as "the conversion of research findings from primary research results, through a series of stages and forms, to impact on health outcomes by way of EB care" (Stevens, 2009, p. 28). As new knowledge is transformed through the five stages—discovery, evidence summary, translation, integration, and evaluation—the outcome is quality improvement of care (Stevens, 2009, pp. 28–30). Discovery is primary research, whereas the evidence summary is the available body of knowledge. As noted by Stevens (2009), the rigorous evidence summary step has moved professional practice from the old paradigm of research utilization to evidence-based care (p. 29).

When systematic reviews of research are available, more is known about the body of knowledge and the evidence is stronger for clinical application, based on the unique needs of the patient population. The Agency for Healthcare Research and Quality (AHRQ) has provided guidance in this area for comparative effectiveness reviews across the health professions. The AHRQ (2014) Effective Health Care Program funds individual researchers, research centers, and academic organizations to produce effectiveness and comparative effectiveness research to improve the quality, safety, efficiency, and effectiveness of healthcare through three primary products: research

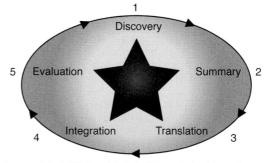

ACE Star Model fo Knowledge Transformation

1 Discovery
2 Summary
3 Translation
4 Integration
5 Evaluation

Figure 5.1 ACE Star Model of Knowledge Transformation. Source: Copyrighted material (Stevens, 2012). Reproduced with expressed permission. Stevens, K. R. (2012). ACE Star Model of EBP: Knowledge Transformation. Academic Center for Evidence-Based Practice. The University of Texas Health Science Center San Antonio.

reviews (comparative effectiveness reviews and technical briefs), original research reports, and research summaries (p. 1).

Evaluating the effectiveness has led to the development of rating scales by some organizations to assist practitioners. In 2009, the American Association of Critical-Care Nurses revised their rating scales for their practice alerts for nurses to support their practice (Armola et al., 2009, pp. 407–408). Since that time, the American Association of Critical-Care Nurses has added additional evidence-based research resources to their Web site for practicing nurses, including a toolkit and practice protocols. However, individual changes in practice do not guide a practice across a profession or professions, hence the focus on dissemination and utilization of current information. This new research utilization effort is called **translational research** (or *translation science*) and is the drive to get the best evidence into practice. Titler (2010) has differentiated between translational research and evidence-based practice (EBP) as follows: "EBP is the process of integrating evidence into healthcare delivery, whereas translation science is the study of how to promote adoption of evidence in healthcare" (p. 36). However, the stages of translational research are described by Grady (2010) as "work in two directions: to continuously develop and reevaluate an intervention across diverse settings and populations and to proactively integrate data from real-world settings into the inception, design, and development of new basic and applied research studies (pp. 164–165).

All of this points to the need for the nurse, both within the discipline and with interdisciplinary colleagues, to seek out the best available information for care of the patient. Fawcett and Garity (2009) identify three valuable questions about information for evidence-based nursing practice:

● Where is the information?
● What is the information?
● How good is the information? (p. 20)

In the ACE Star Model, Stevens (2009) describes the process with evidence summary as the synthesis of the primary research and the body of knowledge leading to translation into practice guidelines and then integrated in practice and evaluation of outcomes (pp. 28–30). Proficiency in critiquing or evaluating research or the evidence summaries is central to the ability to translate and integrate the evidence in professional practice.

When the body of knowledge is evolving and when evidence summaries and systematic reviews are not yet available, individual research studies may provide insight to improvements in care. However, a word of caution is in order: A single study provides information but not compelling evidence unless supported by a body of reseach. But to evaluate the study, a thoughtful critique of the research is required.

ONLINE CONSULT

Academic Center for Evidence-Based Practice at
http://www.acestar.uthscsa.edu

SKILLS FOR A THOUGHTFUL CRITIQUE

Consider both the objective process of critiquing a research study and the subjective process of evaluating its application to practice. An objective analysis looks at the content available to the reader. This analysis is required to have the information for making a judgment as to whether the information is applicable to your practice area and setting.

Objective Evaluation

A research **critique** is an objective analysis of a published research report. The reader must critically consider all components of the report—problem, purpose, supporting literature, theoretical framework, definitions, study questions or hypotheses, design, population and sample, data collection methods and procedures, analysis, and interpretation of findings (Box 5.3). Evidence summaries will have done this across studies for an understanding of the knowledge on a specific area. As practice for understanding the process and terminology, consider an individual research report you have found in the literature. The ultimate goal of a research critique is to evaluate applicability of appropriate scientific findings to one's own professional practice and knowledge base.

A thoughtful critique is based on critical thinking skills used to address the steps of the research process. When publishing research reports, researchers must provide the essential information gained from the study within the given space. This can create a challenge for the reader attempting to glean the vital information for a critique. A published research report is frequently organized into the following sections: abstract, introduction, review of literature, theoretical framework, methods, results, discussion, and references.

Preliminary information provides valuable information for the reader. First, the title of the study should clearly reflect the problem area and attract the reader's interest. Information provided about the researcher includes

---

BOX 5.3 Areas to Address in a Thoughtful Critique*

Areas to address while doing a thoughtful critique of a research study as a component of evidenced-based practice include:
● Title and abstract
● Introduction, problem, and purpose
● Literature review
● Theoretical framework
● Research questions or hypotheses
● Methods: design, ethics, sampling, data collection
● Results and analysis
● Discussion and recommendations
And now, are the findings applicable to use in your practice?

---

*Further information on the areas to address in a research critique is provided on the Intranet site.

background and qualifications in the practice area and for conducting the research study. The abstract briefly reviews the problem, purpose, methodology, findings, and conclusions, summarizing the content and also capturing the reader's attention.

Next comes the introduction to the research report. The opening paragraphs outline the background of the problem, including its purpose and significance to nursing and the care of patients. The **research problem** is the central question that the research has been designed to answer. It is the "what" that is being done in the study to describe, explain, predict, or control some phenomenon of concern to nursing. The research problem contains the major variables and the population of concern to the researcher. The author may also identify specific research aims in this introductory section.

Next, a **literature review** pertinent to the research problem is provided. The literature review is a report and comparison of all pertinent prior investigations on the topic, variables of interest, theoretical models, and methods used. Unlike the library research done for a paper, a research literature review concentrates on primary references. A *primary* source is the actual report of an investigation or development of an instrument or theory written by the researcher or theorist. Using the primary source eliminates the chance of error in interpretation that could occur through analyses by others or loss of the context of the original work.

The literature review should provide a critical appraisal and synthesis of what is already known on the topic. Thus, the literature review supports the study and how the investigation proposes to contribute to the existing body of nursing knowledge. A review of literature may be conducted electronically with the availability of online databases, resources, and articles. Caution is recommended on the use of research reports found in chat rooms, on personal Web pages, or other sources that have not been subjected to a thoughtful peer review process before being accepted for publication.

The theoretical framework may be described in a separate section or may be included with the literature review. As discussed in Chapters 2 and 3, a theoretical framework or model is the way the researcher views the concepts and their interrelationships; it may be described in words or displayed symbolically. This underlying view drives the research in describing, explaining, predicting, or controlling the phenomena, as in the case of empirical research studies.

At this point, the researcher may present specific questions to address in the study or hypotheses to be tested. Specific research questions must flow from, and relate back to, the main research problem or purpose. **Hypotheses** are predictions about the variables that the investigation is testing with a subject group. Hypotheses may be null (statistical), predicting no relationship; conversely, the researcher may state research (alternative) hypotheses that do predict a difference and, in some cases, the direction of the difference (increase, decrease, greater, less). Both null and research hypotheses can be either simple (stating a prediction between two variables) or complex (stating a difference between more than two variables). Hypothesis testing uses inferential statistics, inferring from the sample

to make generalizations about the population. Both research questions and hypotheses must be consistent with the framework that provides the theoretical guidance for the investigation. The variables to be investigated should be readily apparent in the stated research questions or hypotheses.

The next major section in a published research report describes the methodology. This section contains information on the research design, research subjects (including ethical considerations and sampling), and data collection and procedures used. The **research design** is the overall blueprint for the study. The design specifies the setting for the study, the subjects (sample group), the experimental or nonexperimental treatment or grouping methods, the data collection methods, and procedures or protocol. The research design is selected to address the variables of concern to answer the research questions or test the hypotheses. Study designs may be experimental or nonexperimental. Qualitative research studies are also useful in aiding the understanding of a phenomenon that is relevant to your practice area.

Experimental designs are classified as true experiments, quasi-experiments, and pre-experiments, with varying degrees of control, manipulation, and randomization. Nonexperimental study designs may be used to answer the research questions with less human subject involvement or intervention; such designs are ex post facto, correlational, survey, case study, needs assessment, secondary analysis, and evaluation studies. Additional designs you may see in the literature are methodological (studies on research tools or instruments) and meta-analysis, which uses many previous studies to determine the overall effect. The design must "fit" the research problem, purpose, and theoretical framework. You may refer to a nursing research text for more information on these various designs.

The researcher provides definitions for all major variables included in the study. Both theoretical and operational definitions may be provided in the introduction or the review of the literature. Theoretical, or in some cases conceptual, definitions are the general description of a term—that is, the term as defined in a specific theoretical framework or the dictionary. Researchers must provide operational definitions of the major variables of interest, especially when quantitative research methods are used. An **operational definition** is the description specific to the use of the variable in the study. It is precisely what the researchers are looking at and how they are measuring it. For example, consider the term *stethoscope*. Every nurse knows it is an acoustical instrument used to measure heart rate apically or blood pressure peripherally. But the type of stethoscope must be specified in the operational definition, for example, bell-diaphragm combination, electronic, or pediatric. The specification ensures controls in quantitative methods, describing exactly what the researcher used and enabling others to reproduce the study results given a similar set of circumstances or apply the findings to a specific practice setting.

Generally, the researcher provides operational definitions of the study variables in the section on methodology. **Variables** are concepts and constructs defined and manipulated, controlled, or measured in a research study. Independent variables are variables manipulated by the researcher, such as the cause, treatment, or difference between the groups (for example, the type of dressing used). Dependent variables are the outcome variables that the researcher is measuring and analyzing. The researcher wishes to see whether or not the change in the independent variable (type of dressing) caused a difference in the dependent variable (healing time or bacterial colony count). Uncontrolled or confounding variables (such as nutritional status) must also be considered because they can have extraneous and unwanted effects on the dependent variable (healing time). The researcher often attempts to control the extraneous effects by selecting a population or study procedures that meet specific criteria, to reduce the chance of occurrence of the unwanted influences. In the methods section, special attention is given to the descriptions of the subjects. Ultimately, this allows the readers to determine the applicability of results to practice with their specific patient group. Ethical considerations specific to the sample should also be described.

Sampling is the use of a subset (sample) of the population as a feasible group to study, ultimately generalizing the findings to the population. The population is the total group to which the researcher wishes the results of the research to be generalized. For example, not all cardiac patients in a rehabilitation program can be interviewed in person. Yet the researcher would like the study results to be applicable to all patients similar to the subjects interviewed in the study, so that the information will add to the body of nursing knowledge. Samples may be selected by probability (based on statistical chance of selection) or they may be nonprobability samples. Types of probability samples are random, systematic, stratified, and cluster. Nonprobability samples include convenience, purposive, snowball, quota, and expert samples. Each type of sample has advantages and disadvantages that must be considered. At this point, look for the sample size. Smaller sample sizes are associated with qualitative methods. On the other hand, minimum sample sizes are necessary with some statistical procedures in quantitative methods and analysis.

Specific research methods are described as **data collection procedures**. *Data* are the measures or responses obtained from the subjects in the study. Analyzed data become information. Research methods may be quantitative or qualitative. Quantitative methods focus on numerical data that can be obtained from subjects using any one or a combination of measurement instruments. Qualitative methods focus on information gathered from individuals and groups, often in their natural environment, to explore their unique qualities in depth and generate theory on a little-known topic or construct. The different research methods can use similar or different instruments to obtain or measure data.

Instruments are the measurement tools for collecting data. They include paper-and-pencil instruments (such as questionnaires, diaries, or scales), biophysiological instruments (such as a stethoscope, sphygmomanometer, pulse oximeter, electrocardiograph, or electroencephalograph), interview guides, videotapes and audiotapes, and others, depending on the specific investigation and variables. Important considerations for use of any instrument, including an observer as data collector, are the reliability and validity of the measurement. Researchers report the reliability and validity tests before they discuss the findings of their study.

Instrument reliability describes whether the instrument provides consistent measurement. The reliable instrument measures the variable consistently over time. The need for instrument reliability is apparent in examples of a calibrated scale that dependably provides a reading of the patient's weight or the test that consistently estimates the patient's stress level. The types of instrument reliability that are reported in studies are test-retest (stability of the measure over time), internal consistency or alpha (statistical measure on items or parts of a test), equivalent forms of tests, and interrater (equivalence among data collectors).

Instrument validity considers whether the instrument measures what it is intended to measure, such as body surface area and not weight. Types of instrument validity include content, construct, and criterion-related. A panel of experts may assess the content validity of an instrument, ensuring that it adequately addresses the variable or area of interest. Construct validity is described with prior research on the instrument and may be reported as findings from a factor analysis or other statistical test. Criterion-related validity is important when the variable cannot be measured directly, such as family and visitor contacts, cards and gifts, and discussions (as another criterion) to discover social support for a study on the psychosocial stress of the hospitalized patient.

Once the data collection methods have been described, the researcher describes methods used to analyze the data and reports the results in the findings or results section. Methods for analysis of the data are based on the specified research methods and the type of data involved. For numerical data, statistics are used in the analysis of quantitative research methods. **Descriptive statistics** are used to summarize and describe data through graphic displays of the information (percentages and frequency counts), measures of central tendency (means, medians, modes), and measures of dispersion (ranges, variances, and standard deviations). **Inferential statistics** are used to test hypotheses, make predictions, and infer from the sample (statistic) to the population (parameter). Depending on the variables, data, and sample size and distribution, inferential statistics used include nonparametric tests (chi square, Spearman rho, median test) and parametric tests (t-test, analysis of variance [ANOVA], Pearson r correlation coefficient). The results are reported for each research question or hypothesis in an objective manner.

Finally, the researcher presents his or her interpretation of the results in a discussion section. Conclusions should be consistent with the theoretical framework used to guide the study. The discussion also includes the researcher's identification of limitations and recommendations for using the findings in practice, teaching, administration, and further research.

Guidelines to assist with a thoughtful critique of a research study are available on the Intranet site.

Subjective Evaluation: Incorporating Evidence-Based Practice

At this point, the reader must determine the applicability of the results to the individual practice area. A research critique is an objective assessment of the information presented in the report against some criterion, such as the critique questions. The subjective evaluation for use of the findings in one's own practice area is made after the objective critique of the value of the study's process and results. If the critique is positive, you must decide whether the results are applicable in your practice area. If so, consider what other information is known on the topic. Remember, it is a professional responsibility to implement information found to be beneficial to patients, rather than to continue to practice on the basis of tradition.

Reading professional journals and keeping abreast of current knowledge are essential in contemporary nursing practice. Acquiring critique skills is integral for good clinical decisions. Access to quality journals and the depth of reading must also be considered. Look carefully at the professional journals to which you subscribe and the journals that are available at your work site or online. Do they contain research reports? If so, are you reading research studies and systematic reviews as well as the narrative and practice articles? Consider different levels of reading, from skimming the information to a careful analysis of the content or a comparison with other literature to synthesize the information known on the topic. At what level are you reading? Critiquing a research article is at the level of analytic reading rather than merely looking for articles of interest to your practice area. Make time, on a consistent basis, to look for and evaluate research in the professional literature.

As a valuable resource for the implementation of evidence-based practice, alternative sources beyond traditional research articles are available to assist the clinician. These sources provide an integration of findings, as translational science on a specific research topic through sources such as published meta-analyses, systematic reviews, practice guidelines, online reviews, and Internet searches. As noted by Stevens (2009), systematic reviews have been greatly advanced and produce new knowledge. Since they combine findings from all studies, identify bias and limit chance effects, and increase reliability and replication of the results (p. 28).

As mentioned previously, national clinical guidelines have been available since the 1990s. The National Guideline Clearinghouse provides archives of current practice guidelines that have been reviewed, revised, or deleted within the past five years, organized by health conditions and national organizations. The AHRQ also provides useful information for clinicians on current research and quality measures for application in evidence-based practice. The Cochrane Collaboration also provides evidence-based practice information from leading international and interdisciplinary sources.

ONLINE CONSULT

Agency for Healthcare Research and Quality (AHRQ) at http://www.ahrq.gov/

The Cochrane Collaboration at http://www.cochrane.org/

National Guideline Clearinghouse at http://www.guideline.gov/

Once you have obtained the information from the professional literature or resources, the issue is implementation and sharing. Are you sharing the information with colleagues? This can be done informally among your colleagues or formally presented at a unit conference. Having access to "user-friendly" databases or a library is essential for acquiring information on a clinical issue. Investigate what is available in your environment. Attending "brown bag lunches" and participating in a journal club focused on research studies are ways of making this activity more enjoyable and rewarding.

Obtaining new information is the intended aim of attending a clinical conference, regardless of whether you need continuing education units for relicensure or recertification. Quality of programs and significance of the topics to your practice area must be considered for evidence-based practice. Selecting EBP concurrent sessions is a good way to hear current research information. Attendance at an interdisciplinary grand rounds in an institution committed to research is also a valuable experience. Research questions specific to nursing or interdisciplinary collaboration may become available. Your work setting may have a nursing or interdisciplinary research committee. Participating on a research committee can be a challenging and rewarding experience. Nurses can collaborate on different stages of the research process. In addition, the practice problems specific to your setting can emerge, be developed, and be investigated when professionals start the discussion and raise the issues. It can be an extremely stimulating and enjoyable experience.

ELIMINATING BARRIERS TO EVIDENCE-BASED NURSING PRACTICE

Barriers to evidence-based nursing practice should be diminished or removed. Such barriers are a real and perceived lack of educational preparation, administrative support, resources, and time. In this time of diminishing resources, the use of the most reliable and accurate information is crucial. Trial-and-error strategies as the basis for a patient intervention waste valuable resources and are unconscionable if there is contrary evidence. We need an increasing sense of professional commitment to practice based on evidence of effective outcomes for our patients.

Negative attitudes toward research or researchers must be replaced with greater collaboration among clinicians, researchers, administrators, and educators. And this needs to take place among professionals within the discipline and among disciplines. Inclusion of the patient is also a consideration. The patient or significant others may have spent a great deal of time searching for information as "solutions" to the current healthcare problem. Some of the information gleaned from Internet searches or discussions with others may have merit, while other information may be inappropriate or inaccurate. The important consideration is involvement of colleagues and patients in the quest for evidence-based practice.

Clinicians have firsthand awareness of problem areas but must be assisted in accessing the current knowledge base, looking at problems in the domain of nursing that address the need for improved patient outcomes, having the professional commitment to go the extra mile and take time to get involved with research activities, basing their nursing interventions on the current evidence of efficacy, and receiving some form of recognition for their efforts. In addition, these clinicians can be a rich source for identification of areas for change.

The support and encouragement of the chief nurse administrator or executive are a must to ensure that the organizational climate, resources, and philosophy of practice are present in the practice setting. Moving to evidence-based practice will not be an easy transition without a dynamic person spearheading the process. Clinicians must keep an open mind and make a professional commitment to identify problems and search the current knowledge base for information. Researchers must collaborate with clinicians to address nursing questions and avoid speaking or talking in "researchese," thus providing clear practice implications in publications and presentations. Educators must also assist in the development of critique and EBP skills.

Commitment must be made to the ongoing nature of building knowledge and basing practice on evidence of efficacy. Our knowledge base has been evolving since the time of Nightingale and before. It will continue to evolve because of the nature of the information and our focus on people in a dynamic environment. The profession needs more extensive research that is generalizable to and supportive of nursing as a major player in healthcare issues. We need more replications to add reliability and validity to instruments and information for translational research. And the need for interprofessional research is critical when scopes of practice are close or overlap to better address improved patient outcomes. Constant updating and modification of any protocol is needed as more information becomes available. Gaining critique skills and learning the language of EBP are components of this process.

EVIDENCE-BASED PRACTICE: *Consider this....*

Brown (2014) has identified the following considerations for evaluating the clinical significance of a clinical guideline:

- Importance of expected health benefits
- Likelihood of health benefits
- Side effects and risks
- Practicality and acceptability to patients (p. 325)

Suppose you have selected an AHRQ EBP guideline with the systematic review of the literature and suggested guidelines and tools for implementation that are appropriate for your setting.

Question: How will you use this information and include an evaluation process to promote quality improvement?

Source: Brown, S. J. (2014). *Evidence-based nursing: The research practice connection* (3rd ed.). Boston, MA: Jones and Bartlett.

KEY POINTS

- Evidence-based practice, a core competency for health professionals, is defined as the use of clinical expertise and interventions that are based on evidence of efficacy for patient outcomes and the preferences of the patients served.
- Research is a process for generating scientific knowledge and utilizing the knowledge on which to base practice. Using evidence of efficacy for practice is a vital professional attribute and a responsibility.
- Nursing research began with Florence Nightingale and has become vital to both professionals and consumers in investigating the domain of nursing, testing theories and interventions, and demonstrating the efficacy and efficiency of nursing actions.
- Ethical considerations in research must include the four basic human rights:
  - Beneficence ("Do no harm")
  - Full disclosure
  - Self-determination
  - Privacy and confidentiality

Continued

KEY POINTS—cont'd

- A professional nurse should be an active consumer of nursing research, promoting use of current and valid scientific knowledge and identifying the questions to be addressed in further research. Professional accountability demands that one read the literature, attend educational sessions, use critique skills, participate in investigations, and apply and promote evidence-based interventions.

- Empirical research is based on the strict rules of the scientific method, with the following steps:
  - Identification of the problem
  - Statement of the purpose
  - Review of the literature
  - Description of the theoretical framework
  - Definition of terms
  - Statement of hypothesis(es)
  - Selection of the research design, population, and sample
  - Approval by the IRB
  - Collection of data
  - Analysis and interpretation of data
  - Presentation of findings and recommendations

- Knowledge transformation is defined as "the conversion of research findings from primary research results, through a series of stages and forms, to impact on health outcomes by way of EB care" (Stevens, 2009, p. 28).

- Grady (2010) describes translational research "to continuously develop and reevaluate an intervention across diverse settings and populations and to proactively integrate data from real-world settings into the inception, design, and development of new basic and applied research studies" (pp. 164–165).

- A critique is an objective analysis of a research report. The reader must critically consider all components of the report.

- A research problem is the main issue or central question that the researcher addresses in the investigation. Specific research questions or hypotheses flow from the main research problem.

- The literature review is a report and comparison of all pertinent prior investigations on the topic, variables of interest, theoretical models, and methods used.

- Variables are concepts and constructs defined and manipulated, controlled, or measured in a research study. Independent variables are manipulated by the researcher.

- Hypotheses are predictions about the variables that the researcher is testing with a subject group.

- The research design is the overall blueprint and methods for the study.

- Research methods may be quantitative or qualitative. Quantitative methods focus on numerical data that can be obtained from subjects through any one or a combination of measurement instruments. Qualitative methods focus on information gathered from individuals and groups, often in their natural environment, to explore in depth their unique qualities and generate theory on a little-known topic or construct.

- Sampling is the use of a subset (sample) of the population as a feasible group to study and ultimately generalize findings to the population.

- Instruments are the measurement tools for collecting data. Important considerations for use of any instrument are the reliability and validity of the measurement.

- Statistics are used in analyzing quantitative research methods. Descriptive statistics are used to summarize and describe data. Inferential statistics are used to test hypotheses, make predictions, and infer from the sample to the population.

Thought and Discussion Questions

1. Describe activities present in your practice setting that demonstrate the use of evidence-based practice.

2. Develop a plan to encourage or promote evidence-based practice in your nursing practice environment. Select a clinical protocol or problem. Use the following six phases of the research utilization process to organize your plan: (1) identification of clinical problems and access to research bases, (2) evaluation of the knowledge and the potential for application in the organization, along with policy and cost determinants, (3) planning for implementation and evaluation of the innovation, (4) clinical trial and evaluation, (5) decisions to adopt, modify, or reject innovations on the basis of evaluation, and (6) if the innovations are adopted, planning for their extension to other units (Horsley et al., 1978). Describe who will be involved in the process and how the new practice or protocol will be implemented. Finally, identify evaluation criteria.

3. Identify practice issues that can be developed into a nursing research problem for investigation.

4. Find the requirements for the IRB at your college or institution. Be prepared to participate in a discussion of the requirements for the preparation of a research proposal for consideration by the IRB.

5. Look further at PHI and current privacy issues. Be prepared to participate in a discussion as scheduled by your instructor.

6. Review the Chapter Thought located on the first page of the chapter and discuss it in the context of the contents of the chapter.

Interactive Exercises

Go to the Intranet site and complete the interactive exercises provided for this chapter.

REFERENCES

Agency for Healthcare Research and Quality (AHRQ). (2014). *What is the Effective Health Care Program?* Retrieved from http://www.effectivehealthcare.ahrq.gov/index.cfm/what-is-the-effective-health-care-program1/

American Association of Colleges of Nursing (AACN). (2006a). *Essentials of doctoral education for advanced nursing practice.* Retrieved from http://www.aacn.nche.edu/DNP/pdf/Essentials.pdf

American Association of Colleges of Nursing (AACN). (2006b). *Position statement on nursing research.* Retrieved from http://www.aacn.browsermedia.com/publications/position/nursing-research

American Association of Colleges of Nursing (AACN). (2008). *The essentials of baccalaureate education for professional nursing practice.* Retrieved from http://www.aacn.nche.edu/Education/pdf/BaccEssentials08.pdf

American Association of Critical-Care Nurses. (2010). *Practice alert: Family presence during resuscitative and invasive procedures.* Retrieved from http://www.aacn.org/wd/practice/content/family-presence-practice-alert.pcms?menu=practice

American Association of Critical-Care Nurses. (2013). *Ethical foundations for critical care nursing research.* Retrieved from http://www.aacn.org/wd/practice/docs/research/ethical-foundations-critical-care-nursing-research.pdf

American Nurses Credentialing Center (ANCC). (2014). Practice standards. Retrieved from http://www.nursecredentialing.org/Pathway/AboutPathway/PathwayPracticeStandards

Belmont Report. (1979). Ethical principles and guidelines for the protection of human subjects of research, 79 *Fed. Reg.* 12065.

Brown, S. J. (2014). *Evidence-based nursing: The research practice connection* (3rd ed.). Boston, MA: Jones and Bartlett.

Declaration of Helsinki. (1990). Recommendations guiding physicians in biomedical research involving human subjects. *Bulletin of Pan American Health Organization, 24*(4), 606–609.

Fawcett, J., & Garity, J. (2009). *Evaluating research for evidence-based nursing practice.* Philadelphia, PA: F.A. Davis.

Greiner, A. C., & Knebel, E. (Eds.). (2003). *Health professions education: A bridge to quality.* Washington, DC: Institute of Medicine.

Grady, P. A. (2010). Translational research and nursing science. *Nursing Outlook, 58,* 164–166.

Horsley, J. A., Crane, J., & Bingle, J. D. (1978). Research utilization as an organizational process. *Journal of Nursing Administration, 8*(7), 4–6.

Kerlinger, F. N., & Lee, H. B. (2000). *Foundations of behavioral research* (4th ed.). Belmont, CA: Wadsworth Thompson Learning.

Lindeman, C. A., & Krueger, J. C. (1977). Increasing the quality, quantity, and use of nursing research. *Nursing Outlook, 25,* 450–454.

National Institute of Nursing Research (NINR). (2012). *FAQ: General information. What is nursing research?* Retrieved from http://www.ninr.nih.gov/site-structure/faq#.Uu6k1WeYbmQ

National Institute of Nursing Research (NINR). (2013). Mission and strategic plan. Retrieved from http://www.ninr.nih.gov/aboutninr/ninr-mission-and-strategic-plan#.Uu2wi2eYbmI

Nightingale, F. (1859). *Notes on nursing: What it is, and what it is not.* London, UK: Harrison and Sons. (Commemorative edition printed 1992, Philadelphia: J. B. Lippincott.)

Porter-O'Grady, T. (2006). A new age for practice: Creating the framework for evidence. In K. Mallock & T. Porter-O'Grady (Eds.), *Introduction to evidence-based practice* (pp. 1–29). Boston, MA: Jones and Bartlett.

Protection of Human Subjects, 45 CFR 46 (2009). Title 45 Code of Federal Regulations Part 46 (45 CFR 46), §46.102, 110. Retrieved from http://www.hhs.gov/ohrp/humansubjects/guidance/45cfr46.html

Sigma Theta Tau. (2005). *Evidence-based nursing position statement.* Retrieved from http://www.nursingsociety.org/aboutus/PositionPapers/Pages/EBN_positionpaper.aspx

Silva, M. (1995). *Ethical guidelines in the conduct, dissemination, and implementation of nursing research.* Washington, DC: American Nurses Association.

Stevens, K. R. (2005). *Essential competencies for evidence-based practice in nursing.* San Antonio, TX: Academic Center for Evidence-Based Practice.

Stevens, K. R. (2009). *Essential competencies for evidence-based practice in nursing* (2nd ed.). San Antonio, TX: Academic Center for Evidence-Based Practice.

Titler, M. G. (2010). Translation science and context. *Research and Theory for Nursing Practice: An International Journal, 24,* 35–55.

U.S. President's Commission for the Study of Ethical Problems in Medicine and Behavioral Research. (1982). *Compensating for research injuries: The ethical and legal implications of programs to redress injured subjects* (Vol. 1). Retrieved from http://www2.gwu.edu/~nsarchiv/radiation/dir/mstreet/commeet/meet16/brief16/tab_b/br16b1a.txt

United States Department of Health & Human Services (USDHHS). (2004). *Protecting personal health information in research: Understanding the HIPAA privacy rule* (NIH Pub. No. 03–5388). Retrieved from http://privacyruleandresearch.nih.gov/pr_02.asp

BIBLIOGRAPHY

Academic Center for Evidence-Based Practice, UTHSCSA (2012). Welcome to ACE. Retrieved from http://www.acestar.uthscsa.edu/

American Nurses Association. (1997). Position statement: Education for participation in nursing research (retired). Retrieved from members only archive, http://nursingworld.org/MainMenuCategories/HealthcareandPolicyIssues/ANAPositionStatements/Archives/rseducat14484.aspx

American Nurses Association. (1985). *Human rights guidelines for nurses in clinical and other research* (Pub. No. D-46 3M 9/87R). Kansas City, MO: American Nurses Association.

American Nurses Association Commission on Nursing Research. (1981). *Guidelines for the investigative function of nurses.* Kansas City, MO: American Nurses Association.

Crane, J. (1985). Research utilization: Theoretical perspectives. *Western Journal of Nursing Research, 7,* 261–268.

Munhall, P. (2011). *Nursing research: A qualitative perspective* (5th ed.). Boston, MA: Jones and Bartlett.

Munhall, P. L., & Chenail, R. (2008). *Qualitative research proposals and reports: A guide* (3rd ed.). Boston: Jones and Bartlett.

Long, L. E., Burkett, K., & McGee, S. (2010). Promotion of safe outcomes: Incorporating evidence into policies and procedures. *Nursing Clinics of North America, 44,* 57–70.

Peterson, S. J., & Bredow, T. S. (2012). *Middle range theories: Application to nursing research* (3rd ed.). Philadelphia, PA: Lippincott Williams & Wilkins.

Walsh, N. (2010). Dissemination of evidence into practice: Opportunities and threats. *Primary Health Care, 20*(3), 26–30.

ONLINE RESOURCES

Academic Center for Evidence-Based Practice (ACE)
http://www.acestar.uthscsa.edu

Agency for Healthcare Research and Quality (AHRQ)
http://www.ahrq.gov/

The Cochrane Collaboration
http://www.cochrane.org/

Federal Guidelines for the Protection of Human Subjects
http://www.hhs.gov/ohrp/humansubjects/guidance/45cfr46.html

Federal Opportunities for Research Funding
http://www.grants.gov

National Institute of Nursing Research
http://ninr.nih.gov

National Institutes of Health
http://www.nih.gov/

Office for Human Research Protections (OHRP)
http://www.hhs.gov/ohrp/

U.S. Department of Health & Human Services: Health Information Privacy
http://www.hhs.gov/ocr/hipaa/

Sigma Theta Tau International: Research Grant Opportunities
http://www.nursingsociety.org/Research/Grants/Pages/grantsbydate.aspx

U.S. Department of Health & Human Services
http://www.hhs.gov

Critical Abilities in Professional Nursing Practice

Six critical abilities in professional nursing are reviewed in this section. The first critical component addresses *communication skills*, which are vital to professional practice and are in constant need of refinement. The content is presented by Lynne Ornes in Chapter 6, "Effective Communication," with a discussion of communication models, essential ingredients of effective communication, nonverbal communication forms, and specific communication techniques, including communication skills for interdisciplinary practice.

Along with effective communication, **critical thinking** is essential to professional nursing practice. In Chapter 7, "Critical Thinking," Genevieve M. Bartol discusses aspects of critical thinking in nursing, along with further development of critical thinking and analysis skills. Effective communication and critical thinking are required in collaborative practice situations. Chapter 8 focuses on **working with groups,** including the characteristics and roles of groups and group leaders and the skills needed for collaboration, coordination, negotiation, and dealing with conflict and difficult people.

The next critical component for professional practice is the **teaching and learning process.** Chapter 9 presents a discussion of learning theories and learning readiness, along with information on writing behavioral objectives, teaching skills and methods, and preparing outcome evaluations. The Intranet lesson focuses on helping patients locate reliable Web sources.

Leadership and management skills are essential in professional practice, especially in organizational settings. Chapter 10 looks at organizational characteristics and the skills needed for effectively managing and leading in organizational settings, including a discussion of selected theories and delegation principles. Organizations continue to redefine themselves, and effectively dealing with **change** is critical. Chapter 11 includes theories on change and innovation, along with the characteristics of agents for change in individuals, families, groups, and organizations.

Section II concludes with Chapter 12, on **professional ethics,** by focusing on informed consent, advanced directives, the persistive vegetative state, organ procurement and donation, genomics, and impaired practice.

● Lynne Ornes

Effective Communication 6

"A wise old owl sat on an oak; the more he saw the less he spoke; the less he spoke the more he heard; why aren't we like that wise old bird?"

Charles M. Shulz

Chapter Objectives

On completion of this chapter, the reader will be able to:

1. Describe and understand the various communication models.

2. Explain the various forms of communication, such as verbal and nonverbal communication.

3. Evaluate the use of therapeutic communication in the healthcare setting.

4. Differentiate between ways the nurse receives information from the patient.

5. Discuss the various types of barriers to communication.

6. Identify past life experiences that influence communication skills.

7. Describe how structured communication tools can be used to reduce errors in the healthcare system.

8. Evaluate his or her current communication skills with patients and colleagues and propose refinements as a part of advancing his or her career in nursing.

Key Terms

Communication	Receiver	Cultural Variations
Communication Models	Relationships	Kinesics
Source	Transactions	Facial Expressions
Encoder	Contexts	Physical Appearance
Message	Metacommunication	Therapeutic Communication
Channel	Verbal Communication	Active Listening
Decoder	Nonverbal Communication	Collaboration
Environment	Proxemics	SBAR

Communication is a comprehensive and complex process. The word *communication* is similar to words like love, health, and freedom; intuitively, each of us thinks that we know what it means, but in reality people base their definitions on their own life experiences, cultures, and surroundings. For the nurse, communication is an essential element not only in the relationship with the patient but also in working effectively with the interdisciplinary health team. The process of interactions between humans can be verbal or nonverbal, written or unwritten, planned or spontaneous. It is therefore essential for communication to be defined within the context of nursing. Communication consists of "all the cognitive, affective, and behavioral responses used to convey a message to another person" (Watson, 1979, p. 33). Within this context there is no such thing as "no communication" between individuals. All behavior, whether verbal or nonverbal, has both a meaning and a message value.

Effective communication within the nurse-patient relationship is not necessarily a natural process; it is a learned skill. Clear and appropriate communication is essential for providing effective nursing care and presents a unique challenge to nurses today. Society is composed of many different cultures using many different languages. "U.S. census data show that between 1990 and 2000, the percentage of Americans (older than age five) speaking a language other than English at home rose from 13.8 percent to 17.8 percent" (Ku & Flores, 2005, p. 435). For example, in the aftermath of the September 2001 terrorist attack in New York, one of the biggest challenges faced by the Red Cross workers was communicating with individuals who spoke so many different languages. When a nurse is giving care to a patient, the nurse's message must be understandable to the patient and vice versa. Nurses must be aware not only of what they are saying in their words but also of what their body language is saying to their patients and to other members of the interdisciplinary health team.

The 21st century poses an additional challenge to nurses in communicating via technology. Nurses use many different types of communication in their care of patients—in person, the written word, telephone, fax, and e-mail. Finding effective ways to overcome communication barriers, discussed later in this chapter, gives nurses the opportunity to bridge culture gaps within their community and provide care to a larger number of individuals. This chapter will cover various techniques of communication and offer tools to assist you in your professional relationships with others.

COMMUNICATION MODELS

An overview of basic **communication models** is presented first to help you understand the complex process of communication in the healthcare setting. Later, various communication models that are useful in health communication are described.

Basic Components

Whether or not sources of communication are effective depends on a combination of factors (Berlo, 1960). All types of communication require the following components:

- *Source:* The individual who decides what message is to be sent

- *Encoder:* The person who interprets the message
- *Message:* The content
- *Channel:* The medium or way chosen to convey the message
- *Receiver:* The one who receives the message
- *Decoder:* The one who interprets the message sent

Additional factors have been added to the basic components, including the following:

- *Feedback:* The message the receiver returns to the source
- *Interpersonal variables:* Factors that influence communication
- *Environment:* The setting for source-receiver interaction

In intrapersonal communication, the source and the encoder are the same person. The message is then communicated by either verbal or nonverbal language. The message may be sent to any or all of a person's five senses. The receiver is also the decoder. According to Berlo (1960), in effective communication, the receiver is the most important component in the communication process. If the source does not reach the receiver with the intended message, the source might just as well have talked to himself or herself. Feedback is confirmation that the message was received by the receiver and been understood. Examples of interpersonal variables are culture, gender, and age. The environment refers to the setting in which the communication takes place. Is it private? Are there distractions, such as music or talking from others, which is interfering?

In written communication, the reader receiver is most important. In spoken communication, the listener receiver is most important. When the source chooses a "code" for a message, he or she must choose one that is familiar to the receiver. An example of poor communication in the healthcare setting is when a nurse gives information to a patient using a code that consists of the jargon or terms known only within the profession. The patient can receive the information but does not have the knowledge to decode the message.

Human communication is a two-person process in which both individuals influence and are influenced by each other.

Source-Message-Channel-Receiver Model

David Berlo (1960), a professor at Michigan State University, developed the source-message-channel-receiver (SMCR) model of the communication process (Fig. 6.1). This paradigm emphasizes the importance of a thorough understanding of human behavior as a prerequisite to communication analysis. The SMCR model represents a communication process that occurs as a source formulates messages based on the source's communication skills, attitudes, knowledge, and sociocultural system. These messages, which have unique elements, structure, content, treatment, and codes, are then transmitted along channels. Channels are the various senses, such as seeing, hearing, touching, smelling, and tasting. The receiver interprets

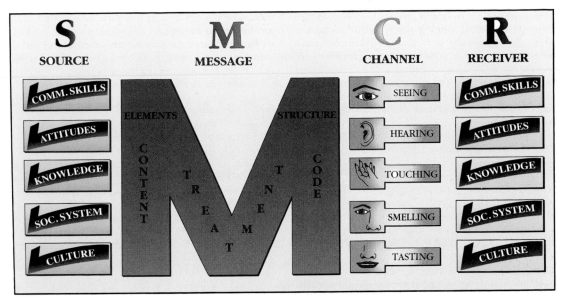

Figure 6.1 Source-message-channel-receiver (SMCR) model of communication. (From Berlo, D. K. [1960]. *The process of communication: An introduction to the theory and practice* [p. 7]. New York: Holt, Rinehart & Winston, with permission.)

messages on the basis of his or her own communication skills, attitudes, knowledge, and sociocultural system.

The strength of the SMCR model is that it demonstrates the complex process of communication and shows that communication is not a static event. It incorporates the sociocultural context of both sender and receiver as a critical component in the communication process. However, the model lacks the important component of feedback (Berlo, 1960). The next model includes this factor in its concepts.

Health Communication Model

Northouse and Northouse (1998) constructed the health communication model (HCM) (Fig. 6.2), which specifically applies to transactions between participants in healthcare about health-related issues. The primary focus of the HCM is on the communication that occurs within the various kinds of relationships in healthcare settings. This model also takes a broader systems view

of communication and emphasizes the way in which a series of factors can affect the interactions in the healthcare setting. Three major factors illustrate the health communication process: relationships, transactions, and contexts.

Relationships

From a systems perspective, the HCM illustrates four major types of **relationships** that exist in the healthcare setting:

- Professional-professional
- Professional-client/patient
- Professional–significant other
- Client/patient–significant other

When an individual is involved in health communication, he or she is involved in one of these types of relationships. In this model, the term *health professional* refers to any individual who has the education, training, and

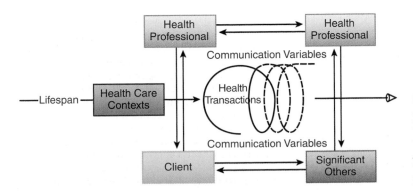

Figure 6.2 Health communication model. (From Northouse, P. G., & Northouse, L. L. [1998]. *Health communication strategies for the health professional* (3rd ed.) [p. 16]. Norwalk, CT: Appleton & Lange, with permission.)

experience to provide health services to others. Health professionals include a wide range of individuals such as nurses, health administrators, social workers, physicians, and occupational and physical therapists (Northouse & Northouse, 1998). Each of these professionals brings unique characteristics and beliefs to healthcare settings that affect the way he or she interacts with the patient and with the other members of the interdisciplinary healthcare team.

Patients are the people who are the focus of the healthcare services being provided. The term *patient* also encompasses the characteristics, values, and beliefs that these individuals bring to the healthcare setting. Just as the personal characteristics of the nurse and other professionals influence their interactions, the characteristics of patients influence their interactions with others. Within the social network of the patient, the patient's significant others include family members and friends who have been found to be essential in supporting patients as they maneuver through the healthcare system. Significant others are all of the people who are significant in patients' lives but are not health professionals.

The patient's self-esteem, emotional stability, and sense of identity will define how the patient relates to the healthcare professionals as well as those significant individuals in his or her life.

Northouse and Northouse (1998) realized that, too often, health professionals overlook the important role played by family members and other significant individuals in enhancing the health of the person. Their model includes this aspect because as patients live longer with chronic health problems, significant others assume an even more central role as patient advocates and are more involved in the direct care of the patient. This concept is also true when the nurse is visiting the patient in the home. The dynamics within the family and the support of the significant others around the patient can help the patient realize the full potential of a healthy lifestyle.

Transactions

Transactions, the second major factor in the HCM, are the health-related interactions between the nurse or other health professional, the patient, and the patient's significant others. These transactions about health can include both verbal and nonverbal communication behaviors, which are equally important and are most effective when they are compatible with each other. Northouse and Northouse (1998) represent these health transactions with a circle from which an unending spiral emerges, signifying that communication is not static but is an interactive process that occurs at various points in a person's life. This continuous feedback allows the message to be changed in accordance with the situation.

Contexts

Contexts, the third major factor in the model, is defined as the settings where the health communication takes place and includes the properties of these settings. At one level, context can refer to the healthcare setting, such as a

hospital room or the patient's home. For example, if the professional is communicating with the patient in an ambulatory clinic, there may be many distractions and infringements of privacy. Each particular healthcare setting affects the dynamics of the transactions that take place. At another level, however, healthcare contexts can refer to the number of participants within the particular healthcare setting. Communication can take place in a one-to-one situation or in small groups. The number of participants present influences the overall interactions in the setting.

The health communication model is based on the assumption that communication is ongoing and dynamic. It is transactional, in that each participant affects the other participants, and it has both a content and relationship dimension that are inextricably bound together in the interactions. It is a model that incorporates the thoughts, feelings, attitudes, and current roles of the participants and demonstrates that all of these things can affect the accuracy of the communication.

FORMS OF COMMUNICATION

In order to share information, people express messages in a complex composite of both verbal (spoken or written) and nonverbal behaviors. Individuals express themselves through language, gestures, voice inflection, facial expressions, and use of space. Within the nurse-patient relationship, information exchanged between two individuals must be interpreted not only by the nurse but also by the patient. The healthcare provider should be aware of styles of communication and should have observational skills that enhance the encounter.

Metacommunication

Metacommunication is a broad term used to "describe all of the factors that influence how the message is perceived" (Arnold & Boggs, 2011, p. 163) and has long been recognized as being of enormous value in the nurse-patient therapeutic relationship. Metacommunication includes all of the things taken into account when the receiver is interpreting a message, such as the role of the communicator, the nonverbal messages sent, and the context in which the communication is taking place. These messages may be hidden within verbal messages or conveyed by nonverbal expressions or gestures. An example is the "play fighting" observed in children and animals. Bateson noted that for an organism to "play" at fighting, it must be able to both appear that it is fighting and simultaneously appear not to be actually fighting but merely simulating the act of fighting (Mitchell, 1991).

In the nurse-patient relationship, metacommunication conveys messages about how to interpret both verbal and nonverbal communication clues. For example, a nurse can convey a message of caring by saying to the patient, "That's important. Let's talk about it." If the nurse sits in a chair and uses nonverbal cues such as maintaining eye contact, smiling, having a relaxed posture, and listening intently, the verbal and nonverbal messages are congruent. If the same verbal message is delivered while the nurse fidgets and looks at the clock, the nurse may provide a nonverbal message that he or she does not have time or is not willing to listen. Metacommunication is the message conveyed when both verbal and nonverbal communication are perceived together.

Nurses must make sure that their verbal and nonverbal messages to the patient are consistent and congruent in order to be sure that the patient interprets the messages clearly. Suppose you walk into a room and ask a patient whether he is in pain and he answers no, but you observe that he is thrashing in bed, clutching his incision, and has deep grimaces on his face. How would you interpret this behavior? A nurse who is skilled in communication would realize that the verbal answer and the nonverbal cues are inconsistent and would clarify the situation. If the nurse points out the incongruent form of communication that he or she observed, the patient may admit that he is in pain (Arnold & Boggs, 2011).

Metacommunication is the message conveyed when both verbal and nonverbal communication are perceived together.

Verbal Communication

Verbal communication takes place when people use words to share experiences with others. Without the use of spoken language, individuals are severely limited in their means of sharing with others what they are feeling. The choice of words that a person uses is based on language, educational background, age, race, and socioeconomic background, as well as on the situation in which the communication takes place.

According to the individual's background and experience, interpretation of words may also vary. One cannot assume that words have the same meaning to everyone who hears them. "Language is useful only to the extent that it actually reflects the experience it is designed to portray" (Arnold & Boggs, 2011, p. 164). If a person speaks a different native language, consider the difficulty that person will have expressing his or her thoughts in English. This could also apply to a small child or an Alzheimer's patient.

Keep in mind that the intended meaning of the message may be represented in the emphasis placed on a particular word. The pitch and tone of a word can suggest mood and can either support or contradict the content of the verbal message. When the patient is explaining something to the nurse, the nurse must consider that certain phrases and words may have entirely different meanings for the patient and the nurse.

Potter and Perry (2013) state that the six most important aspects of verbal communication are (1) vocabulary, (2) denotative and connotative meanings, (3) intonation, (4) pacing, (5) clarity and brevity, and (6) timing and relevance.

Vocabulary

Vocabulary consists of the words or phrases that a person chooses and uses to communicate a message. Communication is unsuccessful if the receiver cannot translate or understand the sender's words and phrases. Nurses work with individuals of various ages, developmental stages, cultures, and educational backgrounds, as well as individuals who have physical problems that distort their communication skills.

Nurses must be very aware of their use of nursing or medical jargon. Consider the nurse who is instructing a patient before an operation. If the nurse says, "You are to be NPO after midnight and you are to void prior to the pre-op injection," what will the patient be able to decipher from this instruction? At the same time, the nurse must not "talk down" to or patronize the patient. The nurse must respect the patient and understand the best way to provide the information in a manner that can be understood readily.

Meaning

A single word may have several different meanings. The denotative meaning is the meaning that is shared by individuals who use a common language. The word *football* may be understood by all individuals who speak English but denotes a different meaning to individuals of different countries. The word *code* denotes a cardiac arrest to members of the healthcare profession but has different meanings outside the health community. The connotative meaning is the interpretation or the way one's feelings, thoughts, experiences, or ideas about a word influence the meaning of the word. When a family is told that their loved one is in "serious condition," they may interpret that phrase to mean that their loved one is near death. To the nurse, however, the term may merely describe the nature of the illness. Nurses should be extremely cautious to use words and phrases that will not be misinterpreted, especially when explaining a patient's condition.

When a nurse is giving instructions to a patient, the nurse must use terms and phrases that the patient understands. The best way to ensure that the patient has understood the instructions is have the patient repeat the instructions to the nurse. At that time, any questions can be answered, and the nurse can be assured that the patient has the correct information.

Intonation

Intonation is the cadence and tone of the spoken word. The intonation of words in a message can readily change the meaning. Take the phrase "He is." If spoken one way it can be a sentence, but with a different tone it can be a question. Emphasizing the "he" or the "is" also changes the meaning of the phrase. Tone of voice can dramatically affect a message's meaning, and emotions directly influence tone of voice. Emotions such as anger, enthusiasm, and concern may be gleaned from the tone of voice that one uses. Nurses must be aware of this fact to avoid sending an unintended message. The nurse must also realize that the patient's intonation may reflect the patient's emotional state, even if the patient's words do not.

Pacing

Pacing is the speed and rate of the spoken word. Communication is more successful when words are spoken at an appropriate speed or pace. Talking too rapidly or too slowly may express an inadvertent message. When communicating important information to a patient, the nurse must speak slowly and clearly and must pause at appropriate points to give emphasis. This approach allows the patient time to absorb the message and to understand it more clearly. Pacing is optimum if the nurse thinks out the message before delivering it.

The nurse should also be aware of the pace of the patient's spoken word. The speech may be slow and slurred if the patient has some type of neurologic problem or is under the influence of drugs or alcohol. The patient who is scared and nervous may speak very rapidly. Cultural variables may also influence the pace of the words; a person from the southern part of the United States may speak more slowly than someone from the Northeast. It is important for the nurse to be aware of these differences and be able to interpret the meanings of a person's pace of speaking.

Clarity, Timing, and Relevance

The nurse should use words and phrases that express an idea simply and directly. Using examples tends to make a message clearer. Timing and relevance are likewise critical in communication. The patient must be ready to hear what the nurse has to say. If a patient is distracted by pain, the nurse must realize that it is not the right time to give detailed instructions. Often the best time to communicate is when the patient has expressed interest in a particular topic. Choosing this timing tends to make the patient more attentive.

Nurses should also demonstrate credibility, which is defined as a sense of trustworthiness, sincerity, reliability, and integrity. The nurse must be dependable and believable. If the patient asks the nurse a question that the nurse does not know the answer to, it is much better for the nurse to say, "I do not know the answer to that but I will find out for you" than to give erroneous information. When a nurse establishes credibility in a nurse-patient relationship, the communication is more reliable and can have more substantial meaning for both the patient and the nurse.

Nonverbal Communication

Nonverbal communication is communication without words; it includes messages that are created through body motions, facial expressions, the use of space and sounds, and the use of touch. Birdwhistell (1970) studied the area of body movement and suggested that 65 to 70 percent of the social meaning of an interaction is transmitted by nonverbal communication. Although nonverbal communication does not include language, it can be either vocal or nonvocal. For example, if a patient is moaning in pain, she is giving a nonverbal cue that the nurse should ask more questions about her condition.

Nonverbal communication can be intentional or unintentional. If a nurse is giving important information to a patient, the nurse should intentionally have a serious facial expression. A patient who is giving the nurse information in an apparently relaxed and gleeful manner but whose face shows expressions of fear and uncertainty demonstrates unintentional nonverbal communication. A prime example of nonverbal communication is Holly Hunter's role in the 1993 movie *The Piano*. For the entire length of the movie, she does not speak one word, yet her nonverbal communication in the role is so effective that it earned her an Oscar for the best actress performance. Monitoring subtle nonverbal communication clues accounts for the vast majority of communication between individuals.

Most Americans are only dimly aware of their use of nonverbal language, although they use it every day. We are constantly communicating our real feelings in nonverbal ways (Hall, 1959). Arnold and Boggs (2011) categorize four areas in which nonverbal behaviors are used: (1) proxemics; (2) cultural variations; (3) kinesics, which includes body language and facial expression; and (4) appearance.

Proxemics

Proxemics refers to how individuals use and interpret space in the communication process. Some areas of proxemics address questions of territoriality, personal space, and distance relevant to the healthcare setting. Each culture has expectations for appropriate distance, depending on the context of communication. Personal space, or one's own territory, is important because it gives one a sense of identity, security, and control. A person may feel threatened or simply irritated when his or her personal space is invaded.

When people enter the healthcare setting, they are required to give up much of their privacy and personal space. They are required to give personal and intimate information to strangers and may undergo procedures that further compromise their sense of privacy and personal space. Although nurses and other health professionals may not be able to eliminate these problems of personal space, the healthcare professional should respect the patient's territory, belongings, and right to privacy. The patient should be given as much control over the situation as possible. For example, the patient should be allowed to decide whether the door to the room is left open or closed and where personal items are placed. The patient's body should be exposed as little as possible to minimize the discomfort involved with procedures that invade his or her privacy.

Cultural Variations

Cultural variations are learned subconsciously through the observations of behavior of significant individuals in the patient's culture. Communication patterns vary in different cultures, even for such conventional social behaviors as smiling, a handshake, and direct eye contact. For many Hispanic individuals, smiling and shaking hands are considered an integral part of sincere interaction and trust, whereas an Asian individual might perceive this behavior to be inappropriate (Galanti, 2014).

Sometimes a nonverbal gesture—a body movement usually with the hand—is totally acceptable in one culture and truly offensive in another one. For example, a nurse may mean to signal to a Brazilian patient that things went well by making an "OK" circle with the thumb and index finger; in Brazil, however, this movement is considered an obscene gesture (Arnold & Boggs, 2011).

Cultural taboos can inhibit nonverbal behaviors. Different cultures have different rules about eye contact. In many Western cultures, looking directly into another person's eyes is interpreted as being interested and attentive. The use of eye contact is one of the most culturally variable nonverbal behaviors, however. Although most nurses have been taught to look directly at the patient when speaking, individuals from other cultures may attribute other culturally based meanings to this behavior. Asian, Native American, Middle Eastern, and Hmong patients may consider eye contact impolite or antagonistic, and they may divert their own eyes when talking to a nurse or physician. In some cultures, showing respect to the nurse dictates that the patient should cast the eyes downward. Navajo patients believe that making direct eye contact is disrespectful and harmful to the spirits of both parties (Galanti, 2014).

In some cultures, touching—coming into physical contact with another person—is one of the most powerful means of nonverbal communication, but the nurse must give careful consideration to issues surrounding touch. Touch can take a variety of forms and can convey a range of meanings, but it is a powerful tool in healthcare when it communicates caring and respect. Touch can ease a patient's sense of isolation and can make procedures seem less invasive. Care must be taken, however, to understand individual cultural customs about touching, which can vary dramatically. For example, the cultures of Muslim and Orthodox Jewish men dictate that they do not touch women outside their families. Such men may be very uncomfortable even shaking the hand of a female healthcare provider (Arnold & Boggs, 2011).

Unfortunately, there is no precise formula to determine when or when not to touch a patient, and no universal meaning can be given to a touch. In order for patients to perceive touch positively in a therapeutic relationship, Northouse and Northouse (1998) suggest that nurses use the following guidelines:

- Use a form of touch that is appropriate to the particular situation. There are many types of touch that can be used in various ways. The nurse should use touch that is fitting to the situation. For example, if a woman has just been told distressing information (e.g., that her child is diagnosed with leukemia), she may respond positively to the nurse's hand being placed on her arm. However, this type of touch may not be therapeutic or well received by a male adolescent who has just been told that he has diabetes and who is in the process of venting anger. It is better to let him get the anger out than to try to console him.
- Do not use a touch gesture that imposes more intimacy on a patient than he or she desires. To some people, certain gestures may imply a level of intimacy or degree of closeness. When the touch suggests a degree of closeness that is not equally shared or agreed on by both parties, distress may occur. The patient may be offended if his or her personal space is violated.
- Observe the patient's response to the touch. Assessment of a touch is especially important in the initial meeting with a patient, when the nurse does not know how the patient will respond. The nurse should observe the patient's nonverbal behaviors. For example, if the patient pulls away or displays a tense facial expression, he or she may be having a negative reaction or response to the touch. On the other hand, if a patient appears relaxed and more comforted after the touch, it is likely that he or she is receiving the touch positively.
- In healthcare situations in which both the nurse and the patient are comfortable with touch and the use of touch is assessed for therapeutic effect, touch can be a very valuable mode of human communication.

Kinesics

Kinesics, commonly referred to as body language, is an important component of nonverbal communication (Arnold & Boggs, 2011). Kinesics is also defined as involving the conscious or subconscious body positioning and actions of the individual giving the message. Some dimensions of kinesics are posturing and gait, gestures, and facial expressions. Body stance can convey a message about the nurse or the patient. If the patient is in a slumped, head-down position, the nurse may assess that the patient may have low self-esteem, whereas an erect posture and decisive movements may suggest confidence and self-control. Rapid, diffuse, or agitated body movements may indicate anxiety.

Facial Expressions

Facial expressions, the various movements in the face, provide emotional undertone and feeling whether or not they are accompanied by verbal communication. Throughout life, individuals respond to the expressive qualities of another face, often without realizing it. Mehrabian (1981), in studying the impact of words, vocalization, and facial expressions, noted that the power of the facial expression supporting the verbal content far outweighs the impact of the actual words.

Facial expression is important in conveying a message; it either reinforces or changes the verbal message that the listener hears. When the verbal message is inconsistent or different from the individual's facial expression, the nonverbal expressions assume more prominence and meaning and are generally perceived as more trustworthy and meaningful than the spoken word (Mehrabian, 1981).

The face is the most expressive part of the body, adding obvious and subtle cues to the real focus of the message. Common facial expressions are surprise, sadness, anger, happiness and joy, disgust and contempt, and fear (Arnold & Boggs, 2011). A patient's facial expression should be part of the nursing assessment. For example, if a patient frowns after receiving information, he or she may be experiencing confusion or anger. The nurse can intervene by saying, "I see that you are frowning. Is something wrong?" The question would encourage the patient to clarify his or her response.

In the healthcare profession, it is very important for the nurse's facial expression to be congruent with the verbal message given to the patient. When a nurse walks into a patient's hospital room, the patient will "search" the nurse's face for clues before the nurse can even speak. For example, if the patient asks the nurse, "Do I have cancer?" the slightest change in the nurse's facial features can reveal the nurse's answer. Although it is difficult to control all facial expressions, the nurse should try to avoid showing overt shock, revulsion, dismay, and other distressing reactions in the patient's presence. If the nurse comes into a patient's room with an expression of anger, stress, or disgust, the patient and his family may perceive the nurse to be uncaring.

Appearance

The nurse's **physical appearance**, including dress, grooming, posture, gestures, and ease of movements, makes an important impact on the patient and conveys the nurse's attitudes about himself or herself and others. Studies have shown that spoken words account for only 7 percent of the message. Tattoos and body art, although very popular these days, can be frightening and offensive to some patients (Cardillo, 2009; Rizk & Bofinger, 2008).

The business world has been aware of the "dress for success" rule and has noted the role clothes play in projecting the image of the serious professional. Nursing is no different; the patient reacts to the way a nurse is dressed. In the past, nurses wore white uniforms and caps in designs that represented their various schools of nursing. In today's healthcare environment there is no standard uniform for the professional nurse—a fact that does tend to confuse the layperson. What nurses wear is usually determined by the area of the hospital in which they work or the role they have in the community. Mangum, Garrison, Lind, Thackeray, and Wyatt (1991) surveyed patients, nurses, and administrators to determine whether or not different styles of nursing uniforms are associated with the professional image of nursing. In their summary, they noted that the nurse is judged primarily by what is worn and presented at the bedside. The nurse should make a conscious effort to dress in a professional way.

Therapeutic Communication

Therapeutic communication, a term coined by Ruesch (1961), is defined as a purposeful form of communication between the health professional and the patient that allows them to reach health-related goals through participation in a focused relationship. "Therapeutic communication differs from ordinary communication in that the intention of one or more of the participants is clearly directed at bringing about a change in the system and manner of communication" (Ruesch, 1961, p. 460). This type of communication differs from a social communication because there is a specific purpose or planned direction to the communication. The nurse uses therapeutic communication to promote a psychological setting that allows positive change, growth, and healing for the patient. As the professional caregiver, the nurse comes to know the patient as an individual who has unique health needs, responses, and patterns of living. With this knowledge, the nurse uses a goal-directed approach when communicating with the patient.

Therapeutic communication can take place in a variety of clinical settings, ranging from the acute care system to nursing homes. As healthcare delivery moves to a community focus, therapeutic communication can take place in nontraditional healthcare settings such as patients' homes, schools, and ambulatory care settings. Therapeutic conversations in healthcare settings are designed to help patients maintain healthy habits, learn about their illness, and learn ways of coping. The communication is goal oriented and patient centered, has rules and boundaries, and uses individualized strategies (Arnold & Boggs, 2011).

Therapeutic Communication Techniques

A number of techniques are used in therapeutic communication (Box 6.1). Nurses should familiarize themselves with and make it a habit to use these techniques both in and outside of therapeutic situations.

Active Listening

Effective therapeutic communication between the nurse and patient begins with **active listening** (Bush, 2001). Listening actively means that the listener is communicating interest and attention to the patient. The goal of active listening is to comprehend and understand fully what the other person is trying to communicate.

Two important techniques used by the nurse in active listening are restatement and reflection (Craven & Hirnle, 2009). Restatement takes place when the nurse listens carefully to the patient and then restates some or all of the content back to the patient to ensure that the nurse has the correct understanding of what the patient has said. When the content is restated, the patient has the opportunity to hear what he or she has said and therefore gains an understanding of how the nurse has perceived what he or she has communicated. The nurse listens to the patient for both content and emotions expressed through nonverbal facial expression, body posture, and emotional status.

Reflection is the process of identifying the main emotional themes in the conversation and directing them back to the patient (Box 6.2). The nurse listens for the underlying feeling that the patient is conveying and then shares this with the patient in a nonjudgmental, open manner. This process allows the patient to explore his or her own ideas and gives the patient a clearer understanding of the feelings being experienced.

BOX 6.1	Therapeutic Communication Techniques

- Active listening
- Restatement
- Reflection
- Asking appropriate questions
- Focusing
- Encouraging elaboration
- Looking at alternatives
- Use of silence

BOX 6.2 **Reflection and Restatement**

Patient: I don't want to eat anything today. I can't even begin to think about food.
Nurse: You don't want to eat, and you can't think about food. (Restatement)
Patient: All I can think about is what the doctor will tell me about the biopsy. (Patient is wringing her hands and almost crying.)
Nurse: The news about the biopsy result is worrying you and makes you unable to eat. (Reflection)
Patient: Yes, I'm very nervous that it will mean that I have to have more surgery. I'm really frightened.

Questions

Questions are an important part of all phases of therapeutic communication because they allow the nurse to obtain information from the patient. The nurse needs to ask pertinent questions, but not to the point that the patient feels that he or she is being interrogated.

Arnold and Boggs (2011) suggest that questions can be divided into three categories: open ended, close ended, and circular. Open-ended questions are stated in such a way that the patient is able to elaborate beyond a simple yes or no answer. This gives the patient a way to "tell a story." Think of such a question as an essay question on a test. It gives the patient a chance to express thoughts about a problem or health need. Open-ended questions often begin with words like "How," "Why," and "Can you describe." Examples of open-ended questions are, "What brought you to the hospital?" and "Can you tell me about your being diagnosed with diabetes?" These questions are general, rather than specific, and are open to the patient's interpretation.

Closed-ended questions require specific answers and limit a patient's response. These types of questions are best used in emergency situations, and it may take more of them to get the desired response. In this situation the nurse wants to obtain information quickly, and the patient's emotional reactions are secondary. Examples of closed-ended questions are, "When did the pain start?" and "How long has it been since you saw the doctor?"

Circular questions focus on the impact of the illness or injury and how it will affect the family and significant others. Circular questions differ from open-ended questions because the nurse is intentionally asking specific questions to elicit responses from the patient or a family member. The nurse uses circular questions as a type of family interviewing strategy. The nurse can use the information that the family or others provide as a basis for additional questions about the patient or other family members. For example, the nurse asks family members about the care of a terminally ill patient (the mother) in their home. From the family's response, the nurse may receive multidimensional information about the family that could not be learned by asking specific questions. This approach provides a basis for open discussion of the patient and the family's circumstances.

Other Therapeutic Communication Techniques

Other techniques the nurse may use in therapeutic communication are focusing, encouraging elaboration, and looking at alternatives. Focusing means asking goal-directed questions that help keep the patient focused on the subject at hand. The nurse is also conveying that he or she is helping the patient discuss the main areas of concern. The nurse can also encourage elaboration. This technique allows the patient to describe the concerns or problems under discussion in a more detailed manner. The nurse can look attentively at the patient and use short responses such as "I see" and "Go on" to allow the patient to continue to explore feelings. Looking at alternatives allows the nurse to help the patient increase the patient's perceived choices. This technique should not be used until the patient has a clear understanding of the current situation. Sometimes the patient has to deal with emotions such as anger and denial before alternatives come into play.

Probably one of the most difficult techniques the nurse must learn is the use of silence, that period when no words are being spoken between the nurse and the patient. For Americans in particular, it takes experience to become comfortable with pauses in the conversation. Most people have a natural tendency to try to fill up the empty spaces with words. By contrast, many Native Americans consider silence essential to understanding and respecting what the nurse has said. In traditional Chinese and Japanese cultures, silence may mean that the speaker wants the listener to consider the importance of the content before continuing. British and Arab people may use silence as a sign of respect for the individual's privacy, whereas French, Spanish, and Russian individuals may consider silence a sign of agreement. Among some African Americans, silence is used to respond to what is perceived as an inappropriate statement (Andrews & Boyle, 1999).

In therapeutic relations, silent moments give the nurse and the patient time to observe each other, digest what messages have been communicated, and think of things to say. Silence can be used deliberately and thoughtfully and can be a powerful listening tool. On the other hand, long silences may be very uncomfortable. By pausing briefly before continuing a conversation with a patient, the nurse gives the patient a chance to reflect and come up with questions of his or her own.

Barriers to Communication

In the therapeutic communication setting, the nurse must be aware of certain responses that may lower the patient's self-esteem and limit full disclosure of patient information. Among the responses that tend to block or present barriers to communication (Box 6.3) are the following:

- Giving false reassurance is the use of clichés or comforting phrases in order to attempt to reassure the patient. These types of responses invalidate the patient's feelings or fears. Expressions such as "Everything will be okay" and "Don't worry" send a message to the patient that the nurse is not interested in the patient's true feelings.

BOX 6.3 **Communication Barriers**

- Giving false reassurance
- Offering advice
- Probing
- Stereotyping
- Providing social comment
- Changing the subject
- Using jargon

- Offering advice is telling the patient what to do or making a decision for the patient. The nurse should avoid offering personal opinions to the patient. Avoid phrases such as "should do" or "ought to do." These types of responses tend to center the interaction on the nurse's needs and perspective rather than on the patient's. If a patient asks a nurse for specific advice, the nurse can use a reflective statement and explore the various choices the patient has in that situation.
- Probing is asking questions out of curiosity rather than for information needed to assist the patient. Many of these questions begin with the word "Why." These types of questions from the nurse tend to put the patient in a defensive mode and also violate the patient's privacy.
- Stereotyping is the process of attributing characteristics to a group of people as though all people in that group possess those features. Stereotyping groups patients in a category and does not value or recognize their individuality. Stereotypes lead the nurse to make false conclusions about the patient, and if they are based on strong emotions, stereotypes can be identified as prejudices. It is important for the nurse to convey acceptance of the patient as a unique individual.
- Providing social comment refers to the use of polite, superficial comments that do not focus on what the patient is feeling or trying to express to the nurse. The nurse can use social comments at the beginning of an interaction to make a connection with the patient. However, the nurse should focus on a therapeutic interaction with the patient when talking about issues or concerns that affect the patient's health. Socialization is inappropriate when a more serious approach to the patient's situation is suitable.
- Changing the subject when the patient is trying to communicate about another topic is rude and shows a lack of sensitivity. Changing the subject tends to block communication; the patient may withhold information about important issues and fail to express his or her feelings openly. If the nurse does have to change the subject, the reason for this change should be given to the patient.
- Using jargon—medical terminology that is used among nurses and other health professionals—when addressing the patient can cause confusion and anxiety. It may also be frightening to some patients. Nurses should try to use common terms with which the patient is familiar. If nurses need to use jargon,

they should make sure that they carefully explain what the terms mean.

COMMUNICATION WITH COLLEAGUES

Healthcare is provided in a complex environment and requires a team approach to deliver effective, safe, and quality care to patients. In 2010, Congress passed and President Obama signed into law comprehensive healthcare legislation. This legislation represents the greatest change in healthcare since the 1965 creation of the Medicare and Medicaid programs and is expected to provide insurance coverage for an additional 32 million uninsured Americans (Institute of Medicine, 2010). The nursing profession will be asked to increase teamwork and collaboration with other disciplines to enhance safety, quality, and efficiency of the healthcare system (Buerhaus et al., 2012).

Nurses must communicate effectively with a diverse group of professionals and unlicensed personnel in caring for patients. When members of the healthcare team communicate ineffectively with one another, delivery of healthcare to the patient suffers. Nearly 70 percent of all medical errors are a direct result of communication breakdown and are avoidable (Greenberg et al., 2007). Effective communication has been shown to influence patient safety. This finding has prompted several healthcare organizations, including the Institute of Medicine and the Agency for Healthcare Research and Quality (AHRQ), to call for improvement in communication skills among healthcare workers, and they have provided strategies toward that end. Furthermore, The Joint Commission has included in its 2015 National Patient Safety Goals for Hospitals a goal to "improve the staff communication" (http://www.jointcommission.org/assets/1/6/2015_HAP_NPSG_ER.pdf).

Given that communication is a part of everyday work and an important requirement of patient safety, organizations must recognize the value of teamwork and work toward improving communication within the team. In a team approach, each person recognizes the boundaries of each discipline and values the contribution that every person makes. Methods of teamwork must be adapted in the workplace to create an environment in which all levels of staff work together and respect each other's opinions.

To achieve this atmosphere, team training can be provided. The U.S. Department of Defense, with assistance from the AHRQ, developed a program known as TeamSTEPPS (http://teamstepps.ahrq.gov/), which stands for Team Strategies and Tools to Enhance Performance and Patient Safety. TeamSTEPPS is an evidence-based model that gives instruction to healthcare professionals on how to improve communication and teamwork skills. The goal is to improve patient safety. Communication is an important principle in this model. Because nurses are the managers of patient care and are with the patient in healthcare settings 24/7, they obtain a great amount of information that must be communicated to other healthcare providers. Nurses realize how important it is to communicate in a clear fashion by thinking about the information that needs to be shared and using a communication technique that other individuals will be able to hear and accept.

Professional Collaboration

To work effectively in a team, nurses must understand the concept of professional collaboration in the context of today's workplace. The Quality and Safety Education for Nurses (QSEN) Institute defines teamwork and collaboration as the ability to "function effectively with nursing and interprofessional teams, fostering open communication, mutual respect, and shared decision-making to achieve quality patient care" (http://qsen.org/competencies/graduate-ksas/#teamwork_collaboration). **Collaboration** is a complex process that requires individuals to be willing to share information about the patient from their own area of expertise. Each discipline that cares for the patient has its own knowledge, skills, and clinical experiences. Respect for each other's knowledge, skills, background, and clinical decision-making is the backbone of a positive collaborative arrangement. It is also important to find the common ground between disciplines because there may be differing patterns of communication (Grover, 2005). Individuals caring for the patient bring unique contributions from the various disciplines. Consider the following observation:

> *Collaboration is significantly more complex than simply working in close proximity to one another. It implies a bond, a joining together, a union, and a degree of caring about one another and the relationship. A collaborative relationship is not merely the sum of its parts, but it is a synergistic alliance that maximizes the contributions of each participant resulting in action that is greater than the sum of individual works.* (Evans, 1994, p. 23)

Therefore, the challenge is to make the most of each encounter and interaction so that the best knowledge and ability of each team member are recognized and valued. In addition to communication, other characteristics of collaboration include accountability and mutual respect. Each person must be accountable for his or her actions and accept the results of his or her decisions or actions. However, in the interest of the care of the patient, no profession stands alone, and the use of good collaborative skills is essential (Lindeke & Sieckert, 2006). Collaboration allows the nurse to identify the contributions of the other disciplines and permits the integration of this information into the healthcare plan for the patient. One study showed that as many as 85 to 95 percent of healthcare workers do not feel able to speak up when they see mistakes being made in patient care (Maxfield, Grenny, McMillan, Patterson, & Switzler, 2005).

Nurses must make a concerted effort to have a collaborative relationship with team members, not just to work in cooperation with them (Silva & Ludwick, 2002). They must value the other team members' suggestions and different perspectives. Using insights from other disciplines and healthcare workers also helps enhance problem-solving skills. Collaboration with other members of the healthcare team is essential for the nursing profession to provide excellent healthcare to all patients.

Workplace collaboration can be reflected on every level of healthcare and is required to achieve cost-effectiveness, quality improvement, and efficiency. Improving patient care and creating gratifying work roles are added benefits.

Barriers to Communication with Colleagues

The many barriers to effective communication among colleagues in healthcare include lack of time to communicate properly; stressful work environments of high patient acuity and staffing shortages; gender, generational, education, or cultural differences; and communication styles (e.g., nurses may give a more narrative description of a patient's condition, whereas physicians may be more action oriented and want the problem to be stated so that action can be taken) (Boaro, Fancott, Baker, Velji, & Andreoli, 2010; Flicek, 2012; Nadzam, 2009). In addition, advances in technology have increased the ways in which messages are delivered, including text pagers, cell phones, and patient inbox messaging, which can add to the complexity of communicating effectively (Flicek, 2012).

Mutual respect is of utmost importance among all members of the healthcare team and must be valued by each individual. In addition, all hierarchy must be eliminated because a healthcare system that is hierarchal in nature does not encourage collaborative practice. Hierarchy is also a barrier to communication. For example, some old-school male physicians may still think that the nurse (traditionally a position dominated by women) should be subservient and have no contribution on a professional level.

In collaboration there is no implied supervision; it is a two-way exchange of information. The relationship between individuals who are collaborating is nonhierarchical. The power is shared and is based on the knowledge and expertise that each individual brings to the setting, not on role or title (Henneman, Lee, & Cohen, 1995). When there is true collaboration in the workplace, the responsibility for the patient is shared; the professionalism of all is strengthened when each member of the group has participated and has obtained success. The unique perspective that each profession brings to a situation tends to result in creative and practical solutions, and in turn, the patient's well-being is of utmost importance. To practice effective communication in the workplace setting, each individual must be willing to participate equally.

Strategies to Increase Communication in Teamwork
Structured Communication Tools

The use of structured communication tools can help organize information, decrease hierarchy, and eliminate differences in communication style. Standardized tools provide strategies to improve the quality of communication between team members and prevent medical errors (Boaro et al., 2010). Several tools are available. The **SBAR** (**S**ituation-**B**ackground-**A**ssessment-**R**ecommendation) system is a format used to structure and standardize communication between healthcare workers, especially during critical situations. Noncritical situation handoff and intershift reporting tools include the formats of "I PASS the BATON," developed by TeamSTEPPS, and ISHAPED, developed by the Institute for Healthcare Improvement (IHI).

SBAR

The SBAR format provides a framework for communication between members of the healthcare team about a patient's condition. It is particularly useful for reporting changes in a patient's status. Other common uses of SBAR include "handoffs," or changes of services. An example of a handoff occurs when a patient is being transferred from the emergency department and admitted to a bed on the inpatient unit.

SBAR is easy to remember and useful for framing any conversation, especially critical ones, requiring a clinician's immediate attention and action. It allows users to organize information in a focused way to set expectations for what will be communicated and how it will be communicated between members of the team, which is essential for developing teamwork and fostering a culture of patient safety. Nurses should organize factual data when presenting information to other team members. The following is a breakdown for each SBAR element:

- Situation: What is going on with the patient?
  Mrs. Adams called me to her room to say that she feels dizzy and her heart is racing.
- Background: What is the clinical background or context?
  Mrs. Adams is a 72-year-old diabetic patient who has a history of hypertension.
- Assessment: What do I think the problem is?
  I think the problem is very likely related to Mrs. Adams' heart and cardiovascular system.
- Recommendation: What would I do to correct it?
  I think you should come to the unit to see Mrs. Adams to examine her. We can also perform an electrocardiogram.

Intershift Report

Handoffs and intershift reports occur two to three times a day or more. Intershift report is a face-to-face handoff between the oncoming and off-going nurses. Ineffective handoffs have been identified as a barrier to patient safety and quality by providing the potential for miscommunication, patient harm, and neglect (Thomas & Donahue-Porter, 2012). Use of structured communication tools assists healthcare workers to give complete and accurate information.

"I PASS the BATON"

"I PASS the BATON" is a tool that was developed for the TeamSTEPPS program to standardize communication in patient care handoffs (Rawlings, 2011). It also can remind clinicians of the key information and factors to include during their medical handoffs. This tool promotes a culture that encourages staff to clarify, question, and confirm information communicated about the patient. The components of "I PASS the BATON" are as follows:

- Introduction
  Introduce yourself and your role/job to the patient.

- Patient
  Name, identifiers, age, sex, location
- Assessment
  Presenting chief complaint, vital signs, and symptoms and diagnosis
- Situation
  Current status and circumstances, including code status, level of (un)certainty, recent changes, response to treatment
- Safety Concerns
  Critical laboratory values and reports, socioeconomic factors, allergies, alerts (e.g., falls, isolation)
- THE
- Background
  Comorbidities, previous episodes, current medications, family history
- Actions
  What actions were taken or are required, and brief rationale
- Timing
  Level of urgency and explicit timing, prioritization of actions
- Ownership
  Who is responsible (nurse/doctor/team), including patient/family responsibilities
- Next
  What will happen next; any anticipated changes; what is the plan, including any contingency plans

Further explanation of this tool can be found online at http://www.ahrq.gov/professionals/education/curriculumtools/teamstepps/instructor/fundamentals/index.html.

ISHAPED

The ISHAPED tool was developed by the INOVA Health Systems in Falls Church, Virginia, with help from the Picker Institute, for use during a handoff or intershift report. The IHI chose the Picker Institute to develop systems to promote patient-centered and family-centered healthcare. This tool is to be used at the bedside so that the patient is involved in the report. Again, it assists healthcare workers to communicate key information while giving the opportunity for the receiver to clarify, question, and confirm information. ISHAPED is an acronym similar to SBAR. Its components are Introduction, Story, History, Assessment, Plan, Error Prevention, and Dialogue.

The ISHAPED tool can be adapted to any clinical setting or system. The process should include the following steps:

1. The handoff happens at the bedside: S, H, A components occur outside of the room; I, P, E, D components occur in the room.
2. Clinical judgment and common sense are used to determine whether a bedside component is inappropriate for a particular patient.
3. The written ISHAPED handoff template is completed by the off-going nurse and given to the oncoming nurse.

Additional information and tools are available at http://www.ihi.org/resources/Pages/Tools/ISHAPEDPatient CenteredNurseShiftChangeBedsideReport.aspx.

Other Techniques

The TeamSTEPPS approach teaches other strategies that promote teamwork and thereby increase patient safety. A technique using CUS words presents a method in which a team member can resolve conflict, advocate for patients, and give mutual support. Techniques of face-to-face gathering of the team for a review of the plan before the event, problem solving during the event, or process improvement after the event are strategies that can promote every team member being on the same page.

CUS Words

CUS words were developed in the TeamSTEPPS program to provide another framework for conflict resolution, advocacy, and mutual support. CUS words are signal words, similar to "danger," "warning," and "caution." Using CUS words, nurses can signal the need to stop, address real or potential risks, and avoid patient safety events. CUS words are **C** = I am **c**oncerned, **U** = I am **u**ncomfortable, and **S** = there is a **s**afety issue. They catch the listener's attention. When CUS words are spoken, the team member or members will understand clearly not only the issue but also the magnitude of the issue. The process of this technique is as follows:

- First, state your **c**oncern.
- Then state why you are **u**ncomfortable.
- If the conflict is not resolved, state that there is a **s**afety issue. Discuss in what way the concern is related to safety. If the safety issue is not acknowledged, a supervisor should be notified.

Briefs-Huddles-Debriefs

Under the construct of Leadership, the TeamSTEPPS program outlines three techniques used to promote teamwork. These are the brief, huddle, and debrief.

Brief is defined as a short planning session before the beginning of an event (AHRQ, 2012). The "briefing" can be used to discuss who is on the team, assign roles and responsibilities, establish expectations, and review the plan. If there is a "checklist," as with some procedures or in the operating room, these can also be completed at this time.

Huddle is defined as an informal, unplanned team meeting. There can be several reasons that a team would use a huddle, including reinforcing a plan already in place for the treatment of a patient, refocusing team members to the plan of care, providing updated information requiring adjustment of the plan, and assessing the need to change plans. Huddles also afford team leaders an opportunity to informally monitor patient and unit-level situations that occur (AHRQ, 2012).

Debrief is defined as a feedback or informal information exchange session that occurs shortly after an event (AHRQ, 2012). It is designed to improve team performance and effectiveness, focusing on what went well, what did not go well, and what can be done in the future to improve performance.

Nurses will be increasingly challenged to become skilled team players as the delivery of care becomes more complex. With various team members coming from different perspectives, effective communication is essential to positive patient outcomes and will result in creative and practical solutions (Pagana, 2011). Take the time and effort to learn from others' perspectives and to encourage new team members to share their experiences. Basic therapeutic techniques of communication are essential; nurses must be aware of the variables of gender, hierarchy, and collegiality and have basic mutual respect for each member of the health team. Nurses should continue to demonstrate that the nursing profession is unique and that nurses bring a different perspective to the patient's care. The attitudes and skills associated with collaborative relationships can be learned if all parties are willing to participate.

ONLINE CONSULT

The *American Communication Journal* at
http://www.acjournal.org/

EVIDENCE-BASED PRACTICE: *Consider this....*

Kalisch, Lee, and Rochman describe nursing teams on acute care patient units, noting that a higher level of teamwork and perceptions of adequate staffing lead to greater job satisfaction with current position and occupation. Teamwork and perceptions of adequate staffing were reported as the major contributors to job satisfaction on acute care units (p. 945).

Question: How will you use this information as a nurse or nurse-manager to improve communication and collaboration on your unit?

Source: Kalisch, B. J., Lee, H., & Rochman, M. (2010). Nursing staff teamwork and job satisfaction. *Journal of Nursing Management, 18*, 938–947.

KEY POINTS

- Effective communication within the nurse-patient relationship is a learned skill and is essential for providing effective nursing care.

- Communication models illustrate the complex process of communication with the basic components: the source/encoder, the message, the medium, and the receiver/decoder.

- The health communications model uses a broad systems view of communication and emphasizes the way in which a series of factors (relationships, transactions, and contexts) can affect interactions in the healthcare setting.

- When people share information, they express messages in a complex composite of both verbal (spoken or written) and nonverbal behaviors. Individuals express themselves through language, gestures, voice inflection, facial expressions, and use of space.

- Metacommunication is a broad term used to "describe all of the factors that influence how the message is perceived" (Arnold & Boggs, 2011, p. 163).

- Oral communication is the use of words by people to think about ideas, to share experiences with others, and to validate the perceptions of the world.

- Potter and Perry (2013) state that the six most important aspects of verbal communication are (1) vocabulary, (2) denotative and connotative meaning, (3) intonation, (4) pacing, (5) clarity and brevity, and (6) timing and relevance.

- Nonverbal communication is communication without words and includes messages that are created through body motions, facial expressions, use of space and sounds, and use of touch. Arnold and Boggs (2011) categorize areas in which nonverbal behaviors are used: touch, proxemics, nonverbal body clues, facial expression, and clothing.

- For patients to perceive touch in a positive therapeutic relationship, Northouse and Northouse (1998) suggest that nurses use the following guidelines: use touch that is appropriate to the particular situation, do not use a touch that imposes more intimacy on a patient than he or she desires, and observe the patient's response to the touch.

- Therapeutic communication is a purposeful form of communication that serves as a point of contact between the health professional and the patient and allows them to reach health-related goals through participation in a focused relationship. Techniques include active listening, restatement, reflection, focusing, encouraging elaboration, looking at alternatives, use of silence, and use of appropriate questions.

- Barriers to communication are certain responses that may lower the patient's self-esteem, limit full disclosure of patient information, and block communication. These barriers include giving false reassurance, giving advice, probing, stereotyping, providing social comment, changing the subject, and using jargon.

- Collaboration in the workplace depends on working in cooperation with other members of the healthcare team. The power is shared and is based on the knowledge and expertise that each member brings to the setting; mutual respect is of utmost importance for successful communication.

- Several tools have been developed for teams to enhance and improve their communication, including the SBAR, ISHAPED, and CUS words for critical communication and handoffs and briefings, huddles, and debriefings techniques for short team discussions.

Thought and Discussion Questions

1. Contrast various communication models for use in the hospital versus the home setting.

2. Explain how nonverbal communication may be more "powerful" than spoken words.

3. Describe a collaborative relationship that you have experienced in your work setting.

4. Read Coeling and Cukr's (2000) article "Communication Styles That Promote Perceptions of Collaboration, Quality, and Nurse Satisfaction" in the *Journal of Nursing Care Quality 14*(2), 63–74. Form a study group and discuss the various aspects of this evidence-based practice study. How does this affect your workplace issues? What new techniques could you introduce in your workplace?

5. Review the Chapter Thought on the first page of the chapter and discuss it in the context of the contents of the chapter.

Interactive Exercises

Go to the Intranet site and complete the interactive exercises provided for this chapter.

REFERENCES

Agency for Healthcare Research and Quality (AHRQ). (2012). *TeamSTEPPS instructor guide.* Agency for Healthcare Research and Quality, Rockville, MD: AHRQ. Retrieved from http://www.ahrq.gov/professionals/education/curriculum-tools/teamstepps/instructor/index.html

Andrews, M., & Boyle, J. (1999). *Transcultural concepts in nursing care* (3rd ed.). Philadelphia, PA: Lippincott.

Arnold, E., & Boggs, K. (2011). *Interpersonal relationships: Professional communication skills for nurses* (6th ed.). Philadelphia, PA: Saunders/Elsevier.

Berlo, D. K. (1960). *The process of communication: An introduction to theory and practice.* New York: Holt, Rinehart & Winston.

Birdwhistell, R. L. (1970). *Kinesics and context.* Philadelphia, PA: University of Pennsylvania Press.

Boaro, N., Fancott, C., Baker, R., Velji, K., & Andreoli, A. (2010). Using SBAR to improve communication in interprofessional rehabilitation teams. *Journal of Interprofessional Care, 24*(1), 111–114.

Buerhaus, P. I., DesRoches, C., Applebaum, S., Hess, R., Norman, L. D., & Donelan, K. (2012). Are nurses ready for health care reform? A decade of survey research. *Nursing Economic$, 30*(6), 318–329.

Bush, K. (2001). Do you really listen to patients? *RN 2001, 64*(3), 35–37.

Cardillo, D. (2009). Projecting your professionalism. *NSNA Imprint,* 30–31. Retrieved from www.nurse.com

Craven, R., & Hirnle, C. (2009). *Fundamentals of nursing: Human health and function* (6th ed.). Philadelphia, PA: Lippincott-Raven.

Evans, J. (1994). The role of the nurse manager in creating an environment for collaborative practice. *Holistic Nursing Practice, 8,* 22–31.

Flicek, C. L. (2012). Communication: A dynamic between nurses and physicians, *MedSurg Nursing, 21*(6), 385–387.

Greenberg, C. C., Regenbogen, S. E., Studdert, D. M., Lipsitz, S. R., Rogers, S. O., Zinner, M. J., & Gawande, A. A. (2007). Patterns of communication breakdowns resulting in injury to surgical patients. *Journal of the American College of Surgeons, 204,* 533–540.

Grover, S. (2005). Shaping effective communication skills and therapeutic relationships at work. *American Association of Occupational Health Nurses Journal, 53*(4), 177–187.

Hall, E. T. (1959). *The silent language.* Garden City, NY: Doubleday & Company.

Henneman, E. A., Lee, J. L., & Cohen, J. I. (1995). Collaboration: A concept analysis. *Journal of Advanced Nursing, 21*(1), 103–109.

Institute of Medicine. (2010). *The future of nursing: Leading change, advancing health.* Retrieved from http://www.iom.edu/Reports/2010/The-Future-of-Nursing-Leading-Change-Advancing-Health.aspx

Kalisch, B. J., Lee, H., & Rochman, M. (2010). Nursing staff teamwork and job satisfaction. *Journal of Nursing Management, 18,* 938–947.

Ku, L., & Flores, G. (2005). Pay now or pay later: Providing interpreter services in health care. *Health Affairs, 24*(2), 435–444.

Lindeke, L., & Sieckert, A. (2005). Nurse-physician workplace collaboration. *Online Journal of Issues in Nursing.* Retrieved from http://www.nursingworld.org/MainMenuCategories/ANAMarketplace/ANAPeriodicals/OJIN/TableofContents/Volume102005/No1Jan05/tpc26_416011.html

Mangum, S., Garrison, C., Lind, A., Thackeray, R., & Wyatt, M. (1991). Perceptions of nurses' uniforms. *Image: The Journal of Nursing Scholarship, 23*(2), 127–130.

Maxfield, D., Grenny, J., McMillan, R., Patterson, K., & Switzer, A. (2005). *Silence kills: The seven crucial conversations for healthcare.* Vital Smarts, E45. Retrieved from http://www.aacn.org/WD/practice/docs/publicpolicy/silencekills.pdf

Mehrabian, A. (1981). *Silent messages* (2nd ed.). Belmont, CA: Wadsworth Publishing.

Mitchell, R. W. (1991). Bateson's concept of metacommunication in play. *New Ideas in Psychology, 9*(1), 73–87.

Nadzam, D. (2009). Nurses' role in communication and patient safety. *Journal of Nursing Care Quality, 24*(3), 184–188.

Northouse, P. G., & Northouse, L. L. (1998). *Health communication strategies for health professionals* (3rd ed.). Norwalk, CT: Appleton & Lange.

Pagana, K. (2011). *The nurse's communication advantage.* Indianapolis, IN: Sigma Theta Tau International.

Potter, A., & Perry, G. (2013). *Fundamentals of nursing* (8th ed.). St. Louis, MO: Mosby.

Rawlings, T. (2011). Passing the baton to standardize handoffs. *OR Nurse, 5*(4), 48.

Rizk, K., & Bofinger, R. (2008). Florence Nightingale versus Dennis Rodman: Evaluating professional image in the modern world. *Annual Review of Nursing Education, 6,* 189–204.

Ruesch, J. (1961). *Therapeutic communication.* New York: W. W. Norton.

Silva, M., & Ludwick, R. (2002). Ethics Column. Ethical grounding for entry into practice: Respect, collaboration, and accountability. *Online Journal of Issues in Nursing.* Retrieved from http://www.nursingworld.org/MainMenuCategories/ANAMarketplace/ANAPeriodicals/OJIN/Columns/Ethics/GroundingforEntryintoPractice.html

Thomas, L., & Donohoe-Porter, P. (2012). Blending evidence and innovation: Improving intershift handoffs in a multi-hospital setting. *Journal of Nursing Care Quality, 27*(2), 116–124. doi: 10.1097/ngc.obolse318241obsb

Watson, J. (1979). *Nursing: The philosophy and science of caring.* Boston, MA: Little, Brown.

BIBLIOGRAPHY

Brown, G. (1995). Understanding barriers to basing nursing practice upon research: A communication model approach. *Journal of Advanced Nursing, 21,* 154–157.

Buttaro, T. (2008). *Primary care: A collaborative practice* (3rd ed.). St. Louis, MO: Mosby.

Leininger, M., & McFarland, M. (2002). T*ranscultural nursing: Concepts, theories, research and practice* (3rd ed.). New York: McGraw-Hill.

Lindberg, J., Hunter, M., & Kruszewski, A. (1983). *Introduction to person-centered nursing.* Philadelphia, PA: J. B. Lippincott.

Peplau, H. (1952). *Interpersonal relations in nursing.* New York: G. P. Putnam's Sons.

Peplau, H. (1960). Talking with patients. *American Journal of Nursing, 60,* 964–966.

Riley, J. (2008). *Communication in nursing* (6th ed.). St. Louis, MO: Mosby Elsevier.

Salle, A. (1999). Effective communication. In B. Cherry & S. Jacob (Eds.), *Contemporary nursing issues, trends, and management* (pp. 378–402). St. Louis, Mo: Mosby.

Stapleton, S. (1998). Team-building: Making collaborative practice work. *Journal of Nurse-Midwifery, 43*(1), 12–18.

United States Census Bureau. *2007-2011 American Community Survey, Table B16001.*

United States Department of Housing and Urban Development. (2008). *Indiana income limits* [Data file]. Retrieved from http://www.huduser.org/Datasets/IL/IL08/in_fy2008.pdf

ONLINE RESOURCES

The American Communication Journal
http://www.acjournal.org

Institute for Healthcare Improvement
http://www.ihi.org/Pages/default.aspx

The TeamSTEPPS program, available free of charge from the Agency for Healthcare Research and Quality (AHRQ)
http://www.ahrq.gov/teamstepps

The Quality and Safety Education for Nurses (QSEN) Institute
http://qsen.org/

7

Genevieve M. Bartol

Critical Thinking

*"The whole science is nothing more than
a refinement of everyday thinking."*

Albert Einstein, *Physics and Reality* (1936)

Chapter Objectives

On completion of this chapter, the reader will be able to:

1. Explain what the term *critical thinking* means.
2. Describe some important characteristics of the critical thinking process.
3. Discuss the relationships between the nursing process and critical thinking.
4. Apply the components of critical analysis to a given nursing practice situation.
5. Analyze problem-solving skills needed in nursing practice case studies.

Key Terms

Critical Thinking	Hypothesis Testing	Concept Formation
Reflective Thinking	Moral Reasoning	Interpretation of Data
Reactive Thinking	Induction	Application of Principles
Problem Identification	Deduction	Interpretation of Feelings, Attitudes,
Data Collection	Assumption Identification	and Values

The National League for Nursing mandates that schools of nursing demonstrate that critical thinking is taught and measured for accreditation. Thinking is quite simply the action of the mind to produce thought. How, then, does the adjective "critical" modify the word "thinking"? Etymologically, critical is derived from two Greek roots: *kriticos* (discerning judgment) and *kriterion* (standards). Critical also has several connotations. Critical, for example, can also be understood as an inclination to find fault, as an essential element, or as a careful analysis of a problem. There is even plenty of discussion in the literature that the term *critical thinking* should be renamed. Nevertheless, however the term is defined or described, there is general agreement that critical thinking is a core skill that is essential for nursing practice (Robert & Peterson, 2013, p. 85).

The concept of **critical thinking** dates back at least to Socrates in ancient Greece. Dewey (1910, 1933) prompted educators to pay attention to how we think and to teach students how to think. Glaser's (1941) and Black's (1952) writings represent efforts to integrate critical thinking into education (cited in Cassel & Congleton, 1993). Paul (1990) reviewed the efforts to teach reasoning in the 1930s and the 1960s. McPeck (1990) pointed out that before 1980, few schools were concerned with teaching critical thinking, and even fewer theoretical analyses of the concept existed. According to McPeck (1990), he had to search disparate sources to find any sustained published discussions of critical thinking (p. 1) when he researched the topic in 1979–1980. In 1990, Facione and Facione (1996) gathered a panel of 48 educators and scholars, including leading figures in critical thinking theory, to work toward a consensus on the role of critical thinking in educational assessment and instruction.

Facione and Facione (1996) reported that the expert researchers and theoreticians described critical thinking as the purposeful, self-regulatory judgment that results in interpretation, analysis, evaluation, and inference, as well as the explanation of the evidential, conceptual, methodological, criteriological, or contextual considerations on which that judgment was based (p. 129). Rubenfeld and Scheffer (2010) used a Delphi process to arrive at a consensus statement and the components of critical thinking. They determined that critical thinking is "an essential component of professional accountability and quality nursing care" (p. 32). They also identified 10 critical thinking habits of mind and seven critical thinking skills.

As you read this chapter, you will see that despite this statement, the literature is replete with definitions and descriptions of critical thinking. The proliferation of journal articles, monographs, essays, conference papers, and books devoted to exploring critical thinking in nursing testifies to the current interest but also suggests that a closer look at the term is warranted. We generally recognize that the professional practice situations that nurses encounter daily are characteristically complex, rapidly changeable, ambiguous, particular, and rife with conflict. We increasingly accept the fact that patients are dynamic systems within an energy field that includes family, workplace, environment, culture, and life history. We know that nurses base their practice decisions on a broad pool of knowledge derived from a variety of disciplines. The scope and standards of holistic nursing practice define critical thinking as "an active, purposeful, organized cognitive process involving creativity, reflection, problems solving, both rational and intuitive judgment, an attitude of inquiry, and a philosophical orientation toward thinking about thinking" (Mariano, 2013, p. 59).

With the holistic nursing practice definition in mind, we will expand on and detail the context and role of critical thinking in nursing.

CRITICAL THINKING IN NURSING

Nurses have been long taught to use the nursing process to guide their practice. The nursing process provides a structure for using knowledge and thinking to provide holistic care for individuals, families, groups, and communities. The process can be used with all theoretical frameworks and patients in all settings. Although its components may be expressed in slightly different ways, the nursing process is basically a problem-solving method that has served nurses well by helping them use empathic and intellectual processes with scientific knowledge to assess, diagnose, plan, implement, and evaluate nursing care and patient outcomes. When used appropriately, the nursing process involves critical thinking. For example, a nurse observes that a patient who underwent surgery 2 days ago has suddenly become agitated. The nurse will consider several possible reasons for the agitation. He or she will speak with the patient, note anything that occurred before the onset of agitation, and gather assessment data, such as vital signs and signs of bleeding at the surgical site. The nurse will then determine what intervention is needed and evaluate whether the chosen intervention is effective. Using the nursing process in this manner requires active engagement and cannot just be a matter of filling in the columns. Rather, the person using the process must be able to recognize relationships, connections, and patterns that promote continuous bidirectional movement and openness to new possibilities.

New scientific understandings of living systems show that our former mechanistic view of the world is inadequate (Bartol & Courts, 2013). Human beings are complex, highly integrative systems that are embedded in and supporting other systems. Schuster (2002) noted that the commonly used five-column format in nursing care plans was not promoting critical thinking (p. vii). Care plans using this format were lengthy to write, time consuming, and too often simply copied from a book. Furthermore, the column format seemed to promote linear thinking and failed to address the patterns and connections essential to providing holistic nursing care.

Schuster (2002) proposed using a diagrammatic teaching and learning strategy to enable students and faculty to visualize the interrelations among medical diagnoses, nursing diagnoses, assessment data, and treatments. In a three-step process, the major medical diagnoses and the problems that resulted from those diagnoses were identified (step 1), the data were organized into a hierarchy of subordinate concepts (step 2), and the meaningful associations among concepts were indicated with lines and the nursing diagnoses selected (step 3). Schuster called this strategy *concept mapping* and suggested that it promoted critical thinking. This visual map serves as a personal pocket guide to patient care that can be revised as needed throughout the day. The development of this process illustrates the use of critical thinking to promote critical thinking in students of nursing.

The increasing diversity and complexity of nursing practice and the exponential growth of knowledge require nurses who can think critically. Nurses must master the reasoning skills needed to process growing volumes of information. When nurses assess patients, the data they gather need to be organized into meaningful patterns. Responses to treatment and care need to be evaluated continuously to determine whether the nursing diagnosis was appropriate and the intended outcome achieved. In the patient situation described previously, the patient may have injured himself when he bumped into the corner of the bedside table while trying to get to the bathroom without assistance and is bleeding internally from injury to his spleen. Even one additional piece of information related to the patient may change the whole configuration and require a redefinition of the problem. In nursing, situations change so rapidly that reliance on conventional methods, procedure manuals, or traditions to guide judgments about the appropriate nursing action required is insufficient. Although decision trees may serve as reminders for the nurse, they cannot be relied on without using critical thinking. Although the nursing diagnoses categorized by major functional health patterns serve as useful tools and aid in communication with coworkers in planning and implementing nursing care, they are not sufficient. Not even evidence-based practice relieves us of the need for critical thinking. Individual differences must always be considered. Taleb (2010) argues that we must always be alert to the highly improbable and that as we draw on evidence-based practices for a particular condition, we need to keep in mind the problem of the "circularity of statistics" (p. 269). To illustrate further: At one time it was believed that all swans were white. The single sighting of a black swan invalidated that general statement and points to the fragility of our knowledge. There may well be an outlier, and we need to remain open to surprise (Taleb, 2010, p. xvii). Furthermore, the writings of Malcom Gladwell serve to remind us to be alert to how we make judgments (Gladwell, 2005) and how our judgments can change with a change in perspective (Gladwell, 2013). The question always remains whether you have enough data to justify confidence in your decision. Remember, as noted previously, that an additional piece of data may change the whole configuration. We need to always keep in mind our limitations. Furthermore, Gladwell (2005) cautions us that we must understand that we all have not one mind but two, and while our conscious mind may be blocked at one point, our unconscious mind is busy scanning the situation, sifting through possibilities, and processing every conceivable clue (p. 71). Sometimes the direction in which a situation turns is due to factors not directly related to the present problem and completely out of our scope of awareness (Gladwell, 2009, pp. 101–125, 208–292). Although we cannot wait to act until all the data are in, we need to remain open to correction.

Johns (2013) offers a practical guide to developing reflective nursing practice. He explores the value of using structured models of reflection to help the nurse center on the context of care and to promote a caring relationship with patients. The nurse is guided to pay attention to what is unfolding and hence to use reflection as a continual process of assessment or awareness of the shifting and patterns of the patient's experience (p. 213). In what ways has your nursing intervention altered the present state? Has the analgesia you administered made a difference? Or has your lack of presence and concern about another patient tempered the effectiveness of the analgesia you administered? According to Johns, the nurse should use narrative to critically assess his or her own practice.

Then again, Taleb (2013) warns us to be alert to the narrative fallacy in which we become so focused on a single outcome that we fail to imagine other possible outcomes. Quite simply, a critical thinker needs to be able to tolerate ambiguity and remain open to surprises.

By now you realize that critical thinking requires attention to many factors. Complex legal, ethical, organizational, and professional factors are involved in seemingly simple decisions. For example, nurses consider ethical factors (e.g., keeping patient information confidential) and scheduling factors (e.g., when to admit visitors) when they decide not to admit visitors to a unit between 10 a.m. and 12 noon because patients are participating in a support group in the commons room. Visitors passing by the commons room may compromise patient confidentiality.

Nurses make inferences, differentiate facts from opinions, evaluate the credibility of the sources of information, and make decisions, all skills that require critical thinking. Because each of these skills can be learned, at least to some extent, an individual can enhance his or her potential to become an effective critical thinker. We develop critical thinking skills through attention and practice. Even though our skills increase, at no time can we rest assured that we have finished learning and are thus incapable of making the wrong decision (Gladwell, 2009, p. 291; Nance, 2008, pp. 11–24).

Nursing is sometimes described as a boundary discipline because it draws heavily on knowledge from the sciences and humanities. Using information from one subject to shed light on another subject requires critical thinking skills. Nursing is concerned with human beings—highly complex integrative, yet open systems—whose care requires a holistic orientation that attends to cyclic processes and patterns in networks of relationships and not just signs and symptoms. Consequently, nursing curriculums generally include courses from the liberal arts as well as from the sciences. Readers Theater has served to help nurses and physicians heighten awareness of and develop compassion for patients and their families and thus enlarge their perspective (Savitt, 1969). According to oral tradition, it is believed that legislators in early Greece were required to attend the theater for those very purposes.

Conceptually, it may be argued that general critical thinking abilities enhance the ability to make good clinical judgments. Nurses can apply theoretical knowledge to a specific clinical situation, thereby enhancing clinical judgment and decision-making skills. The ability to apply learning from a broad range of disciplines enables nurses to expand and modify existing knowledge to accommodate new situations as well as simplify or speed up the task of learning and performing in new situations. For example, orthopedic nurses use critical thinking when applying knowledge of physics (principles related to levers, fulcrums, and balance in positioning and moving patients), biology (characteristics of a bone in the early stages of healing), and psychology (ways of helping patients manage the anxiety related to increasing mobilization) when safely transferring a patient recovering from a serious car accident. Because educational programs cannot provide students with all of the clinical experiences and all of the information they need to handle every future nursing situation they will encounter, students must learn to be critical thinkers.

Critical thinking includes analyzing and evaluating the soundness of the written information and expressed opinions we encounter. We cannot assume that because the information is published it is valid. We need to identify the strengths and weaknesses in the author's argument and the evidence that is presented. We need to examine any assumptions that the author may have made. We need to consider the patient's context as well as our own for those times when a convenient shortcut is needed (Gladwell, 2002, p. 257).

Definitions

What is critical thinking? Some nursing educators would argue that it is really the same as the nursing process (Jones & Brown, 1993; Kintgen-Andrews, 1991; White, Beardslee, Peters, & Supples, 1990; Woods, 1993). Others insist that although the nursing process requires critical thinking, critical thinking is much more. It is generally maintained, however, that critical thinking is a valuable skill or set of skills capable of being learned and enhanced (Facione & Facione, 2000; Robert & Peterson, 2013; Rubenfeld & Scheffer, 2010; Schuster, 2002; Wilkinson, 2001).

Still, critical thinking is often considered a special, even rare, skill. Although the characteristics of critical thinking match those of sound clinical judgments, a review of the nursing literature indicates that there is no general agreement about what critical thinking is. Definitions abound in the nursing literature; Table 7.1 gives a sampling. The definitions have common elements. Critical thinking is viewed as engaging in a purposeful cognitive activity directed toward establishing a belief or map of action. Each definition speaks to the need for a person to process and evaluate information actively, to validate existing knowledge, and to create new knowledge. Each echoes Dewey's (1933) urging to use **reflective thinking** of the kind that turns a subject over in the mind and gives it serious and consecutive consideration (p. 3). All are

consistent with Dewey's definition of reflective thinking as active, persistent, and careful consideration of any belief or supposed form of knowledge in the light of the grounds that support it and the further conclusions to which it tends (Dewey, 1933, p. 9). All suggest using a thought chain (Dewey, 1993, p. 4) that aims at drawing conclusions. Critical thinking is a process that is engaged in not for itself, but rather for the purpose of providing quality patient care. A thought chain refers simply to the process of moving methodically from one thought to another while remaining open to multiple possibilities. Quite simply, one considers, reflects, decides, and yet remains open to changes, always keeping in mind that one additional piece of data can change the whole configuration and send the process in a new direction.

Different elements are also evident in the definitions and descriptions offered in the nursing literature. Some seem to equate critical thinking with reactive thinking (Kataoka-Yahiro & Saylor, 1994; Kintgen-Andrews, 1991). **Reactive thinking** implies a response to what is, and not to what may yet be. Most view critical thinking as a focused, rational analysis of existing knowledge with very specific steps (Bandman & Bandman, 1994; Kataoka-Yahiro & Saylor, 1994; Kintgen-Andrews, 1991). One refers to creating new knowledge (Case, 1994), whereas another implies that only existing knowledge is uncovered (Bandman & Bandman, 1995). Jones and Brown (1993) examine alternative views on critical thinking, arguing that it is both a philosophical orientation toward thinking and a cognitive process characterized by reasoned judgment and reflective thinking (p. 72).

The discussion about critical thinking continues. The many definitions and descriptions suggest that consensus on the role of critical thinking in nursing has not been reached (Paul & Elder, 2008; Robert & Peterson, 2013; Mariano, 2013).

Descriptions

The following statements gleaned from the literature and the author's own thinking are an attempt to provide a fuller description of the role of critical thinking in nursing.

- Critical thinking is directed toward taking action. Although it is often associated with scientific reasoning, which includes **problem identification**, **data collection**, and **hypothesis testing**, it is not limited to that activity. Critical thinking also includes the affective processes of **moral reasoning** and development of values to guide decisions and actions.
- Critical thinking presumes a disposition toward thinking analytically. Uncritical acceptance of all data is antithetical to critical thinking. An attitude that welcomes intellectual skepticism and honesty is essential. Separating or breaking the whole into parts to uncover the nature, function, and relationships is helpful as long as one maintains a sense of the whole.
- Critical thinking embraces thinking about how we think. We need to monitor our approach to the problem and our reasoning process. An error in reasoning may be as serious a barrier to finding a solution as a

ONLINE CONSULT

Refer to the Interactive Exercises from Chapter 5, on a thoughtful critique of research for evidence-based practice, for questions that may help you critically analyze what you read.

TABLE 7.1

Definitions and Descriptions of Critical Thinking

Definition	Source, Date
"The rational examination of ideas, inferences, assumptions, principles, arguments, conclusions, issues, statements, beliefs and actions" (p. 5).	Bandman & Bandman, 1994
"Reflective and reasonable thinking about nursing problems without a single solution and is focused on deciding what to believe and do" (p. 352).	Kataoka-Yahiro & Saylor, 1994
"A process and cognitive skill that functions in identifying and defining problems and opportunities for improvement; generating, examining and evaluating options; reaching conclusions and decisions, and creating and using criteria to evaluate decisions" (p. 101).	Case, 1994
"Reasonable and reflective thinking that is focused on deciding what to believe or do" (p. 152).	Kintgen-Andrews, 1991
"A process that encompasses a holistic perspective of the entire person— composed of skills, abilities, beliefs, attitudes, goals, emotions, and experiences. In addition, critical thinking involves the ability to view the situation from a holistic perspective" (p. 377).	Thurmond, 2001
"Critical thinking is the process of purposeful, self-regulatory judgment. This process gives reasoned consideration to evidence, contexts, conceptualization, methods and criteria" (ERIC Document Reproduction No. ED 315).	Facione, 1990
"Critical thinking is an active, purposeful, organized cognitive process, involving creativity, reflection, problem-solving, both rational and intuitive judgment, an attitude of inquiry, and a philosophical orientation toward thinking about thinking" (p. 59).	Mariano, 2013

miscalculation in determining a proper drug dose. We should critique the process as well as the proposed solution. Bandman and Bandman (1994) identify fallacies or errors in thinking that one should identify, expose, and resist. To illustrate: A nurse reports that all the laboratory tests for a patient came back negative and implies, therefore, that the patient's symptoms must be "all in her head." The fallacy of the appeal to ignorance consists in arguing that the absence of proof against a diagnosis establishes proof that the patient's symptoms are imaginary.

● Critical thinking assumes maturity. Psychology reminds us that our thinking styles evolve as we grow and develop. We think concretely before we think abstractly. The ability to think abstractly is requisite to critical thinking. We accept many beliefs as children simply because an adult told us they were true. Only as we grow do we question and examine those beliefs. We need to reach the place where we have confidence in our reasoning abilities.

● Critical thinking requires knowledge. A broad educational foundation and a healthy intellectual curiosity are prerequisites. A solid educational foundation needs to be informed by common sense and experience as well as knowledge of one's own biases and limitations (Alfaro-Lefevre, 2013). Zealousness in seeking knowledge and understanding through careful observation and deliberate questioning with openness to possibilities is essential (Rubenfeld & Scheffer, 2010).

● Critical thinking requires skills. We need to know how to gather and evaluate data. We need to distinguish facts from opinions and probe the assumptions behind a line of reasoning. We need to know how to draw inferences from facts and observations, evaluating them as tenable or not. Precision is important. Knowing a fact is insufficient; we need to know how that fact was obtained and from where it was derived. We need to identify what data are missing. Throughout the process, we need to suspend judgment until all the evidence is weighed, even as the situation requires tentative action. There are many ways to view a problem. The way we view a situation influences our proposed solutions.

● Critical thinking, however, is more than a set of skills. Syllogistic thinking, inductive and deductive reasoning, analysis, and synthesis are used, but other styles of thinking are also needed. According to Lonergan (1977), imagination is the highest function of the intellect and precedes all other thinking activities. Certainly, critical thinking uses imagination. Using a metaphor such as a computer or a holograph to describe a function of the brain, for example, can provide additional insight into the process. Critical thinking is creative. We reach original solutions by drawing from past experiences and making creative applications to new situations.

● Critical thinking includes feelings because they are inseparable from all thinking and behavior. Feelings cannot be eliminated or viewed as an inconvenience that complicates the activity of critical thinking, but rather are an integral part of all we do. Our feelings can alert us to possibilities and lead us to creative solutions (Bartol, 1986; Lonergan, 1977). To illustrate: A busy staff nurse realized that she could not take time to listen to an elderly patient who began to tell her about his career as a pilot beginning in the 1940s. He was describing in detail the early planes he piloted. Anxious to meet the needs of her other patients, she told the patient that she had to take care of her other patients, but that she knew someone who would very much like to hear what he had to say. With his permission she called her teenage son who aspired to become a pilot and handed the patient the phone. The patient and her son talked for almost 2 hours to the benefit of both.

- Critical thinking frequently involves finding fault. Questions, disagreements, and even arguments may be included in the process. Critical thinking always challenges the status quo. Seeking the truth even if the consequences are contrary to one's assumptions and beliefs is essential.
- Critical thinking considers the complexity and ambiguity of issues. At the same time, critical thinking seeks to identify the essential elements and exclude whatever is irrelevant to the matter being considered. Valid conclusions cannot be drawn or appropriate action taken unless one knows what is to be considered.
- Critical thinking is a contextual activity. We must be aware of our own context and how it influences our thinking. Our social environment, past and present, may bias our thinking, and we must be aware of how this occurs and deal with it appropriately. We do not think in a vacuum.
- Critical thinking is inseparable from language because it is applied to language and expressed through language (Smith, 1990). Attention should be directed to the meaning of words. Words often acquire connotative meanings that over time may differ radically from their original meanings.
- Critical thinking is not always a self-conscious activity. We may not be aware when we are engaging in critical thinking, or even alert to its absence. Moreover, we often unconsciously work on problems and reach solutions without knowing precisely how we arrived at them until we reflect on the process. Intuition is frequently an invaluable guide in highly stressful situations. Gladwell (2005) notes that whenever we are faced with making a decision quickly and under stress, we make the decision unconsciously (p. 12).
- Critical thinking is not an esoteric activity. It is something everyone does to some degree at least some of the time. Written guidelines, decision trees, algorithms, and critical pathways formalize the critical thinking process but cannot contain it wholly. Thinking critically is not just a solitary activity. We expose our beliefs and actions, and the thinking that helped us arrive at those beliefs and actions, to the scrutiny of others. We invite this criticism in different ways—for example, by sharing with colleagues in a discussion or writing a report. We often need others to help us see our errors.

- Critical thinking is a habit that improves with proper use and withers with disuse. In the beginning, we use structure to guide our practice. As we gain proficiency, structure diminishes, but we must continue practicing to improve or even maintain our ability to think critically. Following established protocols in a crisis situation may be helpful but can interfere with recognizing new data.
- Critical thinking includes reflection or contemplation—that is, giving serious thought to a situation with the clear knowledge that even one small additional piece of data may change the whole configuration.

All of these characteristics of critical thinking are present during the process of critical thinking. We may be more conscious of one particular characteristic at a specific point during the process, but the others remain in the background, influencing the outcome. The habit of critical thinking includes drawing from one's unconscious mind (Gladwell, 2005, p. 12).

Measures of Critical Thinking

How do you know if you are thinking critically? Evaluation takes into account the purpose for which the information is gathered, and then a suitable technique is chosen. Many paper-and-pencil objective tests have been designed to measure generic competency in critical thinking, but not specifically in nursing. The Watson-Glaser Critical Thinking Appraisal (W-GCTA), the California Critical Thinking Inventory, and the Cornell Critical Thinking Tests Levels X and Z are the most widely known and used (Norris & Ennis, 1989). The central aspects of critical thinking—**induction, deduction,** and **assumption identification**—are included in all three, but only the California Critical Thinking Inventory (Facione, Facione, & Sanchez, 2000) attempts to measure the disposition toward critical thinking. These tests, however, are limited and are used mostly for research and not primarily to measure achievement. Probably the best way to increase your critical thinking ability is to critique how you are thinking and to practice critical thinking. Rubenfeld and Scheffer (2010) offer a critical thinking inventory that may help you examine and hone your critical thinking skills (pp. 211–214).

DEVELOPING CRITICAL THINKING SKILLS

Critical thinking skills can be developed. Nursing is a practice discipline. A body of knowledge is gained from classes and study and applied in the clinical setting. Information drawn from personal experience in the clinical setting informs this body of knowledge. None of the knowledge in either setting is obtained automatically. Information must be cultivated, organized, and conscientiously arranged by using critical thinking.

Raingruber and Haffer (2001) suggest four strategies that nurses can use to develop critical thinking skills. First, nurses can reflect on accounts of other nurses' clinical experiences. The narratives may be in the form of oral or written accounts and may include anything from a simple story of a clinical event to a detailed case study. Such activities enable you to reach across time and space to broaden your base of knowledge before you encounter those experiences in your clinical practice.

Second, nurses can develop critical thinking skills by applying Brookfield's (1995) three critical thinking processes:

- Securing contextual awareness and determining what needs to be observed and considered
- Exploring and imagining alternatives
- Questioning, analyzing, and reflecting on the rationale for decisions

Third, use mind maps as a visual learning tool. Associations that play a major role in nearly every mental function help you to identify the key elements in a situation and prompt you to generate solutions. For example, you anticipate an assignment in a clinical setting in which you have not previously worked. You are experiencing some anxiety before the assignment. You recall being in a similar situation in the past and take steps to reduce your anxiety. You may call a friend for support, review appropriate material in a nursing text, imagine several scenarios that you may encounter during the assignment, and visualize successfully providing quality care to your patients. Briefly, you would rehearse caring for your patients in your mind in anticipation of providing actual care.

Fourth, you can keep a journal of your clinical experiences, noting your concerns about how you coped with particular situations and your reflections about what you could do to improve the care you delivered. Opportunities to reflect in writing help to clarify meanings and promote increased understanding. Examining your reasoning and actions in writing reinforces learning and enables you to draw on knowledge gleaned from such an activity in future clinical situations. Even examining a brief process recording of the verbal exchange you had with a patient can help you gain insight into your style of communication and what you can do to improve.

Critical thinking can also be enhanced through the arts. In their psychiatric mental health textbook, Frisch and Frisch (2011) use literary excerpts, movie clips, and classic art pieces to stimulate critical thinking and self-exploration. In doing so, the authors encourage the readers to enter the patient's world to understand the process and effects of psychiatric disturbances on an individual's overall health and functioning.

Readers are encouraged to examine how their own personal views and feelings influence their delivery of care.

THE NURSING PROCESS AND CRITICAL THINKING

Nurses can also develop a meaningful concept of information and material needed to practice nursing by using logical steps of the nursing process. Taba (cited in Maleck, 1986) identifies four teaching phases necessary for developing critical thinking. The first three phases—concept formation, interpretation of data, and application of principles—focus on the cognitive domain. The fourth phase speaks to the affective domain and entails interpretation of feelings, attitudes, and values.

1. *Concept formation.* Conception formation is similar to the nursing process. First, the nurse needs to identify known data, determine common characteristics, and prioritize data.
2. *Interpretation of data.* Next, nurses are encouraged to differentiate between pieces of information they gathered, determine cause-and-effect relationships among the information, if any, and draw tentative conclusions.

These first two logical phases or steps in thinking prepare nurses for the third phase.

3. *Application of principles.* Nurses analyze the nature of the problem or situation. It is important to note that nurses do not ask the analytic "why" questions until this application phase. The premature use of why questions produces deductive conclusions rather than inductive alternatives. The question "Why does an infection cause an elevated temperature?" tends to lead to a rote response culled from classroom lectures or the textbook. Conversely, a thought-producing question such as "What factors related to an elevated temperature suggest infection?" encourages nurses to sift and combine cognitive knowledge to understand an important clinical concept. Only after defining the problem are nurses able to isolate the relationship among the data. After these relationships are established, nurses can apply factual information to predict an outcome based on cognitive principles. This approach is not unlike the nursing process. However, avoiding "why" questions and asking about "what factors" help the nurse avoid the trapdoor of drawing premature conclusions.
4. *Interpretation of feelings, attitudes, and values.* The fourth phase involves principles of interpersonal problem solving and analysis of values. This activity, although less concrete than the other three phases, is imperative for determining the nature of attitudes and perceptions developed through one's life experiences. For example, a nurse's concern about a rising temperature in a patient taking haloperidol (Haldol) may be provoked by a past experience with a patient who was taking the drug and developed neuroleptic malignant syndrome. At this point, the nurse needs to gather additional data to confirm or rule out the possibility that the rising temperature is a sign of malignant hyperthermia in the present patient, and not leap to a premature conclusion. Additionally, the nurse must be open to other possible explanations for the elevated temperature. Appropriate action is then taken, including gathering additional data when indicated. Once again, this approach helps prevent the common pitfall associated with using the nursing process: drawing conclusions based on a formula that does not allow for different possibilities. In other words, it avoids the trap of fitting the patient into the textbook model.

These phases have been described in terms of steps, but they can occur almost simultaneously. Sequencing and pacing questions are essential in critical thinking. Sequencing questions is important because the processes of thought evolve from the simple to the complex. Clinical instruction should follow a carefully sequenced set of experiences and questions. As mentioned earlier, asking "why" questions prematurely would only bring premature closure. The principle of pacing allows nurses to match questions to their levels of readiness and cognitive ability. To accommodate pacing, nurses must pursue each question long enough to permit a variety of responses. In this way, they become active participants in the thinking process, and not simply vessels for facts.

A closer look at the nursing process shows that following it appropriately involves critical thinking. The five steps of the nursing process are as follows:

1. Assessment
2. Diagnosis
3. Planning
4. Implementation
5. Evaluation

This process provides a framework for identifying and treating patient problems. The nursing process is an ongoing and interactive cycle that results in dynamic nursing care for all patients. Assessment is the foundation of the process and leads to the identification of both nursing diagnoses and collaborative problems. Nursing diagnosis provides the primary focus for developing patient-specific individualization of patient goals. The planning process allows for individualization of patient goals and nursing care within the context of managed care guidelines. Implementation involves providing nursing actions to treat each diagnosis. Ongoing evaluation determines the degree of success in achieving the patient goals and the continued relevance of each nursing diagnosis and collaborative problem.

The implementation of the nursing process requires complex clinical and diagnostic knowledge and application of critical thinking skills (Box 7.1). One should be able to think outside the box rather than simply apply formulas gleaned from textbook information. Textbook information is often based on the mythical average and can serve only as a general guide; individuals are much more varied. Learning and applying these skills are a continuing challenge for the nurse and require much practice. If the nurse uses the diagnostic reasoning process appropriately, the result will more likely be effective nursing interventions leading to desirable patient outcomes.

Nurses must be critical thinkers because of the nature of the discipline and their work. Nurses are frequently confronted with problem situations; critical thinking enables them to make sound decisions. During the course of a workday, nurses are required to make decisions of many kinds. These decisions often determine the health of patients and even their very survival, so it is essential that the decisions are sound. Critical thinking skills are needed to assess information and plan decisions. Nurses need good judgment, for example, to decide what they can manage and what should be referred to another healthcare provider. Nurses deal with rapidly changing situations in stressful environments. Treatments and medications are modified frequently in response to a patient condition. Routine behaviors are often inadequate to deal with the

---

BOX 7.1 **Critical Thinking with the Nursing Process**

Assessment
- List the significant assessment findings: objective and subjective.
- Cluster the significant assessment data by functional health patterns.
- What general problem does the patient have?
- Develop data clusters for each of the general problems identified.

Nursing Diagnosis
- From the clustered data, develop at least two diagnostic hypotheses using accepted nursing diagnosis labels.
- Evaluate each of the diagnostic hypotheses by writing and comparing the definitions and applicable defining characteristics of each diagnosis.
- Write complete nursing diagnosis statements, by priority.

Planning
- Plan appropriate nursing interventions.

Implementation
- Implement appropriate nursing interventions.

Evaluation
- Evaluate the outcomes.

---

complex circumstances. Familiarity with the routine for giving medications, for example, does not necessarily help you intervene appropriately with a patient who is afraid of injections. When unexpected complications arise, critical thinking ability helps nurses recognize important cues, respond quickly, and adapt interventions to meet specific needs.

Nurses use knowledge from other subjects and fields. Using insight from one subject to shed light on another subject requires critical thinking skills. Because nurses deal holistically with human responses, they must draw meaningful information from other subject areas to understand the meaning of patient data and plan effective interventions. Nurses need knowledge from neurophysiology, social sciences, psychology, and nutrition, for example, to assist patients effectively who are severely depressed.

Case studies offer us excellent opportunities to use critical thinking. The case study presented in Box 7.2 contains data about Mr. Jones, a patient admitted to the same-day surgery unit for repair of a right inguinal hernia. To determine the appropriate care for Mr. Jones, the nurse should organize her thoughts and actions as illustrated. The nurse must use critical thinking in determining appropriate data collection, assessment, nursing diagnoses, and interventions for the care of the patient and his family. Clearly, critical thinking is used in every step of the nursing process as nurses collect, cluster, and analyze data and formulate nursing diagnoses. Critical thinking enables the nurse to provide high-quality care that is appropriate, individualized, creative, sensitive, and comprehensive.

BOX 7.2 Case Study Mr. Jones

Health History and Range of Symptoms
Mr. Jones is a 45-year-old married man, employed as a supervisor with Parrish Construction Company. He is brought by his wife to the same-day surgery unit for a presurgery assessment the day before his scheduled surgery. His breath smells of alcohol.

Chief Concern
"I need to get this surgery over with. We have a big job to do at work, and it will be my butt if it is not completed on schedule. I plan to cut down on my drinking. I know I drink too much sometimes, but it's because of the pain from this thing." (Patient points to area of hernia.)

History of Present Illness
Mr. Jones was sent by the nurse from the construction company to the surgeon, Dr. Judge. Mr. Jones had experienced periodic pain and swelling in his right groin area for at least 5 years and several times has seen the employee health physician, who told him he had a right inguinal hernia that should be repaired. He admits to experiencing decreased appetite and insomnia for the past 10 days.

Social and Family History
Mr. Jones's father died of cirrhosis at the age of 52 years. His mother is 80 years old and has a history of diabetes. Mr. Jones is the youngest of six children. One brother died at birth, another died at age 6 years of a tumor, and a third brother was a heavy drinker. Two sisters are alive and well.

Mr. Jones has been married to his second wife for 9 years; they have no children. His second wife has three boys, aged 12, 14, and 16 years, who live with her first husband and have no contact with Mr. and Mrs. Jones.

Mr. Jones has five children by his first marriage; all are alive and well, living with his first wife. He pays $50 a week for child support for each child. The children visit him every other weekend.

There is no family history of tuberculosis, hypertension, epilepsy, or emotional illness.

Review of Systems
General: No current change in weight and usually feels good, except when the hernia acts up.
Skin: No symptoms.
Eyes: He wears glasses for reading.
Ears: No symptoms.
Nose: No symptoms.
Mouth and Throat: Experiences recurrent episodes of hoarseness. Denies dysphagia.
Neck: No symptoms.
Respiratory System: Denies pain, dyspnea, palpitations, syncope, or edema.
Gastrointestinal System: Reports eating only three "good meals" during the past 10 days. Appetite is good when not drinking. Denies food intolerance, emesis, jaundice, flatulence, diarrhea, constipation, or melena.
Genitourinary System: No symptoms.
Neurological: See "History" and "Interview with Significant Other."

Physical Examination
Mr. Jones is a 45-year-old white man with a dark complexion and a ruddy face who appears chronically ill. He is mildly intoxicated and appears anxious. Weight is 136 pounds; height is 5 feet, 10 inches; temperature is 98.8°F; pulse is 92 beats/minute; regular respirations are 20 breaths/minute and not labored; and blood pressure is 160/90 mm Hg.
Skin: Well hydrated and without lesions.
Head: Normocephalic.
Eyes: PERRLA. Vision corrected with glasses. Visual acuity decreased to 3 mm print at 18 inches on the left and 4 mm print at 18 inches on the right. Extraocular movements full; no nystagmus is noted. Visual fields are intact as tested per confrontation. Conjunctivae are slightly injected. Sclerae clear. Lenses are without opacities bilaterally. Funduscopic examination reveals the discs normally cupped and no vascular changes bilaterally.
Ears: External ears symmetrical, without lesions. Otic canal is clear. Tympanic membrane pearly gray bilaterally. Hearing is within normal limits per watch tick at 6 inches.
Mouth and Throat: Lips, tongue, and buccal mucosa are pink and moist. Teeth are brown, crooked. Gingivae are atrophic. No inflammation of posterior nasopharynx.
Nose: Nasal septum in the midline. Nares are patent bilaterally. Sinuses not tender.
Neck: Full mobility and no significant lymphadenopathy. Thyroid not enlarged, without nodules.
Chest: Bony thorax is without deformity or tenderness. Respiratory movement is full, and diaphragmatic excursion is adequate bilaterally. Lungs are clear to percussion and auscultation.
Cardiovascular: The PMI is in the fifth intercostal space of the LMCL. NSR without murmurs or gallops.
Abdomen: Abdomen is soft and flat. Bowel sounds are heard in four quadrants. Liver is descended 5 cm below the costal margin. No splenomegaly, tenderness, or mass. Surgical scar present in right lower quadrant.
Genitourinary: Normal male genitalia. No hernia palpated.
Rectal: Internal and external hemorrhoids noted at 5- and 7-o'clock positions. Normal sphincter tone. Anal canal free of tenderness. Prostate is in the midline, firm without nodules, not enlarged.

Continued

BOX 7.2 Case Study Mr. Jones—cont'd

Extremities and Back: Muscular development symmetrical. Normal in appearance, color, and temperature. Peripheral pulses palpable and symmetrical. Free of varicosities and edema.

Neurological: Speech is slurred, sensorium somewhat cloudy. Cranial nerves II through XII are intact as tested per gross screen. Moderately tremulous. Biceps, triceps, brachioradialis, patella, and Achilles reflexes are symmetrical but brisk. Babinski's reflexes are down bilaterally.

Significant Laboratory Findings

Blood alcohol level: 0.29 U/L; Stool guaiac: negative; ECG: sinus tachycardia, otherwise WNL; Chest x-ray: no active chest disease; Coulter-S: Hgb 16.0 g/dL (H), HCT 48.2% (H), MCV 101 m3 (H); CL 92 mEq/L (L); Uric acid 8.04 mg/dL (H), SGOT 90 U/L (H); Liver panel: GGT 66 IU/L (H); Urine: bacteria 21, WBC 8–12.

Interview with Significant Other

According to Mrs. Jones, Mr. Jones works out of town from Monday morning to Thursday evening. When he returns home, he begins to drink. He does not drink during the workweek. Mrs. Jones related the following incidents of the past 10 days, which occurred when her husband was intoxicated: ran all of the children out of the home into the rain, scuffled with brother-in-law, and brandished a shotgun after an argument. Mrs. Jones reports that she left her husband in June but returned to him about 4 weeks ago. She has never attended Al-Anon but has reviewed information from the Alcoholism Information Center. This is the second marriage for Mrs. Jones; her first husband and her father were alcoholics.

EVIDENCE-BASED PRACTICE: *Consider this....*

Use of critical thinking in nursing involves careful and effective assessment skills. One of the National Guideline Clearinghouse (2013) guidelines calls for a comprehensive health assessment for adults and children with suspected social anxiety disorders. Social anxiety disorders are defined as: "persistent fear of or anxiety about one or more social or performance situations that is out of proportion to the actual threat posed by the situation" (NGC, 2013, p. 1). Following this, intervention and practices are recommended.

Question: How will you use your critical thinking skills in conceptual care mapping for this individual?

Source: National Guideline Clearinghouse. (2013). *Social anxiety disorder: Recognition, assessment and treatment.* Retrieved from http://www.guideline.gov/content.aspx?id=46234&search=detailed+health+assessment

---

KEY POINTS

- Critical thinking has been defined and described by many scholars. It is multifaceted and involves a combination of logical, rhetorical, and philosophical skills and attitudes that promote the ability to determine what we should believe and do.

- Critical thinking is essential for professional nursing practice. The need for critical thinking in nursing has greatly increased with the diversity and complexity of nursing practice. Reflective thinking is the "active, persistent, and careful consideration of any belief or supposed form of knowledge in the light of the grounds that support it and the further conclusions to which it tends" (Dewey, 1933, p. 9).

- Reactive thinking implies a response to what is, and not to what may yet be.

- Critical thinking is often associated with scientific reasoning, which includes problem identification, data collection, and hypothesis testing, but it is not limited to these activities.

- The central aspects of critical thinking are induction, deduction, and assumption identification.

- Concept formation is similar to the nursing process. First, the nurse needs to identify known data, determine common characteristics, and prioritize data.

- Interpretation of data occurs when nurses differentiate between pieces of information, determine cause-and-effect relationships among variables, and extract meaning from what they have observed.

- Application of principles occurs when nurses analyze the nature of the problem or situation and apply factual information to predict an outcome based on cognitive principles.

- Interpretation of feelings, attitudes, and values requires interpersonal problem solving and analysis of values.

Thought and Discussion Questions

1. Give an example from your clinical practice for five of the descriptive statements of critical thinking.

2. Select a nursing issue, such as an open visiting policy in the surgical intensive care unit or family presence during a code, and engage in a debate with a peer.

3. Select a problem at your place of work. Explore a solution to the problem with the help of a peer with whom you work. Analyze the problem-solving process you used to address the problem.

4. Review the Chapter Thought located on the first page of the chapter and discuss it (online or in class) in the context of the contents of the chapter.

Interactive Exercises

Go to the Intranet site and complete the interactive exercises provided for this chapter.

REFERENCES

Alfaro-LeFevre, R. (2013). *Critical thinking, clinical reasoning, and clinical judgment: A practical approach* (5th ed.). St Louis, MO: Saunders/Elsevier.

Bandman, E. L., & Bandman, B. (1994). *Critical thinking in nursing* (2nd ed.). Norwalk, CT: Appleton & Lange.

Bartol, G. M. (1986). Using the humanities in nursing education. *Nurse Educator, 11*(1), 21–23.

Bartol, G. M., & Courts, N. F. (2013). The psychophysiology of bodymind healing. In B. M. Dossey, L. Keegan, & C. E. Guzzeta (Eds.), *Holistic nursing: A handbook for practice* (6th ed., pp. 705–720). Sudbury, MA: Jones & Bartlett.

Brookfield, S. (1995). *Becoming a critically reflective teacher.* San Francisco, CA: Jossey-Bass.

Case, B. (1994). Walking around the elephant: A critical thinking strategy for decision making. *Journal of Continuing Education in Nursing, 25*(3), 101–109.

Cassel, J. F., & Congleton, R. J. (1993). *Critical thinking: An annotated bibliography.* Metuchen, NJ: Scarecrow Press.

Dewey, J. (1910). *How we think.* Boston, MA: D. C. Heath & Co.

Dewey, J. (1933). *How we think.* New York: D. C. Heath & Co.

Facione, N. C., & Facione, P. A. (1996). Externalizing the critical thinking in knowledge development and clinical judgment. *Nursing Outlook, 44*, 129–136.

Facione, N. C., & Facione, P. A. (2000). *Critical thinking assessment in nursing education programs: An aggregate data analysis.* Millbrae, CA: Academic Press.

Facione, N. C., Facione, P. A., & Sanchez, C. A. (2000) *Test manual: The California critical thinking skills test.* Millbrae, CA: California Academic Press.

Facione, P. (Project director). (1990). Critical thinking: A statement of expert consensus for purposes of educational assessment and instruction. *The Delphi Report: Research findings and recommendations prepared for the American Philosophical Association* (ERIC Doc. No. ED 315 423). Washington, DC: ERIC.

Frisch, N. C., & Frisch, L. E. (2011). *Psychiatric mental health nursing* (4th ed.). Clifton Park, NY: Delmar.

Gladwell, M. (2002). *The tipping point: How little things can make a big difference.* New York: Little, Brown & Co.

Gladwell, M. (2005). *Blink: The power of thinking without thinking.* New York: Little, Brown & Co.

Gladwell, M. (2009). *What the dog saw and other adventures.* New York: Little, Brown & Co.

Gladwell, M. (2013). *David and Goliath: Underdogs, misfits, and the art of battling giants.* New York: Little Brown & Co.

Johns, C. (2013). *Becoming a reflective practitioner* (4th ed.). Oxford, UK: Wiley-Blackwell Publishing.

Jones, S. A., & Brown, L. N. (1993). Alternative views on defining critical thinking through the nursing process. *Holistic Nursing Practice, 7*(3), 71–76.

Kataoka-Yahiro, M., & Saylor, C. (1994). A critical thinking model for nursing judgment. *Journal of Nursing Education, 33*(8), 351–356.

Kintgen-Andrews, J. (1991). Critical thinking and nursing education: Perplexities and insights. *Journal of Nursing Education, 30*, 152–157.

Lonergan, B. (1977). *Insight: A study of human understanding.* New York: Harper & Row.

Maleck, C. J. (1986). A model for teaching critical thinking. *Nurse Educator, 11*(6), 20–23.

Mariano, C. (2013). Holistic nursing scope and standards of practice. In B. M. Dossey, L. Keegan, & C. E. Guzzeta (Eds.), *Holistic nursing: A handbook for practice* (6th ed., p. 59). Sudbury, MA: Jones & Bartlett.

McPeck, J. E. (1990). *Teaching critical thinking.* New York: Routledge.

Nance, J. J. (2008). *Why hospitals should fly: The ultimate flight plan to patient safety and quality care.* Bozeman, MT: Second River Healthcare Press.

National Guideline Clearinghouse. (2013). *Social anxiety disorder: Recognition, assessment and treatment.* Retrieved from http://www.guideline.gov/content.aspx?id=46234&search=detailed+health+assessment

Norris, S. P., & Ennis, R. H. (1989). *Evaluating critical thinking.* Pacific Grove, CA: Midwest Press.

Paul, R. W. (1990). Critical thinking: Fundamental for a free society. *Educational Leadership, 41*, 44.

Paul, R., & Elder, L. (2008). The miniature guide to critical thinking: Concepts and tools. Tomales, CA: Foundation for Critical Thinking Press.

Raingruber, B., & Haffer, A. (2001). *Using your head to land on your feet: A beginning nurse's guide to critical thinking.* Philadelphia, PA: F.A. Davis.

Robert, R. R., & Peterson, S. (2013). Critical thinking at the bedside: Providing safe passage to patients. *MEDSURG Nursing, 22*(2), 85–118.

Rubenfeld, M. G., & Scheffer, B. K. (2010). *Critical thinking tactics for nurses* (2nd ed.). Sudbury, MA: Jones & Bartlett.

Savitt, T. (1969). *Readers Theater.* Iowa City, IA: University of Iowa Press.

Schuster, P. M. (2002). *Concept mapping. A critical-thinking approach to care planning.* Philadelphia, PA: F.A. Davis.

Smith, F. (1990). *To think.* New York: Teachers College Press.

Taleb, N. N. (2010). *The black swan: The impact of the highly improbable.* New York: Random House.

Thurmond, V. A. (2001). The holism in critical thinking: A concept analysis. *Journal of Holistic Nursing, 19*(4), 375–389.

White, N. E., Beardslee, N. Q., Peters, D., & Supples, J. M. (1990). Promoting critical thinking skills. *Nurse Educator, 15*(5), 16–19.

Wilkinson, J. M. (2001). *Nursing process and critical thinking.* Saddle River, NJ: Prentice-Hall.

Woods, J. H. (1993). Affective learning: One door to critical thinking. *Holistic Nursing Practice, 7*(3), 64–70.

BIBLIOGRAPHY

Adams, B. L. (1999). Nursing education for critical thinking: An integrative review. *Journal of Nursing Education, 38*(3), 111–119.

Alfaro-Lefevre, R., & Juall, L. (2005). *The nursing process made easy: Concept mapping and care planning for students.* Philadelphia, PA: Lippincott Williams & Wilkins.

Banfield, V., Fagan, B., & Jones, C. (2012). Charting a new course in knowledge: Creating life-long critical core thinkers. *Dynamics 23*(1), 24–28.

Barnet, S., & Bedau, H. (2004). *Critical thinking, reading & writing: A brief guide to argument.* New York: Bedford/ St. Martins.

Beckie, T. M., Lowry, L. W., & Barnett, S. (2001). Assessing critical thinking in baccalaureate nursing students: A longitudinal study. *Holistic Nursing Practice, 15*(3), 18–26.

Bitner, N. P., & Tobin, E. (1998). Critical thinking: Strategies for clinical practice. *Journal for Nurses in Staff Development, 14*, 267–272.

Bradley, H. E., & Taylor, L. A. (2013). *The American health care paradox: Why spending more is getting us less.* New York: Public Affairs.

Browne, M. N., & Keeley, S. M. (2003). *Asking the right questions: A guide to critical thinking.* Upper Saddle River, NJ: Person Education.

Chafres, J. (2005). *Thinking critically.* Boston, MA: Houghton Mifflin.

DeYoung, S. (2003). *Teaching strategies for nurse educators.* Upper Saddle River, NJ: Prentice Hall.

Gerdeman, J. L., Lux, K., & Jackie, J. Using concept mapping to build clinical judgment skills. *Nursing Education in Practice, 13*(2013), 11–17.

Gladwell, M. (2008). *Outliers: The story of success.* New York, NY: Little, Brown & Co.

Green, C. J. (2000). *Critical thinking in nursing: Case studies across the curriculum.* Upper Saddle River, NJ: Prentice Hall.

Locsin, R. C. (2001). The dilemma of decision-making: Processing thinking critical to nursing. *Holistic Nursing Practice, 15*(3), 1–3.

Nance, J. J., & Bartholomew, K. M. (2012). *Charting the course.* Bozeman, MT: Second River Healthcare Press.

Nosich, G. M. (2004). *Learning to think things through.* Upper Saddle River, NJ: Prentice-Hall.

Patterson, B. J. (2013). Facilitating clinical reasoning in the skills laboratory: Reasoning model versus nursing process-based kills checklist. *Nursing Education Perspectives, 34*(4), 265–267.

Porter, K. A. (1930). The jilting of Granny Weatherall. In *Flowering Judas and other stories* (pp. 80–89). New York: Harcourt, Brace.

Rew, L., & Barrow, E. M. (2007). State of the science: Intuition in nursing, a generation of studying the phenomenon. *Advanced Nursing Science, 30*(1): E15–25.

Zori, S., & Morrison, B. (2009). Critical thinking in nurse managers. *Nursing Economics, 27*(2), 75–80.

ONLINE RESOURCES

Prince George's Community College
http://academic.pg.cc.md.us/~wpeirce/MCCCTR/

The Critical Thinking Community
http://www.criticalthinking.org/

● Rose Kearney-Nunnery

8

Working with Groups

"We communicate in many ways, especially when working with others toward a common goal."

Rose Kearney-Nunnery

On completion of this chapter, the reader will be able to:

1. Explain the techniques for effective communication in group settings.

2. Evaluate personal communication patterns used with patients and colleagues in a group.

3. Describe different types of groups, including their characteristics and roles of group members.

4. Differentiate between effective and ineffective groups and the characteristics of an effective group leader.

5. Evaluate communication patterns in a group for effective functioning in meeting the group's common goals.

Key Terms

Group
Group Process
Group Structure
Group Composition
Group Roles
Group Focus
Professional Groups
Work Groups
Educational Groups

Therapeutic Groups
Effective Groups
Goal Attainment
Member Participation
Cohesiveness
Decision Making
Communication Patterns
Attendance
Creativity

Power
Ineffective Groups
Stages of Group Development
Functional Task Roles
Functional Group-Building
    Roles
Nonfunctional Group Roles
Organizational Group
Virtual Meetings

Communication—verbal, nonverbal, and written—is integral to working with individuals and groups. DeWine, Gibson, and Smith (2000) identify four contexts or environments in which communication takes place: interpersonal, group, organizational, and mass communication. Nurses must be skilled in each of these areas, from the interpersonal situation with a patient or colleague, to small consumer or colleague groups, to larger organizational settings, and, finally, to mass communications with the public.

The concepts of effective group process are important components in professional nursing practice and require understanding of the types of groups, their composition and functions, and the roles played by the members. As nurses, we need to develop skills to use as both leaders and members of various work and professional groups, as well as to apply group process to intervene therapeutically with patients. Working effectively with groups also addresses the American Nurses Association (2010) Standards of Professional Performance concerning communication and collaboration, both with patients and other healthcare providers. Examining the group's characteristics and evaluating the group's effectiveness provide the knowledge and skills needed to accomplish these goals. Note that understanding groups is an initial step in addressing the core competency of working in interdisciplinary teams.

GROUPS

A **group** consists of three or more individuals with some commonality, such as shared goals or interests. Living in society, we are members of many groups—family, work, professional, and social. Each type of group has a specific goal and membership. As nurses, we are involved as participants in work groups and interact with groups of individuals in their healthcare activities. We may also participate in therapy or support groups. We use the principles of group process in all of these activities and in assisting our patients. Some of these groups are structured loosely, with minimal rules, whereas others have clearly defined roles and limits. It is essential for the nurse to understand group processes to communicate, collaborate, and function effectively in the group as both an individual and a professional.

Group Process

Group process is the dynamic interplay of interactions within groups of humans. Interplay includes what is said and done in groups, as well as how members interact with one another and the group leader. A group is actually a social system. Recall from Chapter 2 that systems theory is concerned with holism as opposed to the isolated parts. The basic components of a system are the input, output, boundary, environment, and feedback. A group, as a social system, is composed of people with their unique characteristics and communication styles but focused on the group goals as the output from the system. And as Berlo (1960) pointed out in his classic work on communication, "a knowledge of the composition and workings of a social system is useful in making predictions about how members of that system will behave in a given communication situation" (p. 135). This is particularly applicable to professional practice with the nurses' focus on the importance of working with groups in a variety of practice settings—patient, family, self-help, self-awareness, peer, and task groups.

Group Characteristics

Groups can be classified according to structure, composition, roles, and focus. A particular group often fits more than one classification, especially in terms of its roles. For example, the initial purpose of developing a cancer support group might have been to provide the members with a sense of sharing and support. But this type of group often fills many other functions, such as education regarding medications, traditional and nontraditional treatment programs, and healthcare providers; information sharing about benefits, wills, and finances; and strategy sharing on coping with symptoms and managing daily life.

Group Structure

Groups may be differentiated by **group structure**, such as whether a group is formal or informal. Formal groups are highly structured, with functions specified in job descriptions, contracts, policies, and procedures. Formal groups associated with nursing are the entire nursing staff and the professional standards committee. Each of these groups has particular requirements for membership and specific rules, procedures, and standards of practice. A professional group can also be viewed as a formal group, with requirements for membership, rules that govern meetings, and specific member expectations. An advantage of structured groups is their clear understanding of roles and expectations. This same benefit may become a disadvantage if the group is not open to changing to meet the needs of the members. The leaders of more structured groups tend to have greater power. By contrast, informal groups are more loosely structured, at times disbanding or reconvening according to the needs of the membership. Examples of informal groups are special interest groups and support groups. Informal groups benefit from some degree of flexibility in roles, expectations, and leadership.

Composition of Groups

Groups can also be differentiated by the unique composition of the membership. **Group composition** may be homogeneous or heterogeneous, depending on the characteristics of the members. Members of homogenous groups are similar in some aspect, such as all adolescent male patients or female nurses employed in the intensive care units. A benefit of working with a homogeneous group is the sense of shared connection that the members typically feel from the beginning. This sense may be expressed as "He has the same problem" or "She thinks the same way I do." Heterogeneous groups consist of a mix of individuals, such as patients with various diagnoses or ages, or a work group of both nurses and physicians working with patients in a cardiac intensive care unit. This type of group has a wider range of diversity and therefore usually a greater variety of opinions, beliefs, and needs.

Facilitating a sense of connection among members is a key challenge for the heterogeneous group. With a heterogeneous group, however, group members have the advantage of learning from many different perspectives.

Roles for Members of the Group

A third way to classify groups is in terms of the leader and participant **group roles**. Some groups are led by a professional who is responsible for instituting the rules, establishing the structure, and determining the membership. There are clear expectations for the leader and the participants. An example is an outpatient recovery group, in which a cardiac rehabilitation counselor leads the group, initiates themes for discussion, and often sets criteria for member participation. Other groups have informal leadership as well as rules for members. Peer support groups are an example of this type. Traditionally, the leadership may be shared by members, who are usually working on a common issue. Members are free to attend or not, depending on their own needs and schedules. At times, the group may become engulfed in struggles for leadership, which can compromise the group's effectiveness.

Group Focus

Groups may also be classified according to their focus or approach. The **group focus** can be work-related, educational, therapeutic, or professional. Professional organizations or nursing groups were described in Chapter 1, along with their unique missions and membership requirements. These **professional groups** are generally formal and are directed at professional issues and at the objectives stated in their mission statements. **Work groups** are task oriented, focused on a particular work-related activity, as with a nursing department budget committee and the task of allocating resources. Professional nursing organizations may also have work groups focused on special projects assigned by the leadership of the organization.

Many of us are members of a variety of work groups. Nurses on a particular unit constitute one group, whereas the nursing department as a whole is another functioning work group. Committees that meet monthly are probably commonly viewed as work groups. They may be convened ad hoc (as needed), or they may be more or less a permanent standing group, such as the governance committee, the safety committee, or the quality assurance committee. The membership changes over time, and the structure varies in level of formality. If the group is focusing on one specific issue or task, members may be expected to fulfill assigned roles. At other times there may be a more informal, shifting assignment of roles, as occurs in monthly staff meetings on a care unit. Attendance varies, depending on schedule, patient load, and the issues involved.

Educational groups have a teaching focus, whether members are teaching patients about medications, treatments, parenting skills, or a variety of health promotion activities, or educating their colleagues in areas of expertise. This type of group may actually convene only for an individual session, if held in a clinic or institutional setting, or it may have a series of sessions. An example is a stress reduction class for patients diagnosed with hypertension, which is scheduled on a weekly basis in a clinic or outpatient department. Membership and attendance vary depending on educational needs and appointment schedules. Although the group leader is a professional, the structure is typically less formal and is directed at the learning needs of the audience. Teaching and learning principles, discussed in Chapter 9, are important considerations, along with the group process.

Therapeutic groups vary in nature, depending on the specific treatment or patient needs. This group is led by a professional and is a formally structured group that typically specifies when members can join and when they can leave the group. Examples of these groups are cognitive therapy groups for depressed patients, behavioral therapy groups for anger management, and therapeutic activity groups, such as a music therapy group for patients who have suffered cerebral vascular events. The group leader has special training in the different therapeutic approaches used. Advanced practice nurses (APRNs) can lead groups in specific therapies as defined in practice standards and as recognized by their state practice act.

Effective Groups

Effective groups have an identified purpose or need for the group and a commitment to the process. Once the decision is made to form a new group, several issues are involved in setting up or structuring the group. Arnold (2011) terms this the pregroup phase, in which the following activities occur:

● Alignment of purpose and membership
● Determination of appropriate group size
● Creation of the appropriate environment

The first consideration is the purpose for forming the group. This purpose must be clearly stated for specification of the membership. Once the intended membership is determined, members can be recruited and goals set for the group. The size of the membership must be appropriate to addressing the group goals effectively. As noted by Robert, Evans, Honemann, and Balch (2004) in their guidelines on parliamentary procedure, once a group reaches 12 to 15 people, meetings become more formal and controlled (p. 4). In order to effect change, a professional group must be larger than a work group. A work or therapeutic group becomes less effective when it grows too large, becoming more heterogeneous and unable to focus on the task or treatment aims. For some groups, the leader also spends time interviewing potential members before the initial meeting. This step serves as an orientation to the group as well as a way to determine whether the individual will "fit in."

The room arrangement is another important factor for creating the appropriate environment. When the room is being set up, the goals of the group and interactions needed among members should be considered. A large conference table and chairs may be needed for a work group, whereas placing chairs in a circle to allow individuals to make eye contact without the barrier of a table is imperative in many therapeutic groups. Neither of these arrangements may be feasible or essential in an educational group.

Other factors to consider in creating an effective group include the following:

- The best meeting place and time for meetings
- Fees, dues, or cost factors
- Frequency and length of meetings
- Documentation needed for third-party payers or sponsoring organizations

An effective group will also determine whether there will be a single leader or co-leaders. Those in favor of two-leader groups cite the enhanced ability to examine dynamics, provide feedback, and manage absences of the leader. Those against this style look at the possibility of problems arising between these two individuals in terms of power, equality, and accountability, with the potential for splitting of the group, creating factions, and ineffectiveness. The co-leaders need to understand their role, work closely together, and consistently focus on the purpose of the group. The goal is to form a strong, viable group. Before initiating a group, a nurse should consider all of these concerns.

Evaluating Effectiveness of Groups

Effective groups are those that work toward the stated goals and whose members derive a sense of belonging and acceptance. How these outcomes can be accomplished requires a closer look at behaviors, strategies, and goals. In addition, organizations and third-party payers may determine their own criteria of effectiveness. General factors to consider in determining effectiveness of any group are identified in Box 8.1.

Goal attainment is the initial and most important criterion in determining the effectiveness of any group. It is an evaluation of whether the intended task or goal was accomplished, especially in a work group. In a professional association, goal attainment is focused on the activities related to the organization's mission and strategic initiatives. In a therapeutic group, goal attainment relates to the focus of the group, such as gaining insight, awareness, or skills.

Member participation is another important criterion for assessing the effectiveness of a group. Consider whether all members are included in the discussion and what roles they are playing as group members. On the other hand, think about a situation in which an autocratic leader limits the members' ability to participate in the group discussions.

BOX 8.1 **Factors to Consider in Evaluating Effectiveness of Groups**

- Goal attainment
- Member participation
- Cohesiveness
- Decision making
- Communication patterns
- Attendance
- Creativity
- Power

In an effective group, there is evidence of belonging, camaraderie, and acceptance. But participation does not imply that all members should be in agreement on all issues. "Group think" is the phenomenon by which all members are in constant agreement, which can limit creativity and lead to stagnation.

Cohesiveness among the group members indicates that they are working together toward the group's common purpose or goal. If all members are not focused on the purpose, the original goal for which the group was formed will be difficult to attain, and conflict may arise. To achieve cohesiveness, the group members must be refocused on the original intent for the group, with the leader and members supporting one another in their actions and demonstrating agreement on the common goal.

In an effective group, **decision making** must occur at the group level, with all members being involved in decisions rather than unilateral actions being taken by the leader or a disruptive member. A democratic leader and involved, cohesive members directed toward the common goal usually signify effective group functioning as they actively work toward that goal.

The **communication patterns** among the members provide valuable information on whether there is a common focus, respect, and decision making. Evaluate how the group's decisions are made. The group leader should facilitate effective communication patterns, thus allowing all members to be heard and involved in the group process. In some situations, the leader may ask each member if they have something further to add to the discussion. In an effective group, members are actively involved in a mutual communication process.

Attendance is regular and active in an effective group. Members are punctual and involved, energetically focused on the task or purpose of the group. When a group meeting is arranged in advance, members in an effective group honor their commitments to the meeting rather than making excuses for not attending or demonstrating routine tardiness.

A high level of **creativity** among the members is another sign of an effective group. The group members are spontaneously generating novel ideas for solutions on the common problem. Brainstorming sessions are focused on the goals, and communication is encouraged, with all ideas and contributions from members considered.

Typically, the leadership style in more effective groups is described as democratic, and the interactions among the members are interdependent and collaborative. **Power** is distributed on the basis of the common purpose and abilities of the members to achieve their goal in an effective group. Power struggles disrupt group process, with members focusing inwardly rather than working collaboratively on the group's goals.

Ineffective groups have low levels of productivity. These groups contain much unrest and stagnation, and members feel that they do not belong or that it is not safe for them to share their thoughts, ideas, and feelings. The group members demonstrate an uncaring attitude toward one another, have little spontaneous involvement, or are reluctant participants. The members do not appear to trust one another, seem unwilling to take risks and, in work groups, rarely volunteer for or willingly accept assignments.

The attendance may be uneven, with a high rate of dropouts and tardiness. The leadership style in less effective groups is often described as autocratic or laissez-faire, and the group interactions as independent and competitive.

THE BASICS OF GROUP PROCESSES

Skills in group process are tailored to the developmental stage of the group, and require effective leadership and participation by the members.

The Stages of Group Development

Understanding the expected stages of group development and how to facilitate groups during these stages is essential to nursing practice, whether the nurse is a group member or a leader. As with the developmental stages of individuals, groups go through predictable stages. In his classic work, Tuckman (1965) identified five **stages of group development**: forming, storming, norming, performing, and mourning or termination. Yalom and Leszcz (2005) further describe the storming stage as one of conflict that arises in the group. Arnold (2011) has further clarified the stage of termination as one of adjournment that is more applicable to the professional or work group. An effective group leader must be aware of these stages and must motivate members and modify approaches accordingly.

We can use the traditional stages of the nurse-patient relationship (initial, working, and termination), with the addition of the conflict and norming stages before the working phase, to understand the process of group development better. The stages of group development, along with expected goals and examples of appropriate nursing approaches, are illustrated in Table 8.1. Now, let us consider the five stages of group development: initial or forming, conflict or storming, norming, working or performing, and termination or adjourning.

Forming

In the initial or forming stage, the group is being formed. The members are becoming acquainted with one another, the group, and the purpose and outcomes. Arnold (2011) identifies the major group tasks during this forming stage as establishing the group contract, developing trust, and identification. The leader focuses on orienting the members and determining the structure in terms of time, duration, and frequency of meetings, as well as the goals for the group. Special educational resources may also be provided in order that all group members have a similar basis before the work of the group begins. Cohesiveness of the group is enhanced by clearly stated goals and group norms. Work groups require an introduction, identification of goals and expectations, and orientation to the structure. Patient groups also require this introduction and orientation information, but issues of confidentiality and personal disclosure are important considerations in the forming stage. Another factor to consider is whether members can join or leave at different times or whether all members must begin and terminate together.

Storming and Norming

The next phase is the conflict or storming stage. This is the time when members become more comfortable with the group but may be ambivalent about the need for the group and its intended goals. This ambivalence can be demonstrated by "testing" the authority of the leader

---

TABLE 8.1

Group Stages, Expected Goals, and Nursing Techniques

Stage	Expected Goals	Nursing Techniques
Initial/forming	Sense of trust	Making introductions Structuring group Defining parameters and goals Encouraging the sense of group
Conflict/storming	Sense of commitment	Encouraging verbalizations Allowing interactions and role development Handling confrontations and setting limits
Norming	Sense of purpose	Setting limits, rules, and expectations Encouraging group cohesion
Working/performing	Sense of hope	Facilitating discussion Identifying themes and progress Refocusing as needed Identifying processes
Termination/adjourning	Sense of accomplishment	Summarizing and evaluating goals Facilitating transfer of knowledge and skills Supporting closure

through questioning, skipping sessions, or coming late. These issues must be dealt with openly and clearly so that the group can settle into its work. This becomes the time of norming, with the identification of standards and expectations of behavior. Some level of discomfort or conflict is often expressed overtly or covertly, until the group becomes functional. All groups need this time to set norms such as roles, rules, and structure.

Performing

The working or performance stage involves exactly that—performance of the work of the group. In this stage, the leader becomes less involved in running the group. The members themselves decide what to discuss and how to address the goals and, to some degree, manage the group themselves. Cohesiveness and creativity should be apparent and encouraged. The leader's role is one of facilitator to refocus and clarify as needed, handle problems and conflicts if they arise, and identify the process as it develops. In this process, members may avoid issues or tasks and engage in disruptive reactions and behaviors. By bringing problems and conflict out into the open, the participants can examine these issues and make changes. Some groups establish dates for each stage; others depend on the tasks and type of group.

Adjourning

Termination or adjourning is the formal ending of the group. How long this stage lasts depends on the purpose of the group and its duration. As in the orientation stage, the group leader assumes an active role at this stage. The goals are to assist the members in expressing what has been accomplished and preparing for closure. This can be an emotional stage, with some members striving for continual closeness in some therapeutic groups or the continued camaraderie that is not experienced in the work setting. On the other hand, some work-group members are relieved at having accomplished the intended goals.

The Role of the Group Leader

Role theory is applicable to groups in terms of both leader and member roles. Recall that a group is a social system. As such, the leader and the members will assume selected roles based on expectations, gender, and learning. Roles are simply behaviors and expectations in a specific situation. In the case of the group, the roles of the leader and members reflect the group's identified structure, composition, focus, and associated expected roles. The role of the leader can set the expectations for the group as the social system.

Leadership is an essential consideration for the viability of many groups. One consideration is whether the leader has been selected externally or determined internally through group consensus. This appointment status may affect both the leader and member behaviors within the group. Other factors that may influence the particular leadership style adopted by an individual are the person's personality and skills, the purpose of the group, and the characteristics of the group and the participants or members.

Traditional group leadership styles have been described as democratic, autocratic, or laissez-faire. Group leaders often use a combination of styles or modify their style depending on the group membership or the topic being discussed. With a democratic leadership style, the leader shares the authority and decision-making tasks with members. A democratic leader seeks greater participation by and feedback from group members. One of the benefits of this style is that it typically produces a greater sense of satisfaction among members. On the other hand, the need to have consensus or agreement may impede the progress of the group by monopolizing the discussion.

An autocratic leadership style is one in which the leader makes all pertinent decisions, informs members of the rules, and structures the sessions. This style can facilitate the group effectiveness and goal achievement because the expectations have been clearly delineated and actions controlled. At the same time, it may limit group interaction and lead some members to feel that they are disenfranchised and that their opinions are not valued.

The laissez-faire leadership style is unstructured, allowing members a great deal of freedom and the ability to come and go at will. This style might also involve a change of leader from session to session, which can be effective with a highly functional, goal-directed population but will not work well with poorly focused or unmotivated groups.

Regardless of the leadership style, characteristics of an effective group leader include the ability to understand the dynamics of the group, listen attentively, focus on the goals, and facilitate the progress of the group. Again, effective communication and interpersonal skills are vital attributes of an effective leader. The maintenance of group morale is a major role of the group leader.

Leadership Tasks and Skills

Consider the leadership tasks and skills necessary to manage a group successfully by analyzing the group's purpose, structure, member participation, communication, and goal attainment. One of the first tasks for the group leader is to establish a structure that will promote an effective working relationship. The leader is also responsible for securing a meeting place, deciding the length and frequency of meetings, and determining the goals for the group. These goals must be clearly communicated to the members so that they can assume their roles. At times, goal determination may be delayed to allow members to participate in goal development. The leader must also physically set up the room or ensure that effective arrangements have been made. As discussed earlier, the arrangement of the physical environment is crucial in some groups.

Another critical task for the group leader at this point is to orient the members to the group and its expectations and to allot sufficient time for the group to form before initiating work. The leader can accomplish this by ensuring that the interactions among the members during the initial period of forming remain on a superficial level while the members become acquainted. The stages of forming, storming, and norming may be much briefer in a work group, but the leader must ensure that there is some time for the members to settle in. This may be accomplished in one meeting, but some allowance for introductions and getting to know one another is important, regardless of the group's focus.

Leadership skills are essential to facilitate the group in its deliberation and discussion for decision making. Ensuring participation by all members, avoiding premature closure on the topic, and recognizing the recurring themes are important activities for an effective group leader. The leader can set the tone for the level of communication, whether superficial or personal, as well as set limits on appropriate and unacceptable communication styles. The leader uses techniques such as restatement, reflection, clarification, collaboration, and problem-solving while always attempting to promote open communication among the members. Another useful technique for the leader is role modeling for the group members on how to provide constructive feedback. In this way, the group leader is actually teaching the members effective communication skills.

Attaining group cohesiveness is another skill of the successful group leader. Coming together as a group and focusing on the common goal or purpose are reinforced by the effective group leader. This cooperative and cohesive group esprit de corps can occur and endure when the group leader provides the positive, supportive, and encouraging lead or model for the group. Conflict can arise in any type of group and must be managed. The best resolution entails a "win-win" situation with a solution satisfying to both sides. Conflict is a challenge for the group leader to direct the members in creative problem-solving for both effective and satisfying group process. Nurses commonly face conflict situations in work-group settings and need to keep in mind the four functional problems that Turniansky and Hare (1998) identified—meaning, resources, integration, and goal attainment—as well as the four "must" activities to address these problems with groups in organizations:

- An overall meaning of the activity that sets both a direction and boundaries for the group
- Resources adequate for the task
- Integration in the form of role differentiation and level of morale for the group members to work together
- Enough coordination of the resources and the integration functions to provide for goal attainment. (Turniansky & Hare, 1998, p. 111)

The Conflict Resolution Network (CRN, 2014) also identifies 12 skills useful in a conflict situation (Box 8.2). The CRN is an international organization based in Australia whose purpose is to research, develop, teach, and implement the theory and practice of conflict resolution through a national and international network. Other techniques to use when dealing with difficult people are discussed later in this chapter.

Leaders should avoid using the following ineffective communication techniques: giving advice, giving approval,

---

BOX 8.2 The Conflict Resolution Network's 12 Useful Skills

The Conflict Resolution Network recommends the following 12 skills for dealing with conflict situations:

- The win-win approach
- Creative response
- Empathy
- Appropriate assertiveness
- Co-operative power
- Managing emotions
- Willingness to resolve
- Mapping the conflict
- Developing options
- Negotiation
- Mediation
- Broadening perspectives

Go to CRN's Web site at **http://www.crnhq.org/twelveskills.html** for strategies to address these 12 skills and additional resources and training materials.

---

blaming, and scapegoating. Giving advice and blaming are considered nontherapeutic. Consider that a scapegoat is taking the blame—especially the blame for others. Group leaders must be vigilant not to scapegoat a member or allow other group members to do so, especially a disruptive member. The leader needs to recognize these dynamics and intervene appropriately, creating a safe, open, and productive environment for the group. Giving approval is, perhaps surprisingly, not helpful. Giving approval can interfere with the group process and goal accomplishment by focusing on one individual, which may be interpreted as favoritism. Rather than express approval for an individual's efforts or successes, the leader can reflect back the accomplishment to the person or other members, allowing them to express their feelings. The leader can use the group format as a means of teaching effective communication skills, such as how to listen, give and receive feedback, and express feelings or opinions.

Goal accomplishment has already been identified as a benchmark of success for groups. Giving assignments, such as recording the group's discussion or trying out a particular suggestion from the group, is one helpful measure. The use of assignments communicates the belief that members are capable and that change involves work on the part of group members. In a work group, members are given specific areas to work on or research, with the expectation that the group will reconvene to put these pieces together. Ultimately, the leader is responsible for ensuring that activities in the group remain focused on the common goals that were set for the group.

Another leadership activity is facilitating closure. To provide for group closure, the leader must summarize progress at the end of each session as well as at the official termination of the group. This summarization can be in the form of a debriefing for evaluation of the group's accomplishments, soliciting group feedback. If the members enter and leave the group at various points, the leader may choose to summarize at the start of each session to orient

---

ONLINE CONSULT

Visit the CRN at
http://www.crnhq.org

Identify possible conflict situations in your next work or group session.

Which techniques would you use for effective resolution?

newer and continuing members to current status, goals, and tasks. This approach is also highly effective in educational groups as it serves to reorient learners to prior content. Regardless of the focus of the group, periodic summaries and closure can be essential for the successful functioning of both the group and its members. Group members need an opportunity to acknowledge their accomplishments and be involved in the evaluation of the group process.

Roles of Group Members

Group members demonstrate a variety of roles during particular meetings. These roles may be either functional or nonfunctional for the group process. They may remain similar or constant over the life of the group, or individuals may alter their role from meeting to meeting. It is vital for nurses to recognize the roles assumed in groups and to intervene purposefully when necessary. Consider the last unit meeting you attended. Who led the group? Did anyone stall or disrupt the discussion? Were the topics discussed major issues for the unit or "pet peeves" of one individual? Did all members participate in the discussion? How could you, if you had been the group leader, have changed this meeting?

Functional Group Roles

Functional group roles facilitate the group process and determine the ultimate effectiveness of the group, especially in accomplishing a task or attaining a goal. In any type of group, members may play both functional and nonfunctional roles for various periods. For the effectiveness of

the group process, the goal is for members to demonstrate predominantly functional group roles. For nursing work groups, Tappen (2001) differentiated between **functional task roles** (Table 8.2), which contribute to completion of the task, and **functional group-building roles** (Table 8.3), which support development and meet relational needs. Think about what you have observed in a group meeting.

Observe these roles in any work-group setting, such as a committee or unit meeting. Many functional task and group-building roles are demonstrated by the group leader. The leader may start out as the information giver and standard setter during the forming stage, but then function as an information seeker, gatekeeper, and encourager as the group process evolves in the working stage. The leader may also demonstrate the functional roles of coordinator, energizer, summarizer, and consensus taker to facilitate group process and attainment of the group goals. Other group members will also serve in these functional roles as they become more active and progress toward the achievement of the group's goals. Observe who acts as the procedural technician, helping the leader organize the group and supplying needed equipment and materials. Examine who appears to be the more passive follower in the group, who cracks jokes as the tension reliever, and who records the actions and progress of the group.

Although these roles have been discussed mainly for the work setting, they also apply to professional, educational, and therapeutic group settings. In a professional group, observe the leadership roles shared by the officers, procedural technician roles performed by the aides or room monitors, and the standard setter role taken by the parliamentarian. In an educational group, consider the specific

---

TABLE 8.2	

Functional Task Roles

Initiator/contributor	Makes suggestions and proposes new ideas, methods, or problem-solving approaches
Information giver	Offers pertinent information from personal knowledge appropriate to the group topic or task
Information seeker	Requests information or suggestions from other members appropriate to the group topic or task
Opinion giver/seeker	Offers or requests views, judgments, or feelings about the topic or suggestions under consideration by the group
	Provides the opportunity for values clarification by the group members
Disagreer	Identifies errors in statements made or proposes a different viewpoint
Coordinator	Suggests relationships between the different suggestions or comments made by the group members
Elaborator	Elaborates or expands on suggestions already made
Energizer	Stimulates the group into action toward the goals either by introducing certain issues or topics or by behavior
Summarizer	Summarizes suggestions, actions, and accomplishments that have occurred in the group
Procedural technician	Provides the technical tasks needed for the group functions, such as arrangement of the group, including media, equipment, and work supplies
Recorder	Takes notes to record the progress, suggestions, and decisions of the group

Source: Adapted from Tappen, R. M. (2001). *Nursing leadership and management: Concepts and practice* (4th ed.). Philadelphia, PA: F. A. Davis.

TABLE 8.3

Functional Group-Building Roles

Encourager	Accepts and praises contributions of the group and other group members
Standard setter	Reinforces the standards or processes for effective group functioning
Gatekeeper	Ensures that all members have contributed to the discussion and that the group is not being monopolized by the views of more verbal members
Consensus taker	Seeks the weight of group sentiments or consensus on the issues
Diagnoser	Identifies barriers or blocks to group progress that are occurring
Expresser	Restates or identifies and expresses the feelings of the group
Tension reliever	Uses humor and mediation when group tensions rise and interfere with the group process and accomplishment of tasks
Follower	Consents to whatever is proposed by others in the group. Demonstrates no active participation without great encouragement

Source: Adapted from Tappen, R. M. (2001). *Nursing leadership and management: Concepts and practice* (4th ed.). Philadelphia, PA: F. A. Davis.

content and the size of the audience. Observe the roles taken by the teacher or facilitator, the people who are seated close to the teacher, the people in the back of the room, and the people who are asking most of the questions or cracking jokes. In a therapeutic group, observe the particular role of the leader and how he or she facilitates sharing of the members' feelings and beliefs. Observe the members who verbalize supportive comments versus those who disagree or give further information about similar feelings.

Nonfunctional Group Roles

At times, group members demonstrate nonfunctional roles when they interrupt the group process. An example is the individual who provides negative comments on whatever other group members propose. **Nonfunctional group roles** generally are disruptive to group-building, task accomplishment, and progress toward goal attainment. A group can actually be mobilized to act in response to the unacceptable actions of one member, however, such as speaking up to the individual who repeatedly comes late and then insists on being updated on what already occurred. Tappen (2001) identified the following nonfunctional roles: dominator, monopolizer, blocker, aggressor,

recognition seeker, zipper-mouth, and playboy. Smith (2001) listed similar disruptive roles in a meeting as latecomers/early leavers, silent/shy persons, whisperers/side conversationalists, and talk-a-lots, including loudmouths, know-it-alls, and hostiles.

- The *dominator* or *know-it-all* controls conversations, determines what will be discussed, and may attempt to control or intimidate other members. The dominator is focused on his or her own needs. An example of the dominator in a work group is a unit coordinator at a quality assurance meeting who suggests that the group focus on the number of requests for schedule changes. An example in a therapeutic group is a patient who opens the group by describing her plans with her family for the upcoming holidays rather than addressing the group leader's question on the assigned activity from last week.
- The *monopolizer* or *loudmouth* seeks attention and demands that the group focus on him or her. He or she may repeatedly interrupt others and perceive his or her issues and problems as the most important. A work-group example is the nurse who goes on and on about how he always has to work overtime. In a therapeutic group, an example is a patient who repeatedly interrupts and insists the group listen to her problem.
- The *blocker* interrupts the discussion, often focusing on another topic or personal concerns. The blocker can do this overtly or through side conversations, which can be highly disruptive to the group.
- The *aggressor* or *hostile* attacks during the discussion, making comments that may or may not be relevant to it. Often this individual is focused inwardly on personal needs and demands to be heard, regardless of relevance to the discussion. This member criticizes other group members because they do not have the same insights or experiences from his or her perspective. This individual is readily identified in professional, work, educational, and therapeutic groups by his or her hostile comments. Signs of discomfort or counterattacks may be apparent among other group members.
- The *recognition seeker* consistently attempts to draw the group's attention to his or her personal beliefs, values, and concerns. This individual has a need to stand out among the group members and be heard, respected, and perhaps admired. This member sometimes sounds like the leader but is usually working on personal issues. In a work-group example, this is the nurse who declares, "It's not all shifts that are short-staffed. Mine is the one that's always short-staffed with temps, but I am able to orient them successfully after all."
- The *zipper-mouth* in either a work or a therapeutic group is the silent individual who sits quietly, feeling unlucky to be in the group or even present in the situation. This is not the shy member, who is tracking the meeting content and perhaps needs more time in the group to develop trust, reflection, and opportunity.
- The *playboy* is the joker in the group and does not take the group seriously. Unfortunately, we have all experienced these individuals in a group setting and can easily recognize the disruption they make in the group process. These individuals may also be consistently late without notice or may frequently leave early.

Dealing with Difficult People

The group setting is no different from routine interpersonal interactions. You have probably encountered people who are difficult to work with. Whether a leader or a group member, you will inevitably encounter challenging personalities in the group setting. One of the most effective means of dealing with a difficult member is when the leader, as well as the members, address behaviors destructive to the group process. Awareness of your own reactions, observation of the group behaviors and interactions, and problem-solving are the steps toward effective group process, which can make all the difference between stagnation or dissolution, and meeting group goals.

As with interpersonal communication skills, there are effective ways to deal with difficult and disruptive group members. Consider the suggestions in Box 8.3. The skillful and effective group leader or member can use a variety of these techniques, depending on the group structure, composition, roles, focus, and situational factors. In addition, part of the ground rules can be that any group member may request a break or 10-minute recess. If group members do not ask but look uncomfortable, the leader may ask the group if a break is needed, and this can diffuse a stressful meeting and create a time-out when a situation is getting out of control. Having this as one of the ground rules empowers any member of the group to intervene in a conflict situation. Effective communication techniques and interpersonal skills are critical to success in group process, whether a small working group or a larger organizational setting.

ORGANIZATIONAL GROUPS

Communication issues among the larger **organizational group** and less tangible groups are also worth exploring.

Interorganizational Versus Intraorganizational Groups

Interorganizational groups are those that occur between systems or organizations. Communication is a vital activity to reach out to these other groups or systems. Interorganizational groups may consist of the hospital and the community mental health center, the home health agency, or the various subgroups of a health department. Outpatient hospital groups and inpatient unit groups also fit this category. These groups are often highly structured, with functions specified in job descriptions, policies, and procedures.

Nurses are involved with and provide leadership for effective functioning between or among systems in interorganizational groups. Communication and interpersonal skills are valuable attributes of professional nurses in this process. Along with these skills, a full awareness of each system or organization and its interrelationships is needed. This awareness involves an understanding of each organization's goals and values, hierarchial structure, leadership and management, interpersonal and communication systems, resources and technology, boundaries, and external environments, as illustrated in Chapter 10. In addition, consider the environment in which the different organizations or systems exist. Nursing involvement in interorganizational groups is growing as the complexity of health care and professional practice expands among different systems.

Collaboration among organizational groups is vital for the patient and for effective use of resources.

Intraorganizational groups are those that exist within a single, overall system or organization. The nursing, housekeeping, and physical therapy departments are intraorganizational groups within a hospital system. These groups are somewhat similar in terms of their structure, with specified roles, policies, and procedures. It is imperative for nurses to learn how to interact and negotiate effectively with these intraorganizational groups. An example is how to obtain needed supplies and services from the housekeeping department. Accomplishing this task often depends on the ability of members of each department to collaborate with the others. Activity for patients is a major consideration and incentive to work effectively together. For example, the patient is the focus for physical therapy and nursing departments. A physical therapist has certain scheduling needs based on individual patient progress. The nurse manager has different needs in scheduling staff for treatments, which may be predetermined by patient census, staffing, and care needs. Collaboration in this process is vital for the patient and effective use of resources.

Communication in Organizational Groups

In addition to the verbal and nonverbal interpersonal communication techniques, additional methods of communication are routinely used in large groups and organizations. The information we compile and the method we use to transmit it vary. Considering the purpose of communication in an organization is indispensable. Whether we are involved in health teaching or the transmission of physiological findings, the method and receiver of the information are important. Clear, concise, and timely transmission of information is necessary for an effective process. The time frame and ongoing evaluation are also factors in the initial communication phase as well as in the feedback phase of the process.

BOX 8.3 **Communication Techniques in a Group When Dealing with Difficult Members**

- Make observations and acknowledge contributions.
- Use the communication techniques of reflection and restatement.
- Refocus the discussion if it is getting off track.
- Set limits and adhere to the ground rules agreed upon by the group.
- Focus on potential solutions raised.
- Provide constructive feedback, not corrective feedback, which should be done privately.
- Promote balanced participation from members.
- Assign functional group roles to members displaying nonfunctional behaviors.
- Plan ahead and anticipate for the next group session.

Specifically, information can be sent or received by telephone, fax, e-mail, or texting, depending on the sender's and receiver's access to and skill with the available technology. A classic problem in some organizational settings is fear of technology among some people. Another problem is overuse. Consider the use of e-mail in organizations. The intent is to deliver information efficiently and rapidly to other individuals or groups of individuals in the sender's network while reducing paper and administrative costs. But some people avoid this form of communication, whereas others regularly check for messages, and still others "reply to all" or copy (or blind copy) multiple recipients, creating great volumes of unnecessary messages. If the information is not sent correctly or received appropriately, the message is not communicated and the process is ineffective.

Personal skills in verbal and written communication must be developed continually and refined through specific techniques or technologies. For example, keep in mind that e-mail can be forwarded easily to others, thus communicating with a larger group. The original sender's message will be evaluated by others on the appropriateness of content, format, and presentation (including grammar and appearance). Evaluating the appropriate channels or pertinent audiences and preparing the information in the correct format are vital for effective communication in the organizational setting. And careful proofreading should always take place, remembering that spell-checkers may miss errors—for example, *there* versus *their* and *heal* versus *heel*.

In essence, organizational communication can be thought of as being similar to the rights of administering medications. In organizational communications, these rights are as follows:

1. Information or content
2. Communication channel
3. Format, including use of correct grammar, terms, and language
4. Level of understanding
5. Technology
6. Follow-up

It is a professional responsibility to transmit a correct, credible, properly delivered message. The appropriate communication channel must be selected, using the appropriate chain of command to convey the message. The correct format is essential for decision making. One must decide whether to use an interdepartmental memorandum or a formal letter. The nature of the message dictates the format or type of communication. Correct grammar, terminology, and language are essential to present a professional image. Knowing the level of understanding of your intended audience is vital so that they can process the information. This means using the appropriate reading level and vocabulary. And finally, selecting the appropriate technology is important. Without the appropriate technology, recipients may not even receive your message. And follow-up is a necessary consideration for efficacy.

Virtual Group Meetings

Groups are traditionally viewed as necessitating face-to-face meetings. This situation has changed. Technology now allows groups to meet electronically, whether in real time or asynchronously. Electronic communications have provided the means for **virtual meetings**, by which people connect with others not in the same physical environment. Virtual meetings can be used by work, educational, therapeutic, or professional groups. The group is still focused with a common goal, and members interact with some leadership to organize and maintain the group. Ideas can be exchanged, experiences and information shared, and a common concern discussed. Teleconferencing or Web conferencing may be used alone or along with computer conferencing software that allows sharing of documents and visual presentations. Nursing groups now have Web sites and provide opportunities for students and professionals in groups to "discuss" core issues. Patients can interact with other patients and professionals via e-mail, chat rooms, and scheduled Internet meetings.

Virtual groups meet the same characteristics as face-to-face groups, in terms of group structure (formal or informal), composition (membership), roles (leader as facilitator and participants), and focus (work-related, educational, therapeutic, or professional). The virtual group experiences the same five stages of group development—initial, conflict, norming, working, and termination. The same set of evaluation criteria can be used to assess effectiveness of the virtual group. The role of the leader is more intense as a facilitator in the group process. The leader must employ a variety of group-building roles, time and distance being major considerations.

Like those of distance learning, the advantages of virtual meetings are savings in time and travel and, perhaps, the opportunity for involvement in which the travel distance would have been prohibitive. Because these groups do not meet face-to-face, preparation time and follow-up are more intensive to allow all group members to have equivalent information and participation opportunities.

Disadvantages of virtual meetings include the need for all members to have access to similar technologies and the individual's comfort level with their application. Analyzing the functional and nonfunctional roles of the members as virtual participants can be a bit challenging without the face-to-face assessment of interactions. The functional role of a participant can be identified in the text or content communicated, for example as information giver/seeker or elaborator. The nonfunctional members—dominator, monopolizer, blocker, aggressor, and recognition seeker—may appear to have a smaller impact (after all, members can delete their messages), but the leader must still address the underlying issues. And the issue of "talk-over" must be addressed in teleconference situations when several people want to contribute at the same time. The leader is challenged to have individuals identify themselves prior to providing commentary and share the discussion time on a conference call.

Any group—whether virtual or traditional, organizational, work, professional, educational, or therapeutic—demands the use of skills in observation, interpersonal communication, and group process that are essential characteristics of the involved professional nurse. These skills are tailored to the developmental stage of the group and the unique characteristics of its individual members. Professional nurses function as both members and leaders of such groups, and constant attention to these skills allows them to be integral components of effective groups in the profession and throughout the healthcare delivery system.

EVIDENCE-BASED PRACTICE: *Consider this....*

The American Association of Critical-Care Nurses (AACN) issued a practice alert on assessing pain in the critically ill adult. In addition to listing expected practice and the supporting evidence, they provide the following recommendations:

1. Obtain the patient's self-report of pain using validated pain assessment tools.

2. Perform a pain assessment for patients who are unable to self-report using a validated pain scale.

3. Avoid referring primarily to vital signs for pain assessment.

4. Consider proxy reporting by family members or caregivers who know the patient and can identify behavior indicative of pain. (AACN, 2013, p. 2)

Question: Consider the group process skills you will need for the three groups: (1) nursing staff education, (2) interdisciplinary work group, and (3) family and friends.

Source: American Association of Critical-Care Nurses (AACN). (2013). *Practice alert: Assessing pain in the critically ill adult.* Retrieved from http://www.aacn.org/wd/practice/content/practicealerts/assessing-pain-critically-ill-adult.pcms?menu=practice

KEY POINTS

- A group consists of three or more individuals with some commonality, such as shared goals or interests. Groups to consider in professional nursing practice include professional, work, educational, family, and therapeutic groups, each with specific goals and membership.

- Group process is described as the dynamic interplay of interactions within and between groups of humans.

- Groups are classified according to structure (formal or informal), composition, group roles, and focus (professional, work, educational, and therapeutic).

- The composition of a group may be homogeneous, with the group members sharing similar characteristics, or heterogeneous, with a mix of individuals.

- The issues to be addressed in establishing a group are the need and objectives for change and basic setup activities, including specifying and aligning the group purpose with the intended membership and determining the appropriate environment and group size.

- Effective groups are able to accomplish their goals in a manner that allows all members to participate, whereas ineffective groups become fragmented or dysfunctional.

- Group leaders structure the sessions to promote communication and participation by all members.

- Conflict situations can arise in any type of group, and conflict resolution is a process that requires problem-solving for effective group process.

- Groups go through predictable developmental stages: forming, storming, norming, working, and adjourning. The leader modifies his or her approach according to the group's current stage.

- Traditional group leadership styles are democratic, autocratic, and laissez-faire. Group leaders often use a combination of styles or modify their styles, depending on the group membership or topic being discussed.

- Functional group roles facilitate the group process and the ultimate effectiveness of the group. They include both functional task roles and functional group-building roles. Nonfunctional group roles are disruptive of group-building, task accomplishment, and progress toward goal attainment.

- Organizational groups may be interorganizational or intraorganizational, depending on whether they exist between organizational systems or within an organization.

- Even though technology has provided the opportunity for virtual groups, group process skills are still applicable at a distance in real time or asynchronously.

Thought and Discussion Questions

1. Identify at least three groups of which you are a member. Consider the membership, goals, leader, composition, and focus of each group. What are the similarities and differences? Contrast the leadership styles and skills in the three groups.

2. Be prepared to debate the advantages and disadvantages of heterogeneous and homogeneous groups in an online or class discussion.

3. Observe the members of the next departmental committee or nursing study group you attend.
   - Determine whether the group leader is the designated leader or a member who has assumed this role. If the leader was designated, who made the designation (external or internal designation)? Describe any effect this designation has had on the group function.
   - Describe the roles other members have assumed. Are the group roles different from these individuals' interactions in other settings?
   - Evaluate whether the members appear satisfied with the group's outcomes.
   - Evaluate whether this group or committee meets the characteristics of an effective group.

4. Review the Chapter Thought located on the first page of the chapter and discuss it in the context of the contents of this chapter.

Interactive Exercises

Go to the Intranet site and complete the exercises provided for this chapter.

REFERENCES

American Association of Critical-Care Nurses. (2013). *Practice alert: Assessing pain in the critically ill adult.* Retrieved from http://www.aacn.org/wd/practice/content/practicealerts/assessing-pain-critically-ill-adult.pcms?menu=practice

American Nurses Association. (2010). *Nursing: Scope and standards of practice* (2nd ed.). Silver Spring, MD: Nursesbooks.org.

Arnold, E. (2011). Communicating in groups. In E. Arnold & K. Boggs (Eds.), *Interpersonal relationships: Professional communication skills for nurses* (6th ed., pp. 222–245). Philadelphia, PA: Saunders/Elsevier.

Berlo, D. K. (1960). *The process of communication: An introduction to theory and practice.* New York: Holt, Rinehart, & Winston.

Conflict Resolution Network. (2014). *Conflict resolution skills.* Retrieved from http://www.crnhq.org/pages.php?pID=59

DeWine, S., Gibson, M. K., & Smith, M. J. (2000). *Exploring human communication.* Los Angeles, CA: Roxbury.

Robert, H. M., Evans, W. J., Honemann, D. H., & Balch, T. J. (2004). *Robert's Rules of Order newly revised in brief.* Cambridge, MA: DeCapo.

Smith, T. E. (2001). *Meeting management.* Upper Saddle River, NJ: Prentice Hall.

Tappen, R. M. (2001). *Nursing leadership and management: Concepts and practice* (4th ed.). Philadelphia, PA: F. A. Davis.

Tuckman, B. (1965). Developmental sequence in small groups. *Psychological Bulletin, 63,* 384–387.

Turniansky, B., & Hare, A. P. (1998). *Individuals in groups and organizations.* London, UK: Sage.

Yalom, I., & Leszcz, M. (2005). *Theory and practice of group psychotherapy* (5th ed.). New York: Basic Books.

BIBLIOGRAPHY

Barnard, S. (2001). Running an effective meeting. In S. Barnard, P. J. Casella, C. Coffin, T. Hughes, J. W. Hurst, J. S. Rasey, D. Redding, R. J. Robillard, D. St James, & S. C. Ullery, *Writing, speaking, and communication skills for health care professionals* (pp. 293–304). New Haven, CT: Yale University.

Berne, E. (1963). *The structure and dynamics of organizations and groups.* New York: Grove Press.

Galanes, G. J., Adams, K., & Brilhart, J. K. (2007). *Effective group discussion* (12th ed.). New York: McGraw-Hill.

Lundin, W., & Lundin, K. (1995). *Working with difficult people.* New York: American Management Association.

Merton, R. K. (1957). *Social learning theory and social structure.* New York: Free Press.

ONLINE RESOURCES

Social-Role Theory
http://changingminds.org/explanations/theories/social_role.htm

The Conflict Resolution Network (CRN)
http://www.crnhq.org

MeetingWizard.org
http://www.meetingwizard.org/meetings/effective-meetings.cfm

Mindtools.com
http://www.mindtools.com/index.html

● Rose Kearney-Nunnery

9

The Teaching-Learning Process

"To achieve a lasting change in observed behavior, the value of that change and the intellectual capacity to understand and process the information must first be present."

Rose Kearney-Nunnery

Chapter Objectives

On completion of this chapter, the reader will be able to:

1. Discuss the components of teaching and learning.
2. Examine differences in the ways people learn.
3. Describe methods to assess learning readiness and motivation.
4. Propose different teaching methods for a variety of learning needs.
5. Devise a plan for patient education that contains behavioral objectives, a content outline with appropriate teaching methods, and methods for evaluating learner outcomes.

Key Terms

Behaviorist Perspective
Classical Conditioning
Operant Conditioning
Gestalt Theory
Cognitive Theories
Social Cognitive Theory
Humanism

Andragogy
Transformative Learning
Multiple Intelligences
Teaching
Learning
Affective Domain
Cognitive Domain

Psychomotor Domain
Learning Environment
Cognitive Learning Styles
Readiness
Motivation
Behavioral Objectives

Teaching and learning are integral parts of contemporary nursing practice. Patient teaching has long been an expected nursing role. As a process, teaching and learning are much more than sharing and accepting information. There are many components to consider in order for teaching and learning to be effective.

NURSING PROCESS APPLIED TO THE TEACHING-LEARNING PROCESS

Consider the steps in the nursing process: assessment, diagnosis, outcome identification and planning, implementation, and evaluation. These same steps are applicable to the teaching and learning process.

Assessment and Diagnosis

Think about both the teacher and the learner. They represent more than simply the provider and receiver of information. Communication—verbal, nonverbal, and written—is a vital component in the teaching and learning process. It is a mutual process in which critical thinking is essential for both teacher and learner. Both teacher and learner obtain information, use reasoning skills, make analyses based on the data, and then move to decision making or problem-solving on the learning need or the acceptability of the problem or the information. The learner learns from the teacher, but the teacher also gains awareness and skill from each interaction with learners. In the assessment stage, there is essential information we need to know for an effective teaching-learning process. Some of the following questions arise:

- What are the attributes of each individual teacher and learner?
- Are there literacy, bilingual, or information processing issues to be addressed?
- What are the learning needs of the learner?
- How does the learner learn best?
- What is the readiness for and motivation to learn?
- What changes in behavior or attitude are perceived as being needed by both the teacher and the learner?
- What individual characteristics will enhance or inhibit learning?
- What is the teacher's teaching style?
- What is the cognitive style of the learner?
- What environmental factors will enhance or inhibit learning?
- What activities and resources will enhance learning?
- How can both the teacher and the learner evaluate the effectiveness of the learning process?

Assessing for a learning deficit or teaching need incorporates many factors. Notice that the concentration of the assessment is on the process of teaching and learning, not on specific content to be included in a presentation of information. Determining content is a discrete task performed later in the process, on the basis of the specific attributes and needs of the people and environment. Using this assessment information can lead to a *diagnosis* about the learner's particular teaching need.

Outcome Identification, Planning, and Implementation

Next, developing behavioral objectives with specific outcomes gives direction for a teaching plan and evaluation of the learning. Teaching strategies, methods, and resources to meet the diagnosed learning need, with specific content, must then be identified. The next step is planning for activities in the process, followed by implementation of the plan.

Evaluation

The outcomes of the teaching-learning process are evaluated. The evaluation component focuses on how the learner met the objectives and the specific outcome behaviors from the experience. Outcome objectives should be assessed by both the learner and the teacher. Evaluation is focused on the behavioral objectives specified for the learner earlier in the process. Although the nursing process provides a frame of reference for patient teaching, teaching and learning theories provide direction in the process.

TEACHING AND LEARNING THEORIES

Educators have studied learning theories for many years to understand and improve on the teaching-learning process. There are several schools of learning theories. Major examples of these theories applicable to professional nursing practice are behaviorism, gestalt, social cognitive theory, humanism, andragogy, transformative learning, and multiple intelligences (Box 9.1).

Behaviorism: Classical Conditioning

In introductory psychology courses, classic stimulus-response conditioning and operant conditioning are taught, providing a **behaviorist perspective** on learning. Ivan Pavlov's pioneering research with dogs led to our understanding of **classical conditioning**, in which the reflexive responses in behavior result from some stimulus. In classical conditioning, we saw that the pairing of food (the unconditioned stimulus) with the sound of a bell as a neutral (conditioned) stimulus led to salivation in dogs as an unconditioned response—first as an unconditioned response

---

BOX 9.1 Selected Theories of Learning

- Classical conditioning
- Operant conditioning
- Gestalt theory
- Cognitive development
- Social cognitive theory
- Humanism
- Andragogy
- Transformative learning
- Multiple intelligences

for the sight of the food, and ultimately as a conditioned stimulus with the sound of a bell alone. Using classical conditioning with infants, John Watson provided further insight on learning with his focus on the environment and emotional responses. Watson was a true behaviorist, looking at the development of the emotions of fear, love, and rage through classical conditioning and desensitization in his research with children.

Use of classical conditioning in nursing practice is limited. One situation may be in teaching patients to intervene as needed in response to physiological or emotional cues, auras, or triggers before an allergic, metabolic, or neural response. The individual with diabetes, a severe allergy, or epilepsy can be taught to perceive and make the association with early signs or symptoms that could lead to a larger physiological reaction. Classical conditioning is useful for early intervention to circumvent the reaction chain. Reflexes are important in this scenario to ensure that the individual is in a safe environment and has the resources for prompt treatment. Another example is the use of distraction, focusing, and breathing in certain reflexive situations—for patients in labor, in pain, or experiencing fear, for example.

Behaviorism: Operant Conditioning

Operant conditioning provides further clues to learning, with a focus on purposive behaviors and the role of reinforcement. In Thorndike's Law of Effect, reinforcement of a behavior is more likely to lead to repetition of that behavior. B. F. Skinner's research with rats and reinforcement for learned behaviors provided much additional information. In **operant conditioning**, the behavior is affected by the consequences (reinforcement), but the process is not trial and error (Skinner, 2010, p. 1). This theory introduced positive and negative reinforcers and reinforcement schedules to learning. The work of Skinner led to behavior modification programs and programmed instruction with shaping, reinforcement, and generalization of behavior.

Behavior modification programs are widely used in healthcare and education. They have been used effectively in certain nursing situations, such as nutritional programs that require a lifelong change in behavior. In such situations, old patterns are broken, stimuli are introduced to effect positive outcomes, responses are generalized to specific dietary items, positive and negative reinforcements are applied, and behavior is shaped over time. Another use for behavioral techniques is with adult patients with urinary incontinence. One method of treatment includes bladder retraining with the components of education, scheduled voiding, and positive reinforcement.

Behaviorism focuses on observation and measurement of actions in response to some association or conditioning. Rigorous use of the scientific process in the laboratory setting was a major factor in this perspective. Dissatisfaction with the emphasis on conditioning and reinforcement led to the evolution of other perspectives, including gestalt theory, cognitive theories, social learning theory, and humanism. In these later perspectives, we see an increased focus on the human intellect and human emotions.

Gestalt Theory

Gestalt theory focuses on meaning and thought, holding that learning occurs through perception. In German, *gestalt* refers to the perception of a whole form rather than its component parts. More than 100 laws on this perspective evolved with the identification of major principles concerning the way we perceive objects related to organization, proximity, similarity, direction, simplicity, background, and closure. Gestalt theorists view learning as based on perception of and completion of patterns. Patterns are perceived and reorganized by the person. In terms of learning, this perspective focuses on how the learner perceives the information and the unique environment. Kurt Lewin's field theory provided a major influence in this perspective with the emphasis on the importance of the environmental field. The perception of this environmental field by the person influences how that person, as a system, responds within the larger environmental system.

The classic principle in the gestalt perspective is that the whole is not merely the sum of the parts. This principle is consistent with the holistic view of human beings in professional nursing practice. Consider the importance we place on understanding how the person views the information to be learned. This focus on the person involves teaching materials that are used in addition to perceptual values. Further consider the learning environment and the importance we place on patient teaching in an unrushed, private, and comfortable setting when teaching (or promoting change for) specific health practices, as opposed to the hectic clinic environment where the person is distracted by children playing in the waiting room or verbalizations of discomfort expressed by others in the room. As another example, consider the patient in same-day surgery and the importance of preoperative teaching and the inclusion of significant others rather than the presentation of information when the patient is experiencing the effects from sedation and concerns over surgical outcomes.

Cognitive Theories

Cognitive theories of learning focus on the intellect and the development of knowledge. Recall the example of Piaget's theory of cognitive development from Chapter 2. Schemas were seen as patterns of thought or behavior that become more complex with the addition of more information. *Assimilation* is the acquisition of this information and incorporation into the individual's existing cognitive and behavioral structures. *Accommodation* is the change in the individual's cognitive and behavioral patterns based on the new information acquired. This acquisition of information is learning with the comprehension of concepts, memory, and analysis.

There are many different cognitive theories, mostly focusing on information processing. In nursing practice, use of cognitive theory is readily apparent with our focus on the level of cognitive development and acquisition of healthcare knowledge. We use principles of cognitive development to tailor a teaching plan to the patient's level of development, whether the patient is an elderly diabetic or a child with asthma. We are also concerned about the way learners process information, so that we can tailor our teaching strategies to suit their learning styles. In addition, the use of behavioral objectives with patients provides a focus for developing cognitive skills, moving from recall of knowledge to understanding, application, analysis, evaluation, and creation, as we will see later in the revised taxonomy table (Anderson et al., 2001) that stemmed from the classic work of Bloom's (1956) taxonomy.

Social Cognitive Theory

Cognitive learning through observation and imitation was the basis of Bandura's early theory known as the Social Learning Theory. Through the research of Bandura and his associates, aggressive and socialization behaviors of children were documented after observation of both symbolic and actual models. An important aspect of Bandura's work is the modeling of behavior with television and the effect of visualizing vicarious reinforcement and punishment for behavior. A humanistic, rather than mechanistic, orientation is apparent in this theoretical focus. Bandura (1977) explained the emphasis of vicarious, symbolic, and self-regulatory processes on how humans learn and influence their own destiny. Building on this broader focus on the person, behaviors, and the environment with the concept of self-regulation, Bandura proposed the expansion to the **Social Cognitive Theory** in the 1980s. Since that time, Bandura has incorporated self-efficacy, a theory important to patients in the healthcare setting as well as in normal activities. Self-efficacy is demonstrating a belief in your own competencies to produce a desired outcome. "Efficacy beliefs influence how people think, feel, motivate themselves, and act" (Bandura, 1995, p. 2). Bandura (1995) further identifies four sources of efficacy beliefs: mastery experiences, vicarious experiences, social persuasion, and physiological and emotional states (pp. 3–5). Efficacy can have a powerful effect as individuals take ownership of their individual learning needs. As Bandura (2007) proposes, social cognitive theory highlights distinctly human attributes (p. vii).

Nursing applications of the social cognitive theory are prevalent in the development of psychomotor skills in patients, such as self-administration of medications, procedures, and treatments. We often demonstrate skills to patients and expect them to return the demonstration. We provide positive reinforcement in the coaching function during the process, by making comments such as, "That's good," "That's the way," and "What a nice job." We promote healthful practices with encouragement and the hope for positive results as reinforcement for the new behavior. We show patients videos on a procedure in which they see modeling and reinforcement through a case scenario. These nursing behaviors focus on the individual in the environment as a thinking, feeling, and reacting being. Further, the concept of self-efficacy has long been used in nursing research and practice as we strive for the patient's independence and positive healthcare outcomes. The identified sources of efficacy are consistent with nursing practice with a greater focus on the individual as we promote mastery of skills, use of vicarious experiences in teaching, social persuasion in health promotion activities, and consistently integrate the physiological and emotional states of patients in their plan of care.

Humanism

Humanism has provided a major perspective on learning and one that has led to revision of older models. In this perspective, the focus is totally on the person. Abraham Maslow and Carl Rogers were major influences on this learning theory. As Maslow (1971) stated:

> [T]he humanistic goal . . . is ultimately the "self actualization" of a person, the becoming fully human, the development of the fullest height that the human species can stand up to or that the particular individual can come to. In a less technical way, it is helping the person to become the best that he is able to become. (p. 169)

The full range of human experiences is considered, as personally experienced and interpreted. Maslow's humanistic focus included motivation as a vital concern. Humanism is the basis of Carl Rogers's person-centered counseling. As described by his daughter, Rogers "above all, valued the worth and dignity of the individual and trusted their capacity for self-direction if given the proper environment" (Rogers & Freiberg, 1994, p. iii). Personal growth and autonomy are key to the humanistic perspective.

The humanistic perspective is consistent with the concepts of professional nursing. We focus on the person and assist in empowering him or her for health (whether an emerging state or to a higher level) and advocating for their active involvement in the health promotion process. The environment should be considered in terms of the person and his or her unique environmental setting and culture. Self-direction and insight into personal beliefs, attitudes, lifestyle, and behaviors are fundamental to the learning process. Culture, literacy, and learning or information processing deficits are also vital considerations with this perspective. As viewed in the health models in Chapter 4, cultural perspectives as a way of life must be included in any useful and humanistic teaching-learning plan. In addition, for effective teaching and learning to occur, deficits in learning or information acquisition or processing are humanistic factors that must be discovered, along with an understanding of adaptive patterns. Most consumers of nursing care are adults: parents, couples, individual adult or aging patients, families, community groups, and even professional peers with unique learning needs and characteristics.

Adult Learning Theories

Learning in adults requires the teacher to make adjustments to meet the different characteristics of learners. Adult learners differ from children in that they have past experiences, good and bad, with both teaching and learning.

Malcolm S. Knowles, who was a major force in adult learning in the United States, focused on **andragogy**. The term *andragogical model* was borrowed from European education (Knowles, 1990; Knowles et al., 1985). Expanding the traditional pedagogical learning models used with children to incorporate learning characteristics and needs of adults, this developmental model proposes that the accumulated life experiences of adults give them different teaching and learning needs from younger learners. In the pedagogical model, learners are generally dependent or passive, have few prior experiences to build on, and have external pressures from parents and others to learn something (Knowles et al., 1985, pp. 8–9). Adult learners are self-directing, have experiences that have shaped their identity, have experienced life events or a learning need that triggers their readiness to learn, have internal motivators, and demand an available, knowledgeable resource to assist them with practical problems and identified needs (Knowles et al., 1985).

As Knowles and associates (1985) have pointed out, adult learners often initially assume the comforting and passive learner roles of pedagogy, but then an inner conflict develops with their self-directing nature. The adult's ego system is based on his or her self-concept and accumulated knowledge and experiences, whereas a child is gratified by impressing a parent, teacher, or peer. Knowles's developmental focus is demonstrated further with his identification of life problems by age group in early, middle, and later adult life groups. He specified life problems in the areas of vocation and career, home and family life, personal development, enjoyment of leisure, health, and community living (Knowles, 1990). Recall Bandura's (1995) sources of self-efficacy (mastery experiences, vicarious experiences, social persuasion, and physiological and emotional states) that are consistent with this view.

Adult teaching and learning depend on both physical and psychological climates. Physical climate relates to the learning environment. The setup of the room should not replicate a stilted lecture setting and should promote comfort so that the learners can focus on learning needs and problem-solving. Knowles emphasized the need for adults to feel at ease in the learning environment, which leads to the psychological climate for the adult learner. Knowles identified seven characteristics of the psychological climate conducive to adult learning: mutual respect, collaborativeness, mutual trust, supportiveness, openness and authenticity, pleasure, and humanness (Knowles et al., 1985, pp. 15–17). Knowles viewed the teacher as the catalyst and facilitator. A common thread running through teaching and learning strategies for adults is mutuality—mutuality in diagnosing, planning, learning, and evaluating. One key to successful teaching and learning in adults is their active involvement throughout the process.

On the basis of Knowles's work, Vella further identified 12 principles for effective adult learning. Then, she further considered six concepts from quantum thinking (relatedness, holism, duality, uncertainty, participation, and energy) and reinforced the 12 principles with adult education, especially in the use of dialogue to promote optimal learning:

- Participation of the learners in their needs and resources assessment
- Safety in the environment and the process
- Sound relationships between teacher and learner
- Careful attention to sequence of content and reinforcement
- Praxis (action with reflexion, or learning by doing)
- Respect for learners as decision makers
- Holistic ideas, feelings, and actions
- Immediacy of the learning (relevancy)

- Clear roles and role development (participation in the search for meaning)
- Teamwork and use of small groups
- Engagement of the learners in all domains of what they are learning
- Mutual accountability for the learning. (Vella, 2002, pp. 30–35)

These principles are consistent with our holistic view of patients as unique individuals with respect for their environment. It is critical to promote their empowerment to address their distinctive healthcare learning needs. Content and actions must be meaningful to them for learning to occur.

Transformation Theory

The basis for transformative learning is meaningfulness of experiences, especially for adults who have accumulated knowledge, cultural and environmental patterns, and experiences. Think about the last time you said to yourself, "I'm not going to do that again!"

One of the major theorists in this area is Mezirow (2000), who defines **transformative learning** as follows:

> . . . the process by which we transform our taken-for-granted frames of reference (meaning perspective, habits of mind, mind-sets) to make them more inclusive, discriminating, open, emotionally capable of change, and reflective so that they may generate beliefs and opinions that will prove more true or justified to guide action. (pp. 7–8)

Transformative learning involves three stages: critical reflection of the situation, changing and integrating the new perspective and understanding, and acting on that new understanding. The key is the active and rational process of reflective thinking on past experiences and personal assumptions of the situation. Mezirow (2000) describes this process as reflective discourse: "that specialized use of dialogue devoted to searching for a common understanding and assessment of the justification of an interpretation or belief" (pp. 10–11). This use of dialogue with adult learners is similar to the one described by Vella and can be used effectively in individualized or small group learning environments as adults are actively challenged to find meaningfulness of the information.

Critical reflection involves challenging one's assumptions and beliefs. Do they still hold true, or is there perhaps a better way that is acceptable to the adult learner in his or her unique context? This active and thoughtful process is personally determined. This theory of learning has been described as a "theory in progress" as further research evolves. In addition, a current nursing model has evolved from this theory (Fawcett, 2006, p. 504). Transformation theory is consistent with nursing's view of the person as a thinking, feeling, rational being with past experiences and attributes that influence behavior. But notice that the learners are the active ones in the process. They are assisted with the information for critical reflection, but they must challenge their "habits of mind" and "resulting points of view" that Mezirow (2000) refers to as the two components of one's "frame of reference" (p. 17). Then the person must decide whether to take action on the revised perspective as the transformation. As Kippers and Boden (2012) point out, "at the heart of transformative learning is the notion of partnership" (p. 7). The involvement of the patient in the learning experience must be a partnership for effectiveness.

Adult learning theories have evolved from a humanistic philosophy, focusing on the unique combinations of talents and abilities possessed by an individual based on prior learning, skill sets, and contextual factors.

Multiple Intelligences Theory

Another theory of learning focused on the person proposes **multiple intelligences** (Gardner, 1993a, 1993b, 1999, 2006), all of which are considered equally important and are most often found in combination in individuals to differing degrees. This theory looks beyond cognitive capacity and encourages a view of the individual's cognitive profile. The basis for the theory is Gardner's observations of and work with children, adults, prodigies, and gifted, normal, autistic, brain-damaged, and autistic savant individuals. Gardner (1999) has characterized the seven different multiple intelligences (Table 9.1) according to eight criteria, two each derived from the biological sciences, logical analysis, developmental psychology, and traditional psychological research. From his original work, Gardner (1999) refined his definition of an intelligence as:

A biopsychological potential to process information that can be activated in a cultural setting to solve problems or create products that are of value in a culture. (pp. 33–34)

Gardner (2006) further refers to these *intelligences* as a "set of abilities, talents, or mental skills" (p. 6). The theory of multiple intelligences allows a greater focus on individuals and their unique talents and combinations of abilities in their contextual setting. As Gardner (1999) points out, "what matters is the use of intelligences, individually and in concert, to carry out tasks valued by a society" (p. 208). In addition, "owing to hereditary, early training, or in all probability, a constant interaction between these factors,

some individuals will develop certain intelligences far more than others; but every normal individual should develop each intelligence to some extent, given but a modest opportunity to do so" (Gardner, 1993a, p. 278). Gardner has also thought about two additional *intelligences* that he indicates meet most of the criteria from his theory. Although Gardner (2006) does not seem fully committed to these additions, he names the potential for the naturalist and the existential intelligences as the *8½ Intelligences* (p. 21).

Consider for a moment that you will be caring for two patients following hip replacement surgery and are planning discharge teaching. One patient is an architect who designs custom homes and meets with his customers for at least an hour before he develops the house plans to ensure that he truly understands their desires and ideas. The other is a retired English professor who is concerned about the rehabilitation schedule and the completion of a collection of essays that he must submit to his publisher in six weeks. Your approach to each will differ on the basis of his unique talents and abilities.

The perspective of multiple intelligences is humanistic, focusing on the unique combinations of talents and abilities possessed by an individual. These unique individual abilities are consistent with the practice of nursing dealing with the individual and environmental influences. Given the variety of learning theories, however, application may involve selecting a more eclectic approach. Specific teaching guides involve our consideration of human beings and the environment, given the particular health focus in contemporary nursing practice. Certain principles provide direction in this process.

TEACHING AND LEARNING PRINCIPLES

The philosophical and theoretical structures of any discipline reflect how the teacher and learner are viewed. In nursing, we view both the teacher and the learner as thinking, reasoning, active participants involved in the

TABLE 9.1

Seven Intelligences (Gardner, 1999, pp. 42–43)

Intelligence	Description	Example(s)
Linguistic	Language and verbal	Poets, writers, speakers
Logical-mathematical	Mathematical cognitive skills in logic, mathematics, and science	Mathematicians, scientists
Spatial	Use of mental models of spatial world and manipulate patterns	Sailors, engineers, artists, pilots, architects
Musical	Innate musical sense and talent in performance, composition, and appreciation	Musicians, composers
Bodily kinesthetic	Use of body or parts of the body in problem-solving	Dancers, athletes, craftspeople, mechanics
Interpersonal	Understanding intentions, motivation, and desires of others	Politicians, salespeople, teachers, clergy
Intrapersonal	Understanding of self and one's life course	Self-awareness

teaching-learning process. We believe individuals are influenced by and influence their environment. These environmental influences, including persons, events, and tangible surroundings, must be taken into account when any teaching behavior is considered. In terms of health, teaching in nursing reflects information to promote or maintain the highest level of health attainable. The teacher's and the learner's definitions of health and wellness influence physical, psychological, emotional, and spiritual health as personal determinants of behavior.

Teaching

Although the teaching-learning process is an interactive communication process, its component parts must be considered. With this in mind, several processes can be seen readily as inherent in the teaching-learning process, such as communication and critical thinking. **Teaching** is more than the transmission of information. The information must be received, understood, evaluated, and accepted by the learner. Teaching has been described as "an intentional and reasoned act" (Anderson et al., 2001). Benner (1984) has identified the teaching-coaching function of the expert nurse working with acutely ill patients:

1. Use timing to capture learning readiness and motivation.
2. Assist with integration of learning into lifestyle.
3. Demonstrate an understanding of patient's own interpretation of the situation.
4. Provide interpretations of situations and rationales for new behaviors.
5. Show, through example, coaching behaviors in culturally sensitive issues. (pp. 77–94)

These characteristics demonstrate the active roles of both teacher and learner in the process. Readiness and motivation must be present for both the teacher and the learner during the process. The best teachers are those who truly believe in the information they are sharing and can communicate this belief. They provide the excitement, or at least some reinforcement, for the learner, who wants to know more. The active role of the learner in the process is vital, because passive learning rarely results in persistent change in attitudes or behaviors. The motivation of teacher and learner are also important, as the teacher demonstrates an understanding of the learner's unique characteristics and perspective on the subject or situation. Providing information is the traditional role of the teacher, but doing so in the context of the learner's

reality helps provide a rationale for behavior changes. Finally, coaching through example, with sensitivity, is the essence of expert teaching and nursing.

Teaching is an interactive process, not a unidirectional transmission of information. As Benner demonstrates in her examples of expert nurses, we also learn from those we teach.

Learning

Learning is the perception and assimilation of the information presented to us in a variety of ways. Learning contains the following characteristics:

- Perception of new information
- Initial reaction to the information
- Ability to recall or repeat the information (simple knowledge level)
- Rejection or acceptance of the information (understanding)
- Use of the information in a similar situation (application)
- Critical analysis of the information
- Incorporation of the information into the value system (evaluation)
- Use of the information in various situations and combinations (creation)

An increasing complexity emerges here as the learner moves from receiving and recalling information through:

Understanding

⇓

Application

⇓

Analysis

⇓

Evaluation of the knowledge acquired and *creation* of new applications

We see this process in the patient who accepts information on the importance of breast familiarity, is able to perform the self-examination, does so on a regular basis in combination with mammography and clinical examinations, teaches her daughter or mother the process, and is now investigating regular screening for colon cancer for herself and family members. This patient has moved from simple knowledge to incorporation of knowledge into the value system and behaviors of herself and other family members.

Learning can be enhanced via specific strategies or approaches with learners. Learning is not a linear process of providing information and assessing recall and performance. We must also take into account the person in his or her environment and culture, and the various domains of learning. Consider the difference between the knowledge and the consistent demonstration of behaviors. We may "know" something but either consciously or subconsciously decide not to demonstrate that behavior. For example, a patient may have been prescribed a low-fat diet and can tell you all about foods with high fat content, but may also decide that ice cream is a part of the diet, ignoring its fat content.

Domains

A domain is merely a category. There are three domains of learning or knowledge: affective, cognitive, and psychomotor.

The **affective domain** includes attitudes, feelings, and values. For example, how the patient feels about the importance of or the positive effect on his life of a needed dietary change will influence whether he will make the change. Often, the nursing goal is to incorporate the value of the diet into the person's belief system. Cultural influence, cultural differences in the individual, family, or group, and the nurse's professional influences can all either positively or negatively affect whether the goal is achieved, however.

The **cognitive domain** involves knowledge and thought processes within the individual's intellectual ability. Using the same example of the patient and the low-fat diet, the cognitive domain involves understanding the information received about nutrition, diet, health conditions, and indications. The ability to conceptualize types of foods, gram counts, and dietary needs involves comprehension, application, and synthesis at an intellectual level before the patient performs the actual behaviors.

The **psychomotor domain** is the processing and demonstration of behaviors; the information has been intellectually processed, and the individual is displaying motor behaviors. To continue with the example, psychomotor skills are demonstrated by how the patient has performed on the changed diet, as seen in food diary reporting, preparing and ingesting appropriate foods, and even laboratory reports evaluating bodily functions.

It is important to consider these three domains in the teaching-learning process. Behavioral objectives, teaching content and methods, and evaluation of learning can be very different for the three domains and should be distinct. Remember, to achieve a lasting change in observed behavior (psychomotor domain), the value of that change (affective domain) and the intellectual capacity to understand and process the information for behavioral changes (cognitive domain) must first be present.

Consistent with the philosophical focus of nursing, the **learning environment** is important in any teaching or learning activity. Physical comfort as well as respect and acceptance of the learner are humanistic factors. The consumer of healthcare may also have physical, sensory, or psychological deficits that can interfere with comfort in the learning environment or in the teaching-learning process, as seen in the physiological and emotional source of self-efficacy proposed by Bandura. Comfort measures should be validated with the patient before and during the process. Physical comfort can include such things as the temperature of the room and the height or firmness of the chairs, in addition to specific effects of acute or chronic health problems. Sensory concerns include the extraneous sensory stimuli perceived by the teacher or learner in the learning environment, such as sounds, smells, and sights. In addition, the patient may have sensory deficits—such as visual, hearing, or information processing problems—that may

interfere with learning or may require more resources. Psychological deficits, including fear, problems with cognition, attention span, effects from medications, and worry, can be major inhibitors to teaching and learning. Receptivity of the learner to new and different ideas is vital. Creative measures taken by the nurse as teacher to provide for an environment conducive to learning are essential.

> To achieve a lasting change in observed behavior (psychomotor domain), the value of that change (affective domain) and the intellectual capacity to understand and process the information for behavioral changes (cognitive domain) must first be present.

COGNITIVE LEARNING STYLES

The *cognitive learning process* is a broad area that examines how meaning is perceived, evaluated, remembered, reinforced, and demonstrated. Piaget gave us information on childhood cognition through observations of his own and other children and provided us with the concepts of assimilation and accommodation. Recall that *assimilation* is the acquisition and incorporation of new information into the individual's existing cognitive and behavioral structures, and *accommodation* is the change in the individual's cognitive and behavioral patterns based on this new information. Cognitive learning styles have been discussed with varied research for over 50 years in an attempt to improve teaching and learning outcomes.

In the mid-1980s, Kolb (1981) identified specific learning styles as concrete experience, reflective observation, abstract conceptualization, and active experimentation. And the research and the discussion continue as we seek to understand better how individuals acquire meaning and knowledge. Increasingly we are concerned with the active involvement of the learner in the process, for learning to truly occur. **Cognitive learning styles** or preferences are simply the ways learners perceive, think, organize, use, and retain knowledge. To understand this concept, merely recall colleagues in the same learning environment—those who took copious notes, those who just listened, and those who made notes or drawings on what they interpreted the message in the lecture to be. Understanding the differences in cognitive styles can help teachers and learners make more informed decisions about which learning activities will be useful or productive to learners as individuals and as members of learning groups or communities.

> Stemming from a basis in Jung's theory of the unconsciousness and personality, the Myers-Briggs Inventory was developed and has been used widely in education and business applications for learning styles. This personality inventory uses the following four scales to identify 16 personality types that can be further classified for learning preferences:

- Introversion–Extroversion
- Sensing–Intuition

- Thinking–Feeling
- Judging–Perceptive

Check your style with a similar inventory at
**http://www.humanmetrics.com/
cgi-win/JTypes2.asp**

Teaching and learning strategies have developed to match each learner with the teaching resources most effective for his or her learning style or to develop strategies to adjust to the prevalent teaching style. The main types of learning styles look at preferences for visual learning (reading or watching), auditory (listening or talking), and kinesthetic (doing or participating). For example, some learners are highly visual in the way they perceive information and derive meaning. For these learners, a structured lecture with few visual aids is a less desirable learning environment than one enhanced by visual aids. Others learn better through the written word, either by reading or note taking. Learners who are highly auditory in their learning preference derive greater meaning from just listening to the information. The theory of multiple intelligences can be useful in this situation, to further tailor the learning to the individual's talents.

Assessment data on learning style may be obtained from the patient in a nursing interview rather than formal testing inventories used with larger groups. In essence, good assessment of the learner is vital to ensure the most effective teaching and the most efficient and enjoyable learning.

READINESS AND LEARNING

Readiness is an important concept in learning, regardless of the learner's chronological age. **Readiness** relates to the developmental needs and tasks of individuals. Consider the views of two developmental theorists: Erikson (1963) described readiness as critical periods, whereas Havighurst (1972) referred to readiness as sensitive periods or the "teachable moment." For teaching to be effective and learning to take place, the readiness of the learner must be a prime consideration. A good example is the issue of compliance and noncompliance in the patient group.

Compliance is an often misused and misunderstood concept. We talk about patients being noncompliant when they do not follow their discharge or healthcare teaching instructions. The reasons and background for the behavior in the patient group must first be realized and understood, not assumed. Compliance is yielding to the desire of others, possibly as a result of threats or force. But as we see later in the change process, threats and force do not bode well for a permanent change in behavior. Human behavioral change is more effective when one is personally involved in the process. Specifically, how do learning and readiness apply to receiving and accepting information for a change in lifestyle? Consider the teenager undergoing dialysis who carefully monitors his sodium intake after dialysis but fills up on fast food the day or morning before the scheduled dialysis. Is this truly noncompliance or developmental maneuvering with peer pressure and dietary restrictiveness? Now, consider the adult cardiac patient with a strict dietary sodium restriction. Is noncompliance by this individual due to a stubborn adherence to food preferences, culture, or custom, or perhaps failed health

teaching for change because of a failure to achieve learning readiness?

The learner must be willing to change and accept the learning need. When this occurs, readiness for learning is apparent. This can be seen in terms of King's (1981) theory of goal attainment: Both the nurse and the patient must be focused on and sensitive to the same goal. Readiness for the learning and teaching is then present. Ultimately, the effectiveness of the teaching methods and content is evaluated on the basis of the learning that did or did not take place. Learning readiness involves the following factors: human motivation, understanding or cognitive level, and applicability or acceptability.

Literacy and language issues are an additional consideration in readiness. For the individual with a low literacy level, years of adaptive behavior may disguise the inability to read or process basic information. Likewise, an individual who speaks English as a second language may perceive information differently. In each situation, the individual may be unwilling to indicate to the nurse that he did not fully understand or accept the information presented. In addition, literacy and health literacy are different, with health literacy compounded with new or different health terminology that has different translational or cultural implications. The readiness to learn is inhibited by additional factors in these cases. As recommended by Singleton and Krause (2009), "understanding a patient's level of health literacy requires an assessment of the patient's linguistic skills and cultural norms and the interpretation of these skills and norms into health literacy strategies for the patient's plan of care" (p. 6). In addition, the Joint Commission (2013) has estimated that there are more than 300 languages spoken in the United States and more than 90 million Americans have low health literacy (with difficulty understanding and using health information), thus recommending communicating health information that encompasses language needs, individual understanding, and cultural and other barriers (p. 1).

Motivation

Motivation in humans is a manifestation of internal and external personal and environmental factors that cause people to respond to a situation in the way that they do. Motivation has been classically viewed as needs, drives, and impulses that cause behavior. One view of motivation in humans is Maslow's Theory of Human Motivation, based on the hierarchy of basic needs. Maslow (1954) identified 16 propositions about human desires or motivation that implied a complex interrelationship in human motivation based on internal and external factors as personally interpreted by the individual. Maslow's work indicated that the hierarchy of human needs is based on motivation. But motivation is as intricate as the person, not merely inherent impulses and drives. And even more focused on the individual, Bandura (1995) proposed that efficacy beliefs play a key role in the self-regulation of motivation in that people motivate themselves and guide their actions anticipatorily by the exercise of forethought and form beliefs about what they can do (p. 6).

The concept of motivation, then, considers the person's interpretations of the situation and his or her ability and willingness. Readiness, therefore, involves motivation and understanding. *Understanding* is the cognitive ability to perceive and intellectualize the content and consequences of information. Bandura believes that most actions are under anticipatory control, as humans use symbolic representation to envision future outcomes of behavior. The way the person views these future consequences of behavior becomes the motivation to behave or proceed in the present. This concept relates well to health teaching, in that the patient can be motivated to learn with a realistic anticipation of the situation and consequences. Nurses can recognize patient anticipation in the assessment phase, through interview data, diagnosis of the teaching and learning needs, and development of behavioral objectives. During this process, motivation can be assessed and stimulated by the patient as well as by the professional nurse.

Cognitive Level

A person's cognitive level is a component of understanding; the content provided must be at the person's level of understanding. Piaget's theory of cognitive development describes the differences in learning levels between the sensorimotor infant developing object permanence and the older child who is able to learn abstract mathematical skills through formal operations. Information must be available to the person at his cognitive level for processing and development of knowledge. The person may require concrete examples to envision future consequences or may be able to handle more abstract or even philosophical examples. An important consideration here is the patient's state of health. Current physiological or psychological functioning and medications may interfere with reasoning and understanding as well as with attention span. Readiness for health teaching in this instance may be at different levels, depending on physical and emotional functioning.

Applicability and Acceptability

Another component of readiness for the teaching-learning process is applicability and acceptability of the information. The person must perceive that the information is applicable to him or her, as an individual, a member of the family, or a member of a group. If the person denies that a health problem exists, he or she will not be ready for health teaching in that area. The information is not perceived as personally applicable. *Acceptability* means that the information must be within the person's worldview. Cultural influences are important, because values and belief systems influence understanding and acceptability of information. The health problem and readiness must be seen in the context of the individual's belief system. This is an important relationship, as we see in the health belief model. Cultural assessment data provide important information on the patient's belief system that should be incorporated into the teaching-learning process.

PRACTICAL TEACHING TIPS

Developing behavioral objectives sets the stage for the teaching-learning process. Objectives lead to the planning phase with selection of appropriate teaching strategies

ONLINE CONSULT

Joint Commission Hospitals, Language & Culture at
http://www.jointcommission.org/assets/1/6/ARoadmapforHospitalsfinalversion727.pdf

Think Cultural Health at
https://www.thinkculturalhealth.hhs.gov/

and methods, and evaluation of both the learning outcomes and the teaching process.

Writing Behavioral Objectives

The purpose of writing **behavioral objectives** is to provide a frame of reference for the intended outcomes of the teaching-learning activity for both the teacher and the learner. The use of behavioral objectives gives us a focus on learners and evaluation of their experiences with specific measures for behaviors. Behavioral objectives are the intended outcomes of the learners, not the teacher's goals for the activity.

Think of behavioral objectives in terms of the learner's "who, what, where, when, and how." In viewing the individual components of behavioral objectives, consider those listed at the start of this chapter. Initially, there is the stem statement, "On completion of this chapter, the reader will be able to. . . ." This provides the "who"—the reader of the chapter, and the "when"—after completion of the chapter. The "what" and "how" are the action-oriented outcomes that the learner will demonstrate in the listed behaviors. Behavioral objectives do not address all of the content that will ultimately be included in the teaching plan. Rather, the "what" in the behavioral objectives is the outcome we wish to evaluate after the teaching has occurred. Consider the chapter objectives to determine the "how" and "what" information:

1. Discuss (how) the components of teaching and learning (what).
2. Examine (how) differences in the ways people learn (what).
3. Describe (how) methods to assess learning readiness and motivation (what).
4. Propose (how) different teaching methods for a variety of learning needs (what).
5. Devise (how) a plan for patient education that contains behavioral objectives, a content outline with appropriate teaching methods, and methods for evaluating learner outcomes (what).

This example focuses on the learner at the end of the prescribed learning activity, with action verbs—discussing, examining, describing, proposing, and devising—as their outcome ability, describing "how" they should be able to perform.

The next focus is on the complexity that you as the evaluator (whether learner or teacher) wish to see demonstrated at the end of the activity. This is the degree that can be measured, or the "where." The type and complexity of the outcome behavior are determined by the level of the learning domain.

When developing behavioral objectives, be sure to consider the domains of knowledge. Further, within each domain there is a leveling process, or progress in attainment of increasingly complex skills. From the work of Bloom and other teaching and learning theorists, a revised two-dimensional taxonomy was developed. The revised taxonomy table considers the interrelationship of two dimensions: knowledge and cognitive processes (Anderson et al., 2001). This is the knowledge or the "what" you wish the learner to acquire, and the cognitive process is the demonstration or "how" the learning is evaluated. The taxonomy table allows objectives to be developed that address both knowledge and processes. Consider that the nursing goal for the patient is to be at the procedural knowledge level to apply a dressing change at home but also at the factual knowledge level to evaluate signs of infection or monitor the response to a prescribed medication.

Knowledge Dimension

In this revised taxonomy table, the knowledge dimension represents the four rows of the table with the following knowledge categories:

- Factual, as the basic elements
- Conceptual, or the interrelationships among elements
- Procedural, or demonstration of a set of skills
- Metacognitive, as the highest level of awareness of the thought processes. (Anderson et al., 2001)

Consider the difference of these categories in nursing practice, as in the case of a sterile field. "Factual" is simply the knowledge of the components. "Conceptual" would be the understanding of the interrelationship, as with spillage and contamination of the field. "Procedural knowledge" would be in the performance of a dressing change and maintenance of the field. "Metacognitive knowledge" would occur during practice with an unanticipated occurrence and resolution using critical thinking skills. In patient education, we strive for the procedural level, for the return demonstration of a set of skills, as in the dressing change needed at home and the protection of the surgical or wound site.

Cognitive Processes Dimension

In the revised taxonomy table, the cognitive process dimension is represented in the six columns of the table as the following levels of increasing complexity:

- Remember, as recognizing and recalling
- Understand, as interpreting, exemplifying, classifying, summarizing, inferring, comparing, and explaining
- Apply, as executing and implementing
- Analyze, to include differentiating, organizing, and attributing
- Evaluate, or making judgments based on certain criteria
- Create, or developing a new process (Anderson et al., 2001)

Cognitive processes in this taxonomy build from the simple recall of facts to the extrapolation into a new process. Continuing to use our example, we want the nurse in a preceptor position for a senior student or a new graduate to use cognitive skills through evaluation for the maintenance of the sterile field in all practice applications with the novice nurse or nursing student. In advanced practice, however, the nurse would consistently use all processes in the domain for the specialty area, including the creation of new processes within the selected scope of practice. In the scenario of patient education, the goal would be for the patient to be able to remember, understand, and apply specific skills, and to analyze and evaluate when professional intervention is needed, as in the case of potential infection or a complication.

In the cognitive processes dimension, we first have the knowledge received through recall or recognition. Next, we proceed to an understanding of the information. The final levels of the cognitive domain are applying the information, analyzing, evaluating the information, and finally creating for application of the knowledge in other situations. Consider the levels in the cognitive processes domain with the following action words in your behavioral objectives for teaching a patient about his or her condition:

1. *Knowledge* implies simply that the learner has perceived the information and can report it back to the teacher. Action verbs such as *identifies*, *recalls*, *recognizes*, and *repeats* are useful for behavioral objectives at this knowledge level of the cognitive domains, such as the ability to recall a list of the signs of infection in a learning situation.
2. At the next level, the learner demonstrates *understanding* of the knowledge, based on the four levels of the knowledge dimension. Action verbs for behavioral objectives at this level include *explains* and *compares*, as illustrated by the patient who can explain how to look for redness indicating infection in a surgical wound.
3. The third level of the cognitive domain is *application*, demonstrating the ability to relate the learning to a situation. The following action verbs are appropriate for behavioral objectives for the learner's outcomes at this point: *applies*, *demonstrates*, *employs*, and *uses*. For example, "The patient uses the dressing change skill at home after discharge."
4. Further critical thinking occurs at the next cognitive level of *analysis*. The learner steps back and analyzes the information objectively. Action verbs useful at this level of complexity include *assesses*, *appraises*, *organizes*, and *differentiates*. Now the patient has determined the need to call the physician's office for evaluation of potential complications from the surgery.
5. *Evaluation* occurs at the next level of cognitive processes in which judgment is an essential component. Action verbs appropriate for this level include *evaluates*, *tests*, *monitors*, and *critiques*.
6. *Creation* is the highest level of the cognitive domain, in which the learner manipulates the concepts from the learning in new combinations and situations. Action verbs addressing this level of complexity in the taxonomy include *creates*, *designs*, *devises*, *constructs*, and *generates*.

Both the cognitive and psychomotor domains appear in the taxonomy table with the focus on knowledge and the cognitive process. The psychomotor domain is easily apparent in the application of the knowledge. It is important to include behavioral objectives at the various knowledge levels to measure patient progress from simple to complex skills. For example, suppose you have taught a newly diagnosed diabetic patient to self-administer insulin. As the teacher, you must be able to see how the learner-patient has accomplished this task, beyond the simple return demonstration with saline injections that you observe. At the next level of manipulation of the psychomotor skill, the learner demonstrates the entire procedure of proper injection of insulin, from filling the syringe to disposing of the supplies. Precision of the psychomotor skill is demonstrated when the learner can perform the injection on schedule with a sense of comfort in her ability in the process, expressed with the phrase "Demonstrates skill in the procedure." Articulation, or full use of the skill, is demonstrated when the diabetic patient is able to manage at home with insulin, including testing blood glucose for additional needs during stressful periods. This is reflected in the phrase "Uses results of blood glucose monitoring to regulate. . . ."

The highest level of skill acquisition comes when the individual has a sense of competence and the skill has become a natural part of his routine; the individual can determine signs of hyperglycemia or hypoglycemia and self-test as naturally as she dresses or bathes. The individual has incorporated the process sufficiently to spend a month traveling with a sense of independence, comfort, and control in the process. Action terms reflecting this level include "Independently monitors and effectively regulates administration of insulin." These actions demonstrate Bandura's concept of mastery experiences in self-efficacy.

The affective domain is less apparent in the revised taxonomy table but is inferred in the higher levels of knowledge and cognitive processes. In fact, the creators of the revised taxonomy propose that "nearly every cognitive objective has an affective component" (Anderson et al., 2001). For the affective domain, complexity progresses from receiving to responding, valuing, organizing values, and finally characterizing or standing for certain values transmitted. Consider the newly diagnosed diabetic patient. Acceptance of her condition is vital to developing long-range personal care skills. But this is a difficult domain to measure because values and attitudes are more difficult to assess than knowledge or psychomotor skills. Although action verbs for the affective domain include *receiving, responding, valuing, organizing values,* and *characterizing,* this is a difficult domain of learning to evaluate. We must rely on the individual to communicate her attitudes, feelings, and values honestly through verbal and nonverbal behaviors.

Behavioral objectives are the intended action-oriented outcomes of an educational process. These objectives are tools for teaching, learning, and evaluating. Evaluation data can provide useful feedback on whether the learner has achieved the objective or requires repetition, reinforcement, or revision.

Planning for Learning

Once the assessment of learners and teachers takes place and the behavioral objectives have been developed, we must plan for the specific content and how it will be transmitted to the patient group. But this sounds very directive and controlling. Recall that with the adult learner, the focus is on the holistic individual based on the assessment data and the mutually acceptable objectives.

The assessment data obtained earlier in this process have been used to define and describe the patient, including characteristics, attributes, learning assets and deficits, readiness, and specific needs to be addressed. This procedure was conducted with the patient as an individual, family, or group to diagnose the learning needs and prepare for continuation of the process. Next, behavioral objectives were identified to guide the process and plan for the evaluation of outcomes. Now we must plan the content, teaching strategies and methods of delivery, learning resources, and specific evaluation procedures.

Traditional lesson plans are frequently prepared in a column format. The first column contains the behavioral objectives developed for the learning activity. Subsequent columns contain learning content, teaching strategies or principles, learning resources, evaluation methods, and timing, which can all be viewed easily in relation to the behavioral objectives. A sample format is posted on the Intranet site for this text. This format is actually the plan for the teacher to ensure that the behavioral objectives are addressed with appropriate content, methods, materials, and evaluation methods. It may have to be more flexible based on patient needs.

The learning content is the specific content outline designed to meet the objective. Teaching strategies relate to the objective and the specific content, including variations for the learning setting and patients. Suggested learning resources and materials—perhaps identifying the appropriate tear sheet, pamphlet, learning module, or Web site—are proposed to enhance the teaching strategy and meet the learner's cognitive style, especially if a group or lecture presentation is appropriate for the general audience but may not meet the needs of individual learners. These learning resources may also need to be provided as translations in the native language of the learner for reinforcement in the home environment.

All of the planning so far is the proposal for the teaching-learning activity. Before implementing it, one must specify evaluation methods along with a proposed time frame for the process. Implementation of the teaching-learning process can then proceed using the strategies identified in the plan. Evaluation of the teaching-learning process is essential and is designed to address the behavioral objectives at the level of the taxonomy specified for acquisition of affective, cognitive, and psychomotor behaviors.

Consider the simple example of a 56-year-old female outpatient with unstable hypertension without angina. She has come to the health clinic after being denied health insurance last week because of the prepolicy examination requirement. Blood pressure measurements ranged from 210/105 to 185/100 on two consecutive visits. She has had no serious illness or hospitalizations, but she is leaving town in five weeks to visit family abroad for a month. Today, her doctor prescribed daily antihypertensive medication and a low-sodium diet. The patient has verbalized the need to lower her blood pressure for insurance purposes. She also reported that she has used a salt substitute for the past three days and has continued to play tennis three times a week. Her descriptions of nutritional intake indicate high dietary fat and sodium content in meals prepared at home and selected in restaurants. She volunteers much information about cooking for her family as well as attending gourmet cooking classes at the local college, which she signed up for because she wanted to watch the teacher and ask questions rather than just read the cookbooks.

The assessment data indicate a teaching deficit, learning readiness, and the motivation to adhere to a treatment plan within a confined time frame. You and the patient determine that you will schedule individualized teaching sessions with her for her next four weekly visits. Behavioral objectives for this teaching-learning process might include the following:

1. Explains food selection and preparation techniques to maintain a low-sodium diet.
2. Monitors blood pressure regularly.
3. Uses nisoldipine as prescribed, monitoring for side effects, adverse effects, and toxicity.
4. Makes appropriate food choices and preparations for maintenance of a low-sodium diet.
5. Organizes activities including maintenance of her exercise program.
6. Reapplies for health insurance coverage.

The objectives should be mutually acceptable to both you and the patient.

The learning content addresses the behavioral objectives by teaching food selections and revisions needed with food preparation, periodic assessment of blood pressure, administration of medication, monitoring for side effects and toxicity, and maintenance of a healthy nutritional and exercise program. Teaching strategies are then selected for the individualized cognitive style of the patient, using resources such as videos and written information to take home. Evaluation methods are proposed to address each of the behavioral objectives at the following four weekly visits, specifying the time frame for each activity.

Teaching Strategies and Methods

Teaching strategies and methods are geared toward accomplishing the behavioral objectives in light of the audience. Selection is also based on how the content can best be delivered and addresses the affective, cognitive, and psychomotor domains of learning. Teaching methods generally are lecture presentations, demonstrations, discussions, modeling, role-playing, individualized instruction, programmed instruction, computer-assisted instruction (CAI), other simulations, and group activities. This is the overall plan for the learning experience. The instructional methods that best meet the learner's needs must still be determined.

Selection of a teaching strategy and some combination of teaching methods depends on the patient. For a group of 24, a lecture format followed by breaking out into four small groups to apply the lecture content may be quite appropriate for presenting information on child development and wellness practices. For a group of three new mothers on the postpartum unit, a lecture would be impersonal and less effective than a small-group discussion on plans for returning home with their healthy neonates. In our example of the patient with hypertension, individualized teaching would be most effective, because this individual prefers the interaction with a teacher and has a limited time frame to accomplish the behavioral outcome objectives. The characteristics of the patient group and the intended outcomes, therefore, guide the selection of appropriate teaching methods. For further information on selected instructional methods, refer to Table 9.2.

Enhancing the delivery of content and improving learning on the basis of the cognitive style of the patient require careful selection of learning resources. Teaching aids and instructional technology are frequently used in teaching situations to enhance the content and actively involve the learner in the teaching-learning process. Using assessment data, consider how the patient told you that he or she best learned information in the past. When preparing for larger group presentations, consider how smaller group activities or assignments will address the needs of learners who do not do their best in a large group setting. Remember that adults learn best when actively involved in the process, both intellectually and physically. Think of ways to move the patient from a passive to an active learning situation.

A major consideration is how to enhance the content for the learner's own cognitive style. Some learners are highly perceptive in one or several senses in learning information. They may be highly visual, auditory, tactile, or perceptive in some combination of these senses. Recall the usefulness of understanding multiple intelligences. When you select teaching resources, consider whether the learners are highly visual and obtain and process information mainly through observation of the world around them. These learners do well with visual aids that enhance the content presented in the teaching strategy, such as with presentation graphics or with information presented through pamphlets, handouts, and online searches.

Compare a visual style to the learner whose auditory sense is the most perceptive. Effective auditory teaching aids include video clips, audiotapes, and recordings with well-developed sound presentations. In addition, this learner may do well using the voice notes recorder on a smartphone and reinforce learning through review later. For the individual who prefers to touch and manipulate new information, plan for active involvement in the teaching and learning through demonstrations, models, and samples.

> Adults learn best when actively involved in the process. Think of ways to move the patient from a passive to an active learning situation.

Another consideration is whether the learner prefers to be an individualist or to have other people in the learning environment for interaction and stimulation. Some people learn in a very individualistic way. They prefer to obtain information and then go their own way to process, analyze, and synthesize the material. Having a group discussion to evaluate and apply information directly after it is presented in a lecture is stressful, if not torturous, to

TABLE 9.2

Sample Teaching Methods

Method	Characteristics	Strategies
Lecture	Large group Controlled by the teacher	• To make more learner-centered, provide time for questions/discussion or break-out sessions for discussion • Must address mixed audience of visual, auditory, and kinesthetic learners • Focus on important concepts and provide aids for application of knowledge by learners
Group discussion	Small group Learner-centered as long as it does not revert to a mini-lecture	• Requires good skills in group dynamics by the teacher to keep on the topic and focus the learning • Allows opportunities for application of critical thinking skills, problem-solving, and teamwork by the group • Ideal method for transformative learning • Mixed audience of visual, auditory, and kinesthetic learners is still a consideration on a smaller scale • May include demonstrations for active learning
Computer-assisted instruction	Learner-centered, independent and self-paced activity	• Requires careful design to maintain interest • Requires motivation and persistence by learner • Design promotes individual learner feedback but limited teacher-learner interaction
Simulated environments, games, activities, and role-playing	Learner-centered, with an individual or in small groups	• Requires environmental staging and engaging activity • Role-play may be done with descriptive scripts or be more flexible • Requires development of rapport and group skills • Actively engages learners when the situation is presented in a nonthreatening and nonpersonal manner and viewed as "What if . . ."

this individual, who needs time before sharing thoughts or applying the information. Alternatively, some learners enjoy interactions and learning in a stimulating group environment. A large, impersonal lecture is deadly boring to this learner, who thrives on group discussion to work on questions posed in a case study. But learners are generally not easy to classify; these characteristics can be combined over a wide range. Pure types are rare, and the challenge is to find those teaching strategies and resources that enhance the teaching content and promote learning for each individual. Resources for different cognitive styles are presented in Table 9.3.

In addition to patient teaching, contemporary nursing practice consists of collegial teaching and learning opportunities such as educational programs, lectures, demonstrations, group discussions, professional and clinical conferences, case studies, clinical preceptorships, grand rounds, and chat rooms, just to mention a few. The same steps are involved in this process as with assessment, diagnosis of learning needs, development of behavioral objectives, preparation of a plan with selection of teaching strategies and resources, and evaluation methods. The difference generally lies in the size of the group, which can range from a one-to-one collegial conference to a meeting of the unit staff to a large interdisciplinary group of professionals who are interested in the latest research on a

selected topic. With a large group, it is essential to assess the prevalent characteristics of the learner population. This includes the overall learning need that will become the topic for the presentation. Behavioral outcomes should address what the learners are expected to have gained as knowledge and skills at the end of the program or teaching session, because they will be the ones providing the evaluation data. Teaching strategies may include an interdisciplinary team approach, especially for presentations across disciplines to foster the development of knowledge and collaboration. Although active learning in small groups is highly effective with professional colleagues, this can effectively occur as a small-group breakout phase after the basic information has been presented in a large group presentation format. Highly effective learning resources in this case include multimedia presentations with presentation graphics, video clips, posters, models, photographs, pamphlets, handouts, and reading lists. A word of warning about presentation graphics: Do not read the entire presentation from the screen. Present the pertinent points graphically to engage the audience rather than lose their attention (Box 9.2). In addition, the presentation may be printed as handouts for the audience in which the learner can add additional pertinent notes. After the program or presentation, the teacher or program coordinator receives completed evaluation forms from the program participants

TABLE 9.3

Teaching Methods and Resources to Address the Cognitive Style of the Learner

Cognitive Style	Teaching Methods	Teaching Resources
Highly visual	Small-group discussion, role-playing, simulations, demonstrations, programmed instruction, computer simulations	Multimedia presentations, videos, charts, posters, models, photographs, whiteboards/bulletin boards, publications, handouts, reading lists, CAI with effective graphics, e-mail, chat rooms
Highly auditory	Lecture and discussion, role-playing, simulations, demonstrations	Videos, recordings (prepared audios or self-recorded tapes or notes), CAI with auditory reinforcers, telephone follow-up
Highly tactile	Small-group activities, individualized teaching, role-playing, simulations, demonstrations, games, programmed instruction, computer simulations	Models, bulletin boards, samples, books, pamphlets, prepared handouts, CAI requiring responses to cues, chat rooms, e-mail
Highly interpersonal	Small-group discussion, role-playing, simulations, demonstrations, some computer simulations	Videos, audios, charts, posters, models, photographs, pamphlets, CAI, teleconferencing, chat rooms, e-mail
Highly individualistic	Lecture, simulations, demonstrations, programmed instruction, computer simulations, computer searches	Multimedia presentations, videos, audios, charts, posters, models, photographs, books, handouts, paper and pencils for note taking, CAI, e-mail

BOX 9.2   Tips for Presentations

- Do not read from the screen. Presentation graphics should be used to engage the audience. Use the information on the screen as talking points to keep you on track, not the audience distracted.
- Do not use all capital letters—they imply shouting and are not visually engaging.
- Use a clear font, not a fancy script that is hard to read and distracting for the audience.
- Limit the information on a slide or screen; for example, use only four or five lines on the screen and make sure they are legible from the back of the room.
- Keep it simple. Limit the graphics and displays to important information without distracting background colors or graphics.
- Consider the essential number of slides or displays, in terms of content, allotted time, essential information, and printing costs if you are planning on handouts.
- Carefully proofread to avoid spelling and grammatical errors without reliance on the spell-checker function (e.g., *three*, *their*, and *there* are all in the dictionary).
- If you plan on distributing copies of your presentation as handouts or electronically, make sure the copies are readable, have the same information as your presentation, and include appropriate citations, if applicable.
- Remember your highly auditory learners—speak to them, while assisting your visual learners, who are watching the display rather than you.
- For the active learner, consider a follow-up activity to reinforce the content you presented.

and then develops an overall analysis based on the evaluation data the participants provide.

Evaluation of Outcomes

Evaluating outcomes is a vital component of the teaching-learning process. It may be ongoing and may lead to important information for revisions needed in subsequent sessions. Although evaluation strategies focus on both the teaching and the learning that occurred, the primary focus is on the learner. Is the learner able to demonstrate the outcomes envisioned at the beginning of the process? As in the nursing process, the evaluation phase of the teaching-learning process is used to assess the effectiveness of the process and whether the patient has resolved a knowledge deficit.

Patients are more difficult to evaluate than traditional student learners. Cognitive domain learning activities of students are easily measured with paper-and-pencil tests and computer-adaptive testing that assesses knowledge and cognitive processes. In the patient teaching situation, such tests are rarely used except in research or large group situations. Patient evaluation can be complex, with problems related to timing, access, continuity, measurement, and other factors. In addition, recall that adult learners should be involved in evaluating their own learning. Normally, patient evaluation is done with methods such as return demonstrations, observation, diaries, rating scales, discussion, and electronic communication.

We used different action verbs to address the three domains of learning and levels, or taxonomy, within each. Capturing evaluation data requires specificity in the behavioral outcome objective. The objectives should indicate how you are measuring the outcomes of the teaching-learning process.

The affective domain consists of attitudes, feelings, and values. Evaluation data should show how the learner progressed from receiving to internalizing the values mutually agreed on for the learning. In the case of a newly diagnosed diabetic patient, the teacher and the learner must be able to measure or see attitudinal or value changes through verbal and nonverbal behaviors. The action verbs in the affective domain are *receiving, responding, valuing, organizing values,* and *characterizing specific values.* We need the individual to communicate her attitudes, feelings, and values in verbal and nonverbal behaviors. Methods of evaluation in this area include interviews, discussions, and observations that demonstrate certain beliefs and values. Another means of evaluating affective learning is a reflective diary in which the patient can record feelings and problems that arise between teaching sessions. Analyzing the content of the diaries with the patient can provide useful information on the affective domain as well as knowledge gaps in cognitive processes. And with the availability of electronic communication, cognitive and affective domains can be evaluated via e-mail or electronic postings.

In the cognitive domain, knowledge builds from simple recall to understanding, application, analysis, evaluation, and synthesis or creation of information. Interviews and discussion with patients can be used to evaluate whether the learner can repeat or report back the information as knowledge gains. For understanding, the patient describes, explains, and compares information during the interview. Application of the information can be evaluated as the patient demonstrates and uses the information, providing specific examples of how this was done. Critical thinking and analysis take this one step further, as the patient explains problems and difficulties that arose and steps taken to solve problems without the presence of the teacher. Evaluation by the learner occurs when the patient determines which method worked best. Creation involves manipulating the learning in new combinations and effectively applying the information to a similar problem or situation. The learner has devised a new way of handling a situation on the basis of information obtained in another area. Occasionally, post-tests are used in patient teaching, but test anxiety is a major deterrent to their use for some patients. The evaluation strategies most useful for both teachers and learners to gauge cognitive learning are discussion, questioning, and allowing for description, whether through face-to-face or by electronic means.

Evaluating patient outcomes in the psychomotor domain is easiest through direct observation of skill attainment. At the simplest level of psychomotor skill attainment is the patient's ability to imitate, as seen in a return demonstration. This allows one to assess understanding and the ability to perform a specific skill, such as testing one's blood glucose. But demonstration of a skill in a clinical setting can be artificial, because the patient's own environment often has additional factors not present in the healthcare agency, such as shared bathrooms or medication storage problems in a home with toddlers. Flowcharts, diaries, and checklists are easy for patients to use as reminders and reinforcers in the home, and they can then be discussed at the next clinic visit or teaching session interview. The level of psychomotor skills can be assessed with a checklist or flowchart in terms of following instructions to proper scheduling, precision, and problem-solving in the procedure. The patient can be encouraged to note problems encountered and how they were handled, to demonstrate skills in both cognitive and psychomotor domains. Consider the use of electronic calendars or smart phones in some patient situations. This will provide evaluation data for both the patient, as the learner, and the nurse, as the teacher.

In our example of the patient with hypertension, we implemented an individualized teaching strategy within a limited time frame to accomplish the outcome objectives aimed at the cognitive and psychomotor domains. One method of evaluation would be for the patient to maintain a diary, including daily food intake and exercise, and list daily blood pressure measurements, and medications taken. This evaluation method provides visual data that address the initial five behavioral objectives agreed on by both the patient and the nurse. At each of the four patient visits or teaching sessions, the information in the diary is reviewed and discussed. When both the learner and the teacher are satisfied that these objectives have been met, control of the hypertension problem may be present. A health certificate can then be provided by the primary care provider so that the last objective, reapplication for health insurance coverage, can be attempted with an outlook for success. At the final teaching visit, the patient and the nurse discuss the strategies and resources used during the four-week process, to evaluate the teaching that took place. Electronic communication provides an additional resource for follow-up and evaluation.

Evaluation data can provide useful feedback that objectives have been met or that repetition, reinforcement, or revision is needed. Teaching strategies, like methods and resources, should be evaluated by both the teacher and the learner. Discovering what worked and what may have worked better helps the learner view the process and reinforce the learning while sharing with the teacher ways to improve and strategies for the future. Important factors here are encouragement and openness for honest and constructive evaluation data from both teacher and learner.

ONLINE CONSULT

National Health Information Center at
http://www.health.gov/nhic/

Health Literacy Information at
http://nnlm.gov/outreach/consumer/hlthlit.html

EVIDENCE-BASED PRACTICE: *Consider this....*

In 2010, the Association of Women's Health, Obstetric, and Neonatal Nurses (AWHONN) submitted information on assessment and care of the late preterm infant included in the National Guidelines that included discharge planning including patient education, counseling, and validation of knowledge including signs and symptoms of jaundice and strategies to prevent infection (NGC, 2010, p. 1).

Question: How will you use this information as part of discharge planning for the new family with a late preterm infant? First, consider a mother and child within a traditional family with one older sibling. Second, consider the mother and neonate discharged to a family environment with a maternal grandmother as the leader of the family. Remember to consider your patients as individuals and families and their learning needs.

Source: National Guideline Clearinghouse. (NGC). (2010). **Assessment and care of the late preterm infant. Evidence-based clinical practice guideline**. Retrieved from **http://www.guideline.gov/content.aspx?id=24066&search= discharge+planning#Section420**

KEY POINTS

- There are several schools of learning theories. Major examples of these theories are behaviorism, gestalt, social cognitive, humanism, andragogy, transformative learning, and multiple intelligences.
- Teaching is more than transmitting information. The information must be received, understood, and evaluated by the learner.
- Learning is the perception and assimilation of the information presented to us in a variety of ways.
- Characteristics of learning include:
  - Perception of new information
  - Initial reaction to the information
  - Ability to remember or repeat the information
  - Rejection or acceptance of the information (understanding)
  - Use of the information in a similar situation (application)
  - Critical analysis of the information
  - Incorporation of the information into the value system (evaluation)
  - Use of the information in various situations or combinations (creation)
- There are three learning domains:
  - Affective—attitudes, feelings, and values
  - Cognitive—knowledge and thought processes
  - Psychomotor—demonstration of behaviors
- Cognitive learning styles look at how information is interpreted, influences from others, and reasoning methods. Teaching and learning strategies can then be developed to match the learner's needs and resources.
- Readiness occurs when the learner is willing to change and view the learning need and includes motivation, understanding, and applicability or acceptability.
- The purpose of writing behavioral objectives is to provide a frame of reference for the intended outcomes of the teaching-learning activity for both the teacher and the learner with the focus on the learner and their intended learning outcomes.
- Teaching strategies are geared toward accomplishing the behavioral objectives in light of the audience.
- Evaluating learning outcomes of the teaching-learning process is essential and is designed to address the behavioral objectives at the taxonomic level specified for the acquisition of affective, cognitive, and psychomotor behaviors.
- Evaluation of teaching strategies by the learner provides a further view of the process and reinforces the learning.

Thought and Discussion Questions

1. Explain which theory of learning and learning style is applicable to the way in which you learn best.

2. Remember those two patients following their hip replacement surgeries? One is an architect who designs custom homes and meets with his customers for at least an hour before he develops the house plans to ensure that he truly understands their desires and ideas. The other is a retired English professor concerned about the rehabilitation schedule and the completion of a collection of essays that must be submitted to his publisher in six weeks. Plan for their individualized discharge teaching using the theory of multiple intelligences.

3. Develop a staff conference as a seminar presentation on a clinical topic, with appropriate content for a unit staff of 10 registered nurses, 6 licensed practical nurses, and 15 certified assistive personnel. Propose assessment data on the learners and ways to match cognitive styles and teaching strategies for the group. Be prepared to participate in an online or class discussion, to be scheduled by your instructor.

4. Read the case studies in the Case Study Bank on the Intranet site and be prepared to discuss them in class.

5. Review the Chapter Thought located on the first page of the chapter, and discuss it in the context of the contents of the chapter.

Interactive Exercises

Go to the Intranet site and complete the interactive exercises provided for this chapter.

REFERENCES

Anderson, L. W., Krathwohl, D. R., Airasian, P. W., Cruikshank, K. A., Mayer, R. E., Pintrich, P. R., Raths, R. E., & Wittrock, M .C. (Eds.) (2001). *A taxonomy for learning, teaching, and assessing: A revision of Bloom's educational objectives* (abridged ed.). New York: Longman.

Bandura, A. (1977). *Social learning theory.* Englewood Cliffs, NJ: Prentice-Hall.

Bandura, A. (1995). Exercise of personal and collective efficacy in changing societies. In A. Bandura (Ed.), *Self-efficacy in changing societies* (pp. 1–45). Cambridge, UK: Cambridge University Press.

Bandura, A., Thoresen, C. E., & Plante, T. G. (2007). *Spirit, science, and health: How the spiritual mind fuels physical wellness.* Westport, CT: Praeger.

Benner, P. (1984). *From novice to expert: Excellence and power in clinical nursing practice.* Menlo Park, CA: Addison-Wesley.

Bloom, B. S. (Ed.). (1956). *Taxonomy of educational objectives.* New York: Longman.

Erikson, E. H. (1963). *Childhood and society* (2nd ed.). New York: Norton.

Fawcett, J. (2006). Nursing philosophies, models, and theories: A focus on the future. In A. M. Tomey & M. R. Alligood (Eds.), *Nursing theory: Utilization and application* (3rd ed., pp. 499–518). St. Louis, MO: Mosby.

Gardner, H. (1993a). *Frames of mind: The theory of multiple intelligences* (2nd ed.). New York: Basic Books.

Gardner, H. (1993b). *Multiple intelligences: The theory in practice.* New York: Basic Books.

Gardner, H. (1999). *Intelligence reframed: Multiple intelligences for the 21st century.* New York: Basic Books.

Gardner, H. (2006). *Multiple intelligences: New horizons.* New York: Basic Books.

Havighurst, R. J. (1972). *Developmental tasks and education* (3rd ed.). New York: David McKay.

Joint Commission. (2013). *Facts about patient-centered communications.* Retrieved from http://www.jointcommission.org/assets/1/18/Patient_Centered_Communications_7_3_12.pdf

King, I. M. (1981). *A theory for nursing: Systems, concepts, process.* New York: John Wiley & Sons.

Kippers, S. M., & Boden, C. J. (2012). *Pathways to transformation: Learning in relationship.* Charlotte, NC: Information Age.

Knowles, M. S. (1990). *The adult learner: A neglected species* (4th ed.). Houston, TX: Gulf.

Knowles, M. S., & associates (1985). *Andragogy in action.* San Francisco, CA: Jossey-Bass.

Kolb, D. (1981). *Learning style inventory.* Boston, MA: McBer and Company.

Maslow, A. H. (1954). *Motivation and personality.* New York: Harper.

Maslow, A. H. (1971). *The farther reaches of the human mind.* New York: Viking Press.

Mezirow, J. (2000). Learning to think like an adult: Core concepts of transformation theory. In J. Mezirow & associates, *Learning as transformation: Critical perspectives on a theory in progress* (pp. 3–33). San Francisco, CA: Jossey-Bass.National Guidelines Clearinghouse. (2010).

National Guideline Clearinghouse (NGC). 2010. Assessment and care of the late preterm infant. Evidence-based clinical practice guideline. Retrieved from http://www.guideline.gov/content.aspx?id=24066&search=discharge +planning#Section420

Rogers, C., & Freiberg, H. J. (1994). Freedom to learn (3rd ed.). New York: Merrill/Macmillan.

Singleton, K., & Krause, E. M. S. (2009). Understanding cultural and linguistic barriers to health literacy. *Online Journal of Issues in Nursing*, retrieved from http://www.nursingworld.org/MainMenuCategories/ANAMarketplace/ANAPeriodicals/OJIN/TableofContents/Vol142009/No3Sept09/Cultural-and-Linguistic-Barriers-.aspx

Skinner, B.F. (2010). A brief survey of operant behavior. Retrieved from http://www.bfskinner.org/BFSkinner/SurveyOperantBehavior.html

Vella, J. K. (2002). *Learning to listen, learning to teach: The power of dialogue in adult education*. San Francisco, CA: Jossey-Bass.

BIBLIOGRAPHY

Ginsburg, H. P., & Opper, S. (1988). *Piaget's theory of intellectual development* (3rd ed.). New York: Prentice-Hall.

Knowles, M. S. (1980). *The modern practice of adult education: From pedagogy to andragogy* (Rev. ed.). Chicago, IL: Follett.

Mezirow, J. (1991). *Transformational dimensions of adult learning*. San Francisco, CA: Jossey-Bass.

ONLINE RESOURCES

Joint Commission
http://www.jointcommission.org

Carl Jung
http://www.cgjungpage.org

Howard Gardner
http://howardgardner.com/

Abraham Maslow
http://www.maslow.com

Myers & Briggs Foundation
http://www.myersbriggs.org/

● Rose Kearney-Nunnery

Managing and Leading in the Organization

10

*"I am where I am because
I believe in all possibilities."*

Whoopi Goldberg

Chapter Objectives

On completion of this chapter, the reader will be able to:

1. Apply systems theory to an organizational scenario.
2. Examine the goals, structure, functions, and culture of selected organizations.
3. Differentiate between management and leadership.
4. Analyze factors included in motivational and humanistic management and leadership theories.
5. Examine the various managerial and leadership roles for and skills of nurses in a healthcare organization.
6. Apply methods for appropriate and effective delegation in a healthcare scenario.
7. Inventory your personal knowledge, skills, and abilities in management and leadership for professional nursing practice.

Key Terms

Organization	Management	Executive
Organizational Structure	Motivational Theories	Leadership
Centralization	Theory X	Organizational Culture
Decentralization	Theory Y	Power
Flat Organizational Structures	Hygiene Factors	Negotiation
Tall Organizational Structures	Motivational Factors	Delegation
Organizational Functions	Theory Z	

Max Weber (1947), the renowned German sociologist, described an organization in economic and social terms as "a system of purposive activity of a specified kind" (p. 151). An **organization** is simply an arrangement of human and material resources for some purpose, as in the creation of some institution or agency to meet a stated aim. Organizations range from the single-purpose association to multipurpose, monolithic institutions. They have been studied for years in an effort to improve outputs as the intended mission or purpose. Organizations can be viewed in terms of their structure, function, and people. Most simply, they can be envisioned as the open system described in Chapter 2, with inputs, throughput or transformations, and outputs. But understanding organizations, especially healthcare organizations, becomes more complex as organizations expand, contract, and redefine themselves. Changes in organizations are particularly relevant in light of the need for more operational transparency that occurred following recent and highly visible organizational and executive scandals, along with a view of the global economy.

This chapter examines how organizations are structured, managed, and envisioned to meet their intended mission through management and leadership. Nursing management and leadership in an organization must have a broad environmental, interpersonal, and dynamic vision, beyond patients and equipment in an isolated hospital or agency.

Principles of scientific management, management theory, and leadership have undergone continued investigation and change. Many writers have defined management, but no one definition of management has been accepted universally. The same is true on theories of leadership and the characteristics of a true leader. They discuss the leader and the manager, sometimes interchangeably. Buckingham (2005) looks at the difference in terms of the individual's focus: the leader on the future, the manager on staff, and outcomes for the organization. Use of effective management and leadership theories and skills are critical components of professional practice. Communication, negotiation, and delegation are important factors for both the manager and the leader in the organization. At times, the nurse may function as manager, as leader, or as both manager and leader. However, there are differences between effective management and true leadership.

We will initially consider the organization, since this knowledge is essential to both the manager and the leader for development of skills and abilities in managing and leading. Next, we will consider management theory and applications followed by leadership, since this is often the course that nurses follow in their professional careers—first effectively managing care for patients and care providers and then providing leadership for effective, caring, and innovative care for patients of nursing. Applying these concepts to contemporary nursing practice is vital for the operation of a successful organization and an effective healthcare system.

ORGANIZATIONS AS SYSTEMS

Systems theory provides a useful perspective for viewing the internal and external influences with any organization. In fact, Bertalanffy (1968), who provided the foundations of general systems theory, stated that the only meaningful

way to study an organization is as a system (p. 9). The actual selection of a particular systems model depends on the complexity and uniqueness of the organization. It requires careful assessment of the organization, examining mission and goals, present structure, and the prevailing management and leadership styles being used to guide practice and address organizational goals. Interestingly, Hall and Tolbert (2005) conclude that because organizations are so complex, organizational theories must be used in combination to address the complex phenomena (p. 207).

Healthcare delivery systems are complex open environmental systems. Agency administrative policy and operational structures internally influence and guide the system. The surrounding environmental system of the organization is the healthcare arena that provides the professional, specialization, economic, and additional value structures for the organizational unit and its members. The broader social environment reflects societal norms and values through the real and potential needs of healthcare consumers. Direct or indirect linkages among all system parts are assumed to be essential for effectiveness and continuity. Let us look further at this complex system and the internal environment.

Intricacies of an Organization

A useful perspective for viewing the intricacies of a healthcare organization is to envision it as a system affected by other systems and within the larger healthcare and societal systems (environment or suprasystem). In addition, healthcare organizations focus on people and have the dynamic influence of emerging technology. As a review, consider the principles of systems theory and organizational characteristics in Table 10.1. To understand the organizational system, a careful assessment is needed of the organization's goals and values, hierarchical structure, leadership and management, interpersonal and communication systems, resources and technology, boundaries, and external environments.

Goals and Values

Goals and values are implied in a statement of purpose or philosophy and are the basis of the organization's existence. The institutional mission statement and original or revised incorporation papers contain important information on values—how people within the organization are viewed as customers, staff members, and administrators. Humanistic versus mechanistic values are apparent in these statements of mission, philosophy, and purpose. Organizational values, as the reasons for existence, are provided in vision or goals statements.

Hierarchical Structure

The *hierarchical structure* is the institutional design and lines of authority, as demonstrated by a bureaucratic or organic structure. The system structure is described in formal documents and further interpreted in operation through informal sources, such as technical staff, to determine how tasks are actually accomplished in the organization. The structural design is intended to accomplish the system's mission to provide the intended services through

TABLE 10.1

Systems Theory Components and Organizational Characteristics of a Healthcare Agency

Systems Theory	Organizational Characteristics of a Healthcare Agency
Wholeness	Organizational components of the agency or units and their interactions with each other and their environments, including the healthcare system, community, patient base, external payors, and corporate system (if applicable). The components cannot stand alone.
Hierarchical Order	The organizational structure as defined through functional and reporting hierarchy and demonstrated by the leadership.
Exchange of Information (Openness)	Boundaries among the different organizational units internally and with external boundaries and environments. This includes communication internally and externally.
Progressive Differentiation	Self-organization. The system become increasingly complex to meet the stated organizational goals for the healthcare of individuals and groups. This is the area of rules and management procedures to meet the goal for positive healthcare outcomes.
Equifinality	Patient needs and conditions, as well as provider differences, determine system outcomes. These are the interpersonal relationships and the technology to meet the organizational goals, but they may be met in different ways with individual circumstances in a dynamic open system.
Teleology	The behaviors in the internal environment, with an arrangement of human and material resources, are directed to meet the intended aims. The actions and the behaviors in the organization are directed at the goal for optimal healthcare outcomes. These outcomes are defined in the organizational mission, values, and goals statements and demonstrated by the membership.

leadership and management practices. This structure may be further characterized as complex or simple, centralized or decentralized, tall or flat.

Leadership and Management

Leadership and management styles vary among organizations. As seen later in this chapter, these styles may be directed from the topmost governing board or corporate officers downward. For example, in a bureaucratic organization leadership may come from the board of directors, through the chief executive officer (CEO), and be highly prescriptive. Management in this bureaucratic organization operating under Theory X will also be directive. Alternatively, leadership and management may be more flexible and participatory, as in Theory Z organizations. Leadership will guide the organization and drive the mission. The management style pervasive in the organization should be meeting the organizational goals.

Communication Systems

The *interpersonal and communication systems* are the psychosocial and interdisciplinary relationships unique to the organization—role relationships, attitudes, and values of people and groups within the system. Examine the expected behaviors of each member of the organization and the

interrelationships, in both formal and informal interactions. The organizational culture is a vital consideration here.

Resources and Technology

Resources and technology are the physical resources and collaborative human resources. Physical resources include operating and investment capital, equipment, information systems, services, and tangible assets. Collaborative resources are the additional skills and expertise to provide added input to system functions; this includes the resources for evidence-based practice.

External Environments

Once the system itself is characterized, move outward into the environmental layers of the open system, or the suprasystem. To understand the external environment, we must first reevaluate the organization's mission. As in any business, this provides us with market forces. Is a product being produced or a service being delivered, and to whom? Consider the differences between the environments of local organizations focused on a specific community and those of national or multinational conglomerates. To understand an organization's initial environmental layer, focus first on the immediate output of the system. Suppose we are looking at a home care agency. This type of agency provides home care within specific specialty parameters to an identified service area. In the environment, we initially have the local community with a specific geography, patient population, healthcare provider groups, payment streams, resources, and healthcare needs. This local agency has additional environmental influences from state and federal regulatory bodies and agencies, professional disciplines, and the larger healthcare system.

Now, consider these factors with a larger healthcare agency, which offers more services to a larger patient population, such as a health science center or teaching hospital with a broader service menu and service area. We have to consider the geography, patient population, healthcare provider groups, payment streams, resources, and healthcare needs across the state or perhaps across several states. Services may include not only acute and chronic care but also multispecialty clinics, research and development (R&D), and outreach programs. There are more care providers, including students, faculty, and visiting specialists from various healthcare disciplines. There are also more requirements and regulations from state and federal regulatory bodies and agencies and professional disciplines, just by virtue of the expanded services, funding streams, and service expectations. Coordination with the broader healthcare system must also be considered, as people come from and return to their local areas. External forces also include inputs of energy, information, materials, and myriad technologies received from the environment, transformed, and returned to the environment as outputs.

In an open system, all boundary influences must be identified and relationships evaluated to discover interrelationships and effects. All external layers and interrelating systems are important factors for a true understanding of the influences on any particular open system, as with community support for a local nonprofit agency. They may be positive when speakers at public hearings support county funding. These environmental influences can have unanticipated repercussions on the system, when this previous support interferes with corporate leadership or management decisions.

The healthcare environment can easily be seen as highly complex, dynamic, and uncertain. Changes occur constantly. Change is influenced by consumers, technological advances, government, and third-party payers. The external forces in the broader environment provide inputs into the system and affect internal operations and resultant outputs, such as patient outcomes. Healthcare organizations must respond to external forces in a rapid, dynamic, and innovative manner and cannot remain static. A humanistic philosophy, with its focus on the people in an organization, is needed for a contemporary and innovative healthcare organization. It is the people of the organization that create, define, and fulfill organizational goals with the patient system as the focus. This brings us to an examination of the various structures of organizational systems.

ORGANIZATIONAL STRUCTURES

Mintzberg (1983b) has defined **organizational structure** as "the sum total of the ways in which its labor is divided into distinct tasks and then [how] coordination is achieved among these tasks" (p. 2). Generally, when we think of an organizational structure, we conceive of some type of hierarchy that tells us about positions or roles, responsibilities, status, channels of command or reporting relationships, and tasks to be accomplished. The picture that comes to mind is usually a bureaucratic structure with a multitude of "red tape" with which to contend. This is not always the case. The appropriateness of the structure depends on the organization's purposes (goals and values), how outcomes are best accomplished (leadership and management), the people in the organizational system, the resources and technology used or available, and influences from the external environment(s). These system influences provide us with information on the size and complexity of the organizational structure.

The structure demonstrates the relationships among an organization's components and presents us with its design. Looking at healthcare organizations, we find two general structures: bureaucratic and organic. Mintzberg (1983b) described these two organizational designs at opposite ends of a continuum of standardization (Fig. 10.1). This range gives us a way of viewing organizational structures. At one extreme is the controlled, mechanistic, and standardized classic bureaucracy; at the opposite extreme is the humanistic organization that contains no standardized processes, outputs, or skills across the structure. Healthcare organizations generally fall somewhere between the two extremes, depending on their mission.

Bureaucratic Organizations

The most recognized and traditional organization is the bureaucratic structure. A bureaucracy is a mechanistic model focused on outcomes. Weber (1864–1920) provided the original bureaucratic model, with a high degree of efficiency and control. His work has been translated and interpreted frequently in research on organizations and organizational theory. Merton (1957) further defined a bureaucratic organization as "a formal, rationally organized social structure involving clearly defined patterns of activity in which, ideally, every series of actions is functionally related to the purposes of the organization" (p. 195). The bureaucratic organization has a hierarchical structure with designated lines of authority and control. The mission of the organization is all-consuming. Actions to meet the purposes and directives are taken in lower

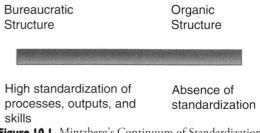

Figure 10.1 Mintzberg's Continuum of Standardization in Organizations. (Adapted from Mintzberg, H. [1983b]. *Structure in fives: Designing effective organizations.* Englewood Cliffs, NJ: Prentice-Hall.)

layers, whereas policy-making, authority, and control reside primarily in the upper layers of the organization. Specific characteristics of a bureaucratic organization are as follows:

1. A clear-cut division of labor
2. Differentiated controls and sanctions
3. Roles assigned on the basis of qualifications and technical efficiency
4. Clearly stated rules and conformity to regulations
5. A premium placed on precision, speed, expert control, continuity, discretion, and optimal returns on input
6. Strict devotion to regulations
7. Depersonalized relationships (Merton, 1957, pp. 195–196)

Examples of bureaucratic healthcare organizations are depicted in Figures 10.2 and Figure 10.3. In these examples, management and control flow downward from the hospital board through the CEO or chief operating officer (COO), who is appointed by the board and is responsible for the organization's mission, whether for-profit or not-for-profit. To accomplish these aims, the executive layer is responsible to the CEO or COO. The executives receive mandates and strategic initiatives from the board through the CEO or COO and decide on priorities, plan implementation, and regulations. Executives, in turn, direct their administrative staffs, and on down the line. Titles and functional areas may vary among organizations but each employee has a specific role in carrying out the organization's mission.

A bureaucratic organization is structured, standardized, controlled, and in many instances, authoritarian. Written and unwritten policies and regulations are prevalent, as are specified channels of command. Efficiency and effectiveness in achieving the organizational mission are organizational values. Bureaucratic organizational structures are seen in the older, traditional, and large authoritarian settings in which control and the ultimate mission of the institution are all-consuming. External influences should be predictable to obtain the most efficient functioning of the organization. Channels of command and productivity are important components of the system. But in recent years, a move toward more flexible and humanistic organizational structures, focusing on environmental influences along with employee involvement and job satisfaction for higher productivity, has led to a transformation to more innovative practices.

Organic Organizations

Organic organizational structures, or adhocracies, have evolved to meet the needs of organizations composed of humans in dynamic and sometimes complex environmental settings. The term *adhocracy* implies that the structure is a design that has been developed to meet the organizational mission and specific goals. Hall and Tolbert (2005) characterize these organizations as closely linked to their environments with a network structure of control, continual adjustment and redefinition of tasks, and a communication context of information and advice replacing the traditional supervisory lines (p. 31). These organizations represent a movement away from the standardized, mechanistic bureaucracies to humanistic forms arising out of behavioral organizational research and management

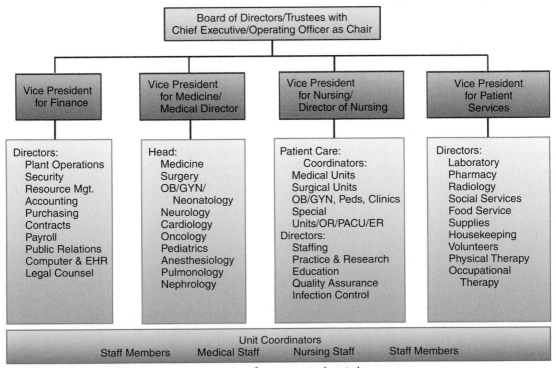

Figure 10.2 Example of flat bureaucratic structure of a community hospital.

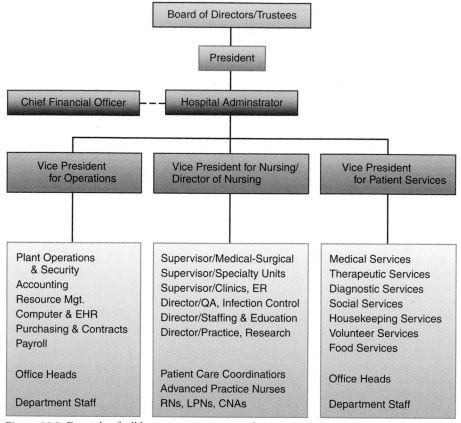

Figure 10.3 Example of tall bureaucratic structure of a community hospital.

theories. Mintzberg (1983b) proposed that this structure is the most useful in a complex and dynamic environment in which experts, managers, and staff from different disciplines cooperate on decentralized project teams to meet a system output goal innovatively. These organic structures focus on dynamic environments and rapid responses to market demands. Several organic designs are seen in healthcare organizations. The most prevalent organic or adhocratic designs are functional, product, and matrix forms.

Functional Structure

A functional structure, like the bureaucracy, focuses on organizational outcomes; but unlike a bureaucracy, it has control and responsibility spread horizontally across the system to meet specific organizational functions. Daft (2007) notes that this structure is most effective when in-depth expertise is critical to meeting organizational goals and the focus is on efficiency. However, the main weakness "is a slow response to environmental changes that require coordination across departments" (p. 102). A functional form can therefore be used in an organization with a specific function, such as a rehabilitative facility. The function of the rehabilitative care across specialty lines is the organization's purpose. The people in the organization have the decision-making authority for their services in the organization. Functional units are thus arranged in specialty areas, as illustrated in Figure 10.4.

The organization is designed to focus on the function of delivering rehabilitative care to the consumer. Two distinct functions are apparent in our example of this functional form: (1) finance and administration of the agency and (2) delivery of rehabilitative health care. An executive director or president oversees the organization with the assistance of two directors. The main organizational function of rehabilitative care delivery is structured as specialty units under the direction of the healthcare director. Fragmentation, duplication of services across specialties, and poor coordination limit this design. This limitation becomes more severe as the organization grows in size and complexity—for example, when services increase and the service area is enlarged.

Product Structure

A product or divisional structure is similar to the functional structure except that the organization is focused only on the product as the outcome, and not also on the means to the outcome. The people and processes in the product structure are grouped accordingly to meet the intended aim with the goals of coordination and patient satisfaction. The product structure promotes flexibility and change with decentralized decision making, a focus on product goals, and coordination across functions (Daft, 2007, p. 104). Consider the example of a large homecare agency (Fig. 10.5). The product is home care services, with

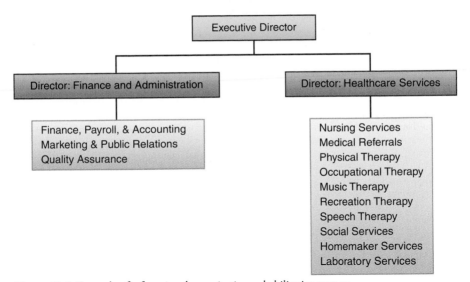

Figure 10.4 Example of a functional organization: rehabilitative agency.

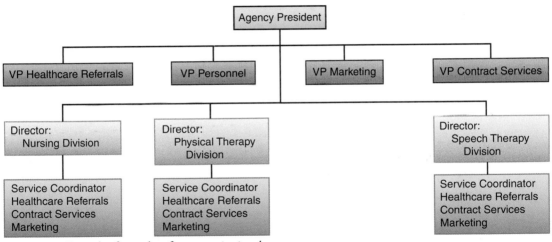

Figure 10.5 Example of a product form organization: home care agency.

attention being given to the needs and desires of the home care patient. The product units are organized in terms of nursing services, physical therapy, and speech therapy. Each unit has a director responsible to the president of the agency for the home care product. Vice presidents are responsible to the president for general functions of healthcare referrals, contractual services, personnel, and marketing. Product units are thus arranged in specified areas (nursing, physical therapy, and speech therapy), with each being directed toward service coordination, referrals, contractual services, and marketing to meet consumer needs.

The product structure works well with an organization whose services and marketing are directed at the consumer. This design is flexible in a dynamic or unstable environment, because consumer needs and satisfaction are of prime concern. Divisions are separated by product—nursing care, physical therapy, and speech therapy. But duplication of services is an immediate problem, especially in healthcare, in which coordination of therapeutic regimens is vital for the consumer.

Matrix Structure

To address the need to coordinate consumer services, another adhocratic design combines the functional and product forms. Multidimensional decision making and responsibility are the features of a matrix organization. In a healthcare agency, this can refer to the product of state-of-the-art care and the function of provision of services to the patient as the consumer. An example of the matrix design is an organization whose mission is directed at research and development and provision of care. Research managers in interdisciplinary areas, such as aging, acute infectious processes, mental health, rehabilitation, and health promotion, are located on one side of the matrix, with specialized healthcare providers on the other side (Fig. 10.6). People as leaders, managers, and workers, along with tangible resources in the environment, are all represented in the matrix cells. Although this design is challenging, it is consistent with the core competency for health professionals identified in Chapter 1 for working in interdisciplinary teams.

Consider the example of home care for an elderly patient following a hip fracture. Care for the patient and the family along the continuum would move from acute care to short-term rehabilitation to home care, with interdisciplinary care providers—including home care coordinators, therapists, and specialists—all contributing to the decision making and service provision. The complexity of this system is initially breathtaking. Both functions and products must be considered in coordination of the services needed by the patient. This is a collegial

structure with integrated functions and products that require multilayered decisions and a good deal of trust and collaboration. The number of people involved in the matrix for decisions varies. Larger organizations may involve only the leadership and managers in the matrix, with traditional departmental structures evolving under each manager. Smaller organizations, such as the earlier example of a home care agency, could realistically involve leaders, managers and providers in the matrix according to the scope of services (product) and resources (human and material as functions).

The matrix design promotes innovative practices as a result of a consumer focus, in the context of current technology, emergent practice problems, research information, and specialty practice. R&D issues are directed at current practice, with experts from each area represented for problem-solving and decision making. This matrix

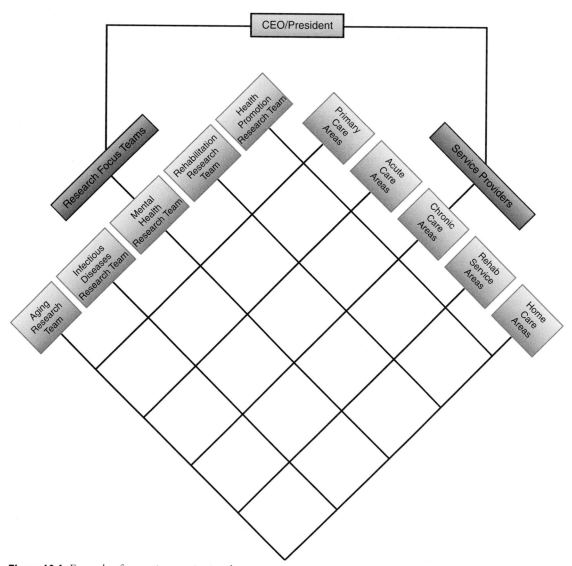

Figure 10.6 Example of a matrix organizational structure.

design is seen more frequently in health settings with a dual focus, such as education and service or research and service. The complexity of the design and problems with integration of all appropriate people and resources are the main disadvantages of the matrix form. Daft (2007) describes its disadvantages more fully as follows:

1. Participants experience dual authority, leading to confusion and frustration.
2. Good interpersonal skills and extensive training of participants are needed.
3. It is time-consuming, with frequent meetings and conflict resolution sessions.
4. Participants must understand and adopt collegial rather than vertical-type relationships.
5. Dual pressure from the environment is required to maintain a balance of power. (p. 111)

Coordination problems are a definite disadvantage of adhocratic designs. Experts and project teams or divisions are focused on innovation and targeting of specific outcomes. This focus may represent only one piece of the mission of the organization, however. Thus, good communication and coordination are critical. But coordination problems are many times outweighed by the advantages of flexibility, innovation, and human involvement.

As an additional note, the organization may have more than one organizational structure, either embedded or mixed. Recall Mintzberg's (1983b) continuum of standardization in Figure 10.1. The healthcare agency may have a formal organizational structure leaning toward a bureaucracy as seen in Figure 10.3. But patient services may have a distinct rehabilitative service with a functional structure seen in Figure 10.4. This will add to the complexity of leadership and management.

Structural Components for Leadership and Management

Organizations are also categorized by how the components are arranged, as centralized or decentralized and flat or tall. Centralized and decentralized organizational structures relate to the lines of control and decision making within the organization. **Centralization** occurs when the span of control or management is in the classic bureaucratic style, governed from the top downward. Authority, control, and decision making occur from the leadership and in upper management, with less participation from the lower levels. **Decentralization** distributes authority downward in an organization, allowing decision making and control at local levels. Reasons suggested for decentralization are to establish a more collegial and participatory model, resulting in employee involvement, performance, and satisfaction. Also, the people who are actually involved in the service are making the decisions about it.

Organizations can also be described as having flat or tall structures, depending on the layers of differentiation for authority, decision making, and coordination. **Flat organizational structures** have a wide base and few layers or tiers for decision making and authority. Decisions, controls, and governance are widely spread across the organization in a horizontal differentiation. **Tall organizational structures** have more tiers and lines of command, with less local decision making at the lower levels. Tall organizations have more management levels, with lines of command resulting in a vertically differentiated hierarchical structure. Compare the organizational structures in Figure 10.2 and Figure 10.3. Both are bureaucratic structures, but decisions and work functions are spread more widely across the organization in flat structures.

Deciding whether a centralized or decentralized, tall or flat structure is best depends on the characteristics of the specific organization. As Hall and Tolbert (2005) have observed, high levels of centralization mean greater coordination but less flexibility and overloaded communication channels as communications flow up and down the hierarchy (p. 62). Many organizations have changed from centralized, tall structures to encourage more employee involvement. But problems can arise when communication, coordination, and monitoring of activities in the organization demand integration for effective functioning. As in his continuum of organizational standardization (see Fig. 10.2), Mintzberg (1983b) suggests that centralization and decentralization be viewed as opposite ends of a continuum rather than absolutes (p. 98). The degree of centralization or decentralization actually should depend on the organization's size, structure, technology, people, and mission to determine where decisions are made best.

ORGANIZATIONAL FUNCTIONS

The purpose or function of the organization is to meet the pre-established goal as outputs from the system. The goals and values described in the institutional mission and purposes statement are the basis for the organization's existence. The mission statement is the overall purpose of the organization, including whether it is a for-profit organization or a not-for-profit organization. Stockholders or shareholders expect to see some return on their investment in a for-profit (or proprietary) organization, and this expectation is reflected in organizational goals. Not-for-profit organizations receive funding from various sources, but there is no sense of ownership. In a not-for-profit organization, profits are generally reinvested in the organization to keep it financially competitive.

Once the mission is understood, the targets to achieve this mission become the issue. Organizational goals are specified for effective and efficient functioning. Mintzberg (1983a) identified four types of goals that demonstrate intent and consistency of behavior in organizations: ideologic, formal, shared, and system.

- *Ideologic goals* relate to the values people in the organization share. An example of an *ideologic goal* in a healthcare organization is access to and provision of high-quality healthcare for people of all ages.
- *Formal goals* are those authorized through the hierarchy from people with authority who have a power base in the organization.
- *Shared goals* are those set and pursued by a particular group in the organization. Involvement of family members in caregiving is an example of a shared goal that a specialty group favors and implements in the organization.

- *System goals* are those set to maintain the system. Mintzberg (1983a) identified system goals as survival, efficiency, control, and growth. System goals relate to continuity of the organization and contain a strong economic component. These survival system goals are driving many healthcare organizations. These may also be the strategic initiatives or priorities for the organization and specified for action within a certain time frame.

Organizations are now recognizing that goals that are too broad can deplete the resources and effectiveness of the intended outcomes and the system goals. We hear of companies and major industries streamlining and getting "back to basics." They seriously consider examining what they know best, and refining and focusing it, rather than diversifying. Linkages with other organizations that can handle the diversifications better may be more beneficial to both the organization and the consumer group. This development has been seen with restructuring in healthcare organizations.

There are three basic reasons for the changes in healthcare structures: environmental influences, changes in the provider system, and changes in consumer needs and demographics. First, external environmental influences have had a major effect on healthcare organizations, as with diagnostic-related groups (DRGs), the prospective payment system (PPS) for healthcare reimbursement, and safety initiatives. Second, specialization and changes in the healthcare provider system have confused consumers and legislators. Disciplinary lines between healthcare providers necessarily have some overlap as we implement cross-training, interdisciplinary practice, and focus on humanistic and holistic values for persons and groups. An example is the core competency of working in interdisciplinary teams. Coordination and collaboration are essential attributes in contemporary practice settings. Third, changes in consumer needs related to increased longevity, chronicity, personal involvement, and health promotion must drive the system to provide safe and effective healthcare services.

Healthcare organizations are now seeing the wisdom of a lesson learned in industry: Not every community hospital needs to offer every specialty service. Community hospitals can offer services that are complementary rather than duplicated and meager. Regionalization can be accomplished by having, for example, maternal and infant or pediatric services in one agency and cardiac diagnosis, surgery, and rehabilitation in another. This arrangement prevents duplication and fosters quality. The population and the health service needs must drive the goals of the organization. A needs assessment provides the information for revision of organizational goals. Important considerations include the specific operations of the organization and the available technology.

Specialized knowledge and expertise of professionals and nonprofessionals are represented in formal and informal **organizational functions**. Formal functions are those defined by the organizational structure. For example, compare the different managerial functions for a unit manager in a vertical, bureaucratic organization with decision making in the upper levels of the hierarchy with those for the unit as a cost and decision center in a more horizontal adhocratic structure. This comparison demonstrates a difference in formal operational functions. Informal functions facilitate goal accomplishment and include effective communication channels and details about how the organizational plans and how tasks are actually accomplished in relation to the available resources. It is essential to be aware of the human factor—that is, the individuals who coordinate the people and resources to meet the goals of the organization, or the managers.

MANAGEMENT

Management, the coordination of resources to achieve organizational outcomes, involves critical thinking, problem-solving, and decision making. Management should not be confused with leadership. A leader mobilizes a group to achieve great things, whereas a manager focuses on directing the group to meet the desired outcomes for the organization through thoughtful and careful planning, direction, monitoring, recognition, development, and representation.

An effective manager must be a good leader but with a focus on the established organizational outcomes; the combination of effective leadership and management skills provides the nurse with the attributes to face the multitude of challenges in the current healthcare system and the various organizational structures. Understanding the foundation of effective management is essential to developing one's own management style.

Management Theories

Management has been studied extensively, with the development of several major theories that are still used to guide current practices. During the 20th century, the major themes were a focus on management science, the process, the people, and even the activities and the intended objectives. Other theories and models are evolving as we attempt to understand and apply the best approaches to "getting things done" efficiently and effectively with the best possible outcomes. The concept of outcomes is an important component in the current view of management, especially in the healthcare arena.

The origins of management theory are often attributed to Frederick Taylor (1911), an engineer who used time-and-motion studies to investigate and then apply efficiency principles with the bottom-line focus on productivity. In this early industrial period, training the right people for the task at hand was vital, and these people were rewarded monetarily as productivity levels rose. The focus was one of efficiency, effectiveness, and quality control. This approach was viewed as "working smarter." These principles have been used effectively with production lines, as in the early days of the automotive industry. Taylor's efficiency and productivity principles persist to this day, with the focus on organizing the proper number of trained people and activities to get a job done in the shortest time. These principles have been followed in the use and examination of nurse-patient staffing ratios and skill mix in hospitals.

In the early 20th century, Henri Fayol (1949) looked further at the process of management and the role and functions of the manager. His universal approach highlighted 14 principles including authority, unity of command (one boss and a chain of command), and communication. The role of the manager in this approach encompassed five functions: planning, organizing, commanding, coordinating, and controlling. During the same period, Max Weber (1947) was addressing organizational structure and the need for consistent rules and tasks in the hierarchical structure of the bureaucratic organization.

Other managerial theories evolved, focused on individuals and the goals of organizations. **Motivational theories** are used to identify and describe the forces that motivate individuals toward a goal. Guided by these theories, an effective manager or leader motivates individuals, thus enhancing their productivity and achieving organizational goals. Classic motivational theories have been proposed by Maslow, McGregor, and Ouchi.

As seen previously, in Chapters 2 and 9, Maslow's (1954, 1970) theory of a hierarchy of human needs was based on his 16 propositions on motivation. Motivation in humans is a manifestation of internal and external personal and environmental factors that cause people to respond to a situation in the way that they do. In these principles, the focus is on the individual in a dynamic, complex, and changing environment. Motivation is as intricate as the person, and an individual's personal basic needs must be satisfied before he or she can focus on higher needs, such as self-esteem in one's position and organizational goals. For a manager, understanding individual motivation is as important as understanding the skills the individual brings to the task at hand.

McGregor (1960) critically reviewed motivation in *The Human Side of Enterprise.* He proposed his classic two "theories" about human nature. The focus during this time continued to be on the human factors of the worker and how to get the work done. In **Theory X**, individuals are viewed as lazy, needing motivation, avoiding responsibility, and requiring constant direction and control by a manager to fulfill their job responsibilities and meet the organizational goals. Rewards and reinforcement are necessary for the individuals, along with a set of rules they must follow. This theory of human nature fits well with the centralized, tall, bureaucratic organizational structure. The role of the manager is one of direction and control.

Alternately, McGregor (1960) postulated **Theory Y**, in which individuals are motivated, self-directed, interested in working toward meeting organizational goals, and willing to accept responsibility without the need for constant direction and supervision. In fact, constant "management" by the supervisor could deter workers from reaping inner rewards from the job. The role of the manager in this situation should be one of coordination, guidance, and support.

Herzberg's (1966) two-factor theory organizes the individual's motivation for his work according to hygiene and motivational factors. **Hygiene factors** are maintenance factors in the workplace, such as salary, supervision, company policy, working conditions, status, job security, and the job's effect on personal life; these factors in the workplace can lead to satisfaction or dissatisfaction and are thus related to the organizational climate. **Motivational factors** are satisfiers within the job that motivate people to higher levels of performance. Motivational factors include achievement, recognition, the work itself, responsibility, and advancement. The manager helps improve job performance by ensuring that both hygiene and motivational needs of the employees are met at some level for both job satisfaction and incentive to achieve the organizational goals.

In the later part of the 20th century, the Japanese style of collaborative management received much attention, with the economic successes viewed within a participatory approach. Ouchi (1981) described this style, **Theory Z**, as an approach in which employees are trusted, empowered, and actively involved in decision making. The components of Theory Z include collective values and decision making, long-term or lifetime employment, slower but predictable promotions, indirect supervision, and a holistic concern for employees (Ouchi, 1981). This participatory style involves indirect supervision with the focus on the group. Ouchi (1981) believed that more creative decision making and more effective implementation occur with the full involvement and consensus of the group (p. 43). There is a "buy-in" by all team members, who are valued as individuals and as important members of the organization. Important values of this theory are trust, fairness, commitment, and loyalty to the organization, which lead to long-term employment and reduced turnover. The use of "quality circles" and "group think" emerged from this theory. Competitiveness in some American organizations is inconsistent with this style of management.

Management by objectives (MBO) and the role of the knowledge worker evolved in the business world from the work of Peter Drucker. Originally from Austria, Drucker profoundly influenced American businesses through his many books and observations on organizations and how they are managed. Drucker focused on the people (both managers and workforce), the organizational functions, and the results achieved in the process in line with the organizational mission. He believed that "since the manager is someone who takes responsibility for, and contributes to, the final results of the enterprise, the job should always embody the maximum challenge, carry the maximum responsibility, and make the maximum contribution" (Drucker & Maciariello, 2008, p. 239). He proposed that management comprises a few essential principles; the first is that "its task is to make people capable of joint performance, to make their strengths effective and their weaknesses irrelevant. This is what an organization is all about, and the reason that management is the critical, determining factor" (Drucker & Maciariello, 2008, p. 23). In addition, Drucker (2002) described the requirement in modern organizations for a manager to be a *knowledge worker* or "**executive**, if by virtue of his position or knowledge, he is responsible for a contribution that materially affects the capacity of the organization to perform and to obtain results" (p. 5). The focus became one of making a contribution to the organization by virtue of one's intelligence, imagination, and knowledge. Recall that applying quality improvement is one of the five core competencies for all health professionals (Greiner & Knebel, 2003). Drucker's works on management cover a wide range of businesses, including hospitals, and look at achievement and contributions of individuals within the framework of organizational settings.

Nursing Management

The core competencies for health professionals are essential characteristics in nursing management. The focus of the nurse manager or nurse *executive* must be on the provision of patient-centered care while fostering the use of evidence-based practice and quality improvement. The complexity of the interdisciplinary team and the use of informatics will depend on the organizational system. All of these tasks involve people and managing resources for the provision of safe and effective care and positive patient and organizational outcomes.

Buckingham (2005) identified four key skills of managers as picking good people, setting clear expectations, praising excellence, and showing you care for your people—but above all, the manager must discover what is unique about each person and capitalize on it (pp. 81–83). But recall that Fayol (1949) identified management functions as planning, organizing, commanding, coordinating, and controlling. The question becomes one of consistency of these functions with the humanistic view of nursing and care of patients.

Planning and organizing are indeed talents of the nurse manager. This is an outcome of the steps of assessment and planning in the provision of nursing care in any organizational context. It is setting clear expectations and requires an in-depth understanding of the organization and the people, the true culture of the organization. At times, it will also involve leading the culture, as with incorporation of evidence-based practice in a particular patient situation and planning for the efficient and effective use of resources.

Commanding in the context of nursing management involves ensuring that the job is done through delegation and supervision, as in the provision of care to patients. It is picking the right people and capitalizing on their talents and requires knowledge of the care requirements, the patients, and external system influences. It also involves recognition of individual talents and "a job well done." All levels of staffing are a vital consideration, including assistive personnel. Delegation is a skill that grows and evolves, as the nurse manager grows from novice to expert. Delegation is a skill critical to both the nurse manager and the leader and one that needs careful and ongoing professional development, as we will discuss later in this chapter.

In a nursing education program, students focus on "total patient care" as they learn the interpersonal, technical, and clinical judgment skills needed in nursing practice. In the final phase of the educational program, they are engaged in obtaining leadership or management skills. This includes assignment and delegation of activities to other healthcare providers, both licensed and unlicensed. Often, these activities are performed with other students rather than within the interdisciplinary team in the acute care setting. Upon graduation and initial licensure, however, nurses are expected to manage the healthcare team effectively and to delegate activities and functions to others for the provision of efficient care to patients. Challenges in the workplace, such as economics, constantly add new

twists. This leads to the need for coordination of resources, including healthcare providers, for accomplishment of the organizational goals and the provision of safe and effective care for patients.

Coordinating is another talent of the nurse manager, as skills in coordination of care have continued to be a component of the practice scope and setting. Controlling in nursing management is ensuring that the care to patients has been provided effectively. Recall, however, that management is the coordination of resources to achieve organizational outcomes and involves critical thinking, problem-solving, communication, and decision-making skills. In addition, remember that Drucker (2002) identifies the executive's vital talents of intelligence, imagination, and knowledge. These talents are also critical for leadership.

LEADERSHIP

Although the effective manager may also provide leadership to the team in terms of accomplishing the goals or objectives for the organization, a leader mobilizes individuals in group to achieve great things. **Leadership** involves action, creativity, motivation, and visioning. It is viewing the possibilities and motivating others to make things happen. As Maxwell (2007) observed, "personal and organizational effectiveness is proportional to the strength of the leadership" (p. 25). There are many theories of leadership, yet no consensus on how these talented individuals make things happen. Much also depends on the environment and the people in that environment. As reported by Sigma Theta Tau (2005), the leader is "someone who influences people, organizations, and situations to bring about transforming change (in clinical, education, administration, research and policy)" (pp. 5–6). What has become critical in leadership situations is the human factor—the leader, the followers, and the consumers. The increasing focus on the human factor has emerged in the research and the evolution of leadership theories and principles.

Leadership Theories

A multitude of studies and manuscripts have emerged on leadership in an effort to make things happen for the success and effectiveness of both the leader and the organization. Often, the basis for the literature contains in-depth research of individuals whose success in their roles has led to the emergence of a highly effective business or organization. Leadership theories have evolved from viewing the individual leader's personal characteristics in the Great Man and trait theories to those addressing environmental influences, as in the contingency theory (see Table 10.2). Understanding subordinates through interaction, coaching, and enabling techniques has emerged from the focus on giving direction to meet organizational goals. In her observations of this new direction in a chaotic world through a focus on quantum physics and patterns in the universe, Wheatley (2006) proposed that the leader's task is to first embody the organization's governing principles (vision, values, beliefs) and then understand that the people in the organization are best mobilized by concepts that invite their

TABLE 10.2

Leadership Theories

Theory	Description
Great Man Approach	One of oldest theories of leadership, this theory proposes that leaders are born with the ability to lead and rise to this role. Examples would be royalty, who are born into the role, and historical figures such as Lincoln, Churchill, and Napoleon.
Trait Approach	Much research has been done on the personality characteristics and qualities that leaders possess. Northouse (2010) identifies the major leadership traits that have emerged in the literature as intelligence, self-confidence, determination, integrity, and sociability (p. 19). These leadership traits have been identified as a focus on the leader and not the constraints in the environment.
Skills and Abilities Approach	Northouse (2010) describes this contemporary conceptual model that evolved out of research in the U.S. Department of Defense, which suggests that leadership can be learned and further developed and applied in an organizational setting and is based on a set of three basic skills: technical, human, and conceptual. Technical skills must be consistent with those of the organization. Human skills include the ability to understand and work with other people. Conceptual skills are those related to visioning and conceptual problem solving. Again, the focus is on the characteristics of the leader.
Situational Approach	This is a directive and supportive approach that is guided by the situation at hand. The focus is first on the situation, including both the environment and the subordinates. Northouse (2010) proposes that "the essence of situational leadership demands that leaders match their style to the competence and commitment of the subordinates" (p. 89). From the situation or environmental context, the leader directs and redirects subordinates to accomplish tasks and meet the intended aims in the organization.
Contingency Approach	This theory matches the leader to the organizational context and setting. There are three basic components in this theory: human relations (especially leader and follower), structure of the work for task accomplishment, and the authority or legitimate power of the leader in their position. This same leader may not be as effective in all settings, since it is contingent on the human relations, the work involved, and the leader's authority in a given environment.
Transformational Leadership Approach	Northouse (2010) describes this approach as a process that changes and transforms people and is concerned with emotions, values, ethics, standards, and long-term goals (p. 171). The transformational leader has the vision and enables others to promote environmental change. The humanistic dimension in this approach is vital, with the leader serving as role model, influencer, and enabler to promote change.
Authentic Leadership Approach	This approach is focused on character-based leadership. One model focuses on problem identification and decision making and another on leadership development for effectiveness. Critical to this approach is a genuine and demonstrated understanding of oneself and others. As Shirley (2006) has indicated, it is the authenticity component—inclusive of character, knowing oneself, and demonstrating relational transparency—that differentiates authentic leadership from other types of leadership (p. 261).

participation and energy to create astonishing complexity and capacity (pp. 130–131). The people in the organization are viewed as critical resources to be involved rather than merely used.

Styles of Leadership

There are three basic leadership styles: bureaucratic, democratic, and laissez-faire. Leaders who are bureaucratic and authoritarian generally issue directives and expect things to happen. The image of the bureaucratic leader that comes to mind is the captain of the ship, who issues orders to the crew members to carry out and then walks away, expecting results. The theories of leadership consistent with this style of leadership are the Great Man and Trait approaches. This leadership style has little to do with contemporary practice, except perhaps in the face of a dire emergency. The people do not feel part of the process and

the solutions for the organization when given authoritarian commands.

The democratic leader involves others in the process, seeking group participation and consensus. People are valued not only for their ability but also for their cognitive input into the situation. These people, as subordinates, are involved and active in discussion and decisions. A focus is directed at group process and group effectiveness, all directed at accomplishment of the task or to address the problem to meet the organizational mission, values, and goals. The more contemporary leadership theories embrace the democratic leadership style.

The laissez-faire leader is a passive leader, expecting the group to progress toward goals with little active involvement on the part of the leader. This type of leader has little relation to our leadership theories. Coaching and empowerment of subordinates toward a common vision, values, and goals are not active endeavors of this type of leader. This leadership style is one of sitting back and letting the group members take on the initiatives toward progress.

As you can imagine, the people in the environment can influence and are influenced by the leadership style. As proposed by the Sigma Theta Tau (2005) Leadership Institute, "leaders failing to be adaptive and innovative in the expression of their roles will simply cease to be effective" (p. 12). The ultimate measure of effective leadership is whether things are happening or changing to address the possibilities.

Leadership Competencies

Recall from our discussion in Chapter 1 that leadership in both the practice setting and in the profession was one of the standards of professional performance (ANA, 2010) for registered nurses. The identified competencies for the nurse include oversight, accountability, vision, good communication, collegiality, commitment, advocacy, and professional involvement. These competencies address the Skills and Abilities approach (Table 10.2), in which leadership skills can be developed and enhanced. In this theoretical approach, there are three basic skills: technical, human, and conceptual.

In healthcare leadership, technical skills comprise two areas, clinical expertise and leadership knowledge. Clinical expertise provides an understanding and appreciation for what is involved in task requirements and for efficiency and efficacy in their accomplishment. Leadership knowledge provides a foundation in the principles needed, along with abilities and evidence of past successful leadership. These two areas of technical skills also provide credibility to the leader in the eyes of peers and subordinates.

Human skills are required to provide effective oversight, share the vision, use effective communication, and promote collegiality and commitment to the project. A keen understanding of the people, use of effective coaching and motivational strategies, and promoting their assets for attainment of the goals are invaluable. Personal skills of the leader, through commitment and professionalism, infuse the group with further confidence and constant focus on the vision, values, and goals.

Conceptual skills allow for dealing with a sometimes chaotic environment and the mental skills needed to envision possibilities and plausible approaches. The leader must be able to deal with ambiguity in the environment and in the vision. For example, when dealing with the group in a brainstorming session, the leader must be able to reframe suggestions within the context of the problem and have the group address options for the progress toward the vision and goals without getting lost in the minutia and while keeping everyone focused.

Bennis (2000) has identified four key competencies of leaders (Box 10.1). Management of attention is a firm focus on the vision and the direction to meet the goals toward that vision. Management of meaning is consistently communicating the message of the goal so that there is clear focus and no diversion. Management of trust is being consistent and transmitting a consistent message so that others are not thinking there are different rules for different people or different days. And finally, management of self is understanding your own strengths and weaknesses. It is building on these strengths and minimizing weaknesses for success toward the vision and goals and taking the next steps.

All of these competencies require time, commitment, and energy. As identified by Tichy and Bennis (2007), "good leaders are able to triage their time and energy and focus on the consequential" (p. 23).

Leadership in Nursing

When we think of leaders in nursing, images come to mind of Florence Nightingale, who made great changes in the care of injured soldiers in the Crimean war and in nursing education, providing a basis for our history of nursing practice, theory, research, and administration. Other nursing leaders that come to mind are our nurse theorists in the late 20th and early 21st centuries, who provided practice paradigms. Still other nursing leaders guide our practice sites as nurse executives, our colleges of nursing as deans, our knowledge base as researchers, and our organizations as officers and elected officials. Leadership is apparent in many venues in nursing and healthcare. But remember that a leader mobilizes individuals in a group to achieve great things through action, creativity, motivation, and visioning to make things happen.

The American Organization of Nurse Executives (AONE, 2012) is focused on representation of leadership through their mission to improve healthcare through innovation and expert nursing leadership with their stated values of creativity, diversity and inclusivity, excellence, integrity, leadership, and stewardship through identified

---

BOX 10.1 Leadership Competencies (Bennis, 2000)

- Management of attention
- Management of meaning
- Management of trust
- Management of self

behaviors of broker, convener, designer, futurist, innovator, maximizer, partner, provocateur, and synthesizer (p. 1). These values and behaviors demonstrate the active role of nursing leadership in the process of creating a new vision for healthcare. These leaders are the drivers of improvements in health and nursing care in patient care arenas. However, leadership is driven not only by the chief nursing executive but also by talented nursing leaders throughout the organization, enabled through their respective roles. The focus becomes leadership in nursing and healthcare.

From a qualitative study with nursing leaders from a variety of leadership positions, essential nursing leadership competencies were identified as a set of five themes:

• Communication proficiency with emphasis on listening skills
• Conflict resolution skills
• Ability to communicate a vision, motivate, and inspire
• Ability to use data and technology in decision making and fiscal savviness
• Courage to be proactive with change and not reactive and crisis driven (Eddy et al., 2009, p. 8)

Each of these themes is consistent with the skills and abilities categorized as technical, human, and conceptual. But notice the identification of fiscal competencies and the need to not be driven by crisis situations. Another characteristic in recent literature is the emotional intelligence (Eason, 2009; Feather, 2008; Goleman, 1995), which includes emotional and impulse control, understanding frustration of both self and others, and maintaining motivation. Malloch (2010) also refers to this as emotional competence propensities. This demonstrates a commitment to the vision, despite challenges that will intervene throughout the process. Effective leadership will be challenged and be challenging, for both leaders and followers.

Kouzes and Posner (2002) propose five practices of effective leadership:

• Model the way.
• Inspire a shared vision.
• Challenge the process.
• Enable others to act.
• Encourage the heart. (p. 13)

These practices are ideal in the healthcare setting. First, as Kouzes and Posner (2002) point out, "titles are granted, but it is your behavior that wins you respect . . . and people first follow the person, and then the plan" (pp. 14–15). Modeling the behavior is the technical ability you present with and your commitment to action. Communicating the vision and creating buy-in and ownership is next in the process. Next, expect obstacles, but the whole idea is a new vision and not business as usual. Encouraging collaboration and helping other to excel in the process requires all of the human skills that nurses have developed. The challenge is not to get lost in details and keep focused on the vision and bring others along in this process. And, finally, celebrate accomplishments, no matter how small, and recognize the achievements of others.

Now, imagine a change you see as needed on an acute care unit in a hospital. Perhaps it is something as ordinary as changes in a fall prevention program for elderly patients. You may think that this is already in place with the quality improvement project that is mandated in policy. But suppose you have noticed a couple of near misses and one actual incident of a patient who fell in the bathroom last month. Perhaps improvements can be made. So first, become the champion for looking at the issue further. There is a good deal of literature and evidence-based practice on the topic. But are there special considerations with the patient population in your area or on your unit? You take the time to look further, and others see you as leading change in this area. Perhaps you have identified that more individual patient information would assist in the process. You propose a new patient profile process that includes home practices and medications that the patient has taken and those that are currently prescribed.

You are sharing a vision with colleagues that there may be more to the picture (your vision). And you are challenging the current fall prevention program, or perhaps some gaps that may not have been noticed. You propose a pilot on your unit and have it approved. The cost and staff time with this new process have been included, and the administration recognized your talent and commitment. Now, you have a plan to implement this additional patient assessment procedure, including identification of risk situations and individuals and staffing adjustments needed during peak periods. But, others will need to be encouraged to follow the plan and evaluate its effectiveness. Everyone is recruited to interact with those patients identified with a potential risk of falls, no matter how remote. At the end of the next month, there are no falls and no near misses, and the patient surveys for your unit demonstrated increased patient and family satisfaction with staff—from nurses to therapists to unlicensed assistants—as caring and helping them to prepare for returning home. Your employee of the month list has changed to employees of the month, and you celebrate your newer and safer environment. You modeled the way, inspired a shared vision, challenged the current practices, enabled others to participate in the process, and celebrated success. You are a nursing leader.

However, healthcare environments and consumers are constantly changing. Leadership challenges will continue to emerge in this dynamic environment. Huston (2008) proposes competencies for the nursing leader in 2020 as follows;

• Global perspective
• Technology skills
• Expert decision-making skills
• Focus on quality and safety
• Political astuteness
• Collaborative skills
• Ability to balance authenticity and performance expectations
• Ability to effectively cope with change and chaos (p. 906)

These skills are expectations for all nursing leaders. Leadership can be found in all environments, the national organization, the school of nursing, the healthcare or community agency, or even in a unit of one of these environments. Empowering groups for positive changes with a vision of the future is a sign of leadership. The ultimate measure of effective leadership is whether things are happening or changing to address the possibilities.

There are several areas of common concern to both leaders and managers. Recall that the leader mobilizes the group and shares a vision, and the manager coordinates the resources to address the goals of that vision. However, understanding the organizational culture, bases of power, negotiation strategies, and delegation skills are critical to achievement of the goals and the vision for the organization.

ORGANIZATIONAL CULTURE

The **organizational culture** is perceptible as the culmination of the norms, attitudes, and values imbedded in the organizational mission and in the expected behaviors of the employees. Daft (2007) views organizational culture as having two dimensions: visible observable symbols (e.g., ceremonies, stories, slogans, behaviors, dress, physical settings) and the underlying values, assumptions, beliefs, attitudes, and feelings of the people (p. 361).

Scrutiny of the organizational culture can provide a sense of the prevailing level of humanism present in the organization—in other words, how people are viewed as employees and consumers. New organizational values and behaviors have emerged as we redefine and recreate organizations for functioning in today's world. We moved from the belief that humans in organizations are lazy and need direction, in McGregor's (1967) Theory X, to the age of humanism. The humanistic perspective is a more positive one that considers the importance of the people in the organization. Still, during times of cost-cutting, a humanistic perspective and recognition of contributions can quickly disappear when the focus turns to head counts or full-time equivalents (FTEs).

Important clues on the involvement, satisfaction, and effectiveness of the people in the organization are reflected in management and leadership styles and the behaviors and attitudes of those in the environment. In healthcare, the organizational culture includes both the consumers and the providers in the agency. The organizational culture is also influenced by the environment—the immediate institutional or agency environment as well as societal expectations and mandates.

As with any set of cultural expectations, the employees are expected to enculturate (adapt and adopt) and espouse the prevailing principles. Failure to enculturate results in being ostracized or terminated. These cultural expectations are the customary ways of thinking and behaving shared by members of the organization, as a form of socialization and allegiance to the norms of the organization. Incorporation of the specific expectations encompasses this organizational socialization process. An example is adopting and using a specific theory that guides the operation of the organization. At the most ideal level, if the nurse cannot view or provide care for patients in accordance with the specific model used at that agency, such as self-care, the best remedy would be to seek employment at another agency more consistent with the nurse's own worldview.

A growing focus on the importance of the organizational climate is apparent from professional groups and associations. In their white paper on the hallmarks of professional nursing practice settings, the American Association of Colleges of Nursing (2002) identified eight key characteristics of the environment that should be evaluated in the organizational climate. Based on a study in 2002, the American Organization of Nurse Executives (McManis & Monsalve Associates, Inc., & AONE, 2003) proposed six critical factors for achieving work environment excellence (p. 5). In 2005, the American Association of Critical-Care Nurses also started a multi-year *Healthy Work Environment Initiative* that includes six standards also applicable to the organizational culture. And consider the value placed on the organizational culture by the American Nurses Credentialing Center (ANCC) Magnet Recognition Program (2014b) and the Pathway to Excellence Program (2014c). Go to the Online Consult and find the five model components of transformational leadership, structural empowerment, exemplary professional practice, new knowledge, innovation and improvements, and empirical quality outcomes and how these evolved from the 14 "Forces of Magnetism" in the Magnet Recognition Program (ANCC, 2014b) and evaluate their contribution to the organizational culture of a hospital system. What these positions and initiatives have in common is the focus on the organizational culture that includes positive leadership, communication, participatory management and local decision making, and collaboration and interdisciplinary relationships. The concepts are particularly appropriate to understanding the people as individuals and groups in healthcare organizations.

Nursing Leadership

The cultural climate generally supports the predominant leadership style. That is why it is so critical that environments have strong nursing leadership. This is emphasized by the AONE as "the importance of forging a supportive, empowering work environment that values and nurtures continuous organizational learning and innovation" (McManis & Monsalve Associates, Inc., & AONE, 2003, p. 8). In addition, part of the requirements for Magnet Recognition is that the nursing leadership meets minimal education requirements, participates in decision-making

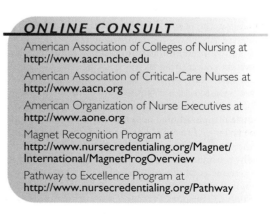

ONLINE CONSULT

American Association of Colleges of Nursing at
http://www.aacn.nche.edu

American Association of Critical-Care Nurses at
http://www.aacn.org

American Organization of Nurse Executives at
http://www.aone.org

Magnet Recognition Program at
http://www.nursecredentialing.org/Magnet/
International/MagnetProgOverview

Pathway to Excellence Program at
http://www.nursecredentialing.org/Pathway

bodies, and meets the expected professional standards for nurse administrators.

Leadership style is a major influence on organizational culture. Nurse leaders must have the qualities to envision the future and assist others in the organization to meet the goals of quality healthcare outcomes for patients. The American Association of Critical-Care Nurses (2006) emphasizes that nurse leaders function as role models in skilled communication for true collaboration, effective decision making, meaningful recognition, and authentic leadership (p. 38). But, as Leininger (2006) points out, nurse administrators "as leaders need to make their practices congruent with changing cultural values, beliefs, and the lifeways in their local workplace, but must also reasonably fit with societal and world-wide trends" (p. 367). These talented leaders must constantly be attuned to both the internal and external environments of the organization.

Communication

Communication of ideas and views is vital in the organizational context. But the prevailing organizational culture may dictate the communication channels and styles. Being able to communicate with patients is quite different from having your ideas heard, considered, and implemented at the organizational level. Portraying yourself as an expert and as a colleague is necessary in both patient and professional interactions within the organization. Whether by ensuring that all committee or group members have the opportunity to express their opinions or by making special efforts to demonstrate recognition and give credit for another's ideas, attention to cultural differences is important. It can make the most of the talents, abilities, and skills of the human resources in the organizational system, especially in management of interdisciplinary teams. We will look further at communication in organizations later in this chapter.

Participatory Management and Local Decision Making

Closely related to leadership style is management focus, whether on individualism and achievement or on collectivism or teamwork as the norms, attitudes, and values of the organization. Management styles have an important influence here. Consider the differences in management with Theory X, which is focused on individual performance, versus Theory Z, which emphasizes collectivism and cooperation. The organizational focus on individualism or collectivism is apparent in promotion and evaluation structures. Administrative policies and procedures provide important clues to the organization's official position. Subgroups or minority groups within the organization may create factions, however. These subgroups may set certain expectations for collectivism and cooperation in behavior or function. For example, the organization may be highly bureaucratic, with expectations and rewards valuing individual performance, competition, and task accomplishment; but if cooperation is the prevailing value in the nursing department, it will be translated into accomplishing outcomes at the upper level of management.

Think about the need for participatory management and decision making. The American Organization of Nurse Executives (McManis & Monsalve Associates, Inc., & AONE, 2003) have described this *empowered collaborative decision making* as follows:

> Nurse empowerment combined with collaborative multi-disciplinary decision-making is an essential attribute of a work environment that values nurses as professionals and provides policy development roles for nursing leaders and staff. (p. 5)

Participatory management and decision making are also a requirement for Magnet Recognition institutions. For eligibility, decentralized, shared decision-making processes must be apparent with nurses in both direct-care and managerial roles involved in decision-making bodies and organizational policy. ANCC (2014b) describes this as a component of transformational leadership, representing the forces of magnetism as the quality of the nursing leadership and the management style.

Collaboration and Interdisciplinary Relationships

One of the core competencies for all health professionals is to work in interdisciplinary teams. As noted in the Institute of Medicine (IOM) report, "teams tend to reduce the utilization of redundant or duplicate services, and they also tend to develop more creative solutions to complex problems because of their members' diverse academic backgrounds and experience" (Greiner & Knebel, 2003, p. 54). Collaboration is a challenge among professionals, especially when scope of practice issues arise, time is limited, and workloads increase. But teamwork is apparent in some organizational climates that foster interdisciplinary practice.

In 2004, the IOM focused on safety and work environment of nurses. They identified two necessary precursors to collaboration: individual clinical competence and mutual trust and respect (Page, 2004, pp. 212–213). These two characteristics seem quite basic, but personalities, a challenging and demanding environment, and incorporation into the organizational culture are issues. The IOM report further identified the characteristics of collaboration, including shared understanding of goals and roles, effective communication, shared decision making, and conflict management (Page, 2004, p. 213). All of these characteristics must be given heed in the culture of a healthcare organization.

Other Concepts in Organizational Culture

In addition to understanding the people and groups in the organizational system, other factors provide information on the organizational culture and the operational climate. The organization's history provides a lasting influence. Discovering the critical decisions made in founding the organization reveals the original intent for the organization and views for the future. Closely related to the founding decisions are the current guiding ideals and mission. The guiding ideals and mission relate to the service orientation.

Consider the difference between missions and the intended consumer groups in not-for-profit and for-profit organizations. This could range from elected fee-for-service care in the for-profit setting to a not-for-profit agency focusing on healthcare to the indigent. The philosophy of the organization provides important information about the current ideals and mission. If revisions have been made over the years, it can be quite helpful to look back at old versions to determine whether the philosophy changed in response to environmental factors.

Looking into the community can also influence the organizational culture. Although nurses are quite mobile and no longer tied to a geographic area, community ties with a rural hospital may provide a profound influence. Remembered history and symbolism of the organization contribute additional information, for example, about an institution designed to provide hospital care for a county that has evolved into a regional referral and tertiary-care center. Remembering the traditions of personalized obstetric care, a local woman's group may provide funding for a special prenatal program for indigent pregnant teenagers.

Finally, institutional arrangements and linkages, such as consortia and cooperating or referral agencies, are frequently quite complex but provide essential information on organizational relationships and interrelationships. These facts are necessary for understanding the culture and influences on the organization. But, as Hall and Tolbert (2005) point out, "culture is not a constant. . . . [V]alues and norms change as the events affect the population involved" (p. 183). The potential for change in the organizational culture requires diligent assessment and communication skills on the part of the nurse manager or leader.

COMMUNICATION UNIQUE TO ORGANIZATION

Communication is vital in complex, highly technological, and dynamic organizations. As was illustrated with organizational functions, the structure of the organization plays an important role in communication channels. Formal channels are easily apparent in highly bureaucratic structures, as dictated by the organizational diagram. But informal communication channels ("grapevines") are sometimes less evident and can be highly effective in such a structure. Consider the need for supplies in some areas of an agency. Ordering can easily be handled through the computerized entry system. But what if some urgently needed item is unavailable through the system? An informal channel may be used to locate a supply from which the item may be "borrowed," to be replaced as soon as the official order is fulfilled. The departmental administrative assistant or clerk who has an informal chain of communication may be able to use his or her knowledge of these informal systems effectively in such a procurement process.

Communication channels are important considerations for effective decision making to achieve quality outcomes. Organizational goals and values must be translated, transmitted, and reinforced throughout the system to meet the institutional mission. The specialized knowledge, skills, and resources represented by people require excellent communication within the system and from external environments to be current and responsive to changes in the knowledge base and technology. Communication is the action component of interpersonal and interdisciplinary roles, behaviors, and relationships in the organization system. The formal and informal communications and interactions are the essence of the organizational culture. The organizational structure is the formal design—with its hierarchy or lines of authority—for the communication channels. Communications may be formally dictated in a linear manner by the bureaucratic structure, or they may be flexible and circular in adhocratic matrix designs. Informal communications must be identified to reveal the actual flow of information, decision making, and goal accomplishment. Communication of information and expectations stems from the pervasive leadership and management styles. Evaluation of the appropriate channels is vital for effective functioning in the organizational setting.

Organizations routinely use methods of communication in addition to the verbal and nonverbal interpersonal communication techniques. Consider the informatics available in organizational settings. We have computer networks, fiber optics, satellite, and teleconferencing technology. Computers manage information storage, inventory, and rapid retrieval, data processing, data analysis, report generation, and even meetings at a distance. The information we compile and the methods we use to transmit it vary with the nature of the communication channel we are using. For example, a general rule in an organization is to limit memos to one page or less and disperse them to the appropriate parties; however, the sender must consider the available and appropriate technology, such as interoffice paper copies or e-mail or messaging.

Considering the purpose of communication in an organization is indispensable. Whether we are communicating with patients or assistive personnel, both the sending method and the receiver of the information are important. Clear, concise, and timely transmission of information is necessary for an effective management process. Recall from Chapter 8 the "rights" of organizational communications: (1) the right information or content, (2) the right communication channel, (3) the right format, including use of correct grammar, terms, and language, (4) the right level of understanding, (5) the right technology, and (6) the right follow-up. The appropriate communication channel must be selected, using the appropriate chain of command to convey your message.

NURSING: POWER, NEGOTIATION, DELEGATION

In the past decades, healthcare organizations have undergone radical change and restructuring. We are now focused on outcomes, patient satisfaction, safety, adequacy of reimbursement for services provided, and the imperative to address health disparities and health literacy.

Systems theory fits well with changes going on in healthcare organizations. But as the system becomes more and more multilayered, the focus shifts to the openness and flexibility of the system boundaries, greater attention to environmental forces, and expanding relationships among organizations. Special attention to external influences is essential for effective leadership and management. This includes a focus on the organization, considering its human resources, information systems, and governance structures for delegation and coordination. Ongoing feedback and evaluation become essential. Professional nurses have major roles in all steps of this process as we now focus on strategic initiatives.

Administrative nursing positions in healthcare systems have been expanded at all levels. Director and supervisor roles, when still apparent in an organizational chart, have been greatly expanded. Nurses have major leadership responsibilities in healthcare organizations. Nurses influence many different types of colleagues. Nurse managers have knowledge of people and the environmental influences on healthcare needs. This is the domain of nursing. In addition, nurses are now well prepared in organizational theory, finance, and policy. We have entered the administrative arena as interdisciplinary care managers, coordinators, and leaders. Strategic planning, public relations, and cost containment have become essential skills. Nurses who have this knowledge have legitimate power in healthcare organizations. But, along with this power comes responsibility, accountability, and the need for effective negotiation and delegation skills.

Power

Max Weber (1947) defined **power** as "the probability that one actor in a social relationship will be in a position to carry out his own will despite resistance, regardless of the basis on which this probability rests" (p. 152). More specific to organizations, Mintzberg (1983a) defines power as "the capacity to effect (or affect) organizational outcomes" (p. 4). This latter definition has much relevance for professional nursing practice, because nurses in healthcare organizations are positioned to effect (or affect) positive healthcare outcomes. These outcomes can be viewed as outputs from the healthcare system, such as patients with improved health status. *Legitimate power* is the authority to effect change within one's position. The professional relationship provides the opportunity for legitimate power, and many nurses now have legitimate power by virtue of their position, role, and expertise. *Informal power* is the assertion of one's will over a situation to achieve a goal without formal or "vested" authority.

Mintzberg (1983a) identified five general bases of power (Box 10.2). These power bases are applicable to professional nursing, especially in organizational settings. First, nurses have demonstrated effective management of resources in decentralized and vertical organizations. They are being vested with responsibility especially with regard to decisions and resources needed for effective organizational functioning. Second, care of patients involves technical skills that must be performed or supervised by nurses. Third, nursing continues to develop its unique body of knowledge needed for evidence-based practice and the health of patients. The fourth base of power involves the legal prerogatives granted and implied under the practice acts, licensure, certification, and professional codes described in Chapter 1. And finally, nurses in interdisciplinary practice have access to colleagues, patients, and influential people on whom they rely for access to the other bases of power. To effect positive healthcare outcomes, skills in negotiation are often necessary.

BOX 10.2 The Five General Bases of Power

- Control of resources
- Control of a technical skill
- Control of a body of knowledge
- Exclusive rights or privileges to impose choices (legal prerogatives)
- Access to people who have and can be relied on for the other four

Source: Data from Mintzberg, H. (1983a). *Power in and around organizations.* Englewood Cliffs, NJ: Prentice-Hall.

Negotiation for power must first be related to the goals of the organization. Nurses have the ability and responsibility to negotiate for legitimate power in organizations. Nurses certainly have access to these power sources if developed, effectively negotiated, and used.

Negotiation

As discussed in Chapter 8, conflict situations can easily arise in a group setting. And the healthcare organization provides the potential for many groups with different compositions, all with the potential for conflict situations to arise. Both the nurse leader and manager will frequently encounter conflict among individuals or groups that necessitates artful use of interpersonal and negotiation skills. Effective conflict resolution requires negotiation and, ultimately, coming to some compromise. This compromise is most effective when the result is acceptable at some level to all parties involved.

Negotiation involves a discussion process whereby individuals or groups with different views on some issue attempt to reach a compromise acceptable to all involved on an area of dispute or conflict. The best scenario is a "win-win" situation with collaboration. In this situation, the solution is satisfying to both sides, who have collaborated, and each side senses some satisfaction and feeling of a "win" situation. Alternately, one side prevails ("win-lose" situation) or both sides experience a compromise that is not really satisfying to either side, thus a "lose-lose" situation.

An effective negotiator should consistently refine and nurture negotiation skills (Box 10.3). First, the negotiator must have excellent *communication and interpersonal skills*. The negotiator must be a skilled communicator, for understanding the concerns of both sides and promoting awareness and collaboration. He or she must focus on the facts (verbal and nonverbal) and try to diffuse emotions with effective communication. Aiken (2004) describes negotiation as a communication process with exchanges of needs and priorities to achieve consensus on critical issues and to gain advantages in the process (p. 439). In this process, power contests may be expected but need to be diffused with a focus on reconciliation of interests on the issue at hand.

As with any nursing care situation, *assessment skills* are needed to understand the interpersonal and situational influences from all sides. For example, consider a conflict situation that arises in the intensive care setting as the group of physicians and nurses attempt to implement a collaborative practice model. The ultimate goal is for the effective care of

BOX 10.3 Attributes of a Skilled Negotiator: CAVEAT

- Communication and interpersonal skills
- Assessment skills
- Vision and application of needed resources
- Endurance
- Awareness
- Trustworthiness

the patient; the negotiator must have an understanding of all of the facts in order to uncover the common ground for all—physicians, intensivists, advanced practice nurses (APRNs), staff nurses, technicians, therapists, associated service providers, and patients. The skillful negotiator must understand what is being said and what is actually occurring in the setting, and should be sensitive to all behaviors, nonverbal and expressed cues, and views. The skillful negotiator must assess not only content but also context, culture, behaviors, and players involved.

The ability to envision what potential outcomes could be and how they would affect each side, individually and collectively, is key. The *vision* of the potential outcomes must be framed for the individuals involved, on the basis of the facts of the situation and the resources available. *Endurance* is a definite prerequisite throughout the process and during the inevitable peaks, valleys, and stalemates that can occur. There are times when the negotiation process must be halted to allow the various individuals or groups to refocus on facts and dilute emotions.

The acute *awareness* of the negotiator must prevail throughout the entire process, from identification of conflict, alertness to all behaviors and actions throughout, to the levels of satisfaction of both parties once the resolution has been agreed upon. This awareness of behavior and situation will have to be restated to all parties on an ongoing basis to focus on the facts continually.

Another important characteristic of the negotiator is *trustworthiness*. All parties must sense the fairness of the negotiator in the process. Building trust is a necessary skill, not only to gain the cooperation of both sides during the negotiation but also to help build trust in the process and the ultimate resolution. The process is often not a smooth, linear activity when one is dealing with people, partiality, and conscious or unconscious behaviors.

Marquis and Huston (2015) identify destructive or manipulative negotiating tactics as the use of ridicule, inappropriate questioning, flattery, demonstrating a sense of helplessness, and aggression or taking over the situation (pp. 503–504). These tactics are ineffective and may delay resolution or even escalate the conflict. Such tactics inhibit the building of trust and negate the collaborative process. The result of the negotiation process must be a compromise acceptable to all at some level of satisfaction. If a compromise cannot be reached, an impasse results. In this situation, the conflict will escalate at some later point, perhaps in a different form or with different players.

Ideally, the negotiation process should take place on neutral ground, or at least in a secure environment acceptable to both parties. Specific terms are used in negotiation tactics, like "reaching a stalemate" (an impasse) and "tradeoffs" (concessions), of which the negotiator must be aware. Marquis and Huston (2015) recommend further that upon resolution of the conflict, the negotiator send a follow-up letter to both parties describing the agreed terms (p. 504). This follow-up serves as reinforcement for both recognition of individual involvement and the results of the process. The correspondence can take the form of a formal memo or an electronic communication commending the participation of both sides in the resolution and restating the agreed-upon conditions. The attributes of a successful negotiator are also essential in delegation activities.

Delegation

Delegation is defined as the "transfer of responsibility of the performance of a task from one individual to another while retaining the accountability for the outcome" (ANA, 2010, p. 10). Further, the National Council of State Boards of Nursing (NCSBN, 2005) views delegation as "a skill requiring clinical judgment and final accountability for patient care" (p. 1).

Delegation activities are required when the novice nurse enters practice on the first day of professional practice. But, as mentioned, educational preparation provides the concepts for the process, although seldom the opportunity to truly develop these critical skills, especially when the new nurse is confronted with long-term interdisciplinary staff who may be entrenched in a certain way of providing care. The new nurse is responsible for the care of a group of patients and works with assistive personnel necessary for the provision of quality care. But delegation is a difficult activity for the novice whose skills are being developed and refined. And the accountability for the delegated act is not consistently internalized, as simple tasks are performed by others for the delivery of care. It is not a matter of simply "assigning" a list of tasks or relying on a nurse manager to make these assignments. Consider the standard practice of routine vital signs taken by assistive personnel like certified nursing assistants (CNAs) or unlicensed assistive personnel (UAPs). We have lost the concept of "monitoring" vital signs when the nurse assumes that the readings will be reported by the assistive personnel in a timely manner. Consider the problems with this arrangement:

- Skill of the assistive personnel
- Accuracy of readings according to a prescribed schedule
- Accuracy and proper functioning of equipment
- Environmental influences and artifacts on both the patient and the assistive personnel
- Report on the findings
- Interpretation of readings
- Nursing judgment on readings, their accuracy, and other variables in the patient's condition
- Alternate comfort measures or positioning that could have an effect on readings

And the list goes on.

Delegation is not the "handoff" of a routine task. Application of the principles of delegation is essential to effective leadership and management as well as for patient safety.

Principles of Delegation

In 2006, the ANA and the NCSBN announced a joint statement on delegation. Subsequently, the ANA (2012) further detailed *Principles for Delegation* to unlicensed assistive personnel. Basic principles of delegation involve awareness of the differences between assignment, delegation, responsibility, and accountability. "Assignment is the distribution of work that each staff member is responsible for during a given work period" (ANA, 2012, p. 5). Delegation "is the transferring to a competent individual the authority to perform a selected nursing task in a selected situation "however, the nurse retains accountability for the delegation (NCSBN, 2005 p. 1). The responsibility for completion of the task has been delegated, but not the accountability for ensuring that the task has been completed correctly by the right person, who has been supervised appropriately. Recall from Chapter 1 that according to the ANA *Code of Ethics for Nurses*, responsibility is defined as "an obligation to perform required professional activities at a level commensurate with one's education and in compliance with applicable laws and standards . . ." (ANA, 2015, p. 45) whereas, accountability is being answerable to self and others for one's own choices, decisions and actions as measured against a a standard . . ." (ANA, 2015, p. 41). The nurse maintains both the responsibility and the accountability for the delegated action. Delegation is required of both the leader and the manager to address the intended goals and, especially with some activities, for necessary care of the patient and to ensure patient safety.

Process of Delegation

NCSBN (2005) envisions delegation as a four-step process: assessment and planning, communication, surveillance, and evaluation and supervision and feedback. The importance of delegation as a process is based on good assessment of the patient, the environment, and providers who are capable and able to be delegated to provide appropriate care for the patient. The process does not stop with delegation. The delegation of a responsibility must be based on this assessment and must be made to the correct person, with monitoring by the nurse, who maintains the accountability for the function. NCSBN (2005) has further provided decision trees in their position paper, located on their public Web site, one as a tool to assist in the process of delegation to assistive personnel and one for accepting assignment to supervise assistive personnel. (See the Online Consult.) These decision trees are also available in Appendix B of the Joint Statement on Delegation by the ANA and NCSBN (ANA & NCSBN, 2006). Both of these decision trees provide specific questions to be addressed for safe practice with delegation. The delegation tree developed by the ANA (2012) clearly illustrates that the nurse assesses the patient, the delegate, the setting, and the task, but that the nurse retains the accountability for the delegation and the patient outcomes. Even when the situation involves the leader delegating a management responsibility to a nurse manager in a situation not involving direct care to a patient population, the leader is accountable for selection the correct manager to achieve the intended and effective outcomes for the situation. Nursing judgment plays a role in the entire process through the evaluation phase. It is vital to remember that nursing judgment cannot be delegated.

In their classic work on delegation, NCSBN (1998) identified five "rights" of delegation (Box 10.4). These five rights were further endorsed in the 2006 ANA/NCSBN Joint Statement. First, the *task* must be the right one for the patient. The nurse must use clinical judgment, not merely assign a CNA a group of rooms for taking vital signs. The *circumstances* must be right for the particular patient and the care needs—again a nursing judgment—as well as for delegation. The right *person* means the right person for the care activity, nurse, technician, or assistive personnel. This person, who will be delegated the care of the patient, must clearly understand what is involved with the care to be given (*direction*). Two-way communication skills are critical. The fifth right is the provision of the correct *supervision* and evaluation of the care and the person who was delegated to provide the care. Once again, supervision and evaluation require the use of nursing judgment.

Where is the patient in a nursing management situation? Consider the patient, fresh from surgery, who has just arrived on the floor: The nurse first makes the assessment of the patient to determine status and care needs. The nurse then decides what type of monitoring of vital signs is needed for the patient's well-being. The assistive person has been trained to take vital signs and has demonstrated this skill (that is, has been certified to perform it). But does this nurse know that the vital signs will be taken accurately and as directed; in other words, is this the right person for the job? If this assistive person is the correct person, then the nurse gives clear, understandable directions, including the reporting cycle back to the nurse for the nurse's clinical judgment. Along with this, the nurse provides the appropriate supervision and evaluation of the care given.

> Delegation involves giving responsibility but not abdicating the accountability for the task or activity.

The manager's or the leader's knowledge of her staff is critical to successful delegation. The education, experience, prior performance, willingness, trustworthiness, and expertise of the person should be considered before appropriate delegation can occur. It is the responsibility of the delegator to make an adequate assessment, which should include how long the individual will need supervision and what type of supervision. Individual Nurse Practice Acts in some states provide specific language and requirements for appropriate delegation by nurses. Be aware of both the provisions in your state practice act and the agency policies and procedures. You must abide by the legal authority in your practice act.

BOX 10.4 The Five Rights of Delegation

The RIGHT
- Task
- Circumstances
- Person
- Direction/Communication
- Supervision/Evaluation

Source: From National Council of State Boards of Nursing. (1998). *The five rights of delegation*. Chicago, IL: Author.

Delegation errors can jeopardize the patient. The correct balance is the key. Delegation is necessary to provide effective care for patients. The nurse must be the one involved with the clinical judgment for the patient's well-being but cannot perform all tasks involved in this process. Delegation is an essential skill of the nurse. Delegation is described in Provision 4 in the *Code of Ethics for Nurses* (ANA, 2015) specifies that "nurses in management and administration have a particular responsibility to provide a safe environment that supports and facilitates appropriate assignment and delegation" (ANA, 2015, p. 17). This environment includes appropriate orientation, mentoring, and protections for patients. Once again, we have the core competencies for the nurse as providing patient-centered care that is based on evidence of efficacy and quality improvement, provided in an interdisciplinary team, and communicated with the assistance of informatics.

As observed by Northouse (2010), "to be effective, organizations need to nourish both competent management and skilled leadership" (p. 11). These competent managers and skilled leaders address the quote provided at the beginning of this chapter by Whoopi Goldberg: "I am where I am because I believe in all possibilities." Change for the good of patients or the healthcare industry can be a result of applying principles of management and theories of leadership in healthcare organizations and addressing innovative possibilities. As we will see in the next chapter, professional nursing practice has an integral role in this process of change and innovation.

ONLINE CONSULT

ANA Principles for Delegation at http://nursingworld.org/MainMenuCategories/Policy-Advocacy/Priority-Issues/ANAPrinciples/PrinciplesofDelegation.pdf (if an ANA member)

ANA/NCSBN Joint Statement on Delegation at https://www.ncsbn.org/Delegation_joint_statement_NCSBN-ANA.pdf

NCSBN Delegation Documents at https://www.ncsbn.org/1625.htm

EVIDENCE-BASED PRACTICE: *Consider this....*

You have read an article on how nursing leaders can promote evidence-based practice as a value in their organizational environments. The article reports that "transformational nursing leaders promote learning cultures, engendering commitment that brings competitive advantages for organizations as new knowledge is transferred to practice" (Halm, 2010, p. 377). The article supported practices of transformational leaders including providing a shared vision, challenging current processes, enabling action by others, and encouraging individual actions. You start thinking about the acute care unit where you are a nurse manager and about the leadership that is needed to foster more evidence-based practice despite staff changes.

Question: How will you use this information to provide leadership and additional focus on the application of evidence-based practice? Identify the skills you will use and those you wish to develop in the nursing staff.

Source: Halm, M. A. (2010). "Inside looking in" or "Inside looking out"? How leaders shape cultures equipped for evidence-based practice. *American Journal of Critical Care, 19,* 375–378.

KEY POINTS

- An organization is simply an arrangement of human and material resources for some purpose, such as creating an institution or agency to meet a stated aim. Organizations can be viewed in terms of their structure, function, and people.
- Organizational structure is the design of the organization, including the type of hierarchy that tells us about positions or roles, responsibilities, status, channels of command or reporting relationships, and tasks to be accomplished. The major organizational structures are bureaucratic and organic (adhocratic).
- Centralized versus decentralized organizational structures involve the lines of control and decision making within the organization.
- Organizations are also described according to the layers of differentiation for authority, decision making, and coordination. Flat organizational structures have a wide base and few layers or tiers for decision making and authority, whereas tall organizational structures have more tiers and lines of command, with less local decision making at the lower levels.
- Organizational functions include goals and operations to fulfill the mission of the organization.
- Management is the coordination of resources to achieve organizational outcomes and involves critical thinking, problem-solving, and decision making.

KEY POINTS—cont'd

- From a focus on the organization and increasing productivity, humanistic theories of management emerged, including the classic motivational theories proposed by Maslow, McGregor, Herzberg, and Ouchi.

- Drucker (2002) proposes that a manager is an executive who is focused on contributing to the effectiveness of organization by virtue of intelligence, imagination, and knowledge (p. 2).

- Leadership involves action, creativity, motivation, and visioning. It is viewing the possibilities and motivating others to make things happen.

- The three basic leadership styles are bureaucratic, democratic, and laissez-faire.

- The organizational culture involves the culmination of the norms, attitudes, and values related to the organizational mission, accompanied by the expected behaviors of people.

- The organizational communication process can also be thought of as containing "rights": (1) information or content, (2) communication channel, (3) format, including use of correct grammar, terms, and language, (4) level of understanding, (5) technology, and (6) follow-up.

- Power is the ability to effect change in people's behavior or in the organization. Legitimate power is the authority to effect change within one's position. Power bases are built on control of resources, technical skills, and a body of knowledge as well as exclusive rights and access to other people with power.

- Effective conflict resolution requires negotiation or coming to a win-win solution.

- Delegation is the "transfer of responsibility of the performance of an activity from one individual to another while retaining the accountability of the outcome" (ANA, 2010, p. 64).

- The five "rights" of delegation are the right task, the right circumstances, the right person, the right direction or communication, and the right supervision or evaluation (NCSBN, 1998).

Thought and Discussion Questions

1. Characterize the organization where you work. Describe the structure, functions, lines of decision making, communication patterns, and sources of power relative to the organizational mission. Be prepared to participate in a discussion (online or in class) to be scheduled by your instructor.

2. Differentiate between management and leadership. Where do the two roles overlap?

3. Interview a member of the administrative team from a large healthcare facility on the various positions held by nurses. Describe their roles, changes that have occurred, areas of legitimate power, and the skills professional nurses need in this setting. Be prepared to participate in a discussion to be scheduled by your instructor.

4. Locate an evidence-based practice summary in your area of clinical interest. Describe how you, as the leader, would plan for practice changes and utilize the practices of effective leadership to describe your strategies in the process. Recall that these five practices are as follows:
   - Model the way.
   - Inspire a shared vision.
   - Challenge the process.
   - Enable others to act.
   - Encourage the heart. (Kouzes and Posner, 2002, p. 13)

5. Observe the start of a shift on a nursing unit. Describe the differences between assignment and delegation. Be prepared to participate in a discussion to be scheduled by your instructor.

6. Review the Chapter Thought located on the first page of the chapter, and discuss it in the context of the contents of the chapter.

Interactive Exercises

Go to the Intranet site and complete the interactive exercises provided for this chapter.

REFERENCES

Aiken, T.D. (2004). *Legal, ethical, and ethical issues in nursing* (2nd ed). Philadelphia, PA: FA Davis.

American Association of Colleges of Nursing. (2002). *AACN white paper: Hallmarks of the professional nursing practice environment.* Retrieved from http://www.aacn.nche.edu/publications/white-papers/hallmarks-practice-environment

American Association of Critical-Care Nurses. (2005). *AACN's standards for establishing and sustaining healthy work environments: A journey to excellence.* Retrieved from http://www.aacn.org/WD/HWE/Docs/HWEStandards.pdf

American Nurses Association (ANA). (2010). *Nursing: Scope and standards of practice* (2nd ed.). Silver Spring, MD: Nursesbooks.org.

American Nurses Association (ANA). (2012). *ANA's principles for delegation by registered nurses to unlicensed assistive personnel.* Silver Spring, MD: Nursesbooks.org. Retrieved from http://nursingworld.org/MainMenuCategories/ThePracticeofProfessionalNursing/NursingStandards/ANAPrinciples/PrinciplesofDelegation.pdf (members only site)

American Nurses Association (ANA). (2015). *Code of ethics for nurses with interpretive statements.* Silver Spring, MD: Nursesbooks.org.

American Nurses Association (ANA) & National Council of State Boards of Nursing (NCSBN). (2006). *Joint statement on delegation.* Retrieved from https://www.ncsbn.org/Delegation_joint_statement_NCSBN-ANA.pdf

American Nurses Credentialing Center (ANCC). (2014a). *Addendum: Changes to the 2014 Magnet® application manual. March 2014.* Retrieved from http://www.nursecredentialing.org/2014-MagnetManualUpdates

American Nurses Credentialing Center (ANCC). (2014b). *The Magnet Recognition® Program: Program overview.* Retrieved from http://www.nursecredentialing.org/Magnet/ProgramOverview

American Nurses Credentialing Center (ANCC). (2014c). *Program overview: Pathway to Excellence® Program: Program overview.* Retrieved from http://www.nursecredentialing.org/Pathway/AboutPathway

American Organization of Nurse Executives (AONE). (2012). *2014-2016 strategic plan.* Retrieved from http://www.aone.org/membership/about/docs/2014-2016%20AONE%20StratPlan.Final.pdf

Bennis, W. (2000). *Managing the dream: Reflections on leadership and change.* Cambridge, MA: Basic Books.

Bertalanffy, L. V. (1968). *General system theory: Foundations, development, applications.* New York: George Braziller.

Buckingham, M. (2005). *The one thing you need to know . . . about great managing, great leading, and sustained individual success.* New York: Free Press.

Daft, R. L. (2007). *Organizational theory and design* (9th ed.). Mason, OH: Thompson South-Western College Publishing.

Drucker, P. F. (2002). *The effective executive revised.* New York: Harper Collins Publishers.

Drucker, P. F., & Maciariello, J. A. (2008). *Management* (rev. ed.). New York: Collins Business.

Eason, T. (2009). Emotional intelligence and nursing leadership: A successful combination. *Creative Nursing, 15,* 184–185.

Eddy, L. L., Doutrich, D., Higgs, Z. R., Spuck, J., Olson, M., & Weinberg, S. (2009). Relevant nursing leadership: An evidence-based programmatic response. *International Journal of Nursing Education Scholarship, 6.* Retrieved from http://www.bepress.com/ijnes/vol6/iss1/art22/

Fayol, H. (1949). *General and industrial management* (C. Storrs, Trans.). London, UK: Pittman & Sons.

Feather, R. (2008). Emotional intelligence in relation to nursing leadership: Does it matter? *Journal of Nursing Management, 17,* 376–382.

Goleman, D. (1995). *Emotional intelligence: Why it can matter more than IQ.* New York: Bantam Books.

Greiner, A. C., & Knebel, E. (Eds.). (2003). *Health professions education: A bridge to quality.* Washington, DC: Institute of Medicine.

Hall, R. H., & Tolbert, P. S. (2005). *Organizations: Structures, processes, and outcomes* (9th ed.). Upper Saddle River, NJ: Pearson Prentice-Hall.

Halm, M.A. (2010). "Inside looking in" or "Inside looking out"? How leaders shape cultures equipped for evidence-based practice. *American Journal of Critical Care, 19,* 375–378.

Herzberg, F. (1966). *Work and the nature of man.* Cleveland, OH: World Publishing.

Huston, C. (2008). Preparing nurse leaders for 2010. *Journal of Nursing Management, 16,* 905–911.

Kouzes, J. M., & Posner, B. Z. (2002). *The leadership challenge* (3rd ed.). San Francisco, CA: Jossey-Bass.

Leininger, M. (2006). Culture care theory and uses in nursing administration. In M. Leininger & M. R. McFarland, *Culture care diversity and universality: A worldwide nursing theory* (2nd ed., pp. 365–379). Boston, MA: Jones & Bartlett.

Malloch, K. (2010). Innovation leadership: New perspectives for new work. Nursing *Clinics of North America, 45,* 1–9.

Marquis, B. L., & Huston, C. J. (2015). *Leadership roles and management functions in nursing: Theory and application* (8th ed.). Philadelphia, PA: Wolters Kluwer/Lippincott Williams & Wilkins.

Maslow, A. H. (1954). *Motivation and personality.* New York: Harper.

Maslow, A. H. (1970). *The farther reaches of the human mind.* New York: Viking Press.

Maxwell, J. C. (2007). *The 21 irrefutable laws of leadership: Follow them and people will follow you* (rev. ed). Nashville, TN: Thomas Nelson.

McGregor, D. (1960). *The human side of enterprise.* New York: McGraw-Hill.

McGregor, D. (1967). *The professional manager.* New York: McGraw-Hill.

McManis & Monsalve Associates, Inc., & American Organization of Nurse Executives. (2003). *Healthy work environments, Vol. 2: Striving for excellence.* Chicago: American Organization of Nurse Executives.

Merton, R. K. (1957). *Social theory and social structure* (Rev. ed.). Glencoe, IL: Free Press.

Mintzberg, H. (1983a). *Power in and around organizations.* Englewood Cliffs, NJ: Prentice-Hall.

Mintzberg, H. (1983b). *Structures in fives: Designing effective organizations.* Englewood Cliffs, NJ: Prentice-Hall.

National Council of State Boards of Nursing (NCSBN). (1998). *The five rights of delegation.* Chicago: Author.

National Council of State Boards of Nursing (NCSBN). (2005). *Working with others: A position paper.* Retrieved from https://www.ncsbn.org/1625.htm

Northouse, P.G. (2010). *Leadership: Theory and practice* (5th ed.). Thousand Oaks, CA: Sage.

Ouchi, W. G. (1981). *Theory Z: How American business can meet the Japanese challenge.* Reading, MA: Addison-Wesley.

Page, A. (ed.). (2004). *Keeping patients safe: Transforming the work environment of nurses.* Washington, DC: Institute of Medicine.

Shirley, M. R. (2006). Authentic leaders creating healthy work environments for nursing practice. *American Journal of Critical Care, 15,* 256–267.

Sigma Theta Tau. (2005). *Resource paper and position statement on: Leadership and leadership development priorities.* Retrieved from http://www.nursingsociety.org/aboutus /PositionPapers/Documents/position_leadership.pdf

Taylor, F. W. (1911). *The principles of scientific management.* New York: Harper & Row.

Tichy, M. N., & Bennis, W. G. (2007). *Judgment: How winning leaders make great calls.* New York: Penguin.

Weber, M. (1947). The fundamental concepts of sociology (A. M. Anderson & T. Parsons, Trans.). In T. Parsons (Ed.), *Max Weber: The theory of social and economic organization* (pp. 87–157). New York: Oxford University Press.

Wheatley, M. J. (2006). *Leadership and the new science: Discovering order in a chaotic world* (3rd ed.). San Francisco, CA: Berrett-Koehler.

BIBLIOGRAPHY

American Nurses Association. (2009). *Nursing administration: Scope and standards of practice* (3rd ed.). Silver Spring, MD: Nursebooks.org.

American Nurses Credentialing Center. (2014). *Transformational leadership: Criteria for nursing excellence.* Silver Spring, MD: Author.

Disch, J. (2009). Generative leadership. *Creative Nursing, 15,* 172–173.

George, B. (2004). *Authentic leadership: Rediscovering the secrets to creating lasting value.* New York: John Wiley.

Grossman, S. C., & Valiga, T. M. (2012). *The new leadership challenge: Creating the future of* nursing (4th ed.). Philadelphia, PA: F. A. Davis.

Hendren, R. (2010). *Six steps to ensure new nurse manager success.* Retrieved from http:// www.healthleadersmedia .com/content/NRS-252808/Six-Steps-to-Ensure -New-Nurse-Manager-Success.html

Houser, B., & Player, E. (2010). *Pivotal moments in nursing: Leaders who changed the path of a profession, Volume I.* Indianapolis, IN: Sigma Theta Tau.

Johansen, B. (2012). *Leaders make the future: Ten new leadership skills for an uncertain world.* San Francisco, CA: Berrett-Koehler.

Locke, E. A. (1982). The ideas of Frederick W. Taylor: An evaluation. *Academy of Management Review, 7*(1), 14.

ONLINE RESOURCES

American Nurses Association
http://nursingworld.org

American Association of Colleges of Nursing
http://www.aacn.nche.edu

American Association of Critical-Care Nurses
http://www.aacn.org

American Organization of Nurse Executives
http://www.aone.org/

Dale Carnegie and Associates
http://www.dalecarnegie.com

Magnet Recognition Program
http://www.nursecredentialing.org/Magnet

National Council of State Boards of Nursing
http://www.ncsbn.org

Peter F. Drucker
http://www.druckerinstitute.com/link/about-peter-drucker/

● Rose Kearney-Nunnery

11

Change and Innovation

*"We must always change, renew,
rejuvenate ourselves;
otherwise we harden."*

Johann von Goethe 1749–1812

Chapter Objectives

On completion of this chapter, the reader will be able to:

1. Differentiate among the theories of change.
2. Apply the stages of change to a patient situation.
3. Given a practice situation, describe the roles and characteristics of an effective change agent.
4. Discuss differences needed in the change process for use with individuals, families, and groups.
5. Describe the process and strategies for effective organizational change.
6. Evaluate his or her personal change quotient.

Key Terms

Change	Unfreezing	Transitions
Planned Change	Moving	Internal Sources of Change
Change Agents	Refreezing	External Sources of Change
Restraining Forces	Innovation	Change Quotient
Driving Forces	Transtheoretical Approach	

In professional practice, we need to focus on the process of planned change, being proactive rather than reactive. In fact, nursing professionals have been challenged to take a leadership role in healthcare. The Institute of Medicine's (2011) seminal report, "The Future of Nursing: Leading Change, Advancing Health," clearly states: "By virtue of its numbers and adaptive capacity, the nursing profession has the potential to effect wide-reaching changes in the health care system (p. S-1). This statement provides a clear directive for change and innovation with nurses as major players in the process.

Change is a part of normal daily life. We talk about changing our hair color, our attitude, someone else's mind, and so on. **Change** can be defined as a process that results in altered behavior of individuals or groups. Change that is accidental, spontaneous, or haphazard is caused by outside forces. On the other hand, intentional or **planned change** involves conscious effort toward some goal as a deliberate and collaborative process. Change is an integral and essential component of professional nursing practice, with nurses as change agents in healthcare settings.

In today's world, change must be viewed as affecting both the individual and the group. One example of planned change would be an individual going on a diet. The result (the change) is a decrease in weight. Such a change may also come about unintentionally, through outside influence. A family crisis or a bout of depression may lead to weight change. Or suppose the individual started eating a lot of chocolate. Gaining weight was not the intention—eating chocolate was—but weight gain was an unintended consequence. In contrast, as a planned change process, the same individual may have gone to Weight Watchers. Improved nutrition and eating practices also influence other family members through food selections and meal preparation in the home, and may even influence friends and colleagues through the individual's example.

Change is a daily occurrence in society. Think about the number of times you have read or heard of global relations, changes in political forces, and changes in healthcare organizations as restructuring. More people are beginning to embrace change since Johnson (2002) published his now classic *Who Moved My Cheese?* comparing the mice and the Littlepeople doing simple things that can either work or immobilize the situation when things change. Still, making change is not an easy process for individuals or organizations.

In professional practice, we need to focus on the process of planned change, being proactive rather than reactive. As we saw in the previous chapter, the ability to embrace change and innovation is a leadership characteristic. Planned changes for individuals or groups in the environment require structural shifts or altered behaviors for improved functioning. Improved functioning involves new (changed) behaviors, attitudes, and relationships. Professional nurses are **change agents** for people and health. Their role is to move for needed, planned change for individuals, families, community groups, and society. Such practice should occur in individual practice as well as on an organizational level.

THEORIES OF CHANGE AND INNOVATION

Understanding the theories of change applicable to individuals, families, groups, and society is the first step in moving from being reactive to unintended change to becoming proactive in creating positive, planned change.

Chinn and Benne (1976) described three classic change philosophies: (1) the empirical-rational nature of man, (2) normative-reeducative philosophy, based on human motivation and norms (attitudes, values, skills, and relationships), and (3) power-coercive philosophy, based on leadership and the application of power (p. 23). The change models that follow reflect the empirical-rational and the normative-reeducative philosophies. These two philosophical orientations focus on the nature of the person or the group in the context of the environment and are consistent with contemporary leadership theories.

Lewin

The classic change theorist was Kurt Lewin, with his normative-reeducative model based on human motivation and norms in the group. Lewin (1951) developed a model based on his Field Theory, a method of analyzing causal relationships and building the scientific constructs for change (p. 45). The mathematical model in his theory merely indicates that human behavior is based on the human being (or group) and his or her environment at that point in time. Lewin (1951) focused on social change, pointing out that "group life is never without change, merely differences in amount and type of change exist" (p. 199). In groups and organizations, multiple influences from individuals and their reactions to the environment cause group behaviors and norms. Field Theory proposes that the status quo, or a state of equilibrium, is maintained when restraining forces and driving forces balance each other. To achieve change, the restraining forces must be weakened and the driving forces strengthened. Consider the illustration of change in Figure 11.1.

Restraining forces in society resist change; they include norms, values, relations among people, morals, fears, perceived threats, and regulations. In essence, these restraining forces are the "old guard" that maintains the status quo. **Driving forces**, on the other hand, support change and include the desire to please or the desire for more novel, effective, efficient, or merely different activities. System imbalance becomes the impetus for change. The process involves weakening the restraining forces and strengthening the driving forces. To do this, Lewin proposed three methods: unfreezing, moving, and refreezing of group standards.

Unfreezing involves disequilibrium, discontent, and uneasiness. Lewin (1951) states that "to break open the shell of complacency and self-righteousness, it is sometimes necessary to bring about deliberately an emotional stir-up" (p. 229). The restraining and driving forces are identified, and comparisons are drawn between the ideal and the actual situation. To bring about change, participants must make the need for change apparent and

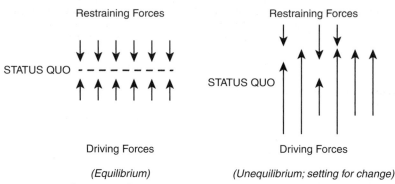

Figure 11.1   Illustration of restraining and driving forces in the change process.

accepted. In many situations, making individuals uneasy and discontented with the environmental system is the initial step in the process. Malcontents want change, whereas individuals who are satisfied and comfortable with the current state of affairs resist changes that will create disequilibrium. Activities are centered on unfreezing the existing equilibrium.

Moving occurs when the previous structure is rearranged and realistic goals are set. The system is moved to a new level of equilibrium. Choices must be made about accepting the change agent and the roles of the group members in the change process. At this stage, group decisions are preferable for moving toward permanent change. This represents the distribution of power among the group members to make them driving forces engaged in the process. The individual involved in the change process acts as a member of a group in which new social values and norms are being established.

A new status quo is established with **refreezing**. Refreezing describes the new level of equilibrium and reinforcement needed for the new patterns of behavior. The focus is on maintaining the goal achieved and highlighting the present benefits over past practices.

Consider Lewin's model with a patient population. The individual with heart disease who is started on a low-salt, low-fat diet has a teaching need to bring permanent change to his diet. You discover through interviews with the patient and family members that the diet at home is highly seasoned and high in animal protein and fats. *Restraining forces* in this situation are cultural values; family traditions; individual and group (family) preferences in food selection and preparation; attitudes toward diet, foods, or food preparation; fears of further illness with changes in diet; and attitudes toward restrictions on personal lifestyle.

Now consider each of these factors in relation to all members of the household and the patient's work, recreation, and social environments. Think about the *driving forces*: fear of further illness without the dietary changes, respect for advice given, support network, educational presentations, role models, and so forth. *Unfreezing* involves the identification of the restraining and driving forces, motivating the patient toward change, and assessing readiness for teaching. *Moving* consists of supporting a positive attitude toward change and providing nutritional

information, including food selection, preparation, and presentation options. *Refreezing* would occur with the patient's stabilization, evidenced through subjective reports (e.g., food diary), objective observations (e.g., health assessment), and laboratory findings in the rehabilitation phase. Valuable nursing theories to support nursing actions include King's Theory of Goal Attainment and Orem's Self-Care Agency. Supporting attitudinal and behavioral changes could occur through follow-up telephone or e-mail service after discharge or interviews at clinic appointments. A similar application could be developed for group change using Lewin's Field Theory or the Health Promotion Model. See Chapter 4 for more information.

Lippitt

As an outgrowth and expansion of Lewin's theory, Lippitt (1973) pointed out that "if we want to understand, explain, or predict change in human behavior, we need to take into account the person and his environment" (p. 3). He identified several complex factors of human behavior that must be considered: motivation, multiple causation, and over-rationalized habits. Looking at both individual and organizational change, he focused further on the change agent and defined seven specific phases (Fig. 11.2) within an idea, similar to Lewin's change model. Thus, Lippitt described more specific activities that are still applicable to the three steps of unfreezing, moving, and refreezing.

Unfreezing, Moving, Refreezing

For *unfreezing*, there is the need to collect data and diagnose the problem and the key people. The driving and

7.	Terminating the Relationship
6.	Maintaining the Change
5.	Choosing the Change Agent's Role
4.	Selecting Change Objectives
3.	Change Agent's Motivation and Resources
2.	Assessment of Motivation and Capacity for Change
1.	Diagnosis of Problem

Figure 11.2   Lippitt's (1973) seven stages of planned change.

restraining people, environmental, and organizational forces are identified, defined, and targeted. Second, the motivation and resources are assessed to identify the desire and capacity for change. This includes the resistance and readiness of the people in the environment. In the third step, the change agent's motivation, commitment, and resources must be assessed for the potential success of the change activity. The skills, efforts, and responsibilities are critical planning pieces in this phase of change.

For *moving*, change objectives must be selected with consideration of activities for progressive change. Lippitt uses the leverage point concept as the starting point at which receptivity for change is apparent and the objectives are initiated. Planning and evaluation are primary activities in this step. Then, following the development of an action plan with evaluation criteria, the change agent and group roles are selected and assigned. Acceptance and selection of an appropriate role is critical in defining the power, outcomes, and strategies of the change agent.

Refreezing, or maintaining the change, occurs through ongoing training, communication, and support of the people in the environment. Communication by both sides, the driving and the restraining forces, advertises the success of the change using actual evaluation results. In many cases, the loudest and most visible of the restraining forces become the change agent's greatest supporters when they accept the merits of the process with evaluation. How many times have you heard someone say, "I never thought it could be done but . . ." or "I was behind that all along but I did not want to show it"? Finally, terminating the helping relationship is necessary on the part of the change agent and major players for the change to become part of the people and the environment, and not just the activity of a select individual or group. Rather, it becomes the new norm of the people or the organization.

Role of Change Agent

A major piece of Lippitt's (1973) model involves the roles for the professional change agent. He proposed four major roles for the change agent:

- Specialist
- Coordinator
- Fact finder and information link
- Consultant

Lippitt views the selection of the appropriate role for the change agent as essential in the moving phase of change. As a *specialist*, the change agent is the expert in the environment on methods and strategies for change. As a *coordinator*, the change agent functions as manager, who plans, organizes, and coordinates efforts and programs for the change. The change agent as a *fact finder and information link* serves as a seeker, clarifier, synthesizer, reality tester, and provider of information, as well as a communications link among all participants in the system (Lippitt, 1973, pp. 60–61).

The *consultant* role is viewed as the most important role for the change agent, both inside the system and with external individuals, groups, and environments. In fact, Lippitt (1973) developed a model of eight specific activity roles within this consultant role, which are viewed along a continuum from advocate through expert, trainer, alternative identifier, collaborator, process specialist, fact finder, and reflector (p. 63). The correct role for the change agent depends on the people, the environment, and how much direction is needed from the agent to implement the change. As the advocate, the change agent as a consultant is highly directive in leading the group toward change. Conversely, the change agent is the least directive as a reflector, helping the group clarify and evaluate their efforts. The change agent must have knowledge, skill, and perseverance in the work-intensive process of change.

Consider, again, our example of the patient who must change to a low-salt, low-fat diet. Under Lippitt's model, first, you need to collect data on meals, food preferences, and preparation at home. You identify, define, and target the environmental forces—family, friends, and cultural and collegial (work or recreational) forces. Second, you assess the motivation, resistance, readiness, and resources of the patient and his family to identify the desire and capacity for change in dietary habits. In the third step, your motivation, commitment, and resources must be realized as the nurse–change agent. Your skills, efforts, and responsibilities are critical in this planning phase. Lippitt's concept of leverage point occurs when the patient and his family are receptive to change and the action plan is initiated with evaluation criteria. Your role as change agent is defined specific to the patient and his needs. Consider the applicability of Orem's three modes of nursing, especially the supportive-educative mode, in relation to his continuum of consultant activities. Your role as change agent may alter rapidly as the patient moves from the hospital setting to the home and clinic settings. Empowerment of the patient and his significant others is critical for success in this type of change. And with the maintenance of the change in diet and health status that occurs through ongoing training in dietary management, communication, support, and reinforcement during the follow-up period, the patient and family are moved into the termination phase. The helping relationship is no longer necessary and the dietary changes have become part of the person and family in their environment.

Havelock

Havelock (1971) used a system and process model to depict an organization with the following major concepts: role, linkages, and communication for transfer and use of knowledge. Using the three major perspectives of problem-solving, research-development-diffusion, and social interaction, Havelock further examined the linkage process to view the change in the broader system (Havelock & Havelock, 1973). His model reflects the empirical-rational nature of humans.

Building on Lewin's stages of change, Havelock added steps highlighting communication and interpersonal activities:

- Perception of need
- Diagnosis of the problem
- Identification of the problem
- Devising a plan of action

- Gaining acceptance of the plan
- Stabilization
- Self-renewal (Havelock & Havelock, 1973)

Unfreezing, Moving, Refreezing

For *unfreezing*, the perception of a need for a change in the system is followed by diagnosis and identification of the problem. At this time, a reciprocal relationship develops between the user (patient) system and a resource system. Linkages with needed resources are made in this initial stage before moving on the change. Havelock and Havelock (1973) stress that the problem-solver must be "meaningfully linked to outside resources" (p. 23).

Moving toward change requires devising a plan of action and gaining acceptance of the plan in the system. This is a stage of searching for a solution and applying that solution to the identified problem, using resource linkages in the environment.

In the final step, *refreezing*, stabilization and the need for self-renewal are specified. First, stabilization in the system is specified to sustain the change (refreezing). Havelock describes self-renewal as being needed to sustain the patient system in the future. This sense of self-renewal is the empirical-rational nature of people where the new values, goals, and activities of the system become the norm.

Role of Change Agent

The importance of and roles for the change agent are also key components of Havelock's model, which lists four roles for the change agent:

- Catalyst
- Solution giver
- Process helper
- Resource linker (Havelock & Havelock, 1973, p. 60)

These roles become increasingly complex. The catalyst serves as the impetus for change. The resource linker brings people, environments, and resources together at the system and macrosystem levels (Havelock & Havelock, 1973, pp. 60–64). For effective functioning within these roles, Havelock further developed a training program for preparing effective change agents.

Havelock's model can also be used with the example of dietary change for our patient with heart disease. Communication and interpersonal activities are core ingredients in the nurse-patient relationship. Identifying the need for altering dietary salt and fat relates to the patient's medical condition. The personal, environmental, social, cultural, and dietary habits are assessed through interview, to define the problem. A reciprocal relationship between the patient system and a resource system occurs through linkages, including meeting with a nutritionist for food selection and preparation options. Informational lists on cookbooks, restaurants, and community associations advocating healthy eating with low-fat, low-salt meals are provided. Using this model, the nurse encourages linkages with outside resources such as the American Heart Association, American Association of Critical-Care Nurses, and collegial relationships with nutritionists, rehabilitation

specialists, and cardiologists. The plan for dietary change is devised in collaboration with the patient system and includes linkages with community resources acceptable to the patient and his family. Recall the concept of cultural competence from Chapter 4 and how it is necessary in this model. Linkages must be retained with the patient after discharge, in the home, clinic, or rehabilitation setting. This follow-up is necessary for stabilizing the diet, given the patient's physiological and psychosocial system influences. The role of the nurse-change agent has moved from catalyst and solution giver in the initial phase of problem identification, to process helper in the planning phase, and then to resource linker. The changes in diet must become a part of the patient's value system. The nurse–change agent then terminates the relationship with the patient, while linkages with external resources provide the patient with self-renewal.

Rogers

As an outgrowth of the change model, Rogers developed the Diffusion of Innovations model. In 1971, Rogers and Shoemaker stated the following:

Although it is true that we live more than ever before in an era of change, prevailing social structures often serve to hamper the diffusion of innovations. Our activities in education, agriculture, medicine, industry, and the like are often without the benefit of the most current research knowledge. The gap between what is actually known and what is effectively put to use needs to be closed. (p. 1)

This is still true today, more than 40 years later. We live in a time of even greater social change. This model was used in nursing in the 1980s to promote research-based practice and is quite appropriate today with the imperative for evidence-based practice. We are not just changing from one practice to another. We want change to be evidence-based, for efficacy related to patient outcomes. Often, this will involve **innovation** or moving to a new, more novel or advanced approach than the one used in the past.

Rogers and Shoemaker (1971) focus on communication and view *change* as the effects of a new idea or innovation being adopted and put into use or rejected. Change may occur at the level of the individual, group, organization, or society. The model was first proposed with four major steps in the process of social change: knowledge, persuasion, decision, and confirmation (Rogers & Shoemaker, 1971, p. 25). Rogers (1983) then extended the Innovation-Diffusion process to five stages:

- Knowledge
- Persuasion
- Decision
- Implementation
- Confirmation

The interest and commitment of key people and policymakers are critical in this model.

Notice how these stages are similar to those in the ACE Star Model of Knowledge Transformation (see Fig. 5.1). Recall that the steps in knowledge transformation were discovery, summary, translation, integration, and evaluation (Stevens, 2009).

Unfreezing, Moving, Refreezing

Developing a sequence of knowledge, persuasion, and decision making is the key activity in the *unfreezing* stage. To develop knowledge, key people and policy-makers are introduced to the innovation to gain understanding. Then comes persuasion to develop attitudes on the innovation. Rogers (1983) uses persuasion to focus on the individual whose attitudes change, either positively or negatively toward the innovation, not on the external force that changes one's mind. The decision to adopt or reject an innovation is the bridge between the unfreezing and moving stages in Rogers' model.

Implementation applies to the stage of *moving*. Revisions, potential adoption, or rejection of the innovation occurs in this implementation phase. Rogers' fifth step, when the innovation changes from being novel to being part of the routine or norm, involves *refreezing* the equilibrium. He calls this step *confirmation*, in which reinforcement is sought and the key people and policy-makers decide to maintain or discontinue the innovation. Rogers (1983) admitted that the research evidence shows no clear distinction between the implementation and confirmation steps. This may be related to the idea of a flexible time span between implementation and confirmation, when the process of refreezing for the innovation occurs. Rogers (1983) describes the final confirmatory stage as "routinization" of the innovation.

Throughout the entire process, five attributes determine the rate of adoption of an innovation by members of a social system:

- Relative advantage
- Compatibility
- Complexity
- Trialability
- Observability (Rogers & Shoemaker, 1971, p. 39; Rogers, 1983, pp. 238–240)

These attributes should be included in all evaluation plans and data on the change. Relative advantage is determined through comparison of the innovation with what was done in the past. The advantage may be effectiveness as well as efficiency, and the process has been described as weighing economic advantages or the cost-effectiveness. Compatibility with the values, beliefs, and needs of the group is the second factor. The complexity (difficulty in use), trialability (experimental trials), and observability (visible evidence) are all considered in the implementation stage and have a direct effect on adoption, revision, or discontinuation of an innovation.

Role of Change Agent

Rogers' model also highlights the roles of the change agent, which occur in the following sequence:

1. Develops the need for change
2. Establishes the relationship with the individual system
3. Diagnoses the problems
4. Motivates the individual system for change
5. Translates intent for change into the actions needed
6. Stabilizes change in system and "freezes" new behavior
7. Terminates the relationship (Rogers, 1983, pp. 315–317)

Like Lippitt, Rogers views the change agent as a professional, skilled in change for effective functioning in the role.

We take a slightly different approach with the application of Rogers' Innovation-Diffusion process model to our example of the patient who needs to change his diet. You have found research studies on effective dietary compliance in cardiac rehabilitation. You now wish to bring this innovation into practice in your organization to use in patient teaching programs. During the initial development of knowledge, key people and policy-makers in nursing service and cardiology are introduced to the teaching program content and methods, along with the results from use with patients in other settings. Next, you need to persuade people of the effectiveness and applicability of this approach—the organization and its resources as well as the patient population. The decision is made to either adopt or reject the new teaching program. If it is decided to try the teaching program with a patient population, the phase of implementation is entered. The teaching program may be revised, adopted, or rejected on the basis of its specificity and acceptability to the patient group and the organization. If the teaching program is found to be applicable and advantageous, it is "confirmed" as the agency procedure or organizational norm. If the procedure is not adopted, the key people and policy-makers must confirm the decision to discontinue the program. These are the steps toward implementing evidence-based practice at the organizational level.

The Transtheoretical Approach

Another model of change arose from a behaviorist perspective and psychotherapy. Prochaska, DiClemente, and Norcross (1992) describe their program of research focused on how people as "self-changers" intentionally change their behavior, both with and without psychotherapy (p. 1102). This led to the emergence of their **Transtheoretical Approach** to change, which they describe as an eclectic model that does not dictate adherence to a specific type of psychotherapy. The empirical basis for this theory provides a broad range of studies on individuals and groups (both inpatients and outpatients), from family therapy to addictive conditions and health-promotion activities. One of the original core concepts of this theory is that people who change or who recover from an addictive condition experience an invariant series of stages for the change to occur (Prochaska & DiClemente, 1984, p. 21). Key components of this model are stages of change and processes for intentional change to occur. Developmental and environmental changes can also occur, but unless individuals see this as an intentional change, they will feel coerced, and reversion to the prior behavior may occur (Prochaska & DiClemente, 1984, p. 80).

Originally, the Transtheoretical Model included five linear stages (precontemplation, contemplation, decision, action, and maintenance) but was then modified based on statistical analysis to four stages, because the individual's decision to make a change included both contemplation and action. The four stages of change—precontemplation, contemplation, action, and maintenance—were envisioned as a revolving door with the potential for relapse (Prochaska & DiClemente, 1984, p. 23).

Further research provided the basis for the refinement of the model, as a spiral with five stages of change, in which relapses were the norm, resulting in regression and the potential for later progression through the five stages (Prochaska et al., 1992, p. 1104). Consider these five stages as described in Table 11.1. Termination with the firm establishment of the changed behavior does not occur until the individual no longer has to make any conscious efforts to avoid a relapse to the prior behavior (Prochaska & DiClemente, 1984, p. 29). The research has indicated that most "self-changers" will "recycle several times through stages before achieving long-term maintenance" (Prochaska et al., 1992, p. 1111).

In addition to the stages of change through which the individual progresses, the model proposes that certain behaviors or processes are more apparent and effective in selected stages of change. A behaviorist philosophy to change is apparent in the 10 proposed processes that occur in the different stages of change as follows:

- Consciousness raising with education and information
- Self-reevaluation as with values clarification
- Self-liberation with a commitment to action
- Counter-conditioning as with alternatives to the behavior
- Stimulus control or counteracting negative stimuli
- Reinforcement management or self-rewards for positive behaviors
- Helping relationships, both social and therapeutic support systems
- Dramatic relief or expressing feelings
- Environmental reevaluation as with the effect of the problem on the environment
- Social liberation and advocacy (Prochaska et al., 1992, p. 1108)

Subsequent research has identified that the most frequently used processes across the various types of intentional change were helping relationships, consciousness raising, and self-liberation, except in the case of overweight individuals who used more self-liberation and stimulus control (Prochaska et al., 1992, p. 1107). These change processes focus on cognitive, affective, and psychomotor behaviors. In the early precontemplation and contemplation stages of change, the cognitive change processes can lead to preparation for change. Active behavioral change processes are critical in the action and maintenance stages, however (Prochaska et al., 1992, p. 1112).

TABLE 11.1

Transtheoretical Model and the Stages of Change

Stage of Change	Behavioral Characteristics		Changes Processes
Precontemplation	Satisfaction with the current situation. The individual indicates no intention to change and may deny the existence of a problem.	↓ ↓	Consciousness raising Dramatic relief
Contemplation	Acknowledges that a problem exists but has not made a commitment to change the negative behavior. An important clue for this stage is a lack of readiness for the change despite thoughtful consideration of the positives and negatives of the situation.	↓ ↓	Environmental reevaluation Self-reevaluation
Preparation	In this stage the commitment to change is made and the individual is intending to take action in the near future.	↓	Self-liberation
Action	Positive actions are now taken for a change in behavior. Individuals in this stage have altered their behavior for a period from one day to six months (Prochaska et al., 1992, p. 1104).	↓ ↓ ↓	Reinforcement management Helping relationships Counter conditioning
Maintenance	The new behaviors have now replaced the prior ones. The individual is committed to the change on an ongoing basis. The theorists describe the "hallmarks" of this stage as stabilizing behavioral change and avoiding relapse, which can last from six months to a lifetime (Prochaska et al., 1992, p. 1104).	↓	Stimulus control

Source: Prochaska, J. O., DiClemente, C. C., & Norcross, J. C. (1992). In search of how people change: Applications to addictive behaviors. *American Psychologist, 47,* 1102–1114.

Unfreezing, Moving, Refreezing

The five stages of change in the Transtheoretical Model are also consistent with Lewin's stages of change. Unfreezing occurs in the stages of precontemplation, contemplation, and preparation, especially with the cognitive change processes. Moving starts with the stage of preparation for the change and then into action. Recall that in the action stage of the Transtheoretical Model, the individual has implemented a changed behavior from one day to six months. Refreezing occurs in the maintenance stage with the stabilization of the behavior.

The Individual as the Change Agent

In this theory, the individual is the agent of change, with external assistance of "helping relationships" in the change process. The focus is clearly on the individual and the potential for relapse and is applicable for individuals as "self-changers," especially given a situation for patient teaching.

Applications of the theory have been noted in the case of both addictive behaviors and for promoting healthier lifestyles. For use with groups, effectiveness depends on whether the individuals are at the same stage of change (Prochaska & DiClemente, 1984). For example, for effectiveness, group members must be homogeneous in terms of their readiness for change as opposed to a group with some individuals in the precontemplation stage (and satisfied with the status quo) and others in the action or maintenance stages.

The focus of the Transtheoretical Approach is on the individual, and the potential for relapse is consistent with the focus of nursing on human beings in their unique environment and with their unique characteristics and needs. They may need additional time to succeed in the changed behavior. As previously noted by the theorists, many need to "recycle" through the stages. As with our example of the patient who must change to a low-salt, low-fat diet, assessment of individual and environmental characteristics is still essential, as is readiness for change. This assessment of readiness will direct your use of change processes to assist the individual through the particular stage of change. For example, with patient teaching as a helping relationship, you may be providing informational materials in the precontemplation and contemplation stages as consciousness raising activities. Also consider the use of active behavioral change activities with food diaries and reinforcement management in the active stages of change. A key component of the self-liberation process in change in the Transtheoretical Approach is the concept of choice, with the component of decision-making and commitment to the decision (Prochaska & DiClemente, 1984, p. 38). And individual differences, self-esteem, and motivation must be considerations in the case of a relapse.

TRANSITIONS

In the area of organizational change, the concept of **transitions**, as a corporate change phenomenon, has emerged with the move to more humanistic organizational theories as these same organizations struggle to survive and thrive in the economic climate. As illustrated in the Harvard Business Essentials publication (2003), "accepting the necessity and inevitability of change enables [businesses] to see times of transformation not as threats but as opportunities— opportunities for reinventing the company and its culture" (pp. 1–2). Numerous consultants as change agents assist corporations through these transitions. Organizational changes fall generally in the areas of mergers, cost-cutting, customer service, or changes in processes of how things get done (Harvard Business Essentials, 2003). In healthcare we have seen all of these types of changes, with process changes an imperative as we focus on safety initiatives and evidence-based practice. Two particular change models reflect the humanistic focus of organizations in transition.

Bridges

Rather than focusing on change as a situation like relocation, Bridges (2009) looks at the psychological processes in stages of transition (Box 11.1), where people must "come to terms with the details of the new situation that the change brings about" (p. 3). These three stages of transition are interacting and nonlinear and may be occurring at the same time at different parts of the organization and with different people.

In the initial stage, this theory focuses on people who have to first "let go" of the comfortable and safe in their day-to-day lives and experience loss. Resistance is to be expected; Bridges (2009) regards this initial stage as an ending in that "before you can learn a new way of doing things, you must unlearn the old way" (p. 23). He describes a grief and mourning process requiring acceptance of and assistance from the people in the organization.

Bridges (2009) describes the second stage as one of great uncertainty, chaos, and the opportunity for innovation. People have given up the old way of doing things but need support in innovation and assistance in the process. He describes Neutral Zone Management as the "only way to ensure that the organization comes through the change intact and that the necessary changes actually work the way they are supposed to" (Bridges, 2009, p. 42). He even recommends the use of transition teams composed of organizational members to monitor the process, progress, and to be the communication channel to the leadership of the organization.

The third stage is the New Beginning, described as a release of new energy in a new direction and with a new identity (Bridges, 2009, p. 57). Again, the humanistic perspective is apparent, with celebrations of the new corporate identity and the people in the new culture actively involved and rejuvenated. Bridges actively speaks to leadership and provides examples of successes

---

BOX 11.1 Bridges' Stages for Managing Transitions

- Ending, Losing, Letting Go
- The Neutral Zone
- The New Beginning

Source: Bridges, W. (2009). *Managing transitions: Making the most of change* (3rd ed.). Cambridge, MA: DaCapo Press.

and pitfalls that occur in the transition. Organizational leadership must focus on the culture, with respect for transition to the new beginning. Checklists are provided to address questions on progress throughout the process.

Bridges's three stages of organizational change can parallel the three stages of unfreezing, moving, and refreezing, but this model focuses on the management and people in the organization for success in the process. As Bridges (2009) points out, "we have learned how self-defeating it is to try to overcome people's resistance to change without addressing the threat the change poses to their world" (p. xi).

Four Quadrants of Change

Another organizational change model focuses on the humanistic factors within the organization, with important considerations of personal transformation. Although not related to particular stages, the Four Quadrants of Change (see Box 11.2) is illustrated as a circle divided into quarters as interacting and vital considerations for success in the organizational change process. The top two quarters represent the individual in the organization but first with psychological, spiritual, and cognitive attributes that must be considered in the transformation process. Quadrant one focuses on the inner development of people, and the recognition that no substantive change is possible without a change in the consciousness of the people (Anderson, Klein, & Stuart, 2000, p. 32). Quadrant two represents the interpersonal and technical skills for motivation and peak performance in the organization (Anderson et al., 2000, p. 32).

At the bottom of the circle, quadrants three and four represent the organizational influences. Quadrant three is the organizational culture and traditions. Quadrant four is the organizational design with technology, policies, procedures, and workflow that determine performance of the organization (Anderson et al., 2000, p. 33). Consideration of all four quadrants is vital in the change process for an organization, but the theorists caution that the humanistic quadrants are vital for an organizational change to succeed. They consider this a personal transformation and a conscious choice because "organizational change is not a question of skills and structure alone, but of identity and worldview" (Anderson et al., 2000, p. 34).

The Role of the Change Agent

In both transitions models, the role of the change agent is the leadership driving the change, with management firmly focused on the organizational culture for reinventing the organization and survival in a humanistic environment. Understanding of human nature and its resistance to change as a loss of the comfortable is necessary for the change agent. The transitions models are focused on organizational change, but the view of change as a transition with the concepts of loss and rejuvenation are still applicable to our example of the patient with a need for a change in diet. The grief, mourning, and loss over past heritage and practices must be considered along with the uncertainty and potential for innovation during the time of transition to the new dietary regime. Perhaps this could be a family cookbook of new recipes and preparations. An important thought is the celebration of the new beginning and whether we help our patients sufficiently celebrate their success with a changed behavior.

The various models of change are summarized in Table 11.2. Selecting an appropriate model to guide practice involves how you look at the world and what is most helpful in driving your skills as an agent in the change process. Moving from the theoretical stages of change to strategies for change and innovation brings the focus to the external influence or change agent.

CHANGE AGENTS

Our second step in becoming a major player in the change process is to develop greater understanding of the roles and attributes of a successful change agent. We have seen the importance of the change agent emerge in the models of Lippitt, Havelock, and Rogers. Recall that in the Transtheoretical Approach, your role as an agent of change will be a part of the "helping relationship." Table 11.3 summarizes the roles and activities of the change agent in these models. In Lewin's original model, change in humans is a function of the person and his or her environment at that point in time. Consider the roles of the change agent in the three general phases of change.

Unfreezing

Good interpersonal and assessment skills are needed to acquire data to weaken restraining forces and enhance driving forces in the present system, and the agent must consider both internal and external system forces. The change agent must then establish a climate that encourages and supports change. Needs assessment, diagnosis, and the establishment of a professional relationship have occurred consistently during the unfreezing phase in all models. Now consider the similarity of this stage to the assessment and diagnosis activities of the nursing process.

ONLINE CONSULT

William Bridges & Associates at
http://www.wmbridges.com

BOX 11.2	The Four Quadrants of Change

- Quadrant 1: Individual/Internal
- Quadrant 2: Individual/External
- Quadrant 3: Collective/Internal
- Quadrant 4: Collective/External

Source: Anderson, B., Klein, E., & Stuart, J. (2000). Why change is a consciousness choice. *The Journal for Quality and Participation, 23,* 32–36.

TABLE 11.2

Comparison of the Stages of Change Represented in Theoretical Models

Theorist	Stages						
Lewin (1951) Force Field	[1] Unfreezing			[2] Moving		[3] Refreezing	
Lippitt (1973) Planned Change	[1] Diagnosis of prob-lem	[2] Assessment of motivation and capacity for change	[3] Change agent's moti-vation and resources	[4] Selecting change objectives	[5] Choosing change agent's role	[6] Maintaining the change	[7] Terminating the relation-ship
Havelock (1971) Linkages	[1] Perception of need	[2] Diagnosis of the problem	[3] Identification of the problem	[4] Devising a plan of action	[5] Gaining ac-ceptance of plan	[6] Stabilization	[7] Self-renewal
Rogers (1983) Innovation-Diffusion	[1] Knowledge	[2] Persuasion	[3] Decision	[4] Implementa-tion	[5] Confirma-tion		
Prochaska et al. (1992) Transtheo-retical Approach	[1] Precon-templation	[2] Contempla-tion	[3] Preparation	[4] Action	[5] Maintenance		
Bridges (2009) Making Transitions	[1] Ending, Losing, Letting Go		[2] The Neutral Zone		[3] The New Beginning		

In the nursing process, health assessment data are collected and problems are identified. Assessing the patient's characteristics, current level of satisfaction with the health problem and condition, and perception of the situation is an essential component of this activity. Diagnostic statements are developed after needs identification. Asking questions and diagnosing the problem for changed behaviors or responses lead to the planning stage of the nursing process.

Moving

The change agent must help the patient set and strive for clear, realistic goals. A good deal of the change agent's time and energy is needed during this phase for strategies to deal with those who are resisting change. Again, interpersonal and motivational skills are critical. The change agent must constantly assess and evaluate resistance, conflict, readiness for change, and motivation in the individual system, and must maintain movement toward the goals and objectives of change.

As in the nursing process, the major activities of the moving stage are implementing plans, goals, and objectives and collecting evaluation data. Patient data are analyzed, interpreted, and acted upon. The nurse actively uses critical thinking, decision-making, interpersonal, and evaluation skills. The same skills are necessary to move toward change. This stage will probably be the most comfortable for the nurse functioning as a change agent, because skills in this area are developed through nursing practice.

Refreezing

Providing rewards and reinforcement for the change is a major part of the change agent's role in the third stage. Evaluation data for reinforcement of change must be used as supportive evidence. Activities for the change agent during this stage are supportive initially, but involvement decreases with the need to terminate and have the patient system totally involved in and responsible for the change without external intervention from the change agent. Recall that in the Transtheoretical Approach, the stage of maintenance may last a lifetime until the individual no longer has to make any conscious effort to avoid a relapse, and the helping relationships may be the social support system.

In the nursing process, the nurse-patient relationship is terminated when objectives are achieved and nursing diagnoses are resolved. The nurse has prepared the person or family for this termination long before discharge orders are written or the person leaves the

TABLE 11.3

Comparing Roles for the Change Agent from Different Theoretical Models

Stages of Change	Lippitt (1973)	Havelock (1973)	Rogers (1983)	Bridges (2009)
Unfreezing	A specialist in the diagnosis and assessment of patient system and change agent as: • Information seeker • Clarifier • Synthesizer • Reality tester • Provider • Problem-solver	A catalyst in the identification of needs, diagnoses, and all aspects of the problem within the roles of: • Clarifier • Synthesizer • Reality tester • Provider • Problem-solver	Range of roles from support to consultant for sharing knowledge, building persuasiveness, and leading the group toward decision making on innovation through activities of: • Needs identification • Establishment of professional relationship with patient system • Diagnosis of problems • Motivation of patient system	The critical ingredient is the match or at least a working understanding of the consistency between the character type of the organization and the change agent. Acceptance and acknowledgment of the grief and mourning process for the loss is vital. The need for detailed information on the plan because the transition must be transmitted and reinforced. Good listening and communication skills are essential with a focus on the person as a member of and part of the organization.
Moving	Communication link viewed within one of eight directive to nondirective consultative roles: • Advocate • Expert • Trainer • Alternative identifier • Collaborator • Process specialist • Fact-finder • Reflector	Solution giver and process helper as: • Clarifier • Synthesizer • Reality tester • Provider • Problem-solver	Range of roles from support to consultant to translate intent for change into the actions needed	The Neutral Zone is a time of uncertainty and uneasiness in the organization and among the people. Once again, excellent communication skills are vital to keeping people informed, on target, and to avoid the development of damaging coalitions, which can inhibit the transition. A transition monitoring team keeps management aware of the progress of the grass-roots members in their transition. Bridges (2009) does point out that role of the team is to monitor progress and should be time limited.
Refreezing	Consultation for: • Maintenance of the change • Termination of the relationship	Resource linker for stabilization and self-renewal as: • Clarifier • Synthesizer • Reality tester • Problem-solver	Range of roles from support to consultant for: • Confirmation of change and stabilizing the adoption to prevent discontinuance and reinforce new behaviors • Termination of relationship	The New Beginning is a time of excitement and celebration for members of the organization in the new ways of the organization. Important roles for both the change agent as the manager of the transition and also for the leadership of the organization with the new culture.

agency environment. Just as discharge planning starts with admission, this last stage must be planned for and worked toward during the entire change process, with the person, family, or group taking increasing responsibility for the new behaviors.

The interventions of a skilled change agent can make all the difference in the planned change process. The essential skills of change agents include the following:

- Vision for the future and creativity
- Ability to look at a situation narrowly and broadly (assessment and critical thinking skills)
- Good interpersonal skills, including those of communication, motivation, assertiveness, problem-solving, and group process
- Flexibility and a willingness to consider alternative views
- Perseverance and a positive attitude
- Integrity and commitment
- Ability to manage conflict and resistance
- A focus on human beings and celebrating their accomplishments

CHANGE IN INDIVIDUALS, FAMILIES, AND GROUPS

As noted earlier, Chinn and Benne (1976) categorized change strategies into three major types: empirical-rational, normative-reeducative, and power-coercive. Power-coercive strategies are based on the application of power by legitimate authority. Nursing concerns are with human beings and their empowerment for healthy behaviors or the creation of optimal health status. Applying power as "the authority" is inconsistent with empowering people. One can alter practices, procedures, or the environment in organizations as a coercive change by imposing major policy, but think of the upheaval this change creates. Coercive change may be necessary in an emergency situation or when the person or family must have major assistance. The problem is that the change may not persist unless the person or group has internalized it into the value system.

The philosophical basis of nursing is consistent with the empirical-rational or the normative-reeducative strategies for change. The empirical-rational strategy assumes that people are rational and have self-interest in change. Power for the individual or group occurs through knowledge. The normative-reeducative approach is based on social norms and the person's interaction with the environment. The normative-reeducative philosophy can be viewed as empowerment with an emphasis on interpersonal skills. Both of these philosophical orientations are consistent with nursing, but their applicability differs according to the nursing model selected for practice. For example, King's Theory of Goal Attainment, Orem's General Theory of Nursing, and Roy's Adaptation Model contain philosophical assumptions similar to the reeducative strategies, with the person viewed as a thinking, feeling, reacting being in the context of his or her environment.

Because nursing looks at human beings and their interactions within the environment, several factors must be considered in the change process. These include resistance to change, empowerment or involvement of the individual, and environmental, cultural, or situational factors.

Resistance to Change

A major concern of the change agent is the person's or group's resistance to change. To handle this resistance, one must evaluate what makes people resist change. People are naturally threatened by change. Change involves loss. It is a threat to their value system and a loss of the comfortable status quo. They feel vulnerable and insecure. Stress is created and must be managed. The need for the change may also be mistrusted or misunderstood. Another innately human characteristic is the fear of failure or being unable to perform the new activities or tasks. This creates more stress. This is the state of relapse in the Transtheoretical Approach in which the individual can then "recycle" through the stages.

Resistance to change can be reduced by several techniques:

- Careful planning
- Allowing sufficient time
- Support and reinforcement
- Involving the person or group

Understanding the full impact of individual or group norms and planning for a change in attitudes can lead to changes in behavior. Recall the adage, "Fools rush in. . . ." Allowing sufficient time for the change to occur and persist is essential. A gradual move toward change is more effective than a radical move. The time needed depends on the physical, psychosocial, cultural, and attitudinal characteristics of the individual or group. Patience, persistence, perseverance, and creativity are essential traits of the change agent. Another strategy for decreasing resistance to change is good communication with key and resource people throughout the entire process. In addition, a good deal of support and reinforcement will be needed. This requires excellent interpersonal skills, verbal and nonverbal, with both individuals and groups.

The involvement of the person or group is needed for lasting change. It is essential to build on their readiness, motivation, self-concept, abilities, and resources throughout the process. Involving people in planning and decision making both reduces resistance to change and creates empowerment. Strategies for involving people include education, training, socialization and persuasion (not imposing), and facilitation. This is a "helping relationship." It would often be easier to make the change yourself as an external force, but the action by the individual is slower and more enduring. Note that education and training involve enlightenment and preparation rather than preaching. This creates the empowerment and sets the stage for a revision of the norm or value system and self-efficacy.

Environmental Assessment

Looking at the situation or environment is critical in the change process. First, one must understand the past or the personal history of the individual, family, or group. You include a past, personal, psychosocial, family, and environmental history in a health history. These are important basic items of information to obtain before doing the physical appraisal in any health assessment. The same thing is needed in the change process. The following questions will help in understanding the situation and people:

1. What types of change has the person or group faced in the past? Information on experience and success with change is valuable to determine whether this person is a novice with change, has embraced change throughout life, or falls somewhere between these experiential extremes.
2. How has the person or group handled change? Stress and coping factors will emerge with this information. You can then discover how to motivate and support behaviors.
3. What resources have been available or used in previous change activities?
4. What is the person's or group's perspective on the applicability of the resources in the environment to the present situation? Human resources are support systems, and can include family, friends, colleagues, clergy, professionals, and even "ideal" role models. These resources may help the person or group. If these are not available or appropriate, linking the person or group with similar resources may be effective. Some people do well in support groups whereas others need more individualized support.

HEALTHCARE ORGANIZATIONAL CHANGE

Both internal and external influences in contemporary healthcare are major considerations for change in healthcare institutions. As Hall and Tolbert (2005) propose, "organizational survival, or the avoidance of death, is . . . the ultimate test of an organization, but at any time, unless death is imminent, what goes on in the organization is based on both environmental pressures and goals" (p. 155).

Everyone within an organization has faced organizational change, from minor changes in policy to restructuring of services. Many have experienced or know a colleague who has experienced a radical reorganization, with restructuring and managerial shifts, layoffs, or ownership changes. With organizational change comes tension and conflict as a natural function of stress on the system, its people, and their daily activities and interactions. Transitions and the sense of loss are important considerations.

Systems theory provides a useful perspective for viewing the internal and external forces of any organization. A healthcare institution or agency is an open environmental system with great complexity. The organization must be considered in terms of the system, as well as the macrosystem and patient system. **Internal sources of change** come from agency administrative, policy, and operational factors guiding the system. Bridges (2000) describes this as the character of the organization. The

surrounding environmental system of the organization is the healthcare arena, which provides the professional, specialization, reimbursement, and additional value structures for the organizational unit and its members. The broader social or macroenvironment reflects societal norms and values through the needs and potential needs of consumers of healthcare. Linkages among all system parts are assumed as necessary for effectiveness and continuity. But look further at this complex system and the internal environment.

When change is proposed for an agency or institutional system, an in-depth look at the organizational environment is needed. Internal sources of change can arise from any one or some combination of these system components. Consider the traditional healthcare agency, the hospital. The associated internal forces can be described as follows:

- Goals and values for healthcare are specified for an organization as a purpose, philosophy, vision, or mission statement. Valuable information on the internal forces is apparent with this organizational view of people, health, and healthcare before translation into departmental or policy statements. Insight can also be obtained from the historical documents on how the institution evolved into a modern healthcare organization.
- The knowledge and skills of the healthcare providers and physical resources in the system are vital considerations. Consider internal forces from the specific equipment, services, and expertise of professional and nonprofessional labor forces in the organizational setting.
- Interpersonal and interdisciplinary relationships with role relationships, attitudes, and values of people and groups within the system must also be considered. Nurses are expected to exhibit behaviors related to the roles of healthcare provider, manager, teacher, researcher, and advocate and to collaborate with members of other healthcare disciplines.
- The organizational design to provide healthcare services must also be considered. In addition to organizational charts, position descriptions, and policy and procedure manuals, informal sources, such as technical and clerical staff, can provide valuable information on the organization's daily operations to illustrate how tasks are accomplished in the organization.
- Governance by a governing board and corporate officers may include paid or volunteer board members, required institutional review boards, and the chief executive team or officers.

External environmental influences are the next factors to consider in terms of impact on the system. **External sources of change** include inputs of energy, information, and materials received from the environment, transformed, and returned to the environment as outputs. One input into the hospital environment is the patient system. The patient enters the hospital with a health deficit and, through the care received while hospitalized (throughput), strives for a higher level of wellness as the intended outcome (output). But, environmental influences add more complexity. External forces are the broader environment providing inputs into the system. As with any open system, however, the external forces affect internal operations, and an exchange of information is returned to the environment as outputs.

External forces have a major impact on the function of the traditional hospital. Suppliers to be considered include physicians, drug and equipment companies, volunteers, and educational facilities. Physicians supply patients. Drug and equipment companies compete for contracts, and organizations seek purchasing power with consortia or multiorganizational contracts. Volunteers provide valuable transportation, recreational, and interpersonal services without which many hospitals could not survive. Educational suppliers provide additional services, with trainees as residents, interns, nurses, therapists, and other preparers of ancillary personnel, as well as the future workforce. And national safety initiatives add additional responsibility and complexity. In addition, new staff members bring different ideas and methods into the system.

Customers are generally thought of as the patient system: inpatients, same-day surgery patients, and clinic patients. But the concept of customer can be seen more broadly to include community initiatives, educational programming, health contracts with business and industry, health maintenance organizations (HMOs), and provider practice groups. Large corporate entities, intraorganizational agreements, health insurers, and second- and third-party payers are major service and economic influences on the patient system. Federal legislation, state laws, local ordinances, regulatory bodies, court precedents, insurers, and professional organizations all have a legal effect on the hospital.

On a broader, macrosystem level, consider changes predicted for the population. The increase in the elderly population, especially frail elders and those with chronic diseases, has a great impact on services that will be needed. The national, state, and local economies, with their associated concerns about costs, are other societal factors that have a profound effect on hospitals and healthcare organizations. All of these factors, individually and combined, influence how the hospital markets and cares for its customers and personnel and meets their organizational mandates and mission. And then, consider the changes in those insured and reimbursement dictates.

But let us return to the change process and activities in the phases of unfreezing, moving, and refreezing. During *unfreezing*, the major change activities include assessment, diagnosis, and establishment of a professional relationship. Assessment must involve in-depth analysis and synthesis of both internal and external forces. As with individuals, families, and groups, methods for data collection include interviews and observation. But with a larger group of people, methods can include questionnaires or surveys for timely and, at times, confidential collection of data.

Like the past and personal change history obtained on a smaller scale with the person, family, or group, an organizational history provides valuable insights. The organizational history can reveal information on development and problem resolution to this point. Methods for gathering an organizational history require not only skillful interviewing of key people but also a careful review of records and documents of the organization.

Consider all environments, including the constraints, demands, and opportunities present. Resources in the environment—people and physical resources—provide major influences on any organizational change. Identifying the driving forces and individuals in the system is essential to building a base of support. Analyze external environments, especially population trends.

Diagnosis of problems becomes more complex as the volume of information and number of people increase. Whether the change agent is selected from within the organization or is an external consultant, he or she will need a high level of skill to achieve organizational change. Clear understanding of both internal and external forces will be necessary, along with a good deal of fortitude to survive the experience. And keep in mind the sense of loss members of the organization may experience in this initial stage of transition.

The *moving* phase in organizational change involves developing strategies to match resources with constraints, demands, opportunities, and history as part of the planning process for change to proceed. Changes in goals and values must be reflected in organizational documents. Key work groups will be needed for decision making and policy formation. People in the organization will need some retraining and educational programs to transmit knowledge of resources and to refine skills. A great deal of time and energy will be needed for the people. Role and status relations will require finesse and great sensitivity. Relating to the variable and altering readiness, resistance, and motivation of many individuals and groups will be quite a challenge.

People must be actively incorporated and empowered in this decision-making and implementation phase. Remember that this may be an opportunity for innovation in moving to a new organizational design or initiative. Involvement of people in the organizational change process necessitates use of excellent leadership and skills in group dynamics, conflict management, and team building. This is especially true when the methods for accomplishment of work activities have undergone major revisions. Communication links with management must be increased and reinforced as organizational members are included rather than alienated from key planners and controllers in the system. Minimizing people's stress and turmoil is a major function of the change agent in this phase.

A formalized evaluation plan must be in place and must be initiated in this moving phase. Data collection and feedback on the process, communicating even small results, are vital and must be ongoing. People in the system need to be continually aware of the result of their efforts. If indicated in the evaluation data, additional resources or linkages must be sought. This is the feedback loop that continues through the phase of refreezing and is essential to any successful organizational change. Evaluation data must be systematically recorded, analyzed, interpreted, and communicated. Evaluation data can be communicated through distribution of short reports, articles, or observations from various sources in newsletters and on bulletin boards, electronically, and in formal and informal discussion groups. Keeping people on track and moving toward new organizational goals and norms requires stamina and a positive outlook despite the inevitable pitfalls and sidetracking that will occur.

> Involvement of people in the organizational change process necessitates use of excellent leadership and skills in group dynamics, conflict management, and team building.

Refreezing the change may take longer than anticipated in the multilevel organizational system. The turmoil and differences that have arisen in the organization environment and the strength of external forces will influence the firm establishment of the change as the new organizational norm. Support and reinforcement are indispensable activities of the change agent, along with ongoing analysis, interpretation, and communication of the evaluation findings. The role of the change agent will naturally become more consultative as termination approaches. At this point, the change should be a part of the expectations of the organization and its members. Ownership of the change is held by the people in the institutional or agency environment and not by key people or the change agent.

Consider the following example of organizational change, extending services from the traditional hospital into the community. Needs assessment, diagnosis of problems, and motivation in agency subsystems must occur in the unfreezing phase for organizational change. In addition to the traditional hospital, this change may involve outpatient departments and clinics, homecare agencies, rehabilitation or nursing home settings, care provider groups, and therapy group practices.

Internal restraining and driving forces are also important. Organizational goals and values for healthcare in the mission statement must change with the move from hospital to home, outpatient, or community care. The physical resources, knowledge, and skills of the healthcare providers must now be broadened, such as intravenous and other therapies requiring periodic skilled in-home nursing care. Extended interpersonal and interdisciplinary relations are needed with a move into the community, along with coordination of services, role relationships, attitudes, and values of people. Nursing roles of healthcare provider, manager, teacher, researcher, and advocate are expanded to include service facilitator and coordinator. The organizational structure is enlarged, with agencies providing both inpatient and community services, and it becomes more flexible and interactive with other environments providing healthcare services. Management is similarly broadened to include overseeing corporations, resulting in buying power, larger constituencies, and overriding governing boards. This translates into more complex goals and policies and comprehensive strategic initiatives provided by the governing board in an effort to reach out into the community.

The design for the provision of care has changed from the image of the traditional 120-bed community hospital. The external forces that drove the need for change include healthcare needs of the patient population, reimbursement policies, provider restrictions, and societal trends. Earlier hospital discharge and high-technology home care have driven service providers from the traditional hospital setting into the community. A good deal of this move into the community environment has been secondary to the reimbursement and insurance restrictions.

Organizational Change Suggestions

Organizations will continue to change and evolve in response to internal and external forces and the needs of patients. This may require more innovative approaches. Recall that innovation is moving to a new, more novel or advanced approach than the one used in the past. Innovation has become a hot topic in top business practices and healthcare organizations as they attempt address consumer needs and capture new markets. In business, Kelley (2001) describes a five-step process (Box 11.3) that has led to new product designs. These steps can be used in the change process when a new, innovative approach is needed.

Understanding the market, client, technology, and constraints is part of the assessment process in the unfreezing step. However, this assessment also involves observing real people and real life. It is stepping back and looking at the situation, putting away preconceived ideas. Look at what is really occurring in the environment. This will allow you to visualize new concepts and individual needs. Evaluating and refining prototypes occurs in the stage of moving when you also implement the new concept. Testing and evaluation occurs throughout this process and leads to refreezing if the innovation is effective, as in Rogers' model of innovation. Consider how you could use this process on a surgical unit.

Look at changes in the patient group. Perhaps you are seeing more patients with limited literacy skills or those of a different cultural group. We know that teaching for care at home must occur before those discharge orders are written. Understanding patients as consumers includes literacy, cultural preferences, and the available technology. You know that time for teaching is a constraint. However, teaching can take more time if the best materials are not available or the methods are ineffective. What are the patients' needs in their real life, at home and in their community? A preconceived idea may be

---

BOX 11.3 **Basic Steps for the Process of Innovation**

- Understand: the market, client, technology, and constraints.
- Observe: real people and real life
- Visualize new concepts and customers
- Evaluate and refine prototypes
- Implement the new concept

Source: Kelley, T. (2001). *The art of innovation.* New York: Doubleday

that the instruction sheet that has been translated into another language is the answer. But perhaps it may be ignored, along with the other forms received before discharge. Look at what is really occurring in the environment and the patient's interactions with family and friends. This will allow you to visualize new concepts and patient needs. Perhaps the patient could benefit from a calendar to help in checking off when medications or dressing changes are due. Perhaps the instruction sheet that had been translated is too "dense" and needs illustrations to promote better understanding. Evaluating and refining your teaching materials as prototypes will help address these new patient groups and assist with the implement of new and more effective materials for discharge.

Nurses have a growing responsibility for more creativity and involvement in change. The American Organization of Nurse Executives (AONE, 2010) has identified the need for nurses to embrace change, stating that "dramatic change and revolutionary thinking are imperative" and indeed are the basis for their guiding principles (p. 1). Nurses function as members of change teams, as change agents, and as developers of organizational systems. This will continue and expand in interdisciplinary practice as their skills in change are recognized and sought. Remember the following steps regardless of the extent of the organizational change:

- *Always do your homework.* Be prepared with information about and knowledge of the organization. Spend the time and acquire the information and background needed before acting or reacting. Then proceed from a solid theoretical base. Understand the change process and all the steps. Review your talents for change strategies.
- *Know your restraining and driving forces.* Take the time to understand or, at minimum, recognize these behaviors. Share information. Make both sides aware of the situation. Take more time to understand behavioral reactions. Cultivate the driving forces and become viewed as the champion for the cause. Use all your skills in interpersonal relationships, and develop more.
- *Be sensitive to environments.* Increase your awareness of what is occurring in society and healthcare. Look beyond your immediate environment. Analyze the internal and external forces and imagine how your environment could be affected by these forces. Use intuition and insight as well as foresight. Be both inspired and inspiring.
- *Maintain a positive attitude and refuse to be diminished by negativity.* Negative colleagues and superiors will always be present. They are an environmental hazard. Someone will always be available to tell you that something never has been or never can be done. If your "homework" background knowledge told you differently, become the agent of change instead of another restraining force. Have courage.
- *Be open and receptive to new ideas.* No matter how you long to keep things as they currently are, be mindful that there may be a better way of doing things. Refuse to be limited by the present, and look to the future and evidence-based practice—a core competency.

Remember, conventional wisdom can be a barrier to needed change.
- *Be open to new people.* Venture out of your discipline. View the situation as larger than nursing care. Collaborate with other health professionals. Discuss. Debate. Interact. Try to recognize when turf issues arise, and negotiate on the basis of facts and what will be best for the patients and the organization while maintaining the integrity of your profession.
- *Involve others.* Try not to do it all yourself. Remember that the most successful and enduring changes occur when others are involved. The change has to become the norm and the expectation of the people in the environment.
- *Refine skills.* Cultivate your change agent skills. Recall the skills and roles of the change agent. Continually develop and refine these skills. Make adaptations necessary for the people and the environments. Look at yourself as objectively as you look at others. If assistance or collaboration is needed, get it.
- *Reassess and evaluate.* Remember to evaluate activity and progress continually. Sufficient time for the change to occur and persistence are necessary components of organizational change. Recall Rogers' (1983) attributes in the diffusion of innovations, which determine the rate of adoption by members of a social system: relative advantage, compatibility, complexity, trialability, and observability. Include these attributes in your evaluation process.
- *Persevere, persevere, persevere.* Have fortitude. Use resources to cope with your stress and frustration levels. Organizational change is not easy. Look for small gains as major steps in the process. Strive for the finish line, but do not look for accolades. Terminate the relationship as the organizational norm takes hold and the organization congratulates *itself* on the accomplishment. Celebrate successes.

The philosophical basis of nursing focuses on the health of human beings as individuals, families, groups, and society in a complex environment. And practice must be based on the latest evidence of efficacy and acceptability. In this role, nurses can be highly effective change agents. How comfortable are you with change? Think about your **change quotient** as your ability to address needed change and to help others as a change agent.

In addition to his work in psychology on multiple intelligences, Gardner (2008) has identified five capacities that individuals need to address the future (Box 11-4). As was illustrated in Chapter 3, the discipline of nursing has a unique body of knowledge. Although we draw on other knowledge disciplines, we have a unique and valued discipline, as has been illustrated in the IOM report on the Future of Nursing. Gardner (2008) identifies the components of synthesis as goals, ideas, approaches, and feedback. The use of evidence-based practice embodies this process. As Gardner (2008) points out, "synthesizing the current state of knowledge, incorporating new findings, and delineating new dilemmas is part and parcel of the work of any professional who wished to remain

BOX 11.4	The Five Minds for the Future

- 1: The Disciplined Mind
- 2: The Synthesizing Mind
- 3: The Creating Mind
- 4: The Respectful Mind
- 5: The Ethical Mind

Source: Gardner, H. (2008). *5 Minds for the future.* Boston: Harvard Business Press.

current with her craft" (p. 6). Creativity is a component of leading change. As noted by Gardner (2008), "rewards accrue to those who fashion small but significant changes in professional practice" (p. 7). Respect and ethics are core components of professional nursing practice. Whether interacting with patients and groups or professional colleagues, respect needs to be present and shared. And as illustrated in Chapter 1, nursing has a distinct ethical code, and some issues that affect daily practice will be discussed in the next chapter.

EVIDENCE-BASED PRACTICE: *CONSIDER THIS....*

You are reading an EBP article on sleep deprivation that addresses individual differences for patients, environmental considerations, and the influences from nursing interventions. One of the recommendations was that "critical care nurses can optimize the sleep environment by restructuring work-flow habits" (p. 33). You start thinking about the acute care unit where you work and the routines during the evening and night. You know staffing is an issue but are concerned about the assessment and documentation of the patients' sleep quality and sleep patterns.

Question: How will you use this information as a change agent to implement a program on your unit for assessment of patients' sleep patterns and restructuring work-flow patterns?

Source: Makic, M. B. F., Rauen, C., Watson, R., & Poteet, A. W. (2014). Examining the evidence to guide practice: Challenging practice habits. *Critical Care Nurse, 34*(2), 28–44.

KEY POINTS

- The classic change model was developed by Lewin (1951), based on his Field Theory. This model contained three phases in the change process: unfreezing, moving, and refreezing.

- Building on Lewin's work, Lippitt (1973) considered human motivation, multiple causation, and habits. He defined seven specific phases in the change process: diagnosis of the problem, assessment of motivation and capacity for change, change agent's motivation and resources, selecting change objectives, choosing the change agent role, maintaining the change, and terminating the relationship. A focus on the change agent emerged with four specific roles and skills.

- Havelock's change model contains the major concepts of role, linkages, and communication. This adds steps to the three stages of change, with heightened communication and interpersonal activities. Havelock and Havelock's (1973) seven steps in the change process are perception of the need, diagnosis of the problem, identification of the problem, devising a plan of action, gaining acceptance, stabilizing the plan, and self-renewal. Four different roles for the change agent are proposed in Havelock's model.

- Rogers' (1983) Diffusion of Innovations model has a five-stage view of change: knowledge, persuasion, decision, implementation, and confirmation. Rogers also considers five factors that influence the rate of adoption of an innovation and that may be used as evaluation criteria in the change process. Seven roles for the change agent are highlighted in this model of change.

- The Transtheoretical Approach to change focuses on the individual as a "self-changer" and is depicted as a spiral with five stages of change: precontemplation, contemplation, preparation, action, and maintenance, with 10 associated change processes that occur in the different stages of change (Prochaska et al., 1992).

- Bridges (2009) looks at the psychological processes of change within the stages of (1) ending, losing, letting go, (2) the neutral zone, and (3) the new beginning.

KEY POINTS—cont'd

- The roles and attributes of a skilled change agent are included in the models by Lippitt, Havelock, and Rogers. General roles for the change agent are assessor or evaluator, communicator, translator, encourager, mediator, and consultant.

- In relation to the activities in the nursing process, the phases of change are consistent with assessment, diagnosis, planning, implementation, and evaluation for resolving the problem or stabilizing the change. They can also lead to the implementation of evidence-based practice in place of traditions from the past.

- The skills of change agents include having a vision for the future and creativity, good assessment skills, good interpersonal skills, flexibility, perseverance, and a positive attitude, integrity and commitment, the ability to manage conflict, and resistance.

- Strategies for reducing resistance to change include careful planning and timing, along with good communication and interpersonal skills.

- Empowerment or involvement of the patient is needed for lasting change. Strategies for patient involvement include education, training, socialization and persuasion, and facilitation.

- Environmental or situational factors relative to individuals, families, and groups provide additional information in the change process. Past experience, stress and coping factors, motivational clues, and resources are important data sought by the change agent.

- To view organizational change, look at internal and external forces with a multisystem approach. And consider the concept of transitions.

- Suggestions for people involved in organizational change include (1) being knowledgeable about the organization, its restraining and driving forces, and the environments, (2) maintaining a positive attitude and being receptive to new ideas and people, (3) involving other people in the change, (4) continuing to refine skills and reevaluating the situation, and (5) persevering throughout the process.

Thought and Discussion Questions

1. Recall a change that has taken place in your family. Using Lewin's theory, identify the restraining and driving forces.

2. Identify some specific sources of internal change in your organization and name the driving forces.

3. Recall a change that has taken place in your organization. Using Lippitt's theory, identify the seven stages of planned change and the roles of the change agent(s) in the process.

4. List at least six specific environmental factors that could influence change in a healthcare organization. Be prepared to discuss these factors in class or online, as scheduled by your instructor.

5. Use Lewin and the Transtheoretical Approach to explain the steps of the process for permanent change to help a new 18-year-old single mother with a normal 7 lb, 9 oz full-term infant (appropriate for gestational age [AGA], Apgar score of 9) develop parenting skills and healthcare, including prevention and health maintenance.

6. Read *Who Moved My Cheese?* by S. Johnson (2002) and determine which character you most resemble and which one you most want to be like. Be prepared to participate in a discussion on your selection of characters, either online or in class as scheduled by your instructor.

7. Review the Chapter Thought located on the first page of the chapter, and discuss it in the context of the chapter.

Interactive Exercises

Go to the Intranet site and complete the interactive exercises provided for this chapter.

REFERENCES

American Organization of Nurse Executives (AONE). (2010). *AONE Guiding Principles for the role of the nurse in future patient care delivery toolkit*. Retrieved from http://www.aone.org/resources/PDFs/AONE_GP_for_Role_of_Nurse_Future.pdf

Anderson, B., Klein, E., & Stuart, J. (2000). Why change is a consciousness choice. *The Journal for Quality and Participation, 23*, 32–36.

Bridges, W. (2000). *The character of organizations: Using personality type in organization development*. Mountain View, CA: Davies-Black.

Bridges, W. (2009). *Managing transitions: Making the most of change* (3rd ed.). Cambridge, MA: DaCapo Press.

Chinn, R., & Benne, K. D. (1976). General strategies for effecting change in human systems. In W. G. Bennis, K. D. Benne, R. Chinn, & K. E. Corey (Eds.), *The planning of change* (3rd ed., pp. 22–45). New York: Holt, Rinehart & Winston.

Gardner, H. (2008). *5 Minds for the future*. Boston, MA: Harvard Business Press.

Hall, R. H., & Tolbert, P. S. (2005). *Organizations: Structures, processes, and outcomes* (9th ed.). Upper Saddle River, NJ: Pearson Prentice-Hall.

Harvard Business Essentials (2003). *Managing change and transition*. Boston, MA: Harvard Business School Press.

Havelock, R. G. (1971). *Planning for innovation through dissemination and utilization of knowledge*. Ann Arbor, MI: Institute for Social Research, University of Michigan.

Havelock, R. G., & Havelock, M. C. (1973). *Training for change agents: A guide to the design of training programs in education and other fields*. Ann Arbor, MI: Institute for Social Research, University of Michigan.

Institute of Medicine (IOM). (2011). *The future of nursing: Leading change, advancing health*. Washington, DC: National Academies Press. Retrieved from http://www.thefutureofnursing.org/sites/default/files/Future%20of%20Nursing%20Report_0.pdf

Johnson, S. (2002). *Who moved my cheese?* New York: G. P. Putnam's Sons.

Kelley, T. (2001). *The art of innovation*. New York: Doubleday.

Lewin, K. (1951). *Field theory in social science*. New York: Harper & Row.

Lippitt, G. L. (1973). *Visualizing change: Model building and the change process*. La Jolla, CA: University Associates.

Makic, M. B. F., Rauen, C., Watson, R., & Poteet, A. W. (2014). Examining the evidence to guide practice: Challenging practice habits. *Critical Care Nurse, 34*, 28–44.

Prochaska, J. O., & DiClemente, C. C. (1984). *The transtheoretical approach: Crossing traditional boundaries of therapy*. Homewood, IL: Dow Jones–Irwin.

Prochaska, J. O., DiClemente, C. C., & Norcross, J. C. (1992). In search of how people change: Applications to addictive behaviors. *American Psychologist, 47*, 1102–1114.

Rogers, E. M. (1983). *Diffusion of innovations* (3rd ed.). New York: Free Press.

Rogers, E. M., & Shoemaker, F. F. (1971). *Communication of innovations: A cross-cultural approach* (2nd ed.). New York: Free Press.

Rose, J. (2009). Quiz on resistance to change. Retrieved from http://www.suite101.com/content/quiz-on-resistance-to-change-a110891

Stevens, K. R. (2009). *Essential competencies for evidence-based practice in nursing* (2nd ed.). San Antonio, TX: Academic Center for Evidence-Based Practice.

BIBLIOGRAPHY

Bennis, W. (2000). *Managing the dream: Reflections on leadership and change*. Cambridge, MA: Basic Books.

Bandura, A. (1977). Self-efficacy: Toward a unifying theory of behavioral change. *Psychological Review, 84*(2), 191–215.

Flower, J. (1996). *The four quadrants of change*. Retrieved from http://well.com/user/bbear/quadrant.html

Levesque, D. A., Prochaska, J. O., Cummins, C. O., Terrill, S., & Miranda, D. (2001). Assessing Medicare beneficiaries' readiness to make informed health plan choices. *Healthcare Financing Review, 23*(1), 87–104.

Lippitt, G. L., & Nadler, L. (1967). Emerging roles of the training director. *Training and Development Journal, 9*, 2–10.

ONLINE RESOURCES

William Bridges & Associates Transition Training
http://www.wmbridges.com

● Rose Kearney-Nunnery

12

Professional Ethics

"When we do the best we can, we never know
what miracle is wrought in our life
or the life of another."

Helen Keller, 1880–1968

Chapter Objectives

On completion of this chapter, the reader will be able to:

1. Examine ethical principles in professional practice.
2. Apply the terminology used in ethical decision making.
3. Analyze ethical dilemmas in contemporary healthcare situations.
4. Apply the components of the ANA Code of Ethics for Nurses to a healthcare scenario.
5. Identify ethical decision making in the practice setting in patient and collegial situations.

Key Terms

Right	Full Disclosure	Code of Ethics
Basic Human Rights	Veracity	Standards of Care
Beneficence	Informed Consent	Advance Directives
Nonmaleficence	Privacy	Euthanasia
Justice	Confidentiality	Human Genome
Fidelity	Utilitarianism	Impaired or Incompetent Colleagues
Self-determination (autonomy)	Deontology	

As a professional nurse, you are confronted by ethical issues on a daily basis. But have you carefully considered all the implications? Are they ethical dilemmas? Dahnke and Dreher (2006) define an ethical dilemma as a problem with options that seem equally unfavorable (p. 4). Let's look at some of the principles and issues in daily practice. In patient situations, think about informed consent, advance directives, a persistent vegetative state, organ procurement and donation, and genomics. In addition, consider ethical dilemmas in interdisciplinary practice, with impaired or incompetent colleagues. However, before looking at specific situations, consider the basis of ethical decision making and professional ethics.

ETHICAL PRINCIPLES

We hear a good deal about human rights. First, consider the concept of rights. A **right** is an agreed-upon entitlement. It is a constant and does not change with the circumstances. Husted and Husted (2008) warn that it is a grave ethical mistake to regard the term *rights* as a political term that can be an ever-changing product of legislation, rather than a more fundamental ethical term. Aiken (2004) describes this blurring of ethical and political use of the term and differentiates among welfare rights, ethical rights, and option rights. Welfare rights are legal rights guaranteed by law, such as freedom of speech. However, legal rights can be changed or modified through legislation. Ethical rights are based on ethical principles like self-determination and autonomy of the individual. Option rights allow some freedom of choice within certain parameters, like choices with advanced directives and not active euthanasia. With this in mind and with our prior focus on the rights of subjects in research, consider more broadly the following ethical and **basic human rights**:

- Beneficence
- Justice and fidelity
- Self-determination and autonomy
- Full disclosure and veracity
- Informed consent
- Privacy and confidentiality

Beneficence is the principle of doing good with the person's best interests as the goal of all actions. This includes the concept of **nonmaleficence** in that we "do no harm" to the individual, family, or group. In healthcare, our role is to help, but the person may be at risk of harm with the treatment. We must be vigilant to protect the person from avoidable harm or error. We will consider this further in the following chapter on safety initiatives in healthcare environments and in the community, as with the use of bar coding to reduce medication errors. Associated with the concept of beneficence are justice and fidelity. **Justice** is fairness to all and avoidance of favoritism. All patients deserve fair access to quality healthcare. The concept of justice embodies health equity and fair distribution of resources. **Fidelity** is loyalty to the person. If we tell a patient we will be back to check on his or her pain relief in ten minutes, we need to be true to that time frame.

Full disclosure and self-determination are associated ethical principles. **Self-determination** or **autonomy** is the sense a person has the right to determine his or her fate. The development of a *living will* or *advanced directives* are examples of self-determination when the patient makes decisions in advance of a critical situation. However, to make life decisions, the person must have complete information, or **full disclosure**. The individual deserves all relevant information about his or her health status to make an informed decision. Full disclosure includes the principle of **veracity**, or providing truthful information. Informed consent incorporates these ethical principles. **Informed consent** occurs when the individual has complete information on all sides of the issue and makes a decision freely and without constraint after careful consideration of both advantages and disadvantages of the action. Think about the patient signing an informed consent form for a procedure. Does that individual understand what is being agreed to, or is he or she in pain and merely signing all forms in the hope that the pain will be relieved? And closely associated with this is the consideration of the significant others. Do they really understand what their loved one wants and is requesting? In addition, will they adhere to the wishes of the significant other in a time of emotional crisis? And think how healthcare professionals are responsible for fidelity to the patient and significant others, especially in stressful, critical, or conflicting situations.

Privacy and confidentiality are also closely associated concepts. **Privacy** means that the person has the right to determine and control the amount of information to reveal about himself or herself. The professional relationship allows the person to provide this private information with the knowledge that it will be respected and remain private. This is **confidentiality**—the information that the person does reveal is respected and not revealed to others except as necessary as part of this professional relationship. This situation can be a delicate one, as in the example of a family history of mental illness, or in any past situation from which the patient feels sensitivity or unease. And how secure is the information from being revealed to others? The patient must have trust in the healthcare professional to feel comfortable to reveal such sensitive information. Again, add the complexity of significant others who may be directly involved in private communications with healthcare providers or be remote and unaware of information shared. Both hard copy and electronic data storage of information are considerations. All of these ethical principles are guided by the way we look at the world. And with our expanding channels of information, including electronic information and health records, the ANA developed a position paper on privacy and confidentiality with nine principles that address patient advocacy and trust in the professional relationship and emphasize that "confidentiality protections should extend to not only health records, but also to all other individually identifiable health information, including genetic information, clinical research records, and mental health therapy notes" (ANA, 2006, p. 1). The International Council of Nurses (ICN, 2008) states that patients should be the primary owners of their health information, and this "includes information related to their health problems, the actions proposed or taken by caregivers, and the consequences of these actions" (p. 1).

As a healthcare provider, you have had required orientation to the Health Insurance Portability and Accountability Act (HIPAA) legislation from 1996. Think about what this legislation means to you: more forms for signature, codes for release of any patient information, even to family members, and additional regulation of healthcare? And what does it mean for the patient? Does she understand that you cannot tell her nephew about her condition, even when he keeps calling the unit? And the ethical question: Have HIPPA regulations provided patient confidentiality or additional burden? Is this a potential burden to the patient or to the healthcare professionals? And are protections in place or being worked around? Think about it.

SYSTEMS OF ETHICAL DECISIONS

Ethics has been defined as a "system of standards to motivate, determine, and justify actions directed to the pursuit of vital and fundamental goals" (Husted & Husted, 2008, p. 315). There are two systems of standards that can be differentiated based on consequence or outcome (utilitarianism) or the obligation for action or inaction (deontology). **Utilitarianism** is focused on the consequence or the outcome. It is based on two basic ideas: happiness and the greatest good for the greatest number. Decisions are made in this framework in terms of means that justify the way of getting there—for the greatest good in the end. Some ethicists further differentiate utilitarianism into rule and act utilitarianism. *Rule utilitarianism* draws on past experiences to formulate personal rules to determine what you consider to be the "the greatest good" for the intended outcome. *Act utilitarianism* is based on the unique situation in the present circumstances for the determination of what is considered "right" and best to reach the intended consequence. As noted by Aiken (2004), this system is oriented toward the good of the population in general, and rules and regulations are not necessarily followed to reach the intended outcome. Think about the times you may have been posed with the question of *who should be in the lifeboat?* Or *who should be saved?* Using the system of utilitarianism focuses on the consequences for the greatest number and the greatest chance of happiness and success, regardless of the means of getting there. With our focus on each individual's unique needs and characteristics, this system does pose limitations when making decisions. Do the "ends" really justify the "means"? Think about it! And who is the one to decide what is the "best" outcome in the situation? Should it be a collaborative decision with the patient as the captain deciding the decision? How will the patient be sure that he or she asks the correct questions and receives the appropriate information upon which to make a critical decision? And further, consider the differences that will be made on past experiences or a unique situation.

ONLINE CONSULT

Official HIPAA site at
http://www.hhs.gov/ocr/privacy/

The second system, **deontology**, is based on obligations as rules and unchanging principles. Based on the writings of the German philosopher Immanuel Kant (1724–1804), this system requires adherence to a set of established rules. The absolute rules are the means to reach the decision. These rules are absolute and unchanging, as is seen in some religious ethical decision-making systems. As with utilitarianism, deontology is divided into two subsets, rule versus act deontology. With *rule deontology*, the ethical standards or rules are made by people—past or present. These rules must be followed and do not change, regardless of the situation or individual factors. In *act deontology*, the highest value is placed on the moral values of the individual. You must make the same decision in any similar situation, regardless of the circumstances. As opposed to rule deontology, with act deontology, you are the one following the rules, based on data you obtain about the situation. But you make the decision and act in a consistent manner, following those rules. You must arrive at the same decision in similar circumstances. Consider this system of ethics and the issue of patient autonomy and self-determination. First, consider who will be making the decisions and which rules and principles are being considered.

CODE OF ETHICS

A professional abides by a certain **code of ethics** applicable to the practice area. Developed within the profession, the code addresses general ethical practice issues. The *Code of Ethics for Nurses* developed by the American Nurses Association (ANA) is the ethical standard for professional nursing practice. As the ANA states, the "The Code is non-negotiable in any setting. . . . [and expresses] the values, virtues, and obligations that shape, guide, and inform nursing as a profession" (ANA, 2015, p. vii). The interpretative statements promote understanding for appropriate application of the code of ethics in professional practice. The ethical principles of human rights, self-determination, privacy and confidentiality, autonomy, and responsibility and obligations are specifically addressed in the code of ethics. Adherence to this specific code may be regulated in your state's practice act. In addition, additional competencies for the nurse prepared at the graduate level are expectations based on preparation, knowledge level, and performance expectations. However, there are other ethical codes, including those of other countries, such as Canada (Canadian Nurses Association, 2008), and globally with the International Council of Nurses (ICN, 2012) *Code of Ethics for Nurses*. As we discussed in Chapter 1, the ANA is one of almost 140 nurses organizations from around the world that are members of ICN. The International *Code of Ethics for Nurses* presents four elements associated with nurses: people, practice, the profession, and coworkers (ICN, 2012). In addition, for each of the elements it illustrates the roles of practitioners and managers, educators and researchers, and national nursing associations. The *Code of Ethics for Registered Nurses* of the Canadian Nurses Association (2008) identifies seven values of ethical nursing practice. Achieving professional status requires ethical standards for expected behaviors with patients, colleagues, and other professionals. Further information on these ethical codes can be found at their Web sites.

Associated with a code of ethics is the concept of standard of care. Aiken (2004) defines **standards of care** as "the average degree of skill, care, and diligence exercised by members of the same profession under the same or similar circumstances" (pp. 38–39). Definition of practice and specific practice standards are further specified within the professional community through major nursing associations. The ANA has specified a variety of practice standards for the profession, both general and specific to certain practice areas. The ANA has prepared several specialty standards documents jointly with the particular specialty organization to reflect the expectations for specialized professional practice. These standards are described as "authoritative statements of the duties of all registered nurses, regardless of role, population, or specialty, are expected to perform competently" (ANA, 2010a, p. 2).

The publication *Nursing: Scope and Standards of Practice* (ANA, 2010a), for example, prescribes standards of practice and standards of professional performance. Standards of practice address safe practice and use of the nursing process with the actions of assessment, diagnosis, outcome identification, planning, implementation, and evaluation (ANA, 2010a). Standards of professional performance (Box 12.1) are expected professional roles and behaviors, including ethics, education, evidence-based practice and research, quality of practice, communication, leadership, collaboration, professional practice evaluation, resource utilization, and environmental health (ANA, 2010a, p. 3). Under the area of ethics, the registered nurse is required to adhere to the *Code of Ethics for Nurses with Interpretative Statements* "to guide practice" (ANA, 2010a, p. 47).

Further, standards of specialty practice are provided through the certification process with specialized education, testing, and ongoing learning requirements. Practice standards and expectations have also been developed by the applicable specialty organization. Adherence to standards of practice is designed to promote safe and effective care, but nurses still face ethical dilemmas on a daily basis.

ONLINE CONSULT

ANA (2015) Code of Ethics for Nurses at http://nursingworld.org/MainMenuCategories/EthicsStandards/CodeofEthicsforNurses

ANA Position Statements at http://nursingworld.org/positionstatements.aspx

ICN Code of Ethics for Nurses at http://www.icn.ch/images/stories/documents/about/icncode_english.pdf

Canadian Nurses Association Code of Ethics for Registered Nurses at http://www.cna-aiic.ca/en/on-the-issues/best-nursing/nursing-ethics

Canadian Nurses Association Position Statements at http://www.cna-aiic.ca/en/advocacy/policy-support-tools/cna-position-statements

MAKING ETHICAL DECISIONS

Making ethical decisions is not an easy task. The choice may be between two equally unpleasant options. In the search for assisting with ethical dilemmas, several models for ethical decision making have been proposed and evaluated over the past years. For example, Husted and Husted (2008) have proposed analysis through extremes to clarify relationships and discover the right thing to do when what is wrong is easier to determine (p. 125). Aiken (2004) proposed a five-step model: data collection and interpretation, stating the dilemma, considering choices of action, analyzing the advantages and disadvantages of the options, and making the decision (pp. 104–106). A classic model by Curtain (1978) provides the following steps for the ethical decision-making process:

1. Obtaining background information
2. Identifying the ethical components
3. Identifying the ethical agents or people involved
4. Identifying the options available

BOX 12.1   Standards of Professional Performance: Ethical Competencies (ANA, 2010a)

The ANA (2010a) has identified the following competencies for ethical practice by the registered nurse:
- Uses the *Code of Ethics for Nurses with Interpretative Statements* (ANA, 2001) to guide practice.
- Delivers care in a manner that preserves and protects healthcare consumer autonomy, dignity, rights, values, and beliefs.
- Recognizes the centrality of the healthcare consumer and family as core members of any healthcare team.
- Upholds healthcare consumer confidentiality within legal and regulatory parameters.
- Assists healthcare consumers in self determination and informed decision making.
- Maintains a therapeutic and professional healthcare consumer-nurse relationship within appropriate professional role boundaries.
- Contributes to resolving ethical issues involving healthcare consumers, colleagues, community groups, systems, and other stakeholders.
- Takes appropriate action regarding instances of illegal, unethical, or inappropriate behavior that can endanger or jeopardize the best interests of the healthcare consumer or situation.
- Speaks up when appropriate to question healthcare practice when necessary for safety and quality improvement.
- Advocates for equitable healthcare consumer care.

Source: American Nurses Association. (2010a). *Nursing: Scope and standards of practice* (2nd ed.). Silver Spring, MD: Nursesbooks.org.

5. Applying ethical principles to the issues, like self-determination

6. Making a final resolution or decision to the ethical dilemma

Think about an ethical dilemma that you have encountered in the past. Return to the basic information and ignore the resolution that was reached. Follow Curtain's (1978) six steps and evaluate the resolution that did occur in that situation.

Despite our code of ethics, that provides direction, or the ethical principles we use, ethical dilemmas arise on a daily basis in healthcare situations. These decisions are not easy, and are made even more complex since they are not made in isolation. Other professionals, and most notably the patient, must be part of the decision to address our ethical principles. And often, these decisions remain a part of us as we recall events and considerations. Interestingly, Husted and Husted (2008) have proposed several characteristics of an *unflawed* ethical decision as follows:

• The decision is going to be acted upon
• Will guide actions to a justifiable end
• Affects one's life and character over time
• Provides the belief that the actions will make life better
• Allows changing one's direction during action (p. 16)

Consider the following issues in nursing practice and the ethical dilemmas involved.

Informed Consent. One of the most common ethical situations concerns self-determination with true informed consent. We are not speaking of simply getting the patient to sign a form. This is not a role for the nurse. The issue of informed consent contains many of the ethical principles we have reviewed: beneficence (doing good with the person's best interests as the goal), justice (avoidance of favoritism), fidelity (loyalty to the person, rather than to what we may see as the reasonable treatment), full disclosure (with complete information on the risks, benefits and options), self-determination (to decide for oneself and not for the sake of others), and without constraint after careful consideration of the situation, knowing that one's privacy is being protected in the confidentiality of the patient-professional relationship. This is what we would want for ourselves. So now, look back at the steps in the decision-making model.

Can you identify the six steps of Curtain's model? First, consider whether all background information has been obtained, including culturally appropriate information. Recall that some medical or surgical procedures are acceptable to certain people or cultures and not to others. So, has appropriate background information been obtained, assumed, discussed, or ignored with a focus on our healthcare model? Have all the ethical components of the procedure and the situation been explained appropriately and been given careful consideration by the patient? And have all the ethical agents or people involved been identified, including relevant extended family members? What are the options available to the patient, and have these been explained and are they fully understood? Now is the time to apply the ethical principles to the issues, like self-determination. What do you think? As for your final resolution to the informed consent—was it true to the ethical principle? You see now why this is not as simple as completing a consent for treatment form!

Advance directives. Most healthcare providers are familiar with **advance directives**, in which individuals provide specific written instructions for their wishes relative to their future health, illness, and care at a time when they are able to specify their wishes, in the event that they are unable to communicate these wishes at that time. The ethical principles of autonomy and self-determination are the basis for advance directives, which can take the form of a living will or healthcare proxy and durable power of attorney.

Advance directives have their basis in both law and ethics. Originally enacted in law and revised in the 1980s, the *Uniform Rights of the Terminally Ill Act* provides for the development of a living will specifying personal requests on care and life support in the case of a terminal illness or injury. A healthcare proxy may also be developed to appoint a person to make decisions on care in the event that the person cannot make them. Making decisions in advance of a critical situation allows the person self-determination of their fate. Yet, when not faced with a terminal diagnosis, additional emotions and considerations may be ignored. In addition to self-determination, there are other ethical principles that must also be honored. When developing advance directives, the individual must understand his or her options and have full disclosure and understanding of the terminology, especially when standard forms are used. The individual must understand the options for the different life support equipment and hydration and nutrition. As reported by the ANA (2012), difficulties and confusion about DNR orders still exist despite efforts to assist consumers in making informed decisions (p. 1). This is also the time to address the choice for organ donation. The documents must be witnessed and notarized, and state requirements should be considered, especially if the individual travels or lives in multiple states. The person can change his or her mind, but a revised document must be developed.

The individual must also have full trust in the person identified as the proxy. This is not a time for favoritism, but one of trust that one's wishes will be honored with judgment and fidelity. Consider the person who has been designated as the "proxy." Is that person agreeable to serve in that role? Does he or she feel compelled to serve, or instead comfortable serving and adhering to the patient's wishes? Does he or she have the resources to advocate for the patient when family members with divergent options arrive on the scene? When a patient is transported to the emergency department, does the individual serving as the proxy have access to the legal documents that will need to be part of the patient's record? Privacy and confidentiality are also important concepts in that one's advance directives are just that—private, not public information, even if the family members do not consider themselves as "the public." It is the individual's self-determination to make the advance decisions and have the documents available to the healthcare proxy, healthcare providers, legal counsel, and family. Ultimately, it is the individual's decision and autonomy.

However, recall the concept of option rights: The range of decisions for the individual to make in advance directives vary by state and nation. In the United States, for example, there are differences among states like Oregon that enacted legislation on physician-assisted suicide. As noted by Bosek and Jannette (2013), three other states (Washington, Montana, and Vermont) have now legislated a form of "patient-directed dying" (p. 136). Proposed legislation in Maine "died in committee" in 2013, and Arizona provided language to assist in palliative care and a proposal for access to non-FDA-approved drugs. Many states have specific forms and language that must be included to be considered a legal and enforceable document. Active **euthanasia** or "mercy killing" is not a component of advanced directives in this country. However, in the Netherlands, Belgium, and Luxembourg, voluntary active euthanasia is legal under strict conditions for valid adult consent (Campbell, 2013, p. 107). The *Code of Ethics for Nurses* (ANA, 2015) dictates that nurses should be knowledgeable about advance directives and "should provide interventions to relieve pain and other symptoms in the dying patient consistent with palliative care practice standards and may not act with the sole intent to end life" (p. 3).

Some people feel that advance directives lessen the burden on the family in the case of a crisis. The focus here is on the individual's autonomy and wishes. However, families are made up of individuals who may be facing the dilemmas of beneficence in adhering to the person's best interests, justice in ensuring that all appropriate care is provided, and fidelity in being loyal to the person's wishes. Although the family does not have to "second guess" the individual's wishes, since these decisions have been specified in the advance directives, at an end-of-life event, many conflicting emotions may surface, and healthcare professionals must be supportive to both the individual and the family while upholding legally enforceable directives. Check out some of the online information available to patients, but ensure that patients are accessing reputable and appropriate information.

Additional dilemmas involved with advanced directives include the following:

- The patient and the family are not in agreement.
- The patient/family is not in agreement with the healthcare provider(s).
- There is disagreement about the issues of
  - "Do not resuscitate" orders
  - Hydration versus nutrition
  - Ventilation
  - Dialysis
  - Pain management
  - Religious and cultural differences
  - End-of-life final requests and planning
  - Organ and tissue donation
  - The meaning of palliative care and what it will be like for the patient, the proxy, and the significant others

What others can you identify?

As noted by the ICN (2012b), "the roles of nurses and other healthcare professionals in caring for dying patients continues to be debated, and nurses must be knowledgeable about the current issues and legislation about end stage of life issues" (p. 2). The concepts of hospice care and palliative care continue to evolve and be differentiated. As reported by the ANA (2013), "both the definition and the terminology associated with palliative sedation have been widely debated" (p. 5), and nurses are urged to take a leadership role in patient advocacy and interprofessional collaboration while adhering to the *Code of Ethics*.

The Persistent Vegetative State. Another dilemma that has had major legal and ethical challenges over the past years is the identification of the persistent vegetative state.

ONLINE CONSULT

AARP at
http://www.aarp.org/home-family/caregiving/legal-and-money-matters/

FamilyDoctor.org: Advance Directives and Do Not Resuscitate Orders at
http://familydoctor.org/familydoctor/en/healthcare-management/end-of-life-issues/advance-directives-and-do-not-resuscitate-orders.html

MedlinePlus: Advance Directives at
http://www.nlm.nih.gov/medlineplus/advancedirectives.html

National Alliance on Mental Illness: Advance Directives at
http://www.nami.org/Content/ContentGroups/Policy/Issues_Spotlights/Psychiatric_Advance_Directives_An_Overview.htm

National Cancer Institute: Advance Directives at
http://www.cancer.gov/about-cancer/managing-care/advance-directives

Medline Plus: Organ Transplantation at
http://www.nlm.nih.gov/medlineplus/organtransplantation.html

The pronouncement of "brain death" is well established and has objective data that must be met. However, the persistent vegetative state has been debated in the courts with specified criteria now proposed. But there is still much discussion, debate, and media coverage. Perry et al. (2005) have illustrated the issues and dilemmas involved in the case of Terri Schiavo, a young woman who was in a constant vegetative state and who persisted in this state beyond the limits of a normal period of recovery. As the authors reported, "no patient, even those with traumatic brain injury, has been reported to recover after a full year of being in a persistent vegetative state" (p. 744). As a result of all the legal contests and ethical debates, Schiavo persisted in this vegetative state for 15 years. However, as a result of her condition and the plight of her family, with debates in the legal and medical communities, specific criteria to understand the persistent vegetative state criteria were developed to address both traumatic and nontraumatic brain injuries. So, think about the dilemmas within the family and in the medical community:

- Would or could she recover?
- The criteria for brain death were not met.
- What would this young woman want since there were not advance directives in place?
- What does the family know, want, perceive, and interpret?
- What different perceptions and feelings exist in the family structure?
- What are the benefits and risks of each treatment to the patient, the family, and society?
- What if you were reliant on a feeding tube for existence?
- What about the use of healthcare resources and the chances of meaningful life?

What others can you identify?

ONLINE CONSULT

U.S. News on msnbc.com: "Schiavo autopsy shows irreversible brain damage" at http://www.msnbc.msn.com/id/8225637/

Terri Schiavo Life & Hope Network at http://www.terrisfight.org/

ONLINE CONSULT

U.S. Government Information on Organ and Tissue Donation and Transplantation at http://www.organdonor.gov/

Organ Procurement and Transplantation Network at http://optn.transplant.hrsa.gov/

Organ Procurement and Donation. Although organ transplants have become a common procedure, there are ethical concerns on both sides of the donation situation. Consider the dilemma of "harvesting," access, self-determination, and cultural beliefs, among others. In the case of procurement or harvesting organs, care must be given to the dignity and wishes of the donor. Family issues are also of concern, with grief on the donor's side and hopeful expectation for the other family. Consider the physiological and emotional issues of the patient in failing health who is awaiting an organ donation, and the care concerns and emotions impacting the significant others. Access continues to be an issue, with cost and accessibility to healthcare. In addition, coming from a utilitarian stance is consideration of the greatest good for the greatest number and issues of care and success as the consequence. In the case of deontology, consistent rules are applied for access, regardless of individual considerations. Self-determination applies, as the wishes of both the donor and the recipient. Cultural beliefs are also a consideration. As noted by Spector (2013), organ donation is permitted in many religious groups but not in the case of Jehovah's Witness followers.

Returning to Curtain's steps in the decision-making process, obtaining background information is vital in the assessment process for both the donor and the recipient as the ethical components, ethical agents, and the available options are identified, and the ethical principles are applied in the final decision. Understandably, individuals on a waiting list are in a constant state of unease and rapidly failing health and functioning. In addition to the disease process limiting the person's functioning, the individual and significant others are facing potential mortality if a suitable organ is not available, along with the emotional impact of being a number on a waiting list and thus constantly on alert in case an appropriate donor emerges. The individual may not retain the same placement on the waiting list if his or her condition changes or if another individual emerges with higher priority for a transplant. In addition to the numbers of individuals on waiting lists, there are other complex issues to confront with the type of donation (blood, tissue, organs, and stem cells) and the individuals involved (youth, aged, minorities, religious and cultural groups). Consider the online information available to the donors and individuals in need and their families. Overall, respect for individuals is an issue. How will you reply when renewing your driver's license if you are asked whether you want your donor status indicated on your license? And, what about the response of a family member to this same question?

Genomics. The Human Genome Project has been a significant scientific achievement that provided new information on gene structure, function, and dysfunction. The DNA sequencing of the human body has been a breakthrough in modern science, providing valuable information on the **human genome** or the complete set of the human DNA. We now know what gene is affected in specific genetic diseases such as sickle cell disease and cystic fibrosis. Current research is ongoing on the genetic mutations that occur with various cancers. Use of individual DNA in the criminal system frequently makes news and is the topic of television entertainment series. But what about the individual's right to privacy? Also consider individual responsibility, as more information is known on certain conditions that can be affected by either heredity or environment. And think about tailoring drug doses for individual DNA profiles. This balance of privacy and responsibility presents numerous ethical dilemmas.

Consider the rights of parents and children. Recall that a right is an agreed-upon entitlement. Genetic mapping "can offer firm evidence that a disease transmitted from parent to child is linked to one or more genes . . . and can be used to find the single gene responsible for relatively rare inherited disorders . . . or more common disorders, such as asthma" (National Human Genome Research Institute, 2012, p. 1). So consider knowledge of transmission versus ignorance of a pre-existing genetic trait—from both the parents' and child's perspective.

We continue to gain much needed scientific information from research on human DNA, but the ethical considerations cannot be ignored in the quest for knowledge or medical breakthroughs. And the ethical issues become as complex as the individual human genome. For example, as Huddleston (2013) describes, genetic-informed consent is more than a signed document and the permission to perform genetic testing because, as some have argued, it is not possible to provide informed consent for genetic research when knowledge is advancing so rapidly that we do not know what tests will be possible or what variants may be identified next week (p. 2). Over a decade ago, Pang (2002) noted that advances in genomics are likely to alleviate infectious diseases and chronic disorders but that "attention must be paid to complex ethical, legal, social and economic issues, as well as to public education and encouragement" (p. 1077). And this is still true as the technology evolves. And what about cloning beyond sheep? At the national level, the Ethical, Legal, and Social Implications (ELSI) Research Program has been established to address the ethical challenges with genomic research. Some of the current research priorities include recruitment issues, such as diversity, perceptions of risks and benefits, informed consent, privacy and identifiability of genomic information, data sharing and data security, governance structures, compensation and distribution of benefits, and the role of community and consultation engagement (National Human Genome Research Institute, 2014). These issues are just a peek at the future dilemmas that the scientific and the healthcare communities will confront. As originally stated by Collins et al. (2003), "society must formulate policies to address many of the questions raised by genomics" (p. 845).

One of these questions addressed consumers' fears with genetic testing and involvement in research with the use of genetic information and discrimination in health coverage and employment. The Genetic Information Nondiscrimination Act (GINA) of 2008 was enacted to provide consistent protections throughout the United States to prohibit discrimination in health insurance coverage and employment based on genetic information. For example, this law provides protection against an increase in the overall premium rate for an employer group plan based on genetic information of an individual. The employer can still determine eligibility or premium rates for an individual with the disease but not use the plan to increase rates for all. Think about the incidence of breast cancer in families. In this case, genetic information and family history cannot be used to discriminate for employment or for health coverage based on this information for an individual who does not manifest the disease or condition. If the person does manifest the condition, he or she may be denied coverage or pay additional premiums. However, the employer cannot raise all premiums in an effort to project costs and coverage impacts on the company's plan.

The American Nurses Association, in collaboration with stakeholder groups, published essential competencies for nurses and for curriculum in the area of genetics and genomics in 2006, with revisions in 2008 and further comments on the competencies of graduate nurses solicited in 2010. These competencies address practice standards for registered nurses. In the area of professional responsibilities, awareness of one's own values, advocacy for patients, and competency in the nursing role relative to genetics and genomics are minimum competencies. In the practice domain, the ANA (2008) competencies focus on nursing assessment; identification of patients, valid information, and ethical standards; referral activities, and the provision of education, care and support (pp. 11–13). These competencies include the need for critical analysis, advocacy, and collaboration with patients and other healthcare providers. Awareness of the terminology, current developments, and ethical standards are vital. To demonstrate the effect of this area on current health priorities, federal agencies such as the Agency for Healthcare Research and Quality have included activities in their annual line item budgets related to genomics. Investigate some of the fact sheets provided at the Web site of the National Human Genome Project and the expected professional competencies.

Impaired or Incompetent Colleagues. As an advocate for effective healthcare for patients, a nurse does not want to be faced with **impaired or incompetent colleagues**. Unfortunately, it does happen, and this creates ethical dilemmas. The ICN (2006b) addresses continuing competence as a professional responsibility and a public right and further mandates the "report of practitioners who fail to deliver competent professional practice" (p. 1). This mandate addresses both impaired and incompetent practice of any healthcare professional and is highlighted in the revised ANA *Code of Ethics for Nurses*. The Code states, "nurses must be alert to and take appropriate action in all instances of incompetent, unethical, illegal, or impaired practice or actions that place the rights or best interests of the patient in jeopardy" (ANA, 2015, p. 12).

Again, no one likes to think about working with or being aware of an incompetent or impaired colleague. It is dangerous to both the patient and others. It endangers patients first but also impacts family members, colleagues, managers, organizational leaders and managers, the profession, and the community at large. Chemical dependency is a complex disease. Drug dependency can be a result of prior conditions that required pain management in the nurse's personal life, a complex biochemical and mental health issue, or psychological issues. Drug diversion, or taking drugs from a patient or the institution, whether for personal use or for a friend or family member, is a criminal offense. The patient may be denied effective pain management or only receive partial doses. This situation is a form of harm to the patient both physiologically and economically. But, the health professional is also being harmed. Healthcare providers have controlled access to drugs like opiates in their care of patients, and this can be a powerful inducement at a time of chemical or emotional weakness or even workload stress. It can also be quite frightening to co-workers who notice unusual behavior in a colleague. As described by Wolf (2012), "when substandard, neglectful nursing care is tolerated or ignored, intense moral distress follows" (p. 22).

In a case of impaired practice, discovery is upsetting to the individual, colleagues, and management. And the patient may have experienced harm from the failure to receive their prescribed medications. Administration may be called and intervene, requesting that the employee submit to a drug screen immediately. This confrontation can engender defensive or escapist behaviors. Discovery may also occur when the employee is off duty during an investigation of drug administration or control irregularities, and the employee is called in to meet with administration or an employee assistance representative. Regardless, if diversion of controlled substances is suspected, drug enforcement and control officials may be called, and the employee may face arrest and criminal prosecution. This criminal action will be in addition to an investigation by the Board of Nursing and perhaps immediate suspension of the license and privilege to practice. The impaired professional may be referred to a special rehabilitative program during this process. Angres, Bettinardi-Angres, and Cross (2010) describe that this referral source expects a treatment provider to determine whether the nurse needs a detoxification program and subsequent treatment including follow-up treatment, family services, and after-care (p. 17). Employment and earning potential may be severely affected for the employee and his or her family. The organization is affected operationally, economically, and emotionally. The entire situation is upsetting and harmful to all involved, especially

ONLINE CONSULT

Genetic Information Nondiscrimination Act (GINA) of 2008 at
http://www.genome.gov/10002077#al-2

National Human Genome Research Institute at
http://www.genome.gov/

American Nurses Association at
http://www.nursingworld.org/MainMenu
Categories/EthicsStandards/Genetics-1
/default.aspx

the patient. Consider the principles of beneficence, non-maleficence, justice, fidelity, and veracity. And drug diversion, whether directly from patients or from the organization, impacts both the patient and the healthcare system.

Bettinardi-Angres and Angres (2010) encourage nurses in authority to understand the disease of addiction as a biopsychosocial disease process and chronic health problem and to use an effective and compassionate approach to benefit the addicted nurse, the healthcare profession, and society (p. 31). Impaired nurses can not only injure themselves and their patients through unprofessional practice, but could seriously impact the performance of colleagues in the performance of their role or even injure or kill others in a motor vehicle accident on the way to or from the healthcare setting. The scope of this discussion is not directed at understanding the disease of chemical addiction or dependency but the effect in the organization and on the leadership and management. In cases that are not subject to criminal charges, the employee assistance program may seek to assist the impaired professional. But reporting an impaired professional to the Board of Nursing starts an investigative process with the potential for discipline and is a requirement that has an impact on the employee, the organization, and society. As the nursing leader or manager, you may be faced with such a situation. You will be confronted with reporting requirements, employee rehabilitation potential or termination, and damage control in the situation and interpersonal situations, and you may even be required to provide testimony to state or law enforcement representatives or agencies. The best scenario is to provide employee assistance and intervention before the impaired practice or diversion occurs. This may not be possible given longstanding physiological and emotional issues. But, consider how to react and respond in the situation. The first consideration in knowing the legal requirements in your nurse practice act, as the statue or law, and in the regulations that interpret and explain the law.

Incompetent practice, or failure to meet the standard of care, is also harmful to the patient, colleagues, the organization, and the profession. Consider the reactions of a colleague who observes this situation: disbelief, denial, making excuses, or perhaps blame directed at the situation or the environment. Consider a possible ethical dilemma: protection of the patient or "whistle-blowing" on a colleague. Once again, return to the ethical decision-making model in this situation:

● Obtaining background information
● Identifying the ethical components
● Identifying the ethical agents or people involved
● Identifying the options available
● Applying ethical principles to the issues, like self-determination
● Making a final resolution or decision to the ethical dilemma

First, you will have to collect the facts on what happened. These facts will also be necessary for an incident report or observation that you will need to provide. Next, in your understanding of the situation, a critical determination will be patient safety and your consideration of the principles of beneficence, nonmaleficence, justice and fidelity. Veracity is directed at the patient, the colleague, and the organization as you identify the ethical agents and the people involved. Next, consider your options and what immediate interventions are needed on the part of the patient and the colleague as you function as a professional and a patient advocate. These interventions for beneficience and fidelity to the patient's safety will be of paramount concern. At the same time, your patients will need the appropriate level of care to ensure their care and safety. Your final steps in the resolution will be based on the facts, ethical principles, and your professional obligations and accountability. Advocacy for patients in the case of an impaired or incompetent colleague presents an ethical dilemma that requires intervention and addressing patient safety while facts surrounding a situation are being collected and blame and personal conflict are minimized.

You will encounter other ethical dilemmas throughout practice. As described in the ANA (2010b) position statement on *The Nurse's Role in Ethics and Human Rights*, "clearly articulated ethical positions, astute understanding of human rights, careful discernment of human rights violations and bold acceptance of responsibility converge to provide a backdrop for all nursing activities" (p. 2). Adherence to ethical principles is a part of clinical judgment and professional practice. Your skills in assessment, critical analysis, and nursing process will be invaluable as you confront the situations as they arise.

EVIDENCE-BASED PRACTICE: *Consider this....*

In 2010, the Food and Drug Administration requested that the Institute of Medicine examine when and how to conduct clinical trials ethically in order to evaluate the safety of drugs. The basis for this request is to address both ethical and patient safety concerns especially when patients are involved in clinical trials.

In its report, the IOM (2012) concluded that the FDA's current approach to drug oversight is not sufficiently systematic to ensure that it assesses the benefits and risks of drugs consistently over the drug's life cycle and recommended adopting a framework standardized across all drugs that is flexible enough to make the decision-making process more predictable, transparent, and proactive (p. 1).

Suppose clinical drug trials are currently being conducted in your organization. Read the current information and response provided by the IOM at http://www.iom.edu/Reports/2012/Ethical-and-Scientific-Issues-in-Studying-the-Safety-of-Approved-Drugs.aspx.

Question: How would you apply the ethical decision-making process by Curtain (1987) to this situation with the current information on this topic?

KEY POINTS

- Rights are agreements that may be welfare or legal rights (based on laws that may be revised), ethical or moral rights (based on an ethical system or rules of conduct) and option rights (with differences within the overall legal parameters).

- Basic human rights include beneficence, justice and fidelity, full disclosure and veracity, self-determination and autonomy, informed consent, and privacy and confidentiality.

- Beneficence is the principle of doing good with the person's best interests as the goal of all actions. Associated ethical principles include justice (fairness) and fidelity (loyalty).

- Self-determination is the sense of autonomy, where the person has the right to determine their fate.

- Full disclosure occurs when the individual has complete and relevant information to make an informed decision and includes the principle of veracity or providing truthful information.

- Informed consent occurs when the individual has complete information on all sides of the issue and makes a decision for care (or not) freely and without constraint given careful consideration on both advantages and disadvantages of the action.

- Privacy means that a person has the right to determine and control the amount of information to reveal about himself or herself, while confidentiality means that the information that the person does reveal is respected and not revealed to others except as necessary as part of this professional relationship.

- Standards of care are the accepted practice that is reasonable under a given set of circumstances for a specific profession.

- The two generally established systems of ethical decision making are utilitarianism (based on the consequence) and deontology (based on the consistent obligations as rules and unchanging principles).

- The *Code of Ethics for Nurses* developed by the American Nurses Association is the ethical standard for professional nursing practice in the United States.

- There are various ethical decision-making models. A classic model includes obtaining background information, identifying the ethical components, identifying the ethical agents or people involved, identifying the options available, applying ethical principles, and making a final decision on the dilemma (Curtain, 1987).

- Advance directives are legal documents (living wills and durable powers of attorney) that provide specific written instructions for an individual's wishes relative to the future healthcare and end-of-life decisions at a time when the person is able to specify his or her wishes.

- Active euthanasia is also called "mercy killing," with an active role with the sole intent to end life is not allowable in the *Code of Ethics for Nurses* (ANA, 2015, p. 3).

- The Human Genome Project has been an outstanding scientific achievement that provided new information on gene structure, function, and dysfunction for the human genome (the complete set of the human DNA).

- Advocacy for patients in the case of an impaired or incompetent colleague presents an ethical dilemma that requires intervention and addressing patient safety while facts surrounding a situation are being collected and blame and personal conflict is minimized.

Thought and Discussion Questions

1. Reflect carefully and identify an ethical dilemma and debate each side with a colleague, one of you using the utilitarianism philosophy and the other using deontology.

2. Identify the basic human rights reflected in the ANA *Code of Ethics for Nurses* (2015).

3. What commonalities can you identify in the ANA *Code of Ethics for Nurses* (2015), the Canadian Nurses Association *Code of Ethics* (2008), and the ICN *Code of Ethics for Nurses* (2012)?

4. Review one standard of care from your facility's policy and procedure manual and investigate its basis in the professional literature.

5. Find a peer from a different ethnic or cultural background and share your values on an ethical topic of your choice.

6. Discuss the Chapter Thought in the context of professional ethics.

Interactive Exercises

Go to the Intranet site and complete the interactive exercises provided for this chapter.

REFERENCES

Aiken, T. D. (2004). *Legal, ethical, and ethical issues in nursing* (2nd ed). Philadelphia: F. A. Davis.

American Nurses Association (ANA). (2006). Position statement: Privacy and confidentiality. Retrieved from http://nursingworld.org/MainMenuCategories/Ethics Standards/Ethics-Position-Statements/Privacyand Confidentiality.html

American Nurses Association. (2008). *Essentials of genetic and genomic nursing: Competencies, curricula guidelines, and outcome indicators* (2nd ed.). Retrieved from http://nursingworld.org/MainMenuCategories/EthicsStandards /Genetics-1/Background-Genetics-and-Genomes /EssentialNursingCompetenciesandCurriculaGuidelines forGeneticsandGenomics.pdf

American Nurses Association. (2010a). *Nursing: Scope and standards of practice* (2nd ed.). Silver Spring, MD: Nursesbooks.org.

American Nurses Association. (2010b). *Position Statement: The nurse's role in ethics and human rights: Protecting and promoting individual worth, dignity, and human rights in practice settings.* Retrieved from http://www.nursingworld.org /ethicsrole

American Nurses Association. (2012). *Nursing care and do not resuscitate (DNR) and allow natural death (AND) decisions.* Retrieved from http://www.nursingworld.org/MainMenu-Categories/EthicsStandards/Ethics-Position-Statements /Nursing-Care-and-Do-Not-Resuscitate-DNR-and-Allow -Natural-Death-Decisions.pdf

American Nurses Association. (2013). *Euthanasia, assisted suicide, and aid in dying.* Retrieved from http://nursingworld .org/MainMenuCategories/EthicsStandards/Ethics -Position-Statements/Euthanasia-Assisted-Suicide-and -Aid-in-Dying.pdf

American Nurses Association. (2015). *Code of ethics for nurses with interpretative statements.* Silver Spring, MD: Nursesbooks.org.

Angres, D. H., Bettinardi-Angres, K., & Cross, W. (2010). Nurses with chemical dependency: Promoting successful treatment and reentry. *Journal of Nursing Regulation, 1,* 16–20.

Bettinardi-Angres, K., & Angres, D. H. (2010). Understanding the disease of addiction. *Journal of Nursing Regulation, 1,* 31–35.

Bosek, M. S. D., Jannette, J. (2013). Attitudes of nurses toward patient-directed dying: A pilot study. *JONA'S Healthcare, Law, Ethics, and Regulation, 15*(4), 135–139.

Campbell, A. V. (2013). *Bioethics: The basics.* London, UK: Routledge.

Canadian Nurses Association. (2008). *Ethical practice: The code of ethics for registered nurses.* Retrieved from http://www .cna-aiic.ca/en/on-the-issues/best-nursing/nursing-ethics

Collins, F. S., Green, E. D., Guttmacher, A. E., Guyer, M. S. (2003). A vision for the future of genomics research: A blueprint for the genomic era. *Nature, 422*(6934), 835–847. Retrieved from http://www.genome.gov/11007524

Curtain, L. L. (1978). A proposed model for critical ethical analysis. *Nursing Forum, 17*(1), 12–17.

Dahnke, M., & Dreher, H. M. (2006). Defining ethics and applying the theories. In V. D. Lachman (Ed.), *Applied ethics in nursing* (pp. 3–13). New York: Springer.

Department of Health and Human Services. (2009). GINA: The Genetic Information Nondiscrimination Act of 2008: Information for researchers and health care professionals. Retrieved from http://www.genome.gov/Pages/PolicyEthics /GeneticDiscrimination/GINAInfoDoc.pdf

Huddleston, K. (December 23, 2013). Ethics: The challenge of ethical, legal, and social implications (ELSI) in genomic nursing. *OJIN: The Online Journal of Issues in Nursing, 17*(1). Retrieved from http://nursingworld.org /MainMenuCategories/ANAMarketplace/ANAPeriodicals /OJIN/Columns/Ethics/Ethical-Legal-Social-Implications -in-Genomic-Nursing.html

Husted, G. L., & Husted, J. H. (2008). *Ethical decision making in nursing and health care: The symphonological approach* (4th ed.). New York: Springer.

Institute of Medicine. (2012). *Ethical and scientific issues in studying the safety of approved drugs:* Retrieved from http://www.iom.edu/reports/2012/ethical-and-scientific -issues-in-studying-the-safety-of-approved-drugs.aspx

International Council of Nurses (ICN). (2006). *Position statement: Continuing competence as a professional responsibility and public right.* Retrieved from http://www.icn.ch/images /stories/documents/publications/position_statements/B02 _Continuing_Competence.pdf

International Council of Nurses (ICN). (2008). *Position statement. Health information: Protecting patient rights.* Retrieved from http://www.icn.ch/images/stories/documents /publications/position_statements/E05_Health_ Information_Patient_Rights.pdf

International Council of Nurses (ICN). (2012a). *The ICN code of ethics for nurses.* Retrieved from http://www.icn.ch /icncode.pdf

International Council of Nurses (ICN). (2012b). *Nurses'roles in providing care to dying patients and their families.* Retrieved from http://www.icn.ch/images/stories/documents /publications/position_statements/A12_Nurses_Role_Care _Dying_Patients.pdf

National Human Genome Research Institute. (2012). *Genetic mapping*. Retrieved from http://www.genome.gov/10000715

National Human Genome Research Institute. (2014). *ELSI Research Program*. Retrieved from http://www.genome.gov/10001618#al-2

Pang, T. (2002). Health policy and ethics forum: The impact of genomics on global health. *American Journal of Public Health, 97*(7), 1077–1079.

Perry, J. E., Churchill, L. R., & Kirshner, H. S. (2005). The Terri Schiavo case: Legal, ethical, and medical perspectives. *Annals of Internal Medicine, 143*, 744–748.

Spector, R. E. (2013). *Cultural diversity in health & illness* (8th ed.). Upper Saddle River, NJ: Pearson.

BIBLIOGRAPHY

Blasi, A.E. (2012). An ethical dilemma: Patients & profits v. access & affordability. *Journal of Legal Medicine, 33*, 115–128.

Blennerhassett, M. (2013). Breast cancer screening: An ethical dilemma or an opportunity for openness? *Quality in Primary Care, 21*, 39–42.

Collins, F., & Barker, A. (2007). Mapping the cancer genome: Pinpointing the genes involved in cancer will help chart a new course across the complex landscape of human malignancies. *Scientific American, 296*(3), 50–57.

Greipp, M. E. (1995). A survey of ethical decision making models in nursing. *Journal of Nursing Scholarship, 1*(1–2), 51–60.

Health; End of Life; Patient Directed Dying Act, VT LEG 262460.1. Retrieved from http://www.leg.state.vt.us/docs/2012/Bills/Intro/H-274.pdf

Lea, D. H. (2009). Basic genetics and genomics: A primer for nurses. *OJIN: The Online Journal of Issues in Nursing, 14*(2). Retrieved from http://www.nursingworld.org/MainMenuCategories/ANAMarketplace/ANAPeriodicals/OJIN/TableofContents/Vol142009/No2May09/Articles-Previous-Topics/Basic-Genetics-and-Genomics.html

Lea, D. H. (2009). The Genetic Information Nondiscrimination Act (GINA): What it means for your patients and families. *OJIN: The Online Journal of Issues in Nursing, 14*(2). Retrieved from http://nursingworld.org/MainMenuCategories/ANAMarketplace/ANAPeriodicals/OJIN/TableofContents/Vol142009/No2May09/Articles-Previous-Topics/The-Genetic-Information-Nondiscrimination-Act-GINA.aspx

McCue, C. (2010). Using the AACN framework to alleviate moral distress. *Online Journal of Issues in Nursing, 16*(1). Retrieved from http://nursingworld.org/MainMenuCategories/ANAMarketplace/ANAPeriodicals/OJIN/TableofContents/Vol-16-2011/No1-Jan-2011/Articles-Previous-Topics/AACN-Framework-and-Moral-Distress.html

Sofaer, N., & Strech, D. (2011). The need for systematic reviews of reasons. *Bioethics, 26*, 315–328.

Ulysse, F. G., Balicas, M., & Xu, Y. (2011). Ethical dilemma: Therapeutic nondisclosure. *Clinical Scholars Review, 4*(2), 115–118.

U.S. Department of Health and Human Services. (2010). *Health information privacy*. Retrieved from http://www.hhs.gov/ocr/privacy/

Winters, N. (2013). Whether to break confidentiality: An ethical dilemma. *Journal of Emergency Nursing, 39*, 233–235.

Wolf, Z.R. (2012). Nursing practice breakdowns: Good and bad nursing. *MESURG Nursing, 21*(1), 16–22, 36.

ONLINE RESOURCES

Agency for Healthcare Research and Quality
http://www.ahrq.gov

AARP
http://www.aarp.org/home-family/caregiving/

American Nurses Association
http://www.nursingworld.org

Bioethics Databases
http://bioethics.od.nih.gov/withinnih.html

Familydoctor.org
http://familydoctor.org/familydoctor/en/healthcare-management/end-of-life-issues.html

HIPAA
http://www.hhs.gov/ocr/privacy/

MedlinePlus
http://www.nlm.nih.gov/medlineplus/medlineplus.html

Medline Plus: Organ Transplantation
http://www.nlm.nih.gov/medlineplus/organtransplantation.html

National Alliance on Mental Illness
http://www.nami.org

National Cancer Institute: Advance Directives
http://www.cancer.gov/about-cancer/managing-care/advance-directives

National Human Genome Research Institute
http://www.genome.gov/

Organ Procurement and Transplantation Network
http://optn.transplant.hrsa.gov/

Terri Schiavo Life & Hope Network
http://www.terrisfight.org/

U.S. Government Information on Organ and Tissue Donation and Transplantation
http://www.organdonor.gov/

Quality Care for Individuals, Families, and Groups

This section starts with a focus on **quality and safety** in Chapter 13, and the national initiatives that have driven this process. Theoretical models for quality are discussed, along with strategies for continuous quality improvement, safety, and efficacy in the healthcare environment. In Chapter 14, the focus is on **population health.** The progress of the *Healthy People* initiatives in the United States is presented. Special populations that are highlighted include the aging population, minorities, and those living in rural areas, with the focus on health promotion for the population and health equity.

In Chapter 15, we look at one of the core competencies for health professionals, the use of **informatics**. Health information systems in the clinical setting are discussed along with the implementation of the electronic health record (EHR). Informatics competencies for nurses, informatics nurses, and informatics specialists are described in this evolving specialty in the discipline.

Quality care includes a focus on **healthcare economics** and policy as presented in Chapter 16. Policy and the associated costs are changing dramatically as we focus on safe, effective, and equitable care for individuals and groups. Stemming from a focus on healthcare policy are the political advocacy skills needed by the **politically active nurse** in Chapter 17. These skills include both understanding the legislative process and promoting policy improvements for the health of individuals and groups.

In Chapter 18, Sister Rosemary Donley challenges us to consider our progress on healthcare reform and global and domestic issues that affect healthcare policy, healthcare delivery, and nursing education and practice. The active participation of professional nurses in policy formulation will strengthen the profession and patient care outcomes.

Finally, in Chapter 19, we look at the trends in professional practice and the competencies needed in future professional practice. You are challenged to develop your own personal strategies for your future contributions to professional practice.

● Francoise Dunefsky   ● Rose Kearney-Nunnery

13

Quality and Safety in Healthcare

"Quality is shared and is everyone's responsibility."

Francoise Dunefsky

Chapter Objectives

On completion of this chapter, the reader will be able to:

1. Describe the steps in the processes of continuous quality improvement.
2. Discuss the role of regulatory agencies in promoting safety and evaluating quality in healthcare settings.
3. Discuss the changes in quality improvement and safety standards and expectations and their impact on current professional nursing practice.
4. Differentiate between the cultures of safety and blame.
5. Explain the use of a root cause analysis for a sentinel event.
6. Identify quality improvement factors to be considered at the unit, organizational, and system levels.

Key Terms

Quality
National Patient Safety Goals
National Hospital Quality
    Measures
Transformation
Quality Planning
Quality Control
Quality Improvement
Learning Organization
Total Quality Management (TQM)

Continuous Quality Improvement
    (CQI)
Benchmarking
Quality Assurance
Risk Management
Just-in-time learning
Just Culture
Sentinel Event
Root Cause Analysis
Process Teams

QI Tools
Flow Chart
Cause-and-Effect Diagram
Data Sheets
Check Sheets
Surveys
Indicators
Variation
Work Redesign

In healthcare arenas, we continue to examine the definition of quality and its relationship to costs. This effort has been stimulated by several factors: the necessity to compete in a global marketplace, where production costs are often significantly lower; the ongoing explosion in technological advances; exponentially increasing expenditures for healthcare services; individual and corporate consumer pressures to improve value, and portability of health information; potential reduction of fragmentation of care; and, of critical importance, the safety of healthcare consumers.

Healthcare institutions are attempting to understand and apply principles and techniques previously reserved for the business world. In their codes of ethics and standards of practice, professional groups, including nurses and physicians, have historically expressed the intent of ensuring that individual patients receive optimal care. The impact of structures and processes on these individual and aggregate outcomes was previously not documented nor necessarily understood.

In addition, societal forces are shifting the healthcare paradigm from a paternalistic model of delivering care and services to one that responds to customer demands. Making providers accountable for evaluating the quality of care they deliver, and for communicating that quality effectively to the public, is an emerging task influenced by corporate buyers of services, who want to know what they can expect to receive for their money. Much progress has been made in the last decade to create an infrastructure that can be used to improve the entire system of care for all stakeholders. In fact, the Agency for Healthcare Research and Quality (AHRQ) is now required to report to Congress annually on healthcare quality and disparities. In a recent report, the AHRQ (2014) noted that healthcare quality was fair but improving, with 70 percent of recommended care actually received, but there was variation across states, with hospital care improving more rapidly and ambulatory, diabetes, and maternal and child care lagging (p. H-1).

With its professional commitment to patients, responsibility for coordinating care, and roots in the psychosocial and physical sciences, nursing is poised to play an important role in the ongoing development and implementation of care delivery models that are effective and efficient, meet customer expectations, and ensure excellent clinical outcomes and safety. The dictionary defines **quality** as a "degree of excellence or distinguishing attribute" (*Merriam-Webster Dictionary*, 2014). In healthcare, we previously defined it as being "free of mistakes" or perfect relative to process. The standard of perfection, or 100 percent compliance, was focused within. The current quality movement is evolving a definition of quality that includes "meeting customer needs" and focusing on outcomes, efficacy, and safety. The Institute of Medicine (IOM) uses the following definition: "The degree to which health services for individuals and populations increase the likelihood of desired health outcomes and are consistent with current professional knowledge" (IOM, 2001, p. 232). A new paradigm for clinical practice across disciplines is contributing to nursing's body of knowledge, current standards of practice, nursing care outcomes, and the consistent use of evidence-based practice. Recall that we have previously defined evidence-based practice as "an integration of the best evidence available, nursing expertise, and the values and preferences of the individuals, families, and communities who are selected" (Sigma Theta Tau, 2005, p. 1).

Healthcare providers have consistently looked at clinical care as the measure for quality. Traditionally, the qualifications of clinicians, state-of-the-art technology, and episodic interventions that cure illness and "do no harm" were considered indices of quality. But asking customers how they perceive "quality" has enabled a more complex picture to emerge. The consumer expects expert clinical care. But equally important are safe, timely, courteous, and respectful treatment, easy access to caregivers and information, unfragmented care delivery, reasonable costs, and the ability to maneuver through the system without too many obstacles. Understanding the convergence of the consumer's perspective of quality and use of evidence-based nursing practice, together with an ongoing focus on continuous improvement, are an integral part of meeting our professional commitment.

HISTORICAL PERSPECTIVES

Human societies have always strived for excellence. Reliance on professional associations such as guilds and inspection by consumers are centuries-old methods of judging quality. Societal values, however, are changing the context in which quality is evaluated.

Pre–World War II healthcare delivery in the United States was mostly a cottage industry. This time is referred to as the "charitable era of healthcare." The wealthy and fortunate rural populations relied on services delivered in the home. The poor and urban working classes were sent to hospitals in critical circumstances or died at home. A sudden growth in technology and treatment modalities and the building of hospitals stimulated by the Hospital Survey and Construction Act of 1946, also known as the Hill-Burton Act, began the corporatization of healthcare delivery. This "technologic era" lasted for more than 30 years. Extensive development of policies, procedures, standards of practice, and professional disciplines ensued. It took 20 years before the industrial model of reliance on departmental inspection and supervisory audits became part of the fabric of healthcare. The role of Medicare and federal and state government accelerated this growth.

The early 1970s saw the beginning of formalized measurement of clinical performance and outcomes. Organizations such as the Joint Commission (formerly known as the Joint Commission on Accreditation of Healthcare Organizations, or JCAHO), professional review organizations (PROs), and some state health departments played a major role in the initial movement. Retrospective audits, investigation of problems, and indicator measurements were all attempts to discover less than acceptable performance by an individual, discipline, or department. The objective was to discover the "bad apples," implement a corrective action plan, and monitor its effectiveness through ongoing measurement. It was assumed that quality was a result of the performance of individuals or groups of individuals. The tools of the corrective action plans were education, disciplinary action, and increased resources such as technology and staffing.

A gradual quality paradigm shift began in the second half of the 1980s. The "economic era" of healthcare was emerging. Other industries purchasing healthcare for their employees at rapidly rising costs challenged the healthcare sector to provide "more" and "better" for "less." The Japanese were successfully invading the American marketplace as a result of quality methodologies developed by Deming, Juran, and others. Deming had persuaded the Japanese government and industry that they should focus on quality rather than price and costs. Knowing that this focus would take time and commitment, they infused their businesses with the belief that work is performed by interdependent teams, that individuals want to do a good job, that those who do the work itself know its processes better than anyone else, and that mass inspection and fear do not automatically result in quality.

Juran proposed the notion that by planning for quality, one avoids multiple trial-and-error situations and costly rework, often referred to as "the cost of poor quality." Quality could be cost-effective. Improvement required even higher goals for quality. Reliance on systems analysis and statistical methods and techniques produced better-quality products than did supervision and inspection of individual human behaviors.

During the next 10 years, companies began to recognize that care is delivered by individuals who function as members of cross-functional and interdisciplinary teams, and those individuals and teams are tools for, rather than objects of, improvement. Currently a body of scientific research is emerging that tests the new theories that care is supported by environmental, managerial, support, and governance structures, and that ensuring accepted clinical outcomes is not enough to meet customer needs.

Many individuals and organizations have contributed to the quality journey over the past 30 years. The Joint Commission, the Institute for Healthcare Improvement, and the IOM are but a few organizations that deserve recognition for being driving forces in the implementation of the new quality care models. In 1996, the IOM, a member of the National Academies, began a multiple-phase Quality Initiative; its landmark reports include *To Err is Human: Building a Safer Health System* (2000), *Crossing the Quality Chasm: A New Health System for the 21st Century* (2001), *Keeping Patients Safe: Transforming the Work Environment of Nurses* (Page, 2004), and more recently, in collaboration with the Robert Wood Johnson Foundation, *The Future of Nursing: Leading Change, Advancing Health* (2011). These and other IOM reports

focus on the quality problems and on the multiple levels of system reform needed.

Largely as a result of the IOM's activities and reports, the Joint Commission in 2002 approved **National Patient Safety Goals**. Requirements define performance expectations with respect to structure, process, and outcomes in order that patient safety and quality may be enhanced. The requirements to meet these goals are surveyed in all healthcare organizations seeking their accreditation. Since then, these goals have undergone revision and updating to focus efforts on current issues and strategies, all directed at patient safety in a variety of environments.

In 1998, the Joint Commission began the journey toward the standardization of core measures with the goal of quality improvement of patient outcomes. In 2004, the Joint Commission partnered with the Centers for Medicare and Medicaid (CMS) on the core measures for greater standardization as common measures. These core measures became **National Hospital Quality Measures** identified as integral to improving the quality of care provided to hospital patients and bring value to stakeholders by focusing on the actual results of care with common and consistent measurement (Joint Commission, 2013h). At first, the focus was on metrics through the identification and implementation of these national measures, followed by expansion and enhancement across the national system for demonstrable improvement in healthcare quality and patient safety. Of note is the collaborative work throughout this endeavor between the Joint Commission, CMS, and the National Quality Forum (NQF), as well as other partners. In 2010, hospitals were required to submit data to the Joint Commission on a minimum of four core standards or a combination of applicable core measures or noncore measures, depending on agency size and focus (Joint Commission, 2010, p. 1). (See current core measures, identified in Box 13.1.) Separate systems can now be compared by using core measures in a standardized fashion. By using specific performance measures for diseases such as acute myocardial infarction or stroke and their management, hospitals regardless of geographical location could be easily compared. In addition, the aim was to minimize redundancy in data collection. Initially the work was hospital-based. However, the measures have now been expanded to provide a greater scope of selection options in long-term care, home care, behavioral healthcare, and ambulatory care, so standardized performance improvement is implemented throughout the entire continuum of care.

CMS has well-established "Compare" websites for hospitals, nursing homes, HHAs, and ESRD facilities. In March 2008, it began posting cost in addition to quality information on Hospital Compare about selected inpatient hospital stays provided to Medicare patients. More recently the site has added 10 new measures of patient experiences of care (Hospital Consumer Assessment of Healthcare Providers and Systems, or HCAPs). Consumers now have access to the three critical elements of quality, satisfaction, and pricing information for specific procedures performed at their hospitals when making informed decisions about where to seek care.

Simultaneously with the Compare activities, CMS developed the Roadmap for Implementing Value Driven Healthcare in the Traditional Medicare Fee-for-Service Program. This included promoting efficiency in resource

ONLINE CONSULT

The Joint Commission at
http://www.jointcommission.org/

The Joint Commission's Quality Report at
http://www.QualityCheck.org

The Institute for Healthcare Improvement at
http://www.ihi.org

The Institute of Medicine: Quality and Patient Safety at
http://iom.edu/Global/Topics/Quality-Patient-Safety.aspx

| BOX 13.1 | National Hospital Quality Measures |

Core Measures:

- Acute myocardial infarction
- Children's asthma care (CAC)
- Emergency department
- Heart failure
- Hospital-based inpatient psychiatric services
- Hospital outpatient department
- Immunization
- Perinatal care
- Pneumonia measures
- Stroke
- Substance use
- Surgical care improvement project (SCIP)
- Tobacco treatment
- Venous thromboembolism

Source: Joint Commission. (2014a). *Core measure sets*. Retrieved from http://www.jointcommission.org/core_measure_sets.aspx.
Specifications Manual for National Hospital Inpatient Quality Measures Discharges 01-01-15 (1Q15) through 09-30-15 (3Q15).

use while providing high-quality care, namely paying for value. Initial steps required Medicare to stop paying for certain reasonably preventable Hospital Acquired Conditions (HACs). As of fiscal year 2013 steps have been implemented to move hospitals from a pay-for-reporting to a pay-for-performance program, called Value-Based Purchasing (VBP). Other providers are preparing for the next phase of the VBP implementation.

The role nursing plays in all of the quality and safety work has been pushed to the forefront. The American Nurses Association, through its National Database of Nursing Quality Indicators (NDNQI), has identified acute care patient outcomes that are dependent primarily on nursing care, commonly referred to as "nurse sensitive." On the basis of evidence-based practice, targets are being set for nurse-sensitive outcomes such as patient falls, pressure ulcers, and peripheral intravenous infiltration. National Database of Nursing Quality Indicator (NDNQI, 2014) guidelines now exist on data collection on nurse-sensitive indicators such as nursing care hours per patient day, skill mix, falls, and falls with injury.

One initiative in nursing education was the development and promotion of the Quality and Safety Education for Nurses (QSEN) competencies by the American Association of Colleges of Nursing. These QSEN competencies were developed along with the IOM competencies for all health professionals, patient-centered care, teamwork and collaboration, evidence-based practice, quality improvement, safety, and informatics (see Chapter 1). Knowledge, skills, and attitudes were identified for each of the competencies. Subsequently, these competencies were incorporated into the *Essentials of Baccalaureate Education for Professional Nursing Practice* (AACN, 2008). Baccalaureate program faculty were trained on these QSEN competencies with content now incorporated in the undergraduate curriculum. This movement then spread to the incorporation of QSEN competencies in graduate nursing education. In addition, QSEN Web-based learning modules are available

on each of the six core competencies. The competency for quality improvement has been defined as "the use of data to monitor the outcomes of care processes and use improvement methods to design and test changes to continuously improve the quality and safety of health care systems" (Cronenwett et al., 2007, p. 127; Smith, Cronenwett, and Sherwood, 2007, p. 133). The knowledge required in the area of quality improvements includes the following:

- Care outcomes in the setting
- Interprofessional systems and tensions affecting these outcomes
- Importance of variation and measurement to assess quality of care
- Various approaches for changing processes (Cronenwett et al., 2007)

Check out the knowledge, skills, and abilities required for quality improvement and the other QSEN competencies at http://qsen.org/. Quality improvement is now an expectation in all professional practice arenas, from basic education through professional practice.

What has become evident is the focus on quality improvement and the use of evidence-based metrics.

THEORETICAL MODELS FOR QUALITY

The models used for quality improvement have come from industry. Some have been adapted for healthcare, but all share the common theme of using the scientific process.

Deming's Principles for Transformation

W. Edwards Deming was the first to challenge seriously the managerial notion that quality and increased productivity are incompatible. In doing his research and developing his 14 Points for Management (Box 13.2), he assumed the radical new approach of listening to

BOX 13.2 Deming's 14 Points

1. Create constancy of purpose for improvement of product and service.
2. Adopt the new philosophy.
3. Cease dependence on mass inspection.
4. End the practice of awarding business on the basis of price tag alone.
5. Improve constantly and forever the system of production and service.
6. Institute training.
7. Adopt and institute leadership.
8. Drive out fear.
9. Break down barriers between staff areas.
10. Eliminate slogans and targets in the workplace that urge increased productivity.
11. Eliminate numerical quotas for the workplace and management.
12. Remove barriers that rob people of pride in workmanship.
13. Encourage education and self-improvement for everyone.
14. Take action to accomplish the transformation.

Source: Reprinted from *Out of the crisis* by W. Edwards Deming by permission of the W. Edwards Deming Institute®. Copyright 1986 by The W. Edwards Deming Institute®.

those who actually do the work (Deming, 1982, 1986). Deming contended that the model can be applied anywhere, including service industries. Nursing leaders at all levels of the organization can apply the principles in their quest to implement quality care. The more pervasive the quality culture in the organization, the easier the model application becomes. The stronger and more visible leadership is in its support for quality, the more rapidly a quality culture **transformation** can be implemented.

The 14 Points for Management

Following is a brief description of each of Deming's (1982, 1986) 14 Points of Management:

1. *Create constancy of purpose for improvement of product and service.* Innovation is the foundation for the future. It requires a belief that there is a future and an unshakable commitment to quality and productivity. Resources must be put into education and research so we can constantly improve. The aim is to meet our mission and serve our customers, because otherwise we will not stay in business. We must address day-to-day problems without getting stuck in them. Nurse managers must plan their resources, energy, and time to deal with the future; work better, not harder, to plan new services. Meeting our customers' needs, and training and retraining personnel, will help deal with required change.
2. *Adopt the new philosophy.* Do not accept existing levels of mistakes or staff members who are not adequately prepared to perform. Become the change agent who meets the challenge. Propose, develop, and implement improvements in systems and services.
3. *Cease dependence on mass inspection.* The inspection stage is too late to improve quality. Quality comes from improvement in production processes. Tools, such as 100 percent case review, will not improve care, are time-consuming, and require resources that could be better spent in improving design or systems. Measuring incomplete records, medication errors, or service delays, in and of themselves, will not improve the delivery of care.
4. *End the practice of awarding business on the basis of price tag alone.* The nurse manager has a responsibility to include total cost when recommending the purchase of goods or services. This includes not only the "up-front" price but also the cost of disposables and maintenance, amount of vendor support provided, ease of training in use, labor costs, and cross-functional use. It is a managerial responsibility to make well-prepared, comprehensive recommendations to the executive team. Deming believes that limiting the suppliers we deal with and establishing long-term relationships with vendors creates interdependency, which assists in the achievement of quality.
5. *Improve constantly and forever the system of production and service.* Quality must be built and incorporated during the design phase in order to avoid costly rework. Teamwork is essential in this process, especially in service industries such as healthcare, in which we rely on interdependent, cross-disciplinary teams to deliver the care that is our product. As our customers' needs and available resources change, we are obliged to improve existing systems. Reductions in length of stay, shifts in delivery of care along the continuum, and changing demographics all require us to seek opportunities to "do it better." It is no longer acceptable to think, "We always did it this way and it worked."
6. *Institute training.* Learning must be lifelong and pervasive. The principles of adult learning, and an appreciation for the fact that different people learn by different methods, apply at all layers of the organization, regardless of length of employment. All must understand the institution's mission, values, customer needs, and expectations. What the assignment is, what acceptable work is, and how we prepare people all must be defined. For the manager, this includes knowing which processes are assigned and understanding variation in these processes. We must become learning organizations.
7. *Adopt and institute leadership.* The job of management includes leadership—namely, vision and communication of that vision—not just supervision. The assignment is to work on quality of service, designing for quality and delivering an actual product. The manager must understand the work supervised and must remove barriers that prevent the staff members from doing their work.
8. *Drive out fear.* Fear of reprisal, fear of admitting mistakes, fear of not having necessary new knowledge, and fear of not meeting deadlines or quotas interfere with seeing opportunities for improvement. Errors, complaints, and areas that appear

out of control must be studied and analyzed for opportunities to improve.

9. *Break down barriers between staff areas.* This point has proved especially difficult in healthcare, where the struggle to establish distinct professional domains fostered accountability, review, and disciplinary actions within professions. The emergence of matrix organizations, patient care departments, use of product- or service-line teams, cross-training, and decentralization of services will assist in the implementation of patient care teams focused on the patient rather than the professional. Simultaneously, this will create a new challenge to ensure that no one can hide behind or dominate the team. All professional groups must be held accountable for their professional practice and for quality in service delivery.

10. *Eliminate slogans and targets in the workplace that urge increased productivity.* The assumption that one can improve quality and productivity by trying harder does not take into account that most problems come from systems rather than individuals. The role of management is to improve the system with the results of sound statistical methods.

11. *Eliminate numerical quotas for the workforce and management.* Quotas assume that the target is correct, not too high or too low, and that all can attain them. They have a negative effect on pride in workmanship. Productivity should be studied, analyzed, and understood. Everyone should know what to do and how to do it. A sustained requirement for all to participate in setting goals and figuring out how to reach them is needed.

12. *Remove barriers that rob people of pride in workmanship.* Make clear what the job is and what the expectations are. Improving the system to make it easier for people to work well will help them invest in the organization, reducing turnover and absenteeism.

13. *Encourage education and self-improvement for everyone.* Study and development should not focus only on the immediate needs of the organization or department. Develop the organization and its members for the future as well as for the present.

14. *Take action to accomplish the transformation.* The leaders must adopt the new philosophy with pride. It must be explained often and well to a critical number of individuals. Everyone in the organization must be asked to participate. This requires substantial and sustained commitment and energy.

Obstacles to Quality Transformation

Deming (1982, 1986) also recognized obstacles to the transformation:

- Desire to achieve instant results by hiring a consultant
- Supposition that solving problems creates transformation
- Belief that one can simply transfer systems from another organization

- Belief that the quality department takes care of quality
- Belief that your problems are different
- Poor understanding of statistical methods

Deming (1982, 1986) referred to more serious blocks as "deadly diseases" because of their severity and resistance to eradication:

- Lack of constancy of purpose
- Emphasis on short-term profits
- Evaluation of performance without long-term improvement in mind
- Mobility of management
- Management by numbers only

When considering applying Deming's principles for transformation, the nurse has to acknowledge realities in the organization. It may be necessary to maintain annual performance review, existing merit systems, strict organizational and professional hierarchies, and a focus on monthly budget fluctuations. Nevertheless, the general principles of constancy of purpose, focus on improvement, creating a learning environment, reducing fear, and removing barriers to pride in workmanship can be adopted by anyone in any setting.

Juran Trilogy

Deming offers a framework for how to transform any organization by incorporating quality, but the Juran Trilogy focuses on the tools that organizations can use while doing the work. The two models are complementary and are often used together.

Joseph Juran (1989) defines *quality* as "fitness for use." This definition assumes both freedom from defects and presence of the multiple elements required to meet the total needs of a customer. The freedom from defect does not guarantee that this is the product the customer wants. The patient assumes we can deliver care without errors. Waiting time, ease of access, and cleanliness may be crucial factors in determining whether a patient chooses a particular provider or urgent care center. Patients may opt to seek urgent care services in freestanding facilities with shorter wait times or diagnostic mammographies in zen-like women's health centers.

The Juran Trilogy utilizes three managerial processes: planning, control, and improvement (Box 13.3). The trilogy's proposed procedural steps and tools are unique.

Quality Planning

Planning for programs or services requires that quality is built into them. This stage of **quality planning** follows five distinct steps:

1. Determine who the customers of the program or service are. They can be external customers, internal customers, or both. In healthcare, patients, families, and payers are all external customers. Departments and providers are internal customers of one another. Nursing receives services from dietary or medical records, and those departments in turn are customers of nursing. Independent

BOX 13.3	Juran Trilogy	
A. Quality Planning	1. Determine who the customers are. 2. Determine the needs of the customer. 3. Develop product features that respond to the customer's needs. 4. Develop processes that are able to produce these product features. 5. Transfer the resulting plans to the operating forces.
B. Quality Control	1. Evaluate actual quality performance. 2. Compare actual performance to quality goals. 3. Act on the difference.
C. Quality Improvement	1. Establish an infrastructure. 2. Identify needs for improvement. 3. Establish project teams for each project. 4. Provide the teams with resources, motivation, and training.

Source: Adapted with the permission of The Free Press, a division of Simon & Schuster Adult Publishing Group, from Juran, J. M. (1989). *Juran on leadership for quality.* New York: The Free Press, © 1988 by The Juran Institute, Inc. All rights reserved.

medical staff members are often considered both internal and external customers because of their ability to choose the institution and their influence and provision of services within the institution.

2. Determine the customers' needs. Surveys, focus groups, individual patient interviews, complaint reviews, and market analysis can be used to determine what our customers want.
3. Develop product features that respond to the customer's needs. Consider offering services outside traditional business hours. Weekend day surgery, diagnostic procedures early and late in the day, and respite care are but a few examples.
4. Develop processes that are able to produce those product features.
5. Transfer the resulting plans to the implementation team.

For example, while teaching breast self-examination at a customer-friendly breast clinic, a nurse hears patients express concerns about the time it takes to receive mammography results. In response to complaints, the nurse, working with the department and a local women's group, initiates a formal survey of women who currently use the center and women who do not. The survey reveals that women want to receive test results within 24 hours and to be able to refer themselves for mammography. As a result, the services at the center are redesigned to incorporate these features. The clinic applies for and obtains an expanded license for self-referral. It institutes policies, procedures, and standards to ensure that the improved services are implemented and monitored.

Quality Control

The three steps of **quality control** involve:

1. Evaluating actual quality performance. This requires knowledge of statistical methods of measurement and analysis.
2. Comparing actual performance with quality goals.
3. Acting on the difference. This assumes understanding of common and special cause variation. Variation is part of any process. Constant reaction to it may destabilize an otherwise stable process.

Example
1. Measure the number of women who underwent mammography and received their results within 24 hours.
2. Compare the number to the agreed-upon benchmark.
3. Analyze the discrepancies for special cause variation and develop an improvement plan.

Quality Improvement

Raising performance to unprecedented levels or **quality improvement** requires four steps:

1. Establishing the infrastructure needed to secure ongoing quality improvement. The infrastructure, which may comprise a quality council, departmental teams, and assigned roles, ensures that quality improvement is part of the way business is done.
2. Identifying specific needs for improvement. Data from quality control, feedback from customers, and goals of the organization help determine what needs to be improved and what needs to be prioritized.
3. Establishing a project team for each project. Responsibility must be defined clearly. This includes the objective for improvement and measures of success.
4. Providing resources, motivation, and training for the teams to diagnose causes of lesser quality, stimulate a remedy, and establish controls to hold the gains in improvements.

ONLINE CONSULT

The W. Edwards Deming Institute at
http://deming.org

Juran: The Source for Quality at
http://www.juran.com

Example

The special cause variation for the delay in result reporting of the mammographies appears to be linked to the day of the week (Friday) and the shift (evening). The radiology nursing staff is drastically reduced on Saturdays with only interventional radiology nursing staff covering for the mammography service. After training this staff regarding the necessary skills about results reporting, you resume measuring and see a marked improvement.

Juran's work has shown that most of the potential for eliminating errors and improving the system does not lie in changing workers. The 85/15, rule as it is now commonly referred to, states that 85 percent of problems can be corrected only by changing systems.

Both Deming and Juran have provided the foundation for today's quality movement in industry and in healthcare. The national initiatives aimed at both quality and safety have helped in the transition from quality assurance to quality improvement.

Monitoring and Evaluation as a Goal of Accreditation

The Joint Commission takes the position that improvement requires effective monitoring and that effective monitoring requires good indicators. Quality assurance evolved into quality improvement largely as a result of this position. The monitoring and evaluation process has been revised over time but remains part of the foundation on which many of quality activities are based. The process requires identifying the most important aspects of care for a particular organization or division, selecting indicators that reflect these aspects, taking opportunities to improve care, taking action, and evaluating the effectiveness of that action. Doing the right thing includes efficacy and appropriateness. Doing it well involves availability, timeliness, effectiveness, continuity, safety, efficiency, and providing services with respect and caring.

You may have been involved in survey visits at your agency. The Joint Commission (2013a) describes the accreditation process as designed to help organizations strengthen community confidence in the quality and safety of care, treatment, and services and to organize and strengthen patient safety efforts (p. 1). The process is designed to monitor compliance with standards and ongoing quality improvement. The leaders in the organization are responsible for fostering quality improvement and setting priorities for assessment and improvement. Leaders are defined as the leadership of the board; the executive team, including the nurse executive; the leaders of the medical staff; and department directors. Nurse managers and other leaders in the nursing staff have direct responsibility for quality.

The unique character of the organization and the scope of services must be viewed consistently by all to be clear about who patients are and what these patients need. Key functions in the organization warrant ongoing monitoring and prioritization. The key function in outpatient areas are often very different from those in bedded units, as are the ones from services focusing on prevention, action, or chronic illness. Timeliness as an aspect of care may vary based on the scope of service and aspects of care of a particular service. Interdisciplinary teams develop and select indicators for those aspects of care that have been prioritized. As an example, turnaround time for laboratory results could be an indicator selected to reflect timeliness in an emergency department. Further, the team determines at what level and time evaluations will be triggered. Identifying thresholds that are not met after quarterly reviews is an example of how to implement evaluation. The review of every unexpected return of a patient to the surgical suite within 24 hours after surgery may be another.

Defining data sources and methodology for collection, the actual data collection, and organization all are parts of this process. Once it is determined that further evaluation is needed, other feedback may be taken into consideration. Intensive evaluation should be performed by teams. Actions for improvement are identified and include changes in the system, education, designation of clear authority and accountability, and development of standards. These actions must undergo ongoing evaluation for effectiveness.

In addition to this intensive analysis of the processes of the organization, attention to and report of national accountability measures is now required as part of the accreditation process. The collection of national information on core measures of performance began in 2002. Collaboration on these core measures with other national groups concerned with quality and safety led to the establishment of national quality measures as accountability measures. The Joint Commission (2014b) defines these accountability measures as "quality measures that meet four criteria designed to produce the greatest positive impact on patient outcomes when hospitals demonstrate improvement" (p. 1). The four criteria for these accountability measures are as follows:

1. Are evidence based
2. Have proximity, in that the care is connected to the patient outcome
3. Accurately measure the provision of care
4. Have little or no adverse consequences (Joint Commission, 2014b, p. 1)

These accountability measures are used to compare institutions and to present a national vision on quality of patient care. Consumers can readily check the quality reports of healthcare organizations in their community and region on these measures at http://qualitycheck.org. In the past years, the focus from within departments to processes, the level of accountability, the understanding and application of statistical methodologies, the role of leadership, and accountability to the public have evolved significantly.

Organizational leaders can no longer delegate responsibility to the quality department. Hiding behind professional or departmental boundaries is not acceptable. Leaders of boards, executive and management teams, and the medical staff are all being held accountable for delivery of quality care and for participation in the transformation of the healthcare system. The focus is on continuous quality improvement and safety.

> The right thing includes efficacy and appropriateness. Doing it well involves availability, timeliness, effectiveness, continuity, safety, efficiency, and providing services with respect and caring.

CONTINUOUS QUALITY IMPROVEMENT IN HEALTHCARE

Healthcare organizations strive to embed quality in every service they provide. Their success lies in their ability to incorporate quality as a key component of their strategic mission and to implement a model by which they continually evaluate and improve quality.

Quality as Strategy

The guiding members of any organization are responsible for developing the mission, vision, and core strategies chosen to achieve the vision. Not every business will choose quality as a strategy. Instituting competitive pricing, instilling a customer service focus, promoting access to the product, and creating a niche market are all examples of different strategies. It is not accidental that agencies accredited by the Joint Commission are required to include a quality plan in their strategic plan. To survive and thrive requires a formal, well-thought-out approach with a focus on the communities we serve.

"Doing the right things right" means that we have identified the "right things." They will vary according to the needs of the particular community and the mission and vision of the organization. Not every hospital can or should serve all the healthcare needs of its community. Such needs may be met better by other community agencies or tertiary care centers. Once the healthcare agency defines what the "right things" are, or what the scope of its services is, it must design quality into the structures and processes, monitor and analyze performance, and identify opportunities for improvement in order to ensure that the right things are "done right" and that the desired outcomes result.

A successful strategic plan also requires identification of needed core competencies and methods to address existing gaps. Core competencies define the organizational capabilities as well as the subsequent employee competencies needed to achieve the vision through utilization of the strategic plan. Core competencies are not stagnant; they change with the organization's strategies. The recruitment, retention, development, and performance management of everyone working in or for the organization plays a key role. Creating a **learning organization**, in which skill development is dynamic, is strategic in and of itself. Understanding how to build quality and safety into structures and processes, knowing the tools and measures to be utilized, knowing how to monitor and analyze performance, and understanding team process, group dynamics, and improvement methods all require learning, which must be included in the organizational development strategies.

Quality is everyone's responsibility. It is a business strategy, or centralized philosophy, with accountability at every service level. Because quality is everyone's job, everyone must be educated and must demonstrate competence about quality—the leadership, the providers, and the customers.

Total Quality Management and Continuous Quality Improvement

The terms **total quality management** (TQM) and **continuous quality improvement** (CQI) have been used interchangeably. TQM is mostly linked with industrial models, whereas CQI has received wide acceptance in healthcare. Because the underpinnings of the two terms are the same, CQI is used throughout the remainder of the chapter.

The basic concepts of CQI are that quality improvement is an ongoing process that utilizes proactive and reactive strategies. The process goes beyond meeting preestablished goals or catching up to the competition; rather, it involves exceeding expectations and creating new opportunities. Improvements can be large-scale or incremental. Quality is defined as satisfying the needs of external and internal customers, including anticipating developing needs and introducing new services. Teamwork is the underlying framework. Improvement activities and measurement are always linked, because without measurement we cannot be sure that improvement has occurred.

Additionally, measurement keeps teams focused on concrete opportunities and provides feedback regarding which core strategies helped achieve the vision and mission of the organization. Choosing measures to analyze internal trends may precede the need for external comparisons. **Benchmarking**, the process of comparing with the best of the industry, requires understanding of statistical methods, including the validity and reliability of the tools and measures used in both organizations, understanding systems variation, and sampling methods.

Transition from Quality Assurance to Continuous Quality Improvement

The traditional model of **quality assurance** (QA)—relying on inspection to catch problems and correcting individual performances—has already evolved in many segments of the healthcare industry. The expectation of perfection is gone, but the search for safety and excellence is essential.

To assume that the journey through quality assurance was wasted fails to recognize that many of the tools used in quality assurance are still used in quality improvement, and the journey helped define what constitutes quality care. There are many differences, however. CQI is widely recognized as being broader in scope, involving the leadership and many more people, and blurring boundaries. The Joint Commission uses the term performance improvement (PI) to integrate the concepts and activities of both QA and CQI. The PI standards support the role of leadership in priority setting and systems development, data collection, and data analysis to identify trends, patterns, and opportunities for improvement.

It is important to understand that the evaluation of individual performance must continue. Standards for hiring competent team members are more important than ever. Results of individual performance should be looked at for trends across shifts, units, and departments. Findings can be used for staff and leadership development. Individual competence remains a professional obligation. The shift in focus from individual to team does not change our standards or our accountability to those we serve. Department- or unit-based quality programs remain valuable and should not be demolished. They are an important vehicle for teaching the concepts of CQI and provide needed mechanisms for ongoing measurement and application of standards. They also recognize that much improvement does not require large teams but can occur at the unit level.

Risk management evaluates the legal standards and their application to the delivery of care, the environment of care, and other services and functions. As with quality assurance, it relies on inspection; however, the focus is on how to protect the assets of the organization against liability. Table 13.1 highlights the differences and similarities between quality improvement, quality assurance, and risk management.

An example of how the same problem may be approached differently with the three approaches is in dealing with a medication error. In the environment of quality improvement, the investigation will search for what system weaknesses may have contributed to the error: Is the dispensing system weak? Are high-risk medications kept separate? and so on. At the unit level, quality assurance may investigate the individual nurse's competencies and performance. In the risk management arena, the focus may be on documentation problems that could be discoverable in court in a malpractice claim.

Putting a Continuous Quality Improvement Structure in Place

It is now widely accepted that quality journeys are lengthy and costly. They require a well-developed structure and plan to connect the vision with the implementation. Because CQI is, first and foremost, a management philosophy, the leaders must be competent in its principles and methodologies.

The actual mechanisms of setting up the program are beyond the scope of this chapter. Creating a structure usually involves a quality council and designation of a CQI coach. The coach functions as the facilitator, educator, and expert in tools and techniques. For organizations seeking Joint Commission accreditation, well-established guidelines and widely used tools are readily available. The function of the council is to create integration, prioritize efforts, allocate resources, develop a learning organization, and charter cross-functional teams. The journey is usually expected to take between three and five years, depending on the resources available and the readiness for change.

Leaders and followers alike need to internalize the new beliefs and learn to use the new techniques and tools. Many organizations fail in the quest to implement the new quality organization because the efforts are all focused on the beginning of the journey. **Just-in-time learning**, the process of acquiring knowledge and skills as they are needed and used, tends to eliminate the feeling that CQI may be another managerial gimmick gone awry.

Another common mistake is the failure to prioritize efforts. Improvement activities require resources and should be linked to strategic objectives, serious quality and safety concerns, or identified needs. Quality costs money, especially in the time and effort of human resources, and few organizations can afford to attempt to improve on all

TABLE 13.1

Comparing Quality Improvement, Quality Assurance, and Risk Management

Quality Improvement	Quality Assurance	Risk Management
Broad in scope	Based at unit or departmental level	Often its own, separate department
Organizational leadership designs and sets priorities	Often uses separate department or committee to design and set priorities	Looks at legally acceptable level of care or service
Purpose is improvement	Compares against standards	Purpose is risk reduction
Focus is on customers	Focus is on the organization	Focus is on preventing loss
Uses problems as opportunities for improvement	Continuous ongoing monitoring identifies problems (inspection)	Continuous ongoing monitoring (inspection)
Focus is on the system as a whole	Focus is on individual performance	Focus is on protecting organization's assets

fronts at once. However, safety is of primary concern. Ultimately leaders, including nursing leaders at the unit, organizational, and systems level are responsible for setting priorities and for providing resources that support safety and quality.

A CALL TO SAFETY

We have seen nursing and healthcare change radically in recent years with care that must be framed in the context of safety, evidence-based practice, and patient involvement. This imperative requires acute attention to safety and a new vision of the culture of healthcare.

Health professions and consumers of healthcare were alarmed with the release of reports from the Institute of Medicine (IOM) of the National Academies on the high incidence of medical errors. There was a definite call to improve safety to patients, and the IOM continued this important work identifying rules for healthcare, overall aims, and core competencies for health professionals. Patient safety and effectiveness of outcomes became major national objectives and directed additional attention to nursing. Research by the Agency for Healthcare Research and Quality (AHRQ) has focused on expanding the knowledge base on how the quality of the healthcare workplace affected the quality of healthcare provided, especially in the areas of workload and working conditions, effects of stress and fatigue, reducing adverse events, and the organizational climate and culture. Patient outcomes were now being investigated, along with nursing-sensitive indicators and factors that promote safe and effective practice. In late 2003, nursing itself was the focus of the IOM in their report, *Keeping Patients Safe: Transforming the Work Environment of Nurses.* The IOM's Committee on the Work Environment and Patient Safety provided specific recommendations to both acute care and long-term care organizations on issues of management practices, workforce capability, work design, and the organizational safety culture (Page, 2004, p. 3). At the same time, another report from the IOM, *Patient Safety: Achieving a New Standard of Care*, was released with the focus on data standards for patient safety—i.e., standardized representations of clinical data important to systems that promote patient safety or, in essence, a new health information infrastucture to support safety programs nationally (Committee on Data Standards for Patient Safety, 2004, p. 40).

In subsequent years, the IOM investigated health disparities, the role of the government (including Medicare), rural health, healthcare reimbursement practices, and mental health conditions among other quality improvement initiatives. Of particular note was a study mandated by the United States Congress on preventing medication errors. In July 2006, the IOM report released on *Preventing Medication Errors* presented information available on the incidence of medication errors in acute care settings, long-term care, and in ambulatory care—including errors in the homes of consumers—in an effort to develop an agenda for the nation to reduce preventable errors and adverse drug events and enhance medication safety. Although the incidence rates were approximated based on the data, the report did emphasize that these rates were most likely underestimates, based on available and reportable data and the incidence of adverse events. It was reported, however, that at least 25 percent of all harmful adverse drug events are preventable (Aspden et al., 2006, p. 4).

Based on the ten rules from the earlier *Quality Chasm* report in 2001, the IOM (Aspden et al., 2006) recommended the transformation of the entire system to a patient-centered, integrated-use system with specific action agendas to support the consumer-provider partnership for healthcare organizations; the pharmaceutical, medical device, and health information technology industries; research on safe medication use; and oversight, regulation, and payment.

The IOM (Aspden et al., 2006) focused further on these seven recommendations:

- Consumer empowerment for self-medication management
- Improvement and standardization of resources by governmental agencies
- Implementation of patient-information and decision-support technologies nationwide
- Improved labeling, packaging, and distribution, including studies on use of samples
- Standards for drug information technologies, including design and alert systems
- Funded research on safe and appropriate medication use across settings, especially on error prevention
- Adoption of broad practices, technologies, and professional behaviors focused on safety and error reduction

In the past, errors resulted in incident reports and someone being identified as the cause. Such finger-pointing at an individual or individuals promotes a culture of blame. This culture and associated practices did not generally yield improvements but, rather, loss of opportunities to make improvements and, at times, secretive practices. Consumers, insurers, and the media became concerned for safety and often questioned too much or too little care and testing. Systemic issues in the healthcare environment were now questioned and targeted for improvement. In a report on *Leadership in Healthcare Organizations* addressing the hospital culture and system performance, five key systems were identified for improving safety and quality of care: "using data, planning, communicating, changing performance, and staffing" (Schyve, 2009, p. 19). Further, in a meta-analysis review of the patient safety literature designed to describe the patient safety "culture," Sammer, Lykens, Singh, Mains, and Lackan (2010) identified the following themes as "subcultures":

- Leadership
- Teamwork
- Evidence-based practice
- Communication
- Learning
- Just Culture
- Patient-centered care (p. 157)

We have entered the culture of safety, in which the environment and the entire system is the focus to allow healthcare providers and consumers to address quality improvement. For years, safety investigations in healthcare, with the goal of quality improvement, have investigated a broad range of safety concepts, including information and applications from the aviation industry in their quest to make air travel safer. Crew Resource Management (CRM) is a safety system used by multiple industries in which human error can have devastating effects. The Federak Aviation Administration (FAA) defines CRM as "the effective utilization of all available resources—Hardware, software, and personnel—to achieve safe, efficient flight operations" (Driskell and Adams, 1992, p. 8). It is an integrated training, process improvement, and management system with roots in aviation but recommended by the Joint Commission for preventing patient injury. The purpose is to create a culture of open communication among team members, to provide a framework for an approach to procedures, especially in high-risk, highly chaotic environments, that is standardized, thorough, and routine. The recent reports on healthcare environments demonstrated the change of focus from an individual causative agent to an environmental practice that needed to change. Concerted efforts must now be collaborative among professionals, governmental agencies, suppliers, educators, and regulators, with the consumer involved in the process. We have moved from a culture of blaming isolated individuals to a culture of safety, or a Just Culture. Sammer et al. (2010) have defined a **Just Culture** as "a culture that recognizes errors as a system failure rather than individual failures and, at the same time, does not shrink from holding individuals accountable for their actions" (p. 157). Further, in their position paper endorsing the Just Culture concept, the American Nurses Association (ANA, 2010) stated, "By promoting system improvements over individual punishment, a *Just Culture* in healthcare does much to improve patient safety, reduce errors, and give nurses and other health care workers a major stake in the improvement process" (p. 7). The focus is firmly on safety, positive patient outcomes, evidence-based practice, and continuous quality improvement.

Healthcare Safety Initiatives

Ongoing efforts have been mandated to provide a safer healthcare environment. We have seen the Joint Commission's focus on safety and the quality of patient care move from not only the performance of the entire agency and system with periodic onsite reviews and annual reports to the inclusion of safety statistics and annual performance on specified accountability measures. We have also seen the implementation of various safety initiatives, including physician order entry, bar coding, intensivists, and limitations on abbreviations that lead to errors. In 2004, the Joint Commission (2013c) published the official "DO NOT USE" list in an effort to further reduce medication errors from faulty or misinterpreted orders.

As part of the safety movement, annual healthcare safety goals for the various healthcare agencies have been specified. For example, the goals for acute care hospitals include accurate patient identification, improved staff communication, safe medication practices, using alarms safely, prevention of infections, identification of patient safety risks as in suicide prevention, and prevention of mistakes in surgery (Joint Commission, 2014e). Evidence-based practice is a vital component of these goals and the quest to improve safety.

When an error or adverse event occurs, it is not a matter of completing an incident report but conducting a careful analysis of the event. The Joint Commission (2013g) defines a **sentinel event** as "an unexpected occurrence involving death or serious physical or psychological injury, or the risk thereof . . . [and] signal the need for immediate investigation and response" (p. 1). (See Box 13.4.) The investigation in the case of a sentinel event takes the form of a special analysis. A **root cause analysis** is an intensive questioning into the cause of a problem, with the goals of providing corrective action, eliminating the problem from recurrence, and instilling quality improvements. This type of intensive analysis considers the entire system, not just individuals. It considers what happened, why it happened, and the causative factors, including factors relating to the following:

• Human beings, including communication, leadership, and management practices

ONLINE CONSULT

The Joint Commission: National Patient Safety Goals at
http://www.jointcommission.org/standards _information/npsgs.aspx

---

BOX 13.4 Types of Reportable Sentinel Events in Hospitals (Joint Commission, 2013g)

• An unanticipated death or major permanent loss of function not related to the natural course of the patient's illness or underlying condition
• Suicide of any patient receiving care in a staffed, 24-hour setting within 72 hours of discharge
• Discharge of infant to the wrong family
• Abduction of any patient receiving care, treatment, and services
• Hemolytic transfusion reaction from blood group incompatibilities
• Invasive procedure, including surgery, on the wrong patient, at the wrong site, or using the wrong procedure
• Prolonged fluoroscopy
• Rape, assault (leading to permanent loss of function), or homicide of any patient receiving care or of a staff member, licensed independent practitioner, visitor, or vendor while on site at the healthcare organization
• Severe neonatal hyperbilirubinemia
• Unanticipated death of a full-term infant
• Unintended retention of a foreign body in a patient after surgery or other invasive procedures

---

ONLINE CONSULT

The Joint Commission: Do Not Use List at
http://www.jointcommission.org/about_us /patient_safety_fact_sheets.aspx

- Equipment, both in terms of proper operation and as contributor to the problem
- Environment, especially those that can be controlled

To assist in the process, special teams are involved, software and consultants may be used, and forms and matrices to assist in the analysis are available on the Joint Commission Web site. The result is the development of an action plan to prevent recurrence of the sentinel event. In addition, the Joint Commission (2013g) has policies and procedures for sentinel events and encourages organizations to report sentinel events and the results of the root cause analysis to be shared with other organizations and interested parties in a special newsletter alert.

Notice that the effort is on problem-solving and finding solutions rather than blaming individuals. Recall that a system has inputs, throughputs, and outputs. In this case, the sentinel event was an output from the system as an adverse event. The people involved, the processes that took place, and the equipment and environmental factors are scrutinized. However, the healthcare professionals are still accountable for actions and decisions.

The Joint Commission is one of many organizations that actively promote patient safety. ANA has long focused on safety and quality improvement for the profession and for consumers. ANA's National Center for Nursing Quality (NCNQ®) addresses both the safety and quality of nursing care for patients and the quality of the nurses' work environments. As described, in the mid 1990s, as part of a safety and quality initiative, ANA began research on nursing-sensitive indicators that looks at care and patient outcomes most affected by nursing care. A database has been developed and continues to be tested nationwide on these nursing-sensitive indicators. ANA (2006) has also developed a position paper on the association between patient safety and healthy nursing work hours to ensure that nurses have adequate resources especially in terms of scheduling, sufficient compensation, and appropriate staffing.

A notable leader for quality and safety in healthcare has been the Leapfrog group, formally established after the IOM report on patient safety. This organization is made up of major corporate leaders and employers (such as Aetna, Dow Chemical, FedEx, Toyota, Verizon, and many others) who want the most for their employees, in terms of both safety and purchasing power. They reward best practices and publish "report cards" on provider performance. The Leapfrog Group (2014) has identified four basic quality practices, called "leaps," based on the safety research:

- Computerized physician order entry (CPOE) systems
- Staffing ICUs with intensivists
- Referrals to hospitals with the best results for treating certain high-risk conditions
- Implementation of the Leapfrog Safe Practices, endorsed by the National Quality Forum (NQF)

Hospitals are scored on their safety records and the implementation of these proven safe practices. The major corporate members are also purchasers for healthcare, and they want the best for their purchasing power.

The NQF has endorsed selected safe practices in healthcare as they address the quality of healthcare in the nation. With a broader composition of both public and private partners, including organizations and national, state, and local governmental agencies, the NQF (2014) describes its mission to lead "national collaboration to improve health and healthcare quality through measurement" (p. 1). Current topics of focus include affordable care, effective communication and care coordination, health and well-being, patient safety, person- and family-centered care, and prevention and treatment of cardiovascular disease (NQF, 2014).

The Institute for Healthcare Improvement (IHI) is a not-for-profit organization focused on patient safety and quality improvement worldwide. This organization strives to build awareness through education, collaborative improvement, and system redesign to promote quality improvement for worldwide healthcare community. It focuses on best practices and sharing the information and unifying the healthcare industry on quality improvement. The IHI (2014) identifies its aims to "improve health and health care worldwide" (p. 1).

Many more organizations, groups, and individuals are actively pursuing patient safety at the local, state, national, and international levels. The few that have been described here will lead to other collaborations and initiatives focused on the quality and safety in healthcare.

TOOLS AND TECHNIQUES USED IN QUALITY IMPROVEMENT

An entire body of knowledge has been created in the area of valid techniques to be used for improving quality. Innovation requires team techniques such as brainstorming, boarding, decision matrices, multi-voting, management of conflict, and quality communication.

Process Teams

Not all improvement projects require a process team. If the project or problem crosses functions and disciplines

---

ONLINE CONSULT

Agency for Healthcare Research and Quality at
http://www.ahrq.gov/qual/

American Nurses Association at
http://www.nursingworld.org/MainMenu
Categories/ThePracticeofProfessionalNursing
/PatientSafetyQuality

Institute for Healthcare Improvement at
http://www.ihi.org/ihi

Joint Commission at
http://www.jointcommission.org

Leapfrog Group at
http://www.leapfroggroup.org

National Patient Safety Foundation at
http://www.npsf.org

National Quality Forum at
http://www.qualityforum.org

and cannot be resolved in the day-to-day operations, a process team is usually necessary. These "project" teams focus on improving or developing specific processes and come together to achieve a specific goal, such as analyzing variation, and have a beginning and an end. **Process teams** must be chosen carefully to represent those involved in or affected by the process. If the team is very large, the project chosen may be too big and may have to be broken into steps.

How, then, does one choose an improvement project? Listen to your customers. Repeated complaints or requests for a particular service may require action. Suppose the evening charge nurse in a nonsectarian hospital receives ongoing requests for pastoral services from patients and their families. Each request requires multiple telephone calls and often results in delays. The nurse recognizes that the nursing department cannot address this problem alone. It involves not only the hospital but also the community. The nurse develops a proposal for a process team. Other methods for selecting or recognizing processes to be improved include asking the people in the process, reviewing existing reports, and recognizing excess complexity or long delays.

Process teams require resources. Because resource allocation is a leadership function, many organizations require the development of a proposal and subsequent approval by the quality council. All teams should develop an opportunity statement (what is wrong or needs improving), define the expected output of the project, and include measures of success. Members of the team must include, at a minimum, a team leader who is invested in the process, a facilitator who brings CQI skills, and a recorder or minute taker. Depending on the skills and information systems available, analytical and statistical support may be necessary.

Because process teams are groups, they will need to go through the stages of group development—forming, storming, norming, performing, adjourning. (Refer to Chapter 8 on Working with Groups.) All teams must mature to perform. It is important to recognize that anxiety, testing of boundaries, competition for control, and minimal completion of work are all part of the early stages. Early cohesiveness and work do not start until the norming stage. Real performance and "team" feeling belong to the performing step. Many teams also struggle with the adjourning phase— namely, meeting the final deadlines and dissolving the group.

The process team must adopt a model or method for doing its work. This model is usually organization-wide. There is value in choosing one model, because it minimizes

ONLINE CONSULT

The PDCA cycle at
http://www.isixsigma.com/dictionary/deming
-cycle-pdca/
http://asq.org/learn-about-quality/project
-planning-tools/overview/pdca-cycle.html

relearning and allows different teams to communicate easily. Some common models are the Juran (1989) quality improvement project model and Deming's (1982, 1986) PDCA (Plan-Do-Check-Act) cycle.

Quality Improvement Tools

Quality improvement (QI) tools can usually be divided into four categories, those used for:

● Process description
● Data collection
● Data analysis
● Process improvement

Many excellent texts provide further assistance in this area. The ultimate purpose of all the **QI tools** is to have data that can be used and translated into information. The novice in QI tools and techniques may need assistance from the CQI coach or further study of these techniques.

Process Description Tools

One tool for process description is the **flow chart**, which describes the process in detail, from beginning to end, as accurately as possible. It is a picture of the movement of information, people, or materials. The top-down flow chart (Figure 13.1) takes the major steps in the process, writes them in a horizontal sequence, and illustrates the substeps to be taken under each step. Flow charts show the rework that gets done, the number of substeps or complexity in each area, the number of handoffs between individuals and departments, and when subteams need to be formed from a particular process team. A flow chart that is too detailed makes it difficult to focus and impedes progress or action.

The **cause-and-effect diagram** (Figure 13.2), also called the fishbone or Ishikawa diagram, helps identify the root causes of a problem. Typical categories are equipment, personnel, method, materials, and environment. The main arrow points toward the problem or

STEP 1 →	STEP 2 →	STEP 3 →	STEP 4
Substeps	Substeps	Substeps	Substeps
......	......	......	......
......	......	......	......
......	......	......	......
......	......	......	......

Figure 13.1 Top-down flow chart.

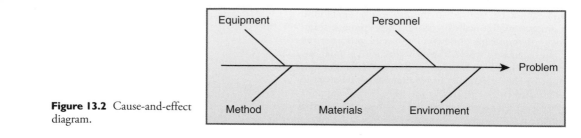

Figure 13.2 Cause-and-effect diagram.

desired result. It is important to remember that cause-and-effect diagrams point only toward possible causes, and more data must be collected to identify the root causes. Cause-and-effect diagrams are most effective after the process has been described, because flow charts help identify what must be included in the diagram.

Tools for Data Collection

Tools for data collection include asking the right questions, and using, among other things, data sheets, check sheets, surveys, focus groups, and interviews. Often, data are collected that turn out to be useless because the question asked was wrong, too broad, or poorly formulated. Data sheets and check sheets are both used to record data (Figure 13.3). They differ in that **data sheets** need further analysis. Ordinarily, a data sheet is completed for each occurrence or event in the study. The data are subsequently aggregated and then sorted according to categories of interest.

Check sheets are used to record multiple events by simply putting a mark in the appropriate box. The best check sheets are those that are easy to use, do not require much interpretation, and visually display the data. An example in which either tool could be used is the study of the delivery time of medications to a patient care unit. With data sheets, every time a medication is taken from the pharmacy, the runner uses a new data sheet. At the end of the study, all the sheets are gathered and analyzed. With the check sheet, the runner could calculate the time it took to deliver the drug and check the appropriate time box on a check sheet. Both data sheets and check sheets may be either in hard or electronic copy.

There are obvious advantages and disadvantages to both tools. Data sheets tend to be more accurate because only one event is recorded on each. Check sheets quickly display trends as they occur without requiring a lengthy analysis. Data sheets and check sheets should be tested before project-wide work is undertaken, so that improvements can be made to ensure that only useful data are collected.

Surveys are a tool for obtaining input from large groups. The response rate and the specificity of the questions affect the usefulness and quality of the information obtained. Focus groups and individual interviews are time-consuming and expensive and may require the use of experienced interviewers, but they enable one to ask open-ended questions and probe deeper, if necessary.

Data Analysis Tools

Tools for data analysis include those that compare categories. Bar and pie charts and the Pareto diagram (Figure 13.4), for example, analyze data within a category, such as numerical and graphic summaries. The Pareto principle, sometimes called the 80/20 rule, was applied to management by Juran. It identifies the few sources of problems that contribute most to the outcome. By ranking problems on a bar graph in descending order, from left to right, Pareto diagrams focus attention on the most common problems and often build consensus about where to concentrate attention and effort.

Analysis of a particular category can include numerical summaries such as average, median, mode, and standard deviation. Graphic summaries—line graphs, histograms, scatter diagrams, and control charts—are especially valuable for working in diverse groups. They provide pictorial display of data, possible analysis and interpretation of patterns, relationships between variables, and the ability to distinguish between common and special cause variation.

Improvement Activities

Criteria-based information and tools are essential in evidence-based practice, performance improvement, and patient safety initiatives. The AHRQ launched its Web site in 2003 as a repository of practical, ready-to-use tools for assessing, measuring, and improving the quality and safety of healthcare.

DEVELOPING A MEASUREMENT PROGRAM

As previously mentioned, improvement and measurement or evaluation are linked. Measurement of the capability of the organization, or its competence, determines the organization's ability to provide, and competence in providing, quality and safe care. Measurement of outcome determines whether the process yielded favorable results. For example, the Breast Care Clinic used as an earlier

ONLINE CONSULT

Agency for Healthcare Research and Quality: Health IT Tools and Resources at **http://healthit.ahrq.gov/health-it-tools-and-resources**

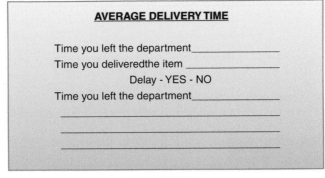

A   **DATA SHEET**

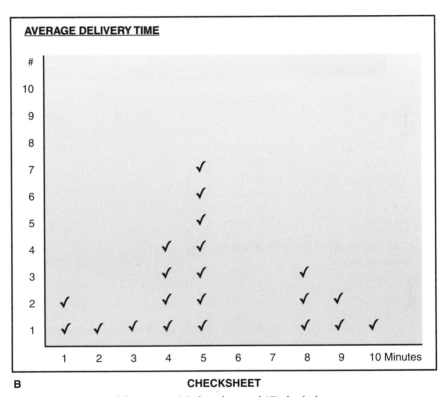

B   **CHECKSHEET**

Figure 13.3 Average delivery time (*A*) data sheet and (*B*) check sheet.

example will not only focus its review on the ability to report examination results within 24 hours and on whether there is a system in place allowing women to self-refer for mammography, it will also measure whether these outcomes actually occur.

Selecting Indicators for Measurement

Indicators are events that are measured. They are categorized by type. They can be structure, process, or outcome indicators chosen in the functions of patient care, services that support the delivery of patient care,

practices, and leadership/governance. *Structure* encompasses the policies or standards regarding how service is delivered and resources made available. *Process* refers to the activities, and *outcome* is the result of activities based on policies, standards, and resources. For example, according to policy, patients receiving conscious sedation shall be monitored by a professional nurse certified in advanced life support (structure), professional nurses competent in advanced life support are hired and credentialed for those services (process), and all patients receiving conscious sedation are monitored according to policy (outcome).

Practice indicators measure professional standards used in the delivery of patient care. Examples of practice

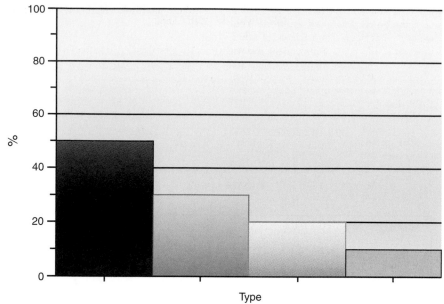

Figure 13.4 Pareto diagram.

indicators include measurement of documentation frequency and content, and utilization of aseptic technique as required. Leadership indicators measure organizational function, namely how the system affects the delivery of care and services.

When standards are clearly written and defined, are valid, and can be measured, indicators are more easily selected and usable. Meaningful indicators are specific, relevant, reliable, valid, and measurable. They use a numerator and denominator, have a target (internal or external benchmark), relate to specific standards, and define where the data or information can be found. For example, the number of individuals monitored by an advanced life support credentialed nurse (numerator) of all the patients receiving conscious sedation (denominator) based on the standard, as documented in the outpatient record.

Many national organizations are currently working on indicators that can be used as external benchmarks, such as the Healthcare Effectiveness Data and Information Set (HEDIS) from the National Committee for Quality Assurance (NCQA). Other professional groups continue to refine and expand the available indicators. Utilizing external performance measures exclusively is not sufficient. Internal performance indicators based on the scope of service, mission, vision, strategic plans, core competencies, organizational culture, and values ensure that overall organizational effectiveness is measured. In turn, external benchmarks compare that performance with the best in the industry. As previously stated, the Joint Commission's work started around the identification, implementation, and use of standardized tools for measuring and improving patient care. By 2004, the implementation of core measures in all acute care hospitals was implemented, with the goal for expansion into other clinical areas

ONLINE CONSULT

National Committee for Quality Assurance: HEDIS at
http://www.ncqa.org/tabid/59/Default.aspx

The Joint Commission at
http://www.jointcommission.org/performance_measurement.aspx

and further study these measures. The focus on understanding quality and safety continues with transparency to consumers.

Understanding Variation

Variation is part of any process. People, equipment, supplies, procedures, techniques, and inaccuracies in the data all contribute to variation in data from an otherwise stable process. *Common-cause variation* is the ongoing, minute variations that are part of nature. *Special-cause variation* is much larger and can be attributed more easily to contributors through statistical methods such as run charts and control charts. These charts can monitor processes because, even though individual data points may be unpredictable, a fluctuating pattern will emerge over time. The normal pattern is bell-shaped, meaning that most points are near the center.

The manager of a process must know when to react to particular data or situations and when it is necessary to improve the entire process. For example, suppose you have monitored medication errors on your unit for many months. When you calculate the number of errors over the number of doses administered, a percentage ranging between 0.01 and 0.02 percent emerges. This is probably the common-cause type of variation. You may want to compare that figure against those of other local institutions, of similar type or size, to evaluate whether this is an acceptable error rate. If, for the first time ever, you see a rise to 0.03 percent, it would be wise to analyze the data further before taking action or deciding to wait. Are all the errors of the same type attributable to a few individuals, or have new systems been introduced? Constant tinkering with systems, without understanding what the causes of the variation are, destabilizes the process. Understanding variation is important. Common-cause variation requires an answer to the question "Is this level acceptable when looked at over time?" Special-cause variation needs careful evaluation to identify the cause and make appropriate, focused interventions. And there is a directive to ensure that these interventions are safe for the consumers of healthcare, whether through actions by healthcare providers or by the consumer once back in the community or home setting.

CONTINUOUS QUALITY IMPROVEMENT IN CONTEXT

CQI in practice requires a number of cost and implementation considerations and varies significantly with the context of the healthcare organization. The rapid changes in healthcare and the added focus on patient safety have required redesign of its delivery. We have a professional obligation to ensure that the way we deliver care is evaluated along the continuum. Despite our frustration with cost containment efforts, we must prudently manage resources to enable us to provide the greatest benefit safely to the largest number of patients possible. We may need to develop new delivery models that optimize the role of the professional nurse, delegate tasks, and meet the needs of our customers.

Case management and work redesign have been used across the country for delivery redesign. Case management requires collaboration in the process of providing options for services that meet an individual's health needs and that promote quality and safe cost-effective outcomes. Critical pathways are tools commonly used in this process. Brainstorming, data-driven decision making, consensus seeking, process flow charting, evaluation of costs, and satisfaction are all tools used in case new quality model.

Work redesign—the process of analyzing how work is done and what system changes need to be implemented to achieve effective and efficient care delivery—also requires quality to be built in up front. Professionals need to participate actively in this evolving course. Reliance on inspection and control will not ensure delivery of quality care. Simultaneously, we cannot insist on doing it the old way. Review of studies on the implementation of redesign activities demonstrate that many focused largely on increasing efficiency and that the changes may not have been managed effectively, resulting in loss of trust in the administration and reduction of clinical nursing leadership (Page, 2004).

> Brainstorming, data-driven decision making, consensus seeking, process flow charting, evaluation of costs, and satisfaction are all tools used in case management as well as in the new quality model.

Continuous Quality Improvement in the Managed Care World

Managed care has received some favor as a methodology for controlling escalating healthcare costs. Buyers of managed care, such as employers and state and federal governments, have something to say about quality, access, choice, and satisfaction with services. The more competitive the environment becomes, the more important demonstrated quality will become, to differentiate between one contract or provider and another. The managed care industry is already developing nationally accepted outcomes and indicators. Report cards on customer satisfaction with individual providers and organizations have gained popularity. Nursing must take an aggressive professional role in ensuring that the data on care delivery reflect direct nursing care delivery, coordination provided by nursing, patient and family teaching, and nursing management along the continuum of care delivery. Recommendations on the need to develop reliable and valid methods to measure nursing care requirements and minimum staffing levels in acute care and long-term care are considered essential (Page, 2004). As more research evolves on the nurse-sensitive indicators, further evidence-based practice can evolve in this area.

Ongoing Role for Regulatory Agencies

Agencies such as the Joint Commission, professional review organizations (PROs), and state and federal government will continue to have a significant role in the assurance that quality, safe healthcare is delivered. Many of the organizations actively collecting benchmarking information. The Joint Commission, in particular, acts as an external change agent with regard to guaranteeing that all providers accept and implement the new paradigm. The hospital associations are helping their members deal with uniform responses to the report cards required by many managed care contracts. Regulators and providers alike are struggling with the implementation of significant change in the delivery of quality healthcare. As noted by Amer (2013), quality "is not a finite goal but rather an ongoing process that is subject to the changing needs of society and the knowledge, expertise, and creativity of the healthcare team and the scientific community" (p. 236). The goal is for continuous quality improvement for patient safety and efficacy of healthcare outcomes.

EVIDENCE-BASED PRACTICE: *Consider this....*

In 2013, the Joint Commission (2013f) issued an alert on medical device safety in the hospital based on research over a 3-year period and identified the following major causal factors from 98 reported events:

- Absent or inadequate alarm system

- Improper alarm settings

- Alarm signals not audible in all areas

- Alarm signals inappropriately turned off

Alarm fatigue was identified as the most common contributing factor (Joint Commission, 2013f, p. 2). The recommendations can be reviewed at **http://www.jointcommission.org/assets/1/18/SEA_50_alarms _4_5_13_FINAL1.PDF**

Question: Have there been any of these events in your hospital over the past year? Who oversees medical device and alarm safety at your organization? What is the level of risk in patient care units, intensive care units, and the emergency department? And, how can you be involved in policy development for promoting medical device alarm safety in your organization?

Joint Commission. (2013f). *Sentinel event alert: Medical device safety in hospitals*, issue 50, April 8, 2013. Retrieved from http://www.jointcommission .org/assets/1/18/SEA_50_alarms_4_5_13_FINAL1.PDF

KEY POINTS

- Rapid changes in healthcare have prompted a new way of doing business.

- Reliance on inspection and control against pre-established standards (the traditional quality assurance model), although of ongoing value, is no longer sufficient.

- Quality models, such as Deming's Principles for Transformation, the Juran Trilogy, and the requirements for accreditation by the Joint Commission provide an excellent foundation for improving quality of care.

- Quality improvement does not just entail correcting problems but also requires ongoing improvement.

- Specific knowledge, tools, and techniques are required to create a new quality and include cross-functional teamwork, lifelong learning, and process improvement.

- Process teams are required for those improvement activities that cross functions and disciplines and cannot be dealt with in the day-to-day operations.

- Variation is part of all processes. It requires statistical analysis before actions that may destabilize the process are taken.

- Benchmarking is the process of comparison with the best practices in the industry.

- Tools for improvement can be divided into four categories: those used for process description, such as flow charts and cause-and-effect diagrams; those used for data collection, such as data sheets and check sheets; those used for data analysis, such as bar and pie charts and the Pareto diagram; and those used for process improvement.

- In the "culture of blame," someone is traditionally identified as the cause of an adverse event. Systemic issues are questioned and targeted for improvement in the "culture of safety," in which the environment and the entire system is the focus to allow healthcare providers and consumers to address quality improvement.

- Sammer et al. (2010) have defined *Just Culture* as "a culture that recognizes errors as a system failure rather than individual failures and, at the same time, does not shrink from holding individuals accountable for their actions" (p. 157).

- The Joint Commission (2013g) defines a sentinel event as "an unexpected occurrence involving death or serious physical or psychological injury, or the risk thereof" (p. 1).

- A root cause analysis is an intensive questioning into the cause of a problem with the goals of providing corrective action, eliminating the problem from recurrence, and instilling quality improvements.

- To improve quality, you must improve the system.

Thought and Discussion Questions

1. You are the nurse manager of an ambulatory surgery unit. Recently, you have seen a sudden rise in the number of surgical patients coming through the unit. Simultaneously, patients, physicians, and other providers have started to complain about long delays during pretesting.
   - Would you attempt to fix this problem by addressing it during a staff meeting? Why or why not?
   - Compare how to address this problem using a process team versus using the staff meeting approach.
   - Describe how you would analyze the process.
   - Explain which tools are appropriate to use for the analysis.

2. A sentinel event has just been identified at your hospital and you have been identified to serve on the team conducting a root cause analysis. Choose a sentinel event from the list provided in Box 13.4. Describe the process for the root cause analysis and suggest learning strategies for staff for continuous quality improvement.

3. To foster professional accountability, discuss how you would plan and implement an interdisciplinary staff education session on Just Culture. Be prepared to participate in an online or class discussion on this topic, to be scheduled by your instructor.

4. Discuss the Chapter Thought located on the first page of the chapter and discuss it (online or in class) in the context of the contents of the chapter.

Interactive Exercises

Go to the Intranet site and complete the interactive exercises provided for this chapter.

REFERENCES

Agency for Healthcare Research and Quality (AHRQ). (2013). *National healthcare quality report 2013*. Retrieved from http://www.ahrq.gov/research/findings/nhqrdr/index.html

Amer, K. S. (2013). *Quality and safety for transformational nursing: Core competencies*. Boston, MA: Pearson.

American Association of Colleges of Nursing (AACN). (2008). *The essentials of baccalaureate education for professional nursing practice*. Washington, DC: Author.

American Nurses Association (ANA). (2006). *Assuring patient safety: The employer's role in promoting healthy nursing work hours for registered nurses in all roles and settings*. Retrieved from http://www.nursingworld.org/MainMenuCategories/Policy-Advocacy/Positions-and-Resolutions/ANAPositionStatements/Position-Statements-Alphabetically/AssuringPatientSafety.pdf

American Nurses Association. (2010). *Position statement: Just culture*. Retrieved from http://www.nursingworld.org/MainMenuCategories/Policy-Advocacy/Positions-and-Resolutions/ANAPositionStatements/Position-Statements-Alphabetically/Just-Culture.html

Aspden, P., Wolcott, J., Bootman, L., & Cronenwett, L. R. (Eds.). (2006). *Preventing medication errors*. Washington, DC: National Academies Press.

Centers for Medicare and Medicaid Services (CMS). (2009). *Roadmap for implementing value driven healthcare in the traditional Medicare fee-for-service program*. Retrieved from http://www.cms.gov/Medicare/Quality-Initiatives-Patient-Assessment-Instruments/QualityInitiativesGenInfo/Downloads/RoadmapOverview_OEA_1-16.pdf

Centers for Medicare and Medicaid Services (CMS). (2013). *Medicare hospital quality chartbook: Performance report on outcome measures*. Retrieved from https://www.cms.gov/Medicare/Quality-Initiatives-Patient-Assessment-Instruments/HospitalQualityInits/Downloads/

Cronenwett, L., Sherwood, G., Barnsteiner, J., Disch, J., Johnson, J., Mitchell, P., . . . Warren, J. (2007). Quality and safety education for nurses. *Nursing Outlook, 55*, 122–131.

Driskell, J. E, & Adams, R. J. (1991). *Crew resource management: A introductory handbook*. Springfield, VA: National Technical Information Service. Retrieved from http://aireform.com/wp-content/uploads/19920800..-CRM-Handbook-contracted-for-FAA.pdf

Institute for Healthcare Improvement (IHI). (2014). *IHI vision and values*. Retrieved from http://www.ihi.org/about/pages/ihivisionandvalues.aspx

Institute of Medicine (IOM). (2000). *To err is human: Building a safer health system*. Washington, DC: National Academy Press.

Institute of Medicine (IOM). (2001). *Crossing the quality chasm: A new health system for the 21st century*. Retrieved from http://books.nap.edu/openbook.php?record_id=10027&page=232

Institute of Medicine (IOM). (2011). *The future of nursing: Leading change, advancing health*. Retrieved from http://books.nap.edu/openbook.php?record_id=12956

Joint Commission. (2010). The evolution of performance measurement at The Joint Commission 1986-2010: A visioning document. Retrieved from http://www.jointcommission.org/performance_measurement.aspx

Joint Commission. (2013a). Benefits of Joint Commission accreditation. Retrieved from http://www.jointcommission.org/benefits_of_joint_commission_accreditation/

Joint Commission. (2013b). Facts about the national patient safety goals. Retrieved from http://www.jointcommission.org/standards_information/npsgs.aspx

Joint Commission. (2013c). Facts about the official "do not use" list. Retrieved from http://www.jointcommission.org/assets/1/18/Do_Not_Use_List.pdf

Joint Commission. (2013d). Facts about ORYX® for hospitals (national hospital quality measures). Retrieved from http://www.jointcommission.org/facts_about_oryx_for_hospitals/

Joint Commission. (2013e). Root cause analysis and action plan framework template. Retrieved from http://www.jointcommission.org/sentinel_event.aspx

Joint Commission. (2013f). Sentinel event alert: Medical device safety in hospitals, Issue 50, April 8, 2013. Retrieved from http://www.jointcommission.org/assets/1/18/SEA_50_alarms_4_5_13_FINAL1.PDF

Joint Commission. (2013g). Sentinel event policy and procedures. Retrieved from http://www.jointcommission.org/Sentinel_Event_Policy_and_Procedures/

Joint Commission. (2013h). Specifications manual for national hospital inpatient quality measures. Retrieved from http://www.jointcommission.org/specifications_manual_for_national_hospital_inpatient_quality_measures/

Joint Commission. (2014a). Core measure sets. Retrieved from http://www.jointcommission.org/core_measure_sets.aspx

Joint Commission. (2014b). Facts about accountability measures. Retrieved from http://www.jointcommission.org/facts_about_accountability_measures/

Joint Commission. (2014c). Facts about patient safety. Retrieved from http://www.jointcommission.org/about_us/patient_safety_fact_sheets.aspx

Joint Commission. (2014d). Improving America's hospitals: The Joint Commission's annual report on quality and safety 2013. Retrieved from http://www.jointcommission.org/annualreport.aspx

Joint Commission. (2014e). National patient safety goals. Retrieved from http://www.jointcommission.org/standards_information/npsgs.aspx

Juran, J. M. (1989). *Juran on leadership for quality: An executive handbook*. New York: Free Press.

Leapfrog Group. (2014). *The Leapfrog Group fact sheet*. Retrieved from http://www.leapfroggroup.org/about_leapfrog/leapfrog-factsheet

Merriam-Webster Collegiate Dictionary. (2014). Retrieved from http://www.merriam-webster.com/dictionary/quality

National Database of Nursing Quality Indicators (NDNQI). (2014). *About NDNQI*. Retrieved from http://www.nursingquality.org/About-NDNQI

National Quality Forum (2014). *About NQF*. Retrieved from http://www.qualityforum.org/about/

Page, A. (Ed.) (2004). *Keeping Patients Safe: Transforming the Work Environment of Nurses*. Washington, DC: National Academy Press.

Sammer, C. E., Lykens, K., Singh, K. P., Mains, D. A., & Lackan, N. A. (2010). What is patient safety culture? A review of the literature. *Journal of Nursing Scholarship, 42*, 156–165.

Sigma Theta Tau. (2005). *Evidence-based nursing position statement*. Retrieved from http://www.nursingsociety.org/aboutus/PositionPapers/Pages/EBN_positionpaper.aspx

Smith, E. L., Cronenwett, L., & Sherwood, G. (2007). Current assessments of quality and safety education in nursing. *Nursing Outlook, 55*, 132–137.

BIBLIOGRAPHY

Barnsteiner, J. (2011). Teaching the culture of safety. *Online Journal of Issues in Nursing, 16*(3), Manuscript 5. Retrieved from http://www.nursingworld.org/MainMenuCategories/ANAMarketplace/ANAPeriodicals/OJIN/TableofContents/Vol-16-2011/No3-Sept-2011/Teaching-and-Safety.html

Barnsteiner, J., & Disch, J. (2012). Second generation quality and safety education for nurses. *Nursing Clinics of North America, 47*, xi–xiii.

Barnsteiner, J., Disch, J., Johnson, J., McGuinn, K., & Swartwout, E. (2012). Diffusing QSEN competencies across schools of nursing: The AACN/RWJF Faculty Development Institutes. *Journal of Professional Nursing, 29*, 68–74.

Centers for Medicare and Medicaid Services (CMS). (2013). *Medicare hospital quality chartbook: Performance report on outcome measures*. Retrieved from https://www.cms.gov/Medicare/Quality-Initiatives-Patient-Assessment-Instruments/HospitalQualityInits/Downloads/-Medicare-Hospital-Quality-Chartbook-2013.pdf

Chassin, M. R., Loeb, J. M., Schmaltz, S. P., & Wachter, R. M. (2010). Accountability measures: Using measurement to promote quality. *New England Journal of Medicine, 363*, 683–688.

Deming, W. E. (1994). *The new economics for industry, government, education* (2nd ed.). Cambridge, MA: MIT Press.

Hughes, R. G. (ed). (2008). *Patient safety and quality: An evidence-based handbook for nurses* (AHRQ Publication No. 08-0043). Rockville, MD: Agency for Healthcare Quality and Research. Retrieved from http://www.ahrq.gov/qual/nurseshdbk/

Institute of Medicine (IOM). (2010b). Quality and patient safety. Retrieved from http://www.iom.edu/Global/Topics/Quality-Patient-Safety.aspx

International Council of Nurses (ICN). (2012). *ICN position: Patient safety*. Retrieved from http://www.icn.ch/images/stories/documents/publications/position_statements/D05_Patient_Safety.pdf

Juran, J. M. (1988). *Juran on planning for quality*.New York: Free Press.

Nace, J. J. (2008). Why *hospitals should fly: The ultimate flight plan to patient safety and quality care*. Bozeman, MT: Second River Healthcare Press.

Orsini, J. N. (Ed.). (2013). *The essential Deming: Leadership principles from the father of quality*. New York: McGraw-Hill.

National Database of Nursing Quality Indicators (NDNQI). (2014). *Frequently asked questions*. Retrieved from http://www.nursingquality.org/FAQ

National Quality Forum. (2012). *National voluntary consensus standards for patient safety measures: A Consensus report*. Retrieved from http://www.qualityforum.org/Publications/2012/06/National_Voluntary_Consensus_Standards_for_Patient_Safety_Measures_A_Consensus_Report.aspx

President's Council of Advisors on Science and Technology (PCAST). (2014). *Report to the president: Better health care and lower costs: Accelerating improve*ment *through systems engineering*. Retrieved from http://www.whitehouse.gov/sites/default/files/microsites/ostp/PCAST/pcast_systems_engineering_in_healthcare_-_may_2014.pdf

QualityNet. (2014). *Hospital inpatient quality reporting (IQR) program overview.* Retrieved from https://www.qualitynet.org/dcs/ContentServer?c=Page& pagename=QnetPublic%2FPage%2FQnetTier2&cid= 1138115987129

Sullivan, D. T., Hirst, D., & Cronenwett, L. (2009). Assessing quality and safety competencies of graduating prelicensure students. *Nursing Outlook, 57,* 323–331.

ONLINE RESOURCES

American Association of Colleges of Nursing
http://www.aacn.nche.edu/qsen/home

National Committee for Quality Assurance
http://ncqa.org

National Database of Nursing Quality Indicators (NDNQI)
**http://pressganey.com/ourSolutions/performance-and
-advanced-analytics/clinical-business-performance
/nursing-quality-ndnqi**

PDCA Cycle
http://www.isixsigma.com/dictionary/deming-cycle-pdca/
**http://asq.org/learn-about-quality/project-planning-tools
/overview/pdca-cycle.html**
**http://www.ihi.org/resources/Pages/HowtoImprove
/ScienceofImprovementHowtoImprove.aspx**

QSEN Institute
http://qsen.org/

The Institute for Healthcare Improvement (IHI)
http://www.ihi.org/IHI/

The Institute of Medicine
http://www.iom.edu

The Joint Commission
http://www.jointcommission.org

The Joint Commission: Quality Check
http://www.QualityCheck.org

● Rose Kearney-Nunnery

14

Population Health

*"Wherever we look upon this earth,
the opportunities take shape
within the problems."*

Nelson Rockefeller, 1908–1979

On completion of this chapter, the reader will be able to:

1. Describe the national initiatives aimed at improving health equity and reducing health disparities.

2. Identify trends and health needs of our at-risk populations.

3. Discuss strategies for reducing health disparities for at-risk population groups.

4. Discuss the characteristics of the aging population.

5. Examine the issues to address in minority health promotion activities.

6. Contrast urban and rural community needs and resources.

7. Identify the role for professional nurses in community and public health initiatives.

Key Terms

Public Health	Determinants of Health	Minority Health
Population Health	Leading Health Indicators	Health Equity
Healthy People	Topical Areas	Social Determinants of Health
Healthy Communities	Foundational Health Measures	Urbanized Area
Health Promotion Strategies	Aging Adults	Rural Area
Health Protection Strategies	Disability	Rural Health
Preventive Services	Chronicity	Community Health Nursing

Initiatives to address the health and wellness of the public have been in existence for hundreds of years. Recently, however, efforts to address the health of population groups locally, nationally, and globally have become more visible. The mission of **public health** continues to focus on protection of the public from health threats. The Committee for the Study of the Future of Public Health (1988) traced the history of public health in the United States over the past 200 years, from the 18th century efforts directed at control of the spread of diseases like cholera through isolation and quarantine; to the implementation of sanitary standards, water purification, immunization, and the establishment of state health departments; to personal clinical care and health promotion activities of private and governmental agencies in the 20th century. Community health nursing has had a vital role in these activities since the early 20th century when Lillian Wald established the Henry Street Settlement with a focus on immigrant populations, which became the Visiting Nurses Service in New York City. The ultimate aim is to treat and promote health in population groups. As noted by Kindig and Stoddart (2003), **population health** does not have a precise definition but is generally a research approach focused on determinants of health (p. 380). This lack of a precise definition was further supported by the IOM (2014) in its workshop summary and implications with the passage of the Accountable Care Act in 2010.

Population health and measures for the determinants of health have become a constant theme as we strive to improve health status and outcomes and address health disparities. Two major community health initiatives began in the last decades of the 20th century in the United States: *Healthy People* and *Healthy Communities*. The focus became the health of the nation as a whole through concentration on wellness and healthful initiatives as a strategic planning process for disease prevention and health promotion.

As a corollary to this movement, we have seen a greater focus on consumer and public protection. In 1998, the President's Advisory Commission on Consumer Protection and Quality in the Industry presented a report with more than 50 objectives identified to address problem areas, including avoidable errors, both underutilization and overuse of services, and variation in services. Measures proposed to strengthen the healthcare industry included use of group purchasers, having informed consumers with access to services, accountability, reducing errors and increasing safety, and addressing the needs of vulnerable populations. Sources of vulnerability were identified as economic status and geographic location; health, age, and functional or developmental status; communication barriers; and unexplained vulnerability associated with race, ethnicity, and sex (The President's Advisory Commission on Consumer Protection and Quality in the Health Care Industry, 1998, pp. 130–132). At the end of the 20th century and into the next decade, the focus on patient safety was highlighted further with the subsequent Institute of Medicine (IOM) reports on the current state of healthcare for consumers and calls for safety improvements.

The nation's population profile is changing. We are older and more diverse. Although we remain a youth-oriented society, the aging of the baby boomers has had a profound effect on the demographics and the health needs of the population. In addition, we are becoming more culturally diverse and must endeavor to celebrate, respect, and embrace our differences while eliminating health disparities. Professional nursing practice has a vital role in utilizing and expanding knowledge of health determinants, promoting health initiatives, and in eliminating health disparities.

HEALTHY PEOPLE

For *Healthy People 2000* (U.S. Department of Health and Human Services, Public Health Service [USDHHS, PHS], 1992), groups at higher risk were identified as part of the design more extensively than in the 1990 objectives according to demographic and socioeconomic dimensions of risk (p. vii). This focus continued as a national commitment with *Healthy People 2010*, which was introduced in 2000, and *Healthy People 2020*, which was introduced late in 2010. *Healthy Communities* was designed to help implement these objectives in community settings. It became an accepted fact that healthy behaviors and prevention are vital for individuals, families, and society.

In *Healthy People 2000*, three general goals were stated as national health promotion and disease prevention objectives (see Table 14.1). This initiative took a major step in that it did not merely look at the health of the nation, but rather, it devised strategies for improvement. The outcome was the specification of 22 priority areas for health promotion and disease prevention. For each priority area, the workgroup formulated objectives with specific targets to measure success in addressing the three major goals. The priority areas were further classified as health promotion, health protection, and preventive services. Recall the discussion on levels of prevention (primary, secondary, and tertiary) in Chapter 4. The terminology from *Healthy People 2000* (USDHHS, 1992) identified **health promotion strategies** as individual lifestyle and personal choices. Health promotion activities are both protective and preventive, but they require consumers to be actively involved in all levels of prevention. **Health protection strategies** consist of environmental or regulatory measures that confer protection on population groups. **Preventive services** comprise counseling, screening, immunization, and chemoprophylactic interventions.

Findings on the 22 priority areas were reported along with identification of problem areas. For example, in the area of health promotion, in terms of physical activity and fitness and nutrition, they found a decline in coronary deaths but overweight prevalence, iron deficiency, and a need for more physical activity. In addition, health disparities were becoming apparent with the identification of increased pregnancy rates in adolescents, marijuana use in adolescents, increased diabetes, and cirrhosis deaths in certain minority groups.

The initiative also looked at specific age groups (infants, children, adolescents and young adults, adults, and

TABLE 14.1

Overall Goals for *Healthy People* Initiatives, 2000, 2010, and 2020

Healthy People 2000 (USDHHS, 1992, p. 6)	Healthy People 2010 (USDHHS, 2000a)	Healthy People 2020 (USDHHS, 2010c, p. 1)
Goals:	**Goals:**	**Goals:**
• Increase the span of healthy life for Americans • Reduce health disparities among Americans • Achieve access to preventive services for all Americans	• Increase the quality and years of healthy life • Eliminate health disparities	• Attain high-quality, longer lives free of preventable disease, disability, injury, and premature death • Achieve health equity, eliminate disparities, and improve the health of all groups • Create social and physical environments that promote good health for all • Promote quality of life, healthy development, and healthy behaviors across all life stages
Priority Areas (22)	**Focus Areas (28)**	**Topical Areas (42)**
Health Promotion • Physical Activity and Fitness • Nutrition • Tobacco • Alcohol and Other Drugs • Family Planning • Mental Health and Mental Disorders • Violent and Abusive Behaviors • Educational and Community-Based Programs *Health Protection* • Unintentional Injuries • Occupational Safety and Health • Environmental Health • Food and Drug Safety • Oral Health *Preventive* • Maternal and Infant Health • Heart Disease and Stroke • Cancer • Diabetes and Chronic Disabling Conditions • HIV Infection • Sexually Transmitted Diseases • Immunization and Infectious Diseases • Clinical Preventive Services *Other* • Surveillance and Data Systems	• Access to Quality Health Services • Arthritis, Osteoporosis, and Chronic Back Conditions • Cancer • Chronic Kidney Disease • Diabetes • Disability and Secondary Conditions • Educational and Community-Based Programs • Environmental Health • Family Planning • Food Safety • Health Communication • Heart Disease and Stroke • HIV • Immunization and Infectious Diseases • Injury and Violence Prevention • Maternal, Infant, and Child Health • Medical Product Safety • Mental Health and Mental Disorders • Nutrition and Overweight • Occupational Safety and Health • Oral Health • Physical Activity and Fitness • Respiratory Diseases • Public Health Infrastructure • Sexually Transmitted Diseases • Substance Abuse • Tobacco Use • Vision and Hearing	• Access to Health Services • Adolescent Health • Arthritis, Osteoporosis, Chronic Back Conditions • Blood Disorders and Blood Safety • Cancer • Chronic Kidney Disease • Dementias, including Alzheimer's Disease • Diabetes • Disability and Health • Early and Middle Childhood • Educational/Community-Based Programs • Environmental Health • Family Planning • Food Safety • Genomics • Global Health • Health Communication and Health IT • Healthcare-Associated Infections • Health-related Quality of Life and Well-being • Hearing/Other Sensory or Communication Disorders • Heart Disease and Stroke • HIV • Immunization and Infectious Diseases • Injury and Violence Prevention • Lesbian, Gay, Bisexual, and Transgender Health • Maternal, Infant, and Child Health • Medical Product Safety • Mental Health and Mental Disorders • Nutrition and Weight Status • Occupational Safety and Health • Older Adults • Oral Health • Physical Activity • Preparedness • Public Health Infrastructure • Respiratory Diseases • Sexually Transmitted Diseases • Sleep Health • Social Determinants of Health • Substance Abuse • Tobacco Use • Vision

older adults) and special populations (low-income, minorities, and people with disabilities) in order to address specific health promotion and disease prevention efforts within these divergent groups. For example, a dramatic decline in the infant mortality rate had occurred; however, continued attention was needed in the area of maternal and infant health. In addition, progress was demonstrated with a decrease in injuries in children with the increased use of child restraint systems in motor vehicles; however, a continued problem area was the asthma hospitalization rate for children, which was identified as a major cause of morbidity. Additional differences were identified for other age groups.

Healthy People 2000 focused also on health disparities. A disparity existed between African Americans and the overall population with respect to average life expectancy, with African Americans having a significantly lower life expectancy (USDHHS, 2000a, p. 12). Disparities also included differential rates in infant mortality, receipt of prenatal care, maternal mortality,homicides, AIDS, lung cancer, breast cancer, coronary heart disease, diabetes complications and related deaths, and immunizations. For Native Americans and Alaskan natives, seven health areas were highlighted: alcoholism and substance abuse, child and family violence, diabetes, women's health, the health of the elderly, maternal and child health, and injuries. Asian Americans and Pacific Islanders were found to have a higher life expectancy than the population as a whole. However, several health problems were particularly noteworthy for these groups, including increasing rates of cerebrovascular diseases and cancer deaths. Elimination of these health disparities became a major initiative in *Healthy People 2010*.

People with disabilities and those in low-income groups were also investigated. Although a decline was found in nonfatal head injuries and spinal cord injuries, there was an increase in other conditions that led to disability, including fetal alcohol syndrome, visual impairments, asthma, and complications of diabetes. An escalating relationship between lower incomes, limitations in activity, health promotion and screening activities, insurance coverage, and chronic conditions was also a finding from *Healthy People 2000*.

During the same period, the American Public Health Association (APHA, 1991) published *Healthy Communities 2000: Model Standards* to assist planners in adapting the *Healthy People 2000* objectives to the needs and resources of individual communities. The conceptual basis of healthy communities included an emphasis on health outcomes, flexible planning, a focus on the entire community with the involvement of local governments and local flexibility, uniform standards and guidelines, and an emphasis on accessibility of programs (APHA, 1991, pp. xvii–xix).

By the final review point for *Healthy People 2000*, most states, the District of Columbia, and Guam had statewide objectives, some with comprehensive strategic plans and assessment projects that addressed the objectives. The strategic planning process continued with a look to revised resources to address the newer national initiatives in *Healthy People 2010*.

The prevention agenda for the nation and the associated objectives for the next decade were introduced in January 2000 as *Healthy People 2010* (USDHHS, 2000a), with two major goals that were more aggressive than the 2000 objectives. For instance, *Healthy People 2000* sought to reduce health disparities, whereas *Healthy People 2010* proposed to eliminate them. Building upon *Healthy People 2000, Healthy People 2010* specified 28 focus areas (Table 14.1) containing objectives and targets for the nation to address the specific trends of the decade, such as diversity and the aging population. *Healthy People 2010* used a systematic approach to health improvement guided by a model with four key elements: goals, objectives, determinants of health, and health status. The objectives were de*signed to* "focus on the **determinants of health,** which encompass the combined effects of individual and community physical and social environments and the policies and interventions used to promote health, prevent disease, and ensure access to quality health care" (USDHHS, 2000a, p. 7).

Specific objectives in each focus area were designed to address the health initiative as subgoals under the direction of a lead government agency. Objectives were both measurable (with specific set targets for which data were tracked) and developmental (for which no baseline data were available). Availability of data and interagency collaboration were essential components of this aggressive and evidence-based project to address the health of the nation.

The midcourse review of *Healthy People 2010* was conducted in 2005 on the status of the objectives and was based on public comments and expert evaluation of the data, apparent trends, and emerging knowledge. Objectives were revised, clarified, and some recommended for deletion if there was not a valid data source. For some developmental objectives, researchers established targets because data were now available for baselines and the objectives could now be measured and tracked. For example, the developmental objective on reducing the number of school or work days missed by persons with asthma now had an established baseline of about six days for persons aged 5 to 64 years, with a target set to reduce the days to two by 2010 (USDHHS, 2006a).

Other developmental objectives were dropped when no data source could be established, as with the objective to increase the number of state prison systems that provide comprehensive education on sexually transmitted diseases. Some developmental objectives were retained if the data source was identified and the objective clarified with the potential for measurement prior to 2010, as with the objective for reducing the proportion of females with human papillomavirus (HPV) infection (USDHHS, 2006b). Other objectives and subobjectives were retained and were being measured or had revisions in language, baselines, or targets.

Reducing health disparities involved addressing the needs of individuals or groups at risk. The needs of these at-risk populations were identifiable in the focus areas and objectives to be addressed. The demographic characteristics identified and targeted for action included gender, age, race and ethnicity, income and educational level, disability, geographic location, and sexual orientation.

A component of the *Healthy People 2010* document was the identification of **leading health indicators**

(Box 14.1). "The leading health indicators reflected the major public health concerns in the United States and were chosen based on their ability to motivate action, the availability of data to measure their progress, and their relevance as broad public health issues" (USDHHS, 2000a, p. 24). These 10 indicators, linked to the *Healthy People 2010* objectives, were designed for the ability to provide a snapshot at a point in time by which to view the health of the nation to "illuminate individual behaviors, physical and social environmental factors, and important health-system issues that greatly affect the health of individuals and communities [and] underlying each of these indicators is the significant influence of income and education" (USDHHS, 2000a, p. 24).

An emphasis on health promotion and disease prevention is evident in these identified leading health indicators. And continued emphasis from the *Healthy People* 2000 results was apparent, as with physical activity and obesity. For example, although the benefits of physical activity have been demonstrated, sedentary lifestyles were still common in the United States, which is a major public health concern. This health indicator targeted perceived barriers to regular, moderate physical activity and sought to prevent conditions associated with lack of activity. Disparities were identified with gender,

age, race, educational level, geography, and socioeconomic status. At-risk groups were identified as females, the elderly, African Americans, Hispanics, low-income individuals, the disabled, and individuals in the southern and northeastern states (USDHHS, 2000b). In addition, increasing trends and associated conditions like heart disease, diabetes, and other chronic illnesses can be directly attributed to overweight and obesity. The interaction with physical activity is evident, along with metabolic and genetic factors, as well as behaviors affecting dietary intake and physical activity; environmental, cultural, and socioeconomic components also play a role (USDHHS, 2000b, p. 19–4). Disparities were reported both within and among population groups related to gender, race, ethnicity, and socioeconomic status. Obesity and overweight continue to be a concern in children and adolescents. Objectives in both this area and under physical activity were directed at these population groups.

The use of tobacco and substance abuse were two additional leading health indicators. Tobacco use, whether by smoking, chewing, or exposure to secondary smoke in the physical environment or in utero, has long been associated with serious complications and consequences. Objectives addressed use of specific products in selected groups, cessation efforts, secondhand exposure, and needed social and environmental changes for limitations or cessation in select populations. Disparities existed by age, gender, race and ethnicity, socioeconomic status, educational level, and geography. Several refinements to the objectives, subobjectives, and baseline data were made for this indicator at the midcourse review, as with revisions of data sources or elimination of subobjectives due to unreliable sources for data. Substance abuse represents more than the use of illicit drugs; it includes adverse drug consequences such as motor vehicle and other accidents, domestic violence, intentional or unintentional overdoses, experimentation with other substances, bingeing, lost productivity, and associated conditions. Substance abuse crosses all ages, genders, racial and ethnic groups, regions, educational levels, and socioeconomic groups.

In *Healthy People 2010*, sexually transmitted diseases (STDs) were described as "common, costly, and preventable" (USDHHS, 2000b, p. 25–7). Although they exist in all gender, racial, ethnic, and socioeconomic groups, differences in responsible sexual behaviors were identified within and among groups for use as targets for intervention activities in the stated objectives. Several developmental objectives were deleted for this indicator at the midcourse review, and refinements in others were based on data and current trends. For example, the objective for a reduction in the proportion of cases of HPV infection was made specific to *females* rather than *humans*, as more became known about data sources and the infection.

"Mental health is a state of successful performance of mental function, resulting in productive activities, fulfilling relationships with other people, and the ability to adapt to change and to cope with adversity" (USDHHS, 2000b, p. 18–3). Although differences have been identified within and among groups, "mental disorders occur across the lifespan, affecting persons of all racial and ethnic groups, both genders, and all educational and socioeconomic groups" (USDHHS, 2000b, p. 18–3). Comorbidities and secondary

---

BOX 14.1 *Healthy People 2010* and *Healthy People 2020*

Healthy People 2010 Leading Health Indicators
- Physical activity
- Overweight and obesity
- Tobacco use
- Substance abuse
- Responsible sexual behavior
- Mental health
- Injury and violence
- Environmental quality
- Immunization
- Access to healthcare

Healthy People 2020 Leading Health Indicators (LHI) (26 LHI organized under the following 12 topics):
- Access to Health Services (2)
- Clinical Preventive Services (4)
- Environmental Quality (2)
- Injury and Violence (2)
- Maternal, Infant, and Child Health (2)
- Mental Health (2)
- Nutrition, Physical Activity, and Obesity (4)
- Oral Health (1)
- Reproductive and Sexual Health (2)
- Social Determinants (1)
- Substance Abuse (2)
- Tobacco (2)

Sources: U.S. Department of Health and Human Services (USDHHS). (2000a). *Healthy People 2010: Volume I* (2nd ed.). Washington, DC: Author.
U.S. Department of Health and Human Services (USDHHS). (2014f). *Leading health indicators.* Retrieved from http://healthypeople.gov/2020/LHI/default.aspx

problems are vital considerations for this indicator, as are treatment opportunities. The midcourse review resulted in revised data, objectives, and targets for this indicator, including a focus on the homeless. New targets were aimed at treatment rather than merely the identification of the proportion of the homeless who are identified with serious mental health problems.

Objectives related to the leading health indicator on injury and violence called for the reduction in injuries, disabilities, and deaths. *Healthy People 2010* noted that "although the greatest impact in injury is human suffering and loss of life, the financial cost is staggering [including costs of] . . . direct medical care and rehabilitation as well as lost income and productivity" (USDHHS, 2000b, p. 15–4). In addition, disparities in rates of injuries by age, racial and ethnic group, and economic status were noted. The four developmental objectives for this indicator became measurable and provided baseline data and targets at the midcourse review, as with bicycle helmet use and protective equipment in school sports activities.

The environmental quality indicator addressed air and water quality and toxic influences in homes, at worksites, and in the community to promote public health and protection. Individuals of certain races and socioeconomic status were identified as being at greater risk for indoor air pollution, inadequate heating or cooling, sanitation, or environmental structural issues including fire hazards (USDHHS, 2000a, p. 8–7). The midcourse review provided data enhancement and refinement, as with the measurability that became available for fish contamination in the nation's lakes and rivers, providing baseline and target data.

Strategies to address the identified increase in infectious diseases included immunization recommendations and programs, both universal and targeted, as well as concentrating on selected infectious processes and antimicrobial resistance. Particular at-risk populations were identified related to age, ethnicity and race, and geography. Updated information on tuberculosis, hospital-acquired infections, and immunization recommendations arose and are available on an ongoing basis with the data provided through the Centers for Disease Control and Prevention (CDC).

Access to quality services was identified as a leading health indicator and continues to be a concern. Consider the implications of this leading health indicator and its target of 100 percent health insurance coverage by 2010. Needless to say, the target was not met. The objectives for this indicator addressed clinical preventive care, primary care, emergency services, and long-term care and rehabilitative services. Disparities have been monitored during the data collection process. At the June 2002 progress review, lower levels of insurance were noted in the Latino, Native American, and Alaskan Native populations. Lower levels of health insurance and ongoing sources of care were also noted in populations with lower levels of family income and education. Racial and ethnic representation in the health professions were also under study with this objective, as a component of cultural competence. Little change has been demonstrated, with minority underrepresentation persistent in the health professions. In *Healthy People 2010* (USDHHS, 2000a), access to quality healthcare services was viewed through selected indicators considered "predictors" of availability and acceptability of

quality services. These indicators or predictors included having health insurance, having a regular provider of ongoing care, and the use of prenatal care as a preventive service (USDHHS, 2000a). The baseline year was 1997, with 83 percent of persons under 65 years of age with health insurance, and we remained at the same percentage in 2010.

At the local levels, *Healthy Communities 2010* was involved with initiatives and data collection. States initiated *Healthy People 2010* plans specific to their population and geography. For example, Alaska implemented a Talking Circle, Arizona had 12 Focus Areas, Michigan concentrated on 25 specific Focused Indicators, and Vermont had specific Goals for Healthy Vermonters.

At the national level, ongoing collaboratives to address the public's health continued. For example, preventing medication errors was included as an issue related to prevention of injury in the focus area of medical product safety. Following an act of the United States Congress, the Centers for Medicare and Medicaid Services (CMS) sponsored a study by the IOM in 2006 with the aim of developing a national agenda for reducing medication errors in hospitals, long-term care and ambulatory-care facilities, and in community and home settings (Aspden, Wolcott, Bootman, & Cronenwett, 2006). Activities to address error reduction and adverse drug events address the *Healthy People 2010* goals to eliminate health disparities and increase the quality and years of healthy life.

The work on *Healthy People 2020* began in 2007 following the midyear review for *Healthy People 2010*. Unlike with the past two projects, for this new initiative, a statement of vision, mission, and goals was developed based on data and public input. The overarching goals were stated as follows:

- Attain high-quality, longer lives free of preventable disease, disability, injury, and premature death.
- Achieve health equity, eliminate disparities, and improve the health of all groups.
- Create social and physical environments that promote good health for all.
- Promote quality of life, healthy development, and healthy behaviors across all life stages. (USDHH, 2014a)

Notice that the focus is now firmly on quality of life for all, across the life span. Now, there were 42 identified **topical areas** (see Table 14.1) with four **foundation health measures** to monitor the health of the nation both for progress and in terms of quality of life issues:

- General Health Status
- Health-Related Quality of Life and Well-Being
- Determinants of Health
- Disparities (USDHHS, 2014b).

A continuing focus remained on most of the focus areas from *Healthy People 2010*—for example, access to health services as well as certain chronic and infectious diseases like arthritis, osteoporosis and chronic back conditions, diabetes, kidney disease, respiratory diseases, and HIV. Selected groups for continued attention remained as well, as with maternal, infant, and child health. Health promotion activities were carried forward with oral health, physical activity, and environmental health. However, additional age groups received added focus, such as early and middle childhood, adolescent health, and older adults, as with *Healthy People 2000*. Thirteen newer focus areas emerged, for example, genomics, global health, and social determinants of health. For the development of the objectives for these goals, specific criteria were established, and each objective must include the following:

- Reliable data source
- Baseline measurement
- Specific improvements targeted to be achieved by 2020 (USDHHS, 2014g)

These objectives were to be relevant, reliable, current, reflective of the population, and measurable. Public meetings were held and comments were requested. The criteria that were set for the objectives were rigorous to include measurability and based on scientific evidence. The model for the process had added complexity from the 2010 objectives and has become an action model looking at assessment, monitoring, evaluation, and dissemination of interventions and outcomes for determinants of health through interconnected variables using a lifespan perspective.

Proposed objectives were also based on the data from *Healthy People 2010*. Some of the 2010 objectives were retained, revised, or moved to a different topical area with data sources identified. For example, in the first topical area on *Access to Health Services*, five of the objectives in this area were retained from *Healthy People 2010* to continue toward the target. Vital areas carried over from the *Healthy People 2010* initiative included the proportion of people with health insurance, those with a usual primary healthcare provider, and access to and use of emergency medical services. Three of the 2010 objectives in this area were also retained but modified for additional specificity to address the targets or had a portion removed from the objective since it was best measured in another topical area of *Healthy People 2020*. Five of the 2010 objectives in this area were moved to other areas in *Healthy People 2020*. Six other 2010 objectives were archived because the previous target had been met, there was inadequate data to address the objectives, or they duplicated measures in other areas (USDHHS, 2008). Two new objectives were added to *Healthy People 2020* focused on evidence-based and primary care, both developmental to assess adequacy of data sources. In late 2010, the Institute of Medicine provided direction for addressing healthcare quality and disparities and appointed a special committee to work toward recommending leading health indicators and objectives for *Healthy People 2020*.

As illustrated in Box 14.1, *Healthy People 2020* was focused on additional metrics with specified targets to assess the health of the public. Moving from the 10 Leading Health Indicators (LHI) in 2010, there were now 26 specific measures organized under 12 topical areas.

At the progress review in March 2014, positive progress was reported on many of the indicators on the *Healthy People 2020* targets as follows:

- 15.4% (4 LHI) met or exceeded the targets
- 38.5% (10 LHI) demonstrated improvements
- 30.8% (8 LHI) demonstrated little or no change
- 11.5% (3 LHI) demonstrated a decline in performance
- 3.8% (1 LHI) had only baseline date (USDHHS, 2014e, p. 2)

The targets were met in the areas of environmental quality (air quality and children exposed to secondhand smoke), number of homicides, and on the physical activity of adults. For example, for adults meeting the recommended aerobic physical activity indicator, the target was 20.1% with the baseline of 18.2% in 2008 and the 2012 measure of 20.6% (USDHHS, 2014e, p. 3). Although the targets were not met in 2014, improvements were demonstrated in the areas of adults receiving colorectal screening, adults with controlled hypertension, childhood immunizations, the number of injury deaths, infant mortality and pre-term births, knowledge of serostatus among HIV-positive individuals, students awarded a high school diploma four years after starting ninth grade, adolescents using alcohol or illicit drugs, and cigarette smoking in adults. For example, the target for adolescents using alcohol or illicit drugs was set at 16.6% with a 2008 baseline of 18.4% and the 2014 measure of 17.4% (USDHHS, 2014e, p. 4). Little or no detectable change was reported in 2011–12 for two LHI in the access to health services, but this may be significantly improved with the implementation of the Affordable Care Act in 2014–15. Little or no improvement was also reported in the areas of diabetes, obesity, intake of vegetables, and adolescent cigarette smoking. Performance declines were reported on two mental health indicators and percentage of visits to a dentist.

One of the most notable factors in this process is the reliance on measurability and the use of scientific evidence. Data were available on a variety of measures and were evolving in other areas. Support of interventions and outcomes with evidence is of prime concern. We are concerned about individuals, families, groups, and communities as we strive to raise the health status of the nation. These activities are especially important in light of our aging population and attendant health challenges.

OUR AGING POPULATION

The term *healthy life* applies not only to longevity but also to functional independence and the perception of healthy days. Older adults are now included back into *Health People 2020* as a distinct area for attention as we focus on the issue of quality of life and *healthy* life expectancy. The major causes of death in people 65 years and older are heart disease, cancer, and stroke. Consider the life expectancy trends reported in Table 14.2. Although life expectancies for both men and women have increased, the years of functional health and independence after age 65 are less than the 12 to 19 actual remaining years of life. In addition, disparities exist by gender and race. On the other hand, trends in limitation of activities of daily living, defined as physically unhealthy days, have declined only marginally for **aging adults** 65 years and

---

ONLINE CONSULT

Healthy People 2020 at
http://www.healthypeople.gov/2020/
aboutdefault.aspx

TABLE 14.2

Life Expectancy (in Years) at Birth, 65, and 75

	1900	1950	1980	1990	2000	2010
At Birth	47.3	68.2	73.7	75.4	76.8	Males 76.2 Females 81.0 Both sexes 78.7
At 65 Years	11.9	13.9	16.4	17.2	17.6	Males 16.0 Females 19.0 Both sexes 17.6
At 75 Years	—	—	10.4	10.9	11.0	Males 11.0 Females 12.9, Both sexes 12.1

Sources: National Center for Health Statistics. (2013). *Life expectancy at birth, at age 65, and at age 75, by sex, race, and Hispanic origin: United States, selected years 1900–2010.* Retrieved from http://www.cdc.gov/nchs/data/hus/hus13.pdf#018

older living in the community with disability percentages showing an increase to 37.9 percent in 2010 (CDC, 2013d, p. 15). The annual trend report for mean number of unhealthy days reported by age group has changed little, especially for the 65 to 74 and 75+ age groups. The rates were 4.8, 5.1, and 4.9 and 6.1, 6.4, and 6.0 for the years 1993, 2003, and 2010 for the 65 to 74 and 75+ age groups, respectively (CDC National Center for Chronic Disease Prevention and Health Promotion, 2012). When considering self-reported activity limitations due to poor physical health, there were 2.4 and 2.9 days in the last 30 days reported by the 65 to 74 and 75+ age groups, respectively (CDC, 2011b). In addition, more activity limitations and physically unhealthy days were reported with lower educational levels, with lower annual household income, and for race/ethnicity other than Asian and white/non-Hispanic (CDC, 2011a, 2011b). The difference between healthy life and unhealthy life is the loss of independence in activities of daily life and increasing dependence on others.

The percentage of the population aged 65 years and older has been steadily increasing, with 13 percent of the population in this age group according to the 2010 census. To look further at this perspective, there were 30 million people in this age group in 1988, with a projected 40 million in 2011 and 50 million in 2019 (National Institute on Aging, 2009, p. 5). And, 72 million older Americans are predicted to be alive in 2030 when the last of the "baby boomers" turns 65 years old (CDC, 2013, p 1). In fact, the population 85 years and older grew dramatically from 1950 to 1990. According to U.S. Census Bureau estimates, there were 5.7 million Americans aged 85 and older in 2010, with the projection that this number will grow to 8.5 million in 2030 and 18.2 million in 2050 (National Institute on Aging, 2009, p. 5). Worldwide, the population over 65 years of age and older was estimated as 524 million in 2010 (8 percent of the global population) with a projection that by 2050 there will be 1.5 billion older people, or 16 percent of the global population (National Institute on Aging, 2011, p. 4). The country with the greatest percentage of people over 65 is currently Japan, but with the rapid population growth by 2050, 65 and older population predictions are expected in China (330 million from 110 million in 2010) and India (227 million from 60 million in 2010) (National Institute on Aging, 2010, p. 5).

Despite Medicare coverage, the growing population of aging Americans, especially those over 85 years, is experiencing differences in purchasing power and socioeconomic status. The affordability of healthcare and medications is a serious concern to our aging population. For example, in 2008, older Americans averaged a 57 percent increase of out-of-pocket expenditures since 1998 and spent an average of $2,844 for insurance, $793 for medical services, $821 for drugs, and $143 for medical supplies (Administration on Aging [AOA], 2009, p. 15). Medicare Part D and new provisions with the Affordable Care Act will reduce some of these escalating expenditures.

However, disposable income is a consideration in retirement. In 2008, approximately 3.7 million elderly persons (9.7%) were living below the federal poverty level, with another 6.3 million classified as "near poor" at 125 percent of the federal poverty level (Administration on Aging, 2010, p. 11). In 2010, this percentage of elderly people living at the federal poverty level had declined to 9 percent, with 26 percent classified in a low income group (Federal Interagency Forum on Aging-related Statistics, 2012, p. 13). There has been some change related to availability of pensions to workers in the second half of the 20th century in addition to Social Security assistance, but differences in income are evident related to socioeconomic status, race, gender, marital status, and geography.

The difference between healthy life and unhealthy life is the loss of independence in activities of daily life and increasing dependence on others for health and routine care. We now see chronic illness rather than acute illness as the major morbidity factor in aging adults. Prevention of disability and promotion of independent functioning are essential and can be aided by healthy behaviors such as smoking cessation, good nutrition, reduction of sodium intake and body weight, reduction in social isolation, regular physical activity, and availability of primary care services.

Approximately one-third of people hospitalized are older than 65 years. In the acute care setting, the average length of stay for individuals over 65 years was 5.6 days, compared with 4.8 days for individuals of all ages (AOA, 2010, p. 13). Even though the average length of hospital stays has shortened, those older than 65 years require a great proportion of our resources, both in and out of the acute care setting. With projections for a dramatic increase in the older population and the associated costs, several national projects and metrics have been initiated to promote healthy lifestyles and lifestyle changes for seniors. As noted by the director of the Centers for Disease Control and Prevention (CDC, 2013d), "more than a quarter of all Americans and two out of three older Americans have multiple chronic conditions, and treatment for this population accounts for 66% of the country's health care budget" (p. ii). For example, think about safety with medications (availability, administration, and interactions) and in the prevention of falls and the associated cost factors.

Theories on and Types of Aging

With the focus on health promotion and quality of life for the growing aging population and the entry of the increased number of baby boomers into this category, research has evolved in several disciplines, all proposing different theories on aging. No agreement on a specific theory has emerged. Research continues, and our knowledge of the aging process grows with biological, sociological, psychological, longevity, medical, and nursing theories on aging. For example, medical theories highlight disease-related influences on physiological functioning of the person, while nursing theories propose functional consequences in which age-related changes are the risk factors.

Interestingly, aging has also been classified as successful, usual, or pathological (Rowe & Kahn, 1987). In *successful aging*, there is a positive interaction between the individual's genes and the environment. Such an interaction results in no serious detriment in functioning from the middle 20s until the early 70s. Minimal measurable changes in functioning are seen, with these individuals as the energetic and functional "survivors" in aging. Successful agers represent only about 5 to 10 percent of the population. These individuals are the aging "stars" we aspire to be—those active, energetic, and involved elders we revere, admire, or respect.

Usual aging occurs in the vast majority of individuals. With usual aging we observe an interaction between the person's genetic endowment and their environment. A neutral or negative environment has positive or neutral genes. Think about diet, cholesterol, and heredity, and individual differences for the person as affected by heredity and the unique environment. This raises concern for the reversible risk factors that occur with aging. The gene-environment interaction leads to obvious functional limitations, but the limitations are not serious enough to affect activities of daily living (ADLs) as long as the person makes compromises and adaptations. An example is the person whose mobility is limited but who adjusts to the limitation and is still able to live independently without assistance in daily life. With usual aging, we may also see genetic diseases, but again, adaptations are made that do not significantly interfere with independent daily functioning. This is the quality of life focus for the increasing numbers of aging adults.

At the opposite extreme is *pathological aging*. Here we see a negative interaction between genetic and environmental factors. Some combination of negative or neutral influences arises from both the individual's genes and the environment. We often see clinical evidence of genetic diseases in these aging individuals. This gene-environment interaction leads to serious functional limitations for the individual, such as being unable to take care of personal needs, inability to perform ADLs, and sometimes the inability to sustain life. These functional limitations require substantial intervention. Prevention of disabilities and quality of life issues in this population are the focus of healthy initiatives.

Characterizing Aging Americans

We have acknowledged that aging adults represent a growing segment of our population, especially those 85 years and older and those who are members of minority groups. As these population proportions increase even more, we will need to consider individual differences, needs of age groups, cultural and ethnic trends, and changing family patterns. Intergenerational issues will involve more than children, parents, grandparents, and great-grandparents. Consider the complexity of a family with two or three older adult groups, those in their middle to late 60s, 80s, and 100s, as well as the family members younger than age 60. The concern also arises as to who will be the caregiver for the frail older adult. Will the 80-year-old be caring for a frail spouse as well as a 99-year-old mother, or will the 60-year-old be caring for both the 80-year-old parents and the 99-year-old grandmother and perhaps be the head of the household also caring for grandchildren? Older women are expected to continue to outnumber men by at least three to two, according to life expectancy projections.

Residential Changes

About 30% (11.3 million) of noninstitutionalized older persons live alone (8.3 million women, 3.0 million men). Half of older women (49 percent) aged 75 years and older live alone.

Living arrangements are an important factor for aging adults. Most aging adults live in the community, usually with a spouse, alone, or with adult offspring. The proportion of people older than 65 who are living in nursing homes is less than 5 percent. And approximately 30 percent, or 11.3 million aging adults, live alone in the community, with 49 percent of women 75 years of age and older living alone (AOA, 2010, p. 1). Decisions about living arrangements should include considerations for optimal promotion of functional independence and health. Opportunities for social interactions and access to resources and caregivers, when needed, are vital considerations.

Various housing options are considered by aging adults. In our more mobile society, being tied to a homestead may no longer be preferable, especially for urban and younger aging adults. Retirement planning may include relocating to a more temperate climate or closer to grandchildren. Instead of the large family home, smaller detached homes, condominiums, town homes, gated retirement communities, continuing care communities, assisted-living apartments, senior homes, and group homes are options, depending on needs, affordability, and accessibility. In addition, a frail elder may relocate again to live with a child or other relative after the death of the spouse, sale of the retirement home, or growing loss of functional independence.

Physical Changes

Characteristics of aging adults continue to be as varied as the individuals themselves. Aging adults come with years of unique experiences that have molded their psychosocial profile. Physically and physiologically, aging adults also differ in development and progression of age-related changes. Aging is progressive and irreversible, but the manner in which these changes occur is variable. Appearance changes and motor activities slow down. But things do not stop without some disease process. Aging adults are more susceptible to disease and environmental factors. Maintaining homeostasis is more difficult.

Age-related changes occur in biological systems. Skin becomes less elastic. Sweat glands, temperature receptors, pigment, and subcutaneous fat decrease. This makes the aging adults more susceptible to temperature extremes (cold and hot), sunlight, and injury. Other senses are affected by aging as well. Visual and hearing acuity diminish. Adaptation of the lens and ocular muscles decreases, with a decrease in depth perception. Glare and driving at night become stressful, especially if the aging person looks at oncoming headlights. The home environment must be well illuminated, but with nonglare lights. For example, reducing the glare with fluorescent lights can also lower the chance of accidents, especially falls. Print may need to be larger and bolder. Eye examinations are important. The loss of the driver's license may be devastating to an aging person, even if his driving is limited.

Moreover, muscle mass and strength decrease, and joints may be stiff with arthritis. Muscle mass may be replaced with connective tissue. Osteoporosis occurs with calcium losses and hormonal changes, and worsens with inactivity. Low-impact, isometric, and routine exercises can prevent further immobility and loss of function. Digestion and slower motility are improved with small meals. Food may taste and smell bland. Herbs and seasoning can be used, but one must beware of hidden sodium content.

Changes in level of consciousness and delirium are not normal signs of aging. Neurological changes do occur but may indicate an underlying pathology or drug interaction. If this situation continues, possibilities should always be investigated further with referrals. Time rather than loss should be the first thought with the delays that may happen; it may take a little more time to remember something, but that does not mean that the memory is lost.

Sexuality and sexual intercourse continue, but adaptation may be needed as well, such as more time for arousal, excitement, and foreplay, or lubrication for vaginal dryness. Impotence should be evaluated for pathology or possible drug side effects. Counseling, erectile aids, reduction in alcohol consumption, and changes in medications are all possible treatments. Sexual activity need not stop because of advancing age, although partner availability may become an issue.

Major Health Problems of Aging Adults

Chronic illness and frailty are primary concerns of aging adults and their healthcare professionals. Diseases common to aging include osteoporosis, diabetes, stroke, depression, arthritis, dementias, cancer, and cardiovascular disease.

Consider the key health indicators of older Americans listed in Box 14.2. The first one, physically unhealthy days, measures the number of days out of the previous 30 days that a respondent's physical health, including physical illness and injury, was self-reported as "not good." A slight but insignificant decline in the mean number of days was reported between 2004 (5.1 days for adults 65 to 74 years and 6.4 days for adults 75+ years) and 2010 (4.9 days for adults 65 to 74 years and 6.0 for those 75+ years of age) for all states (CDC, 2012), but some states had lower scores reported by aging adults, as with respondents in Hawaii, New Hampshire, North Dakota, and Connecticut in 2010. Self-perception of health status was also assessed in 2009, with 41.6 percent of older persons assessing their health as excellent or very good in the overall population, and little difference between men and women over 65 years (AOA, 2010). However, there were differences among racial groups, with older African Americans (25.1 percent), American Indians/Alaska Natives (23.2 percent), and Hispanics (28.0 percent) less likely to rate their health as excellent to very good than their counterpart of older whites (41.8 percent) or Asians (35.2 percent) (AOA, 2010). Another study on disability and activity limitations in 2007 found that 25 percent of older adults living in the community had difficulty performing one or more ADLs (AOA, 2010, p. 14), however, these limitations were increased markedly by age groups 65–74, 74–84, and 85 and older. Older individuals living in the community increasingly report limitations of daily activities as a result of at least one chronic illness. In addition, it has been noted that the presence of a severe disability is associated with lower income levels and educational attainment (AOA, 2010, p. 14).

Consider the difference between disability and chronicity. **Disability** is the inability to do something because of a physical or mental impairment. **Chronicity** is

---

BOX 14.2 Key Indicators of Older Adult Health

Health Status
- Physically Unhealthy Days
- Frequent Mental Distress
- Oral Health; Tooth Retention
- Disability

Health Behaviors
- Leisure Time Activity in the Past Month
- Fruits and Vegetables Consumed Daily
- Obesity
- Current Smoking
- Medication for Hypertension

Preventive Care and Screening
- Flu Vaccine in the Past Year
- Pneumonia Vaccine
- Mammogram Within the Past 2 Years
- Colorectal Cancer Screening
- Up-to-date on Preventive Services

Injuries
- Fall Within the Past Year

Source: Centers for Disease Control and Prevention. (2013b). Healthy people targets. Retrieved from http://www.cdc.gov/aging/help/DPH-Aging/healthy-people.html

ONLINE CONSULT

CDC: The State of Aging and Health in America Report at
http://www.cdc.gov/features/agingandhealth/state_of_aging_and_health_in_america_2013.pdf

related to duration or recurrence of a condition. The individual may have a chronic condition but, with healthy behaviors, he or she can limit, delay, or prevent disability. Hence, health promotion behaviors and empowerment of the individual are essential for taking charge of one's own life. Unlike the irreversible normal changes of aging, risk factors can be reduced and in some cases eliminated.

Risks in aging adults include physical, environmental, psychosocial, and chemical factors. *Physical risks* affect the biological system and related physiological function. Examples of physical risks are limitations in flexibility leading to falls and vision changes, resulting in automobile accidents. *Environmental risks* can be natural or artificial. Natural environmental risks include ultraviolet radiation and weather extremes. Examples of artificial or human-made environmental risks are poor air quality, hazards in housing, and lack of maintenance of equipment. *Psychosocial risks* are a part of everyday life, whether the aging person is isolated or active. Stress levels from illness of self, family members, or friends take an increasing toll on the individual. An inward focus on problems may make the aging person more egocentric and, as a result, more isolated. To address these risks, the special needs of aging adults should be considered.

Needs of Aging Adults

The major needs of aging adults roughly parallel the leading health indicators in *Healthy People 2010* and have been made a distinct topical area for *Healthy People 2020*. Longevity factors that have been supported by research include genetics, gender, environment, physical activity, alcohol consumption, sexual activity, nutrition, and social factors (such as economics, marital status, and family), religious beliefs, purpose in life, and laughter. Positive behaviors must be directed at promoting and maintaining health and functional independence and at reducing risk factors and disability. The aging adult also requires access to affordable healthcare, including transportation and acceptability of the provider to the person.

Family needs and issues are another consideration. Given the proportion of aging adults living in the community and projections for population increases, especially in the group 85 years and older, family needs are a major issue in health promotion and care activities. Much can be found in the literature about family decisions for nursing home placement and the "sandwich generation" of caregivers. But recall that only a small proportion of older adults live in institutional settings, the great majority being cared for in the community. In addition, consider the projected increase in number of aging adults in minority groups and the importance of the extended family in some cultures. Likewise, the growing older population uses many resources, placing a strain on society as a whole.

Lay Caregivers

The fact is that caring for a frail older adult takes a major toll on the caregiver and the family. The number of informal and family caregivers is approaching 40 million nationwide, most of them women caring for relatives, adult children with disabilities, or their grandchildren. The physical and emotional toll on the caregiver can be enormous while the caregiver continues maintaining other family, social, work, and personal obligations. The physical and emotional strains on the caregiver often compromise her health. Financial and economic difficulties can compound the strain on the caregiver.

The concept of respite care, to give the caregiver a break, is ideal but is not always perceived as available, affordable, or even emotionally acceptable. Regardless, the caregiver will need some form of respite, and this must be determined, sought, and used regularly. The reauthorization of the Older Americans Act supported demonstration projects on caregiving and authorized the National Family Caregiver Support Program. This program provides support and resources at the state and local levels for informal caregivers providing care for their older relatives or adults with disabilities. User-friendly Web sites are available to provide information on resources and support for both caregivers and professionals. Tax credits and reimbursable services are available in some areas for lay care of elders. In addition, family leave through the Family and Medical Leave Act (FMLA) also addresses the need for care of spouses and parents with serious health conditions.

Societal Needs

Societal needs and issues are another consideration for aging adults. Public policy issues include the availability and allocation of resources for aging adults as well as the use of these resources. Some people contend that aging adults are using the vast majority of the resources with their chronic health problems. Focusing on the prevention of these health problems in the baby boomers is critical.

Healthcare legislation and financing for aging adults occur mainly through the Social Security amendments and

ONLINE CONSULT

AARP: Caregiving at
http://www.aarp.org/relationships/caregiving/

Administration for Community Living at
http://www.acl.gov/Index.aspx

CDC: Family Caregiving: The Facts at
http://www.cdc.gov/aging/caregiving/facts.htm

Family Caregiver Alliance at
https://caregiver.org/about-fca

National Alliance for Caregiving at
http://www.caregiving.org/

AOA: The National Family Caregiver Support Program at
http://www.aoa.acl.gov/AoA_Programs/HCLTC/Caregiver/index.aspx

The Family and Medical Leave Act of 1993 at
http://www.dol.gov/whd/fmla/index.htm

budget reconciliation acts, which include Medicare and Medicaid funding. With Medicaid, the role, legislation, and funding levels fall within the domain of the state of residence. But what about part-time residents who spend half of the year in a state in which they do not claim primary residence? What about the issue of reverse migration of frail aging adults who, after years of retirement in a satisfactory condition in one state, lose a spouse and become increasingly frail, move to be cared for by their children? Their affluence was spent somewhere else, but when they move near the children, the new community must absorb the cost of chronic health conditions and increasing frailty. Similar situations can have great impact on society and resources.

Elder Abuse

Another area of concern at the individual, family, and societal levels is elder abuse. This includes physical neglect or violence, verbal abuse, psychological or emotional abuse, financial exploitation, and sexual abuse. It may be intended or unintended in active or passive actions of the abuser. Those aging individuals most at risk are the frail elderly who are functionally impaired and depend on others. The Administration on Aging (AOA, 2014a, 2014b) provides information on this serious situation and financially funds the National Center on Elder Abuse. The National Center on Elder Abuse (2014a) has reported that elder abuse perpetrators are frequently family members, both men and women, most often the victim's adult child or spouse. The elders may be in dysfunctional family situations or even in nursing homes, but they often fear being alone more than the abuse or neglect they are experiencing. The National Center on Elder Abuse (2014b) has described the abuse of noninstitutionalized, institutionalized, and disabled elders but cannot determine the exact extent of the problem because many cases are not reported. Assessment, reporting, education, and counseling are responsibilities of providers and members of society. Elder abuse has also been related to caregiver stress. Special efforts being made to address this growing problem include the Older Americans Act and other national legislation for awareness and outreach. "Additionally, a new indicator has been included in the *Healthy People 2020* initiative, increasing the number of states that collect and publicly report incidences of elder maltreatment" (Federal Interagency Forum on Aging-Related Statistics, 2012, pp. 72–73).

Elder abuse is only one aspect of the broader domestic violence problem in this country. The frail elder is certainly not the only one affected by abuse or violence in the environment. Spouses, parents, and significant others are all considerations in cases of domestic violence. In fact, estimates are that almost 15 percent of women and 4 percent of men have been injured as a result of intimate partner violence that included rape, physical violence, and/or stalking (National Domestic Violence Hotline, 2014).

If you suspect that an older person is being abused or neglected, you must call the adult protective services of the state where the elder is located. Proof is not required, and calls are confidential. Some states have separate reporting lines for domestic versus institutional elder abuse. Access the agency to contact in your state at http://www.thehotline.org/help/resources/#tab-id-1

ONLINE CONSULT

Administration on Aging: What is elder abuse? at **http://www.aoa.gov/AoA_programs/elder_rights/EA_prevention/whatisEA.aspx**

National Family Caregiver Support Program at **http://www.aoa.gov/AoA_programs/HCLTC/Caregiver/index.aspx**

National Center on Elder Abuse at **http://www.ncea.aoa.gov/**

National Domestic Violence Hotline at **http://www.thehotline.org**

MINORITY HEALTH

In pursuit of the goal to eliminate health disparities, *Healthy People 2010* identified the following demographic groups within which health disparities occur: gender, race or ethnicity, education or income, disability, geographic location, and sexual orientation. In the area of race or ethnicity, *Healthy People* proposed that the identified disparities were "the result of the complex interaction among genetic variations, environmental factors, and specific health behaviors" (USDHHS, 2000a, p. 12). The following disparities between white and minority populations were documented:

- Higher infant mortality rates for African Americans, Native Americans, and Alaskan Natives
- A higher incidence of cancer and heart disease for African Americans
- Higher mortality from HIV/AIDS for African Americans
- Increased diabetes-related deaths for Hispanic Americans and a higher incidence of diabetes for Native Americans and Alaskan Natives
- A higher incidence of hypertension and obesity in Hispanic Americans
- High death rates from unintentional injuries and suicide for Native Americans and Alaskan Natives
- High rates of tuberculosis in Hispanics, Asians, and Pacific Islanders
- High rates of hepatitis in Asians and Pacific Islanders. (USDHHS, 2000a, p. 12)

Health disparities continued despite the goal for elimination in the *Healthy People 2010* goal. The *Healthy People 2020* goal directed in this area is to "achieve health equity, eliminate disparities, and improve the health of all groups" (UDHHS, 2014a, 1). Clearly, the reasons for the occurrence of the health disparities among ethnic groups are multifaceted and complex and the focus of many different initiatives to address the national goals. A large focus of **minority health** is on the special needs of groups characterized by race or ethnicity. The Office of Minority Health and Health Equity of the CDC (2014) classifies racial or ethnic minority populations as follows:

- American Indian and Alaskan Native
- Asian
- Black or African American
- Hispanic or Latino
- Native Hawaiian and other Pacific Islander

During *Healthy People 2010*, a 2001 study conducted by the Commonwealth Fund documented racial and ethnic disparities in the areas of insurance coverage, health perceptions, incidence of and mortality from chronic conditions, and higher utilization of emergency services and no source of regular care (Collins et al., 2002, p. 39). In a further study on racial and ethnic data-collection processes, the researchers concluded, "minority data collection and reporting was inconsistent and sometimes contradictory" (Perot & Youdelman, 2001, p. 24). Stabilization was recommended. And we continue to investigate the issues and differences among population groups and the needs of the members. The Commonwealth Fund identified that racial and ethnic disparities exist in numerous areas of diagnosis, treatment, and preventive care (even when income, insurance status, and other socioeconomic factors are held constant). California, Florida, and Louisiana have been active in dealing with minority health issues through statutes (Gamble et al., 2006, p. 2) to address their large diverse populations.

Addressing the Disparities

Plans are ongoing to address current and emerging minority issues in order to achieve the goal of elimination of disparities. Federal, state, and local initiatives are actively focusing on the needs of the nation. In 1999, Congress (Public Law 106–129) directed the Agency for Healthcare Research and Quality (AHRQ) to examine priority populations, including minority groups, low-income groups, women, children, the elderly, individuals with special needs, and rural residents. In 2000, Congress passed the Minority Health and Health Disparities Research and Education Act (Public Law 106–525), establishing the National Center on Minority Health and Health Disparities under the National Institutes of Health (NIH). The NIH, along with its Specialty Institutes and Centers, integrated this initiative to eliminate health disparities into the strategic plans for the various agencies, including the National Institute of Nursing Research. Initiatives continue to address not only health habits and access to care but also provider-patient interactions in their research support.

In 2003, the Kaiser Family Foundation, the Robert Wood Johnson Foundation, and national heart organizations, in response to a meta-analysis research on disparities in cardiac care in different population groups, led a national initiative for physician outreach about racial and ethnic disparities in medical care. This research reviewed prior rigorous studies in the literature and documented evidence of racial or ethnic differences in cardiac care, with African Americans less likely to receive certain procedures and care than their white counterparts despite similar patient characteristics (Lillie-Blanton, Rushing, Ruiz, Mayberry, & Boone, 2002). Mixed findings were reported for Hispanic patients.

Then, in their 2005 report, the AHRQ (2005) noted four major themes: disparities still exist, some disparities are diminishing, opportunities remain for improvement, and the information on disparities is improving (p. 3). In 2011, the Offices of Minority Health were established

within the following six governmental agencies as a requirement of the Affordable Care Act:

- Agency for Healthcare Research and Quality (AHRQ)
- Centers for Disease Control and Prevention (CDC)
- Centers for Medicare and Medicaid Services (CMS)
- Food and Drug Administration (FDA)
- Health Resources and Services Administration (HRSA)
- Substance Abuse and Mental Health Services Administration (SAMHSA)

At this time, the CDC Office was renamed from the Office of Minority Health and Health Disparities to the Office of Minority Health and Health Equity (OMHHE) in response to "compelling evidence that race and ethnicity correlate with persistent, and often increasing, health disparities among US . . . and to advance the science and practice of health equity"(p. 2). "**Health equity** is achieved when every person has the opportunity to attain his or her full health potential and no one is disadvantaged from achieving this potential because of social position or other socially determined circumstances" (CDC, 2013a, p. 1). However, the AHRQ (2012) identified that minority populations continued to lag behind whites in areas including quality of care, access to care, timeliness, and outcomes of care and that other problems disproportionally affect minorities such as provider bases, poor communication, and health literacy issues (p. 1). Three new themes were subsequently identified in this report published in 2012 (Box 14.3). As a leading health indicator, social determinants of health are vital considerations. **Social determinants of health** have been defined by the World Health Organization (WHO, 2015) as "the conditions in which people are born, grow, live, work and age; these circumstances are shaped by the distribution of money, power and resources at global, national and local levels" (p. 1). Social determinants of health are a leading health indicator in *Healthy People 2020* (USDHHS, 2014c) and are described as "in part responsible for the unequal and avoidable differences in health status within and between communities" (p. 1).

Providers and communities must address the documented disparities. Doing so requires an understanding of

---

BOX 14.3 | **Themes from National Health Disparities Report (AHRQ, 2012)**

- Health care quality and access are suboptimal, especially for minority and low-income groups.
- Overall quality is improving, access is getting worse, and disparities are not changing.
- Urgent attention is warranted to ensure continued improvements in:
  - Quality of diabetes care, maternal and child health care, and adverse events
  - Disparities in cancer care
  - Quality of care among states in the South

Source: Agency for Health Care Research and Quality (AHRQ). (2012). *2012 National Healthcare Disparities Report.* Rockville, MD. Retrieved from http://www.ahrq.gov/research/findings/nhqrdr/nhdr12/index.html

the evidence and the people. Under the U.S. Department of Health and Human Services, a national partnership was created "to mobilize and connect individuals and organizations across the country to create a nation free of health disparities, with quality health outcomes for all people" with the following aims:

- Increase awareness of the significance of health disparities
- Strengthen and broaden leadership for addressing health disparities at all levels
- Improve health and healthcare outcomes for racial, ethnic, and underserved populations
- Improve cultural and linguistic competency and the diversity of the health-related workforce
- Improve data availability and coordination, utilization, and diffusion of research and evaluation outcomes (DHHS National Partnership for Action, 2011, p. 1).

Resources for health professionals and consumers are available through these governmental agencies (see Online Consult).

Nevertheless, delivery of services to specific minority populations such as the Alaskan Native and Hispanic/Latino groups is influenced by the availability, accessibility, and acceptability of services. Difficulty with communication and other problems may hamper acceptance of early care or access. Acceptability of services may be limited by the patient's healthcare beliefs and practices or other factors. Continuing development in cultural competence is essential for the nurse to address minority disparities. A major resource for professionals can be the faith community specific to the particular minority population.

The projection for an increase in minority populations necessitates immediate action for the health of the nation. Improved data collection has been designed for enhanced practice based on better evidence. Initiatives for cultural competence in the current system, improved communication, and greater diversity of providers are designed to address existing disparities and perceived quality of care and health status. And these initiatives must be reflective of and driven by their local communities. Collaborative efforts are growing at the national, state, and local levels. However, the lack of data on certain populations was noted as a persistent barrier by the CDC (2013c) in their annual report that called for the ongoing need to identify disparities and monitor them over time as a necessary first step toward the development and evaluation of evidence-based interventions that can reduce disparities (p. 186).

RURAL HEALTH

Geographic location has also been identified as a demographic characteristic for which definable health disparities exist. Geographic location, both urban and rural, has also been identified as an area for documenting and addressing health disparities in the plan for *Healthy People 2020*. The National Rural Health Association (NRHA, 2014) identifies the issues with rural Americans facing a unique combination of factors that create disparities in healthcare not found in urban areas, including economic factors, cultural and social differences, educational shortcomings, lack of recognition by legislators, and the sheer isolation of living in remote areas (p. 1). Rural areas have been defined in several ways in the literature and at the federal level. These divergent definitions impeded research and policy-making. Most definitions have been based on population or population density of a specified area. In 2013, criteria based on the 2010 census were released, defining an **urbanized area** with a populated surrounding area of 50,000 or more people, urban clusters with at least 2,500 and less than 50,000 people, and no explicit definition of rural or areas with less than 2,500 people. At the same time, the White House Office of Management and Budget designates counties as metropolitan (area with a population of 50,000 or more people), micropolitan (areas with a population between 10,000 and less than 50,000 people), or neither, with all counties not considered a metropolitan statistical area designated as **rural** (HRSA, 2014). However, the National Rural Health Association (NRHA, 2014a) "recommends that definitions of rural be specific to the purposes of the programs in which they are used and that these are referred to as programmatic designations and not as definitions" (p. 1).

Certain health problems have been identified as particular to people living in rural areas. In fact, *Healthy People 2010* characterized **rural health** issues as follows:

Twenty-five percent of Americans live in rural areas, that are with fewer than 2500 residents. Injury-related death rates are 40 percent higher in rural populations than in urban populations. Heart disease, cancer, and diabetes rates exceed those for urban areas. People living in rural areas are less likely to use preventative screening services, exercise regularly, or wear seat belts. Timely access to emergency services and the availability of specialty care are other issues for this population group. (USDHHS, 2000a, p. 16)

According to 2008 population estimates, 70.5 million people (23% of the population) in the United States lived in rural areas compared with the 233.5 million in urban

ONLINE CONSULT

USDHHS OMH at
http://minorityhealth.hhs.gov/

AHRQ at
https://innovations.ahrq.gov/qualitytools/office-minority-health-resource-center

CCD OMHHE at
http://www.cdc.gov/minorityhealth/OMHHE.html

CMS at
http://www.cms.gov/About-CMS/Agency-Information/CMSLeadership/Office_OMH.html

FDA at
http://www.fda.gov/AboutFDA/CentersOffices/OC/OfficeofMinorityHealth/default.htm

HRSA at
http://www.hrsa.gov/culturalcompetence/index.html

SAMHSA at
http://www.samhsa.gov/minorityfellowship/

areas. And, with *Healthy People 2020*, the term rural was replaced with geography to better reflect disparities in the population for people in both rural and urban areas.

Further complicating matters is the fact that rural communities may share some features but are not all the same. For example, characteristics and problems of rural residents in South Georgia may be quite different from those of rural residents in Montana or New Mexico. It is important to be aware that the large majority of rural residents are not farmers. But for those who are, agriculture is a dangerous occupation with great risk of injury and illness, even for children.

The National Rural Health Association (2014b) characterized the health issues and care for the nearly one-fourth of the population who live in rural areas as follows:

- Death and serious accidents account for 60 percent of total rural accidents compared with 48 percent of urban accidents related to delayed emergency response times (estimated as 8 minutes longer in rural areas).
- Only about 10 percent of physicians practice in rural America.
- Rural residents are less likely to have employer-provided healthcare coverage or prescription drug coverage, and the rural poor are less likely to be covered by Medicaid benefits.
- Rural residents are nearly twice as likely to die from unintentional injuries other than motor vehicle accidents, with a significantly higher risk for death by gunshot.
- Rural residents tend to be poorer, and nearly 24 percent of rural children live in poverty.
- People who live in rural America rely more heavily on the federal food stamp program.
- Abuse of alcohol and use of smokeless tobacco is a significant problem among rural youth.
- The majority of first responders in rural areas are volunteers.
- There are 60 dentists per 100,000 population in urban areas, versus 40 per 100,000 in rural areas.
- Dental care and mental health services are less available in rural areas.
- The incidence of hypertension is higher in rural areas, as well as the incidence of suicide, particularly among adult men and children.
- Medicare payments to rural hospitals and physicians are dramatically less than those to their urban counterparts for equivalent services.
- Medicare patients with acute myocardial infarction (AMI) who were treated in rural hospitals were less likely than those treated in urban hospitals to receive recommended treatments and had significantly higher post-AMI death.
- Rural residents have greater transportation difficulties reaching healthcare providers and hospitals.

The urban setting features a high volume of patients with an emphasis on technology-intensive and inpatient services. The rural setting focuses more on ambulatory care and features a much lower patient volume, usually more elderly patients or those with advanced and chronic illnesses.

The rural health literature addresses a variety of problems. Two recurring concerns seem to predominate: chronic illness (particularly in the elderly) and inadequate prenatal care. Just consider the issue of access in rural areas, especially with challenges related to reliable transportation, limitations in activities of daily living secondary to a chronic illness, and cost factors with additional childcare or loss of income from time off work. Census data indicates a growth in minority populations in rural areas, particularly Hispanic or Latino. Not surprisingly, rural growth is also higher in the more temperate climate areas of the South and the West. Demographic factors such as age, gender, race and ethnicity, socioeconomic status, and educational level are all considerations when rural geography and health status are investigated.

Delivery of services in rural communities is heavily influenced by the availability, accessibility, and acceptability of services. Rural communities have fewer resources. Distance, lack of communication, and other problems may hamper access. Acceptability of services may be limited by the patients' beliefs and practices or other factors. In addition, the rural community health nurse may well be the only health professional in the community, working with very limited resources. Rural residents tend to be religiously and politically conservative, self-sufficient, and wary of outsiders (especially urbanites). Thus, the community health nurse cannot expect to rush eagerly into a rural community with good intentions and gain immediate acceptance. Building rapport with residents of a rural community takes time, and showing respect for their values and beliefs is imperative. In other words, the nurse must be sensitive and must demonstrate cultural competence. A further challenge is presented when the rural residents are also members of an ethnic group that is different from that of the nurse. The rural community health nurse must beware of assuming that these patients (and their problems) are the same as those of their urban counterparts. Their ruralism may be as significant as their ethnic identity.

RURAL HEALTH CLINICS

Under Public Law 95-210, rural health clinics (RHCs) were established in 1977 to provide primary care services for residents of medically underserved areas. Under budget reconciliation acts, requirements for these clinics have resulted in some changes during their inception.

ONLINE CONSULT

Agency for Healthcare Research and Quality: Rural Health at
http://www.ahrq.gov/research/ruralix.htm

CDC Office of Minority Health and Health Equity at
http://www.cdc.gov/minorityhealth/populations/atrisk.html#Geography

Health Resources and Services Administration: Rural Health at
http://www.hrsa.gov/ruralhealth/index.html

National Rural Health Association at
http://www.ruralhealthweb.org/

U.S. Department of Health and Human Services: Office of Minority Health at
http://minorityhealth.hhs.gov/

These clinics are located as permanent facilities or mobile units throughout the nation with most staffed with advanced practice nurses (APRNs). To be certified as a RHC, two general requirements must be met: be located in a nonurban area and be in a designated shortage area. There are certain exceptions that may be applied for to continue as a RHC and receive Medicare designation and payment for services. One of the newer requirements is that the RHC employ a nurse practitioner or physician assistant and have a nurse practitioner, physician assistant, or certified nurse midwife staffing the clinic at least 50 percent of the time that services are provided (DHHS Centers for Medicare and Medicaid Services, 2013, p. 5). In addition to this staffing requirement, the clinics are certified by the Centers for Medicare and Medicaid (CMS) and have specified service and reimbursement components. Federal legislation has also created the Federally Qualified Health Center (FQHC) program, which includes the Migrant Health Center (MHC) and Community Health Center (CHC) programs funded under the Public Health Service Act to provide primary care for medically underserved rural populations. Agencies receiving funding under the FQHC program must provide primary services for all age groups including diagnostic and lab, pharmacy, preventive health and dental, transportation, case management after hours care, hospital/specialty care, and emergency medical services either onsite or through provider arrangements. The RHC program requires similar primary services.

Reimbursement

Reimbursement policy is a major issue for providers of rural healthcare. Although some improvements have occurred, especially in designated health professional shortage areas, urban providers are reimbursed by Medicare at a higher rate than rural providers. Individual states direct Medicaid reimbursements, so these vary. An important consideration is economy of scale, in that certain key services must be available despite the low volume of service in rural agencies compared with their urban counterparts. Home healthcare is also more costly in the rural area because of low volume and longer travel distances.

In 2000, reimbursement for care was changed from cost-based to a prospective payment system (PPS). In addition, there are specific requirements for payments by the patients or their secondary insurance. Each year the allowable payment may change since the per-visit limit is established by Congress based on the Medicare Economic Index. Further information on payment systems is provided in Chapter 16.

Telecommunication

The use of telecommunications technology in healthcare (*telemedicine* or *telehealth*) has greatly increased in recent years. It is being used extensively in some areas to enhance care of rural residents, as with a specialist at an urban medical center consulting on a patient in a remote rural area via telecommunications. This is also occurring globally, providing consultations, preparation of imaging,

or interpretation of findings. There is a tremendous potential for greater access with telemedicine, but it is not without problems. Issues such as reimbursement, liability, patient privacy, and credentials and licensure must be addressed.

Based on pilot programs to provide telehealth to rural areas, the Rural Healthcare Connect Fund was established in 2013 to expand healthcare provider access to broadband services and to encourage the formation of state and regional broadband networks linking healthcare providers. The Rural Healthcare program (FCC, 2014) received federal funding capped at $400 million dollars annually with the following goals:

- Increase access to broadband for healthcare providers (HCPs), especially those serving rural areas.
- Foster development and deployment of broadband healthcare networks.
- Maximize impact of the FCC universal service healthcare funding.

This available funding to healthcare providers includes hospitals, rural health clinics, local health departments, community health centers or health centers providing healthcare to migrant workers and postsecondary educational institutions offering heathcare instruction, teaching hospitals, and medical schools. Linkages to the rural communities are designed to improve both the quality and quantity of healthcare. As with the national *Healthy People 2020* initiative, initiatives with this program will provide greater outreach and improved health for the rural population.

COMMUNITY NURSING IN THE CONTEXT OF HEALTHY PEOPLE

The nature of nursing practice in the community is different, dynamic, and responsive. Community health nursing crosses age, demographic, and specialty groups. **Community health nursing** is built upon the principles of nursing and public health, with the broader focus on the patient in the context of his environment for health promotion and illness treatment and prevention. Community health nursing crosses many traditional boundaries, is holistic, and is not limited to a particular age group, diagnostic category, or narrow set of specialized skills. Although patients include individuals and families, community health nursing may have a group or even an entire community as a client. Patients may be well or ill. Their health risks or needs may be either physical or mental in nature. In addition, spiritual needs are also a consideration, especially with parish- or faith-based nursing care.

Several factors determine the roles, activities, and intervention strategies of an individual community health nurse, working in the context of *Healthy People*:

• Mission, philosophy, and priorities of the employing agency
• Level of prevention at which intervention is aimed
• Definition of patient/client

The mission, philosophy, and priorities of a private agency or a faith-based organization can be quite different from those of an official government agency. The level of funding influences how well the agency is able to implement its priorities, which should be based on identified health needs in the community.

Another factor that influences the functions for the community health nurse is the agency's level of prevention focus. Community health nurses are involved in all three levels of prevention. However, historically these nurses have played a key role in primary prevention efforts. For more than 100 years they have been involved in health promotion and disease prevention. Over the past years, and despite initiatives like *Healthy People*, these traditional services have suffered under-reimbursement, with health departments compelled to provide more direct clinical services. Consequently, many public health nurses have taken on a role that is more illness-oriented. Nevertheless, *Healthy People* priorities clearly reflect a need for community health nurses, especially those in public health agencies, to renew and strengthen their role in primary prevention.

Community health nursing is frequently described in the literature as a synthesis of nursing and public health. Public health is unique because it broadens concerns to the "public" with a population and collaborative focus. The mission of the Public Health Nursing Section of the American Public Health Association (APHA, 2014) is to "advance the health of the population in partnership with the community through evidence-based practice, education, and research" (p. 1). They further state that "in any setting, the role of public health nurses focuses on the prevention of illness, injury or disability, the promotion of health, and maintenance of the health of populations" (American Public Health Association, 2014, p. 2).

In published standards of public health, the American Nurses Association (2013), in collaboration with other public health nursing organizations, identified six standards of public health nursing practice consistent with the nursing process (assessment, population diagnosis and priorities, outcomes identification, planning, implementation, and evaluation) and 10 standards of professional performance (ethics, education, evidence-based practice and research, quality of practice, communication, leadership, collaboration, professional practice evaluation, resource utilization, environmental health, and advocacy). The focus is on promoting and protecting the health of populations. Clearly, an interdisciplinary focus is necessary to address the health of the community and the people who make up that community. An important consideration, as mentioned in *Healthy People*, is the environmental concerns that affect the health of the community. This includes population threats as well as the promotion of health of individuals and groups and a healthier environment for the population. In addition to *Healthy People 2020*, the National Prevention Strategy released in 2011 with the annual report in 2013 documented progress across governmental agencies to address the following four strategic directions:

• Healthy and Safe Community Environments
• Clinical and Community Preventive Services
• Empowered People
• Elimination of Health Disparities (National Prevention, Health Promotion, and Public Health Council, 2013)

The documented multiagency involvement is apparent with interprofessional collaboration vital to advance the health of the public. As noted by Teutsch, Chokshi, Stine, and Fielding (2013), "the public health orientation toward geographic populations and the clinical focus on individuals engaged in care can be difficult to unite in shared accountability'" (p. 1). However, "the aim of population health as a discipline is virtually synonymous with public health: to maintain and improve the health of a defined human population, correct deviations from good health, and reduce health inequities across population groups" (White, Stallones, and Last, 2013, pp. 106–107). These are shared values for clinicians, politicians, policy analysts, and consumers. And nurses practicing in public health or community health settings are a vital part of this initiative to improve the health and environment of the public. Population-focused nursing is fundamental to baccalaureate generalist practice focused on population health and clinical prevention (AACN, 2008), described more specifically in the supplement, *Public Health: Recommended Baccalaureate Competencies and Curricular Guidelines for Public Health Nursing* (AACN, 2013), which requires "an ecological perspective in health assessment, planning, and interventions with individuals, families, and groups" (AACN, 2013, p. 25).

Challenges exist in many areas for professional nursing practice as we address the health needs of national and global populations. Whether talking about the aging member of a minority population, the well elder in the community, the rural child with asthma, or the individual with diabetes, health professionals focus on high-quality lives free of preventable disease, health equity and the elimination of health disparities, environments that promote good health, and quality of life and healthy development as stated in the goals for *Healthy People 2020*.

EVIDENCE-BASED PRACTICE: *Consider this....*

The Agency for Healthcare Research and Quality (AHRQ, 2014) reported that Americans in 2011 made about 421 visits to the emergency department (ED) for every 1,000 individuals in the population, and more than five times as many individuals who visited an ED were discharged as were admitted to the same hospital. In addition, for patients younger than 18 years, the most common reasons for admission to the hospital after an ED visit were acute bronchitis (infants younger than 1 year), asthma (patients aged 1 to 17 years), and pneumonia (infants and patients aged 1 to 17 years); in adults aged 45 to 84 years, septicemia was the most frequent reason for admission to the hospital after an ED visit (AHRQ, 2014, p. 1). They also found that ED visits were potentially preventable in that access to high-quality community-based healthcare can prevent the need for a portion of the ED visits (AHRQ, 2014, p.1).

You are working as a nurse manager in the emergency department in a rural hospital and have noticed an increased number of low-income elderly patients who have been diagnosed with hip fractures.

Question: What are the characteristics of your patient population? What health promotion activities will you discuss at your next staff meeting? And how can these activities be implemented in your emergency department?

Source: Agency for Quality and Research (AHRQ). (2014). *Overview of emergency department visits in the United States, 2011: Statistical brief #174.* Retrieved from http://www.hcup-us.ahrq.gov/reports/statbriefs/sb174-Emergency-Department-Visits-Overview.jsp. Retrieved from http://www.ahrq.gov/news/nn/nn111810.htm

KEY POINTS

- Public health focuses on protection of the public from health threats.

- Population health is an area of inquiry measured by health indicators, such as social, economic, and physical environments, personal health practices, individual capacity and coping skills, human biology, individual development, health services, and demographic forces that shape the composition of populations (White, Stallones, and Last, 2013, p. 106).

- *Healthy People 2010* built upon the information from the prior decade but was developed with the two major goals of increasing the quality and years of healthy life and eliminating health disparities. It uses a framework of 28 focus areas, 467 objectives, and 10 leading health indicators.

- Leading health indicators reflected the major public health concerns in the nation.

- *Healthy People 2020* builds on the work of the 2010 initiative but is guided by a vision, mission, and four goals to address the health of the nation. Objectives under 42 topical areas were developed based on the data from 2010, specific criteria, and input from the public. In addition, four foundation health measures were specified to monitor the health of the nation for both progress and in terms of quality of life issues.

- Proportional increases in the population of aging adults are predicted, with the greatest increase in those 85 years and older. Women currently account for a large proportion of this group. Predictions include an increase in minority groups represented in our aging population.

- Chronic illnesses and increasing frailty are the major causes of morbidity in aging adults. Disability is the inability to do something because of a physical or mental impairment. Chronicity is related to duration or recurrence of a condition.

- Aging adults face physical, environmental, psychosocial, and chemical risk factors. The risks commonly affect many aging adults, creating conditions that interfere with activity. Health-promotion activities are vital in this area to maintain functional ability and reduce the incidence of frailty and disability.

- Evidence that health disparities exist among ethnic groups of all ages has been documented; however, reasons for their occurrence are multifaceted and complex. Minority health is an important initiative for the health of the nation.

- The Office of Minority Health and Health Equity of the CDC (2014) classifies racial or ethnic minority populations as American Indian and Alaskan Native, Asian, Black or African American, Hispanic or Latino, and Native Hawaiian and other Pacific Islander.

Continued

KEY POINTS—cont'd

- Health equity is achieved when every person has the opportunity to attain his or her full health potential and no one is disadvantaged from achieving this potential because of social position or other socially determined circumstances (CDC, 2013a, p. 1).

- Social determinants of health are the conditions in which people are born, grow, live, work, and age and are shaped by the distribution of money, power, and resources at global, national, and local levels (WHO, 2015).

- In 2013, new criteria based on the 2010 census were released, defining an urbanized area as a central city with a densely populated surrounding area of 50,000 or more. Rural areas are generally defined as areas with a population of less than 2,500. However, the White House Office of Management and Budget designates counties as metropolitan (area with a population of 50,000 or more people), micropolitan (area with a population between 10,000 and less than 50,000 people), or neither, with all counties not considered a metropolitan statistical area designated as **rural** (HRSA, 2014).

- Rural health clinics (RHCs) have been established to provide primary care services for residents of underserved areas. Federal legislation has also created the Community Health Center (CHC) and Migrant Health Center (MHC) programs to provide primary care for medically underserved rural populations.

- Community health nursing is frequently described in the literature as a synthesis of nursing and public health. The mission of the Public Health Nursing Section of the APHA has as its mission "advance the health of the population in partnership with the community through evidence-based practice, education, and research" (American Public Health Association, 2014, p. 1).

Thought and Discussion Questions

1. Consider one of the goals of *Healthy People 2020*: "attain high-quality, longer lives free of preventable disease, disability, injury, and premature death" (USDHHS, 2014a). Be prepared to share your impressions on achievement of this national goal in a discussion to be scheduled by your instructor.

2. Another goal of *Healthy People 2020* is to "promote quality of life, healthy development, and healthy behaviors across all life stages" (USDHHS, 2014a). Select one objective in *Healthy People 2020* from one of the following topical areas: Adolescent Health; Early and Middle Childhood; Maternal, Infant and Child Health; and Older Adults. Be prepared to share your impressions on the targets set for this goal and how it is or could be addressed in your community in a discussion to be scheduled by your instructor.

3. What initiatives and training materials are available in your hospital or agency for the recognition and reporting of domestic or child abuse?

4. Determine whether your community is a metropolitan statistical area (MSA), a micropolitan area, or a rural population area. Investigate what public/community health clinics are available to residents in your community.

5. Review the Chapter Thought located on the first page of the chapter and discuss it in the context of this chapter.

Interactive Exercises

Go to the Intranet site and complete the interactive exercises provided for this chapter.

REFERENCES

Administration on Aging (AOA). (2010). *A profile of older Americans: 2010.* Retrieved from http://www.aoa.gov/aoaroot/aging_statistics/profile/2010/docs/2010profile.pdf

Administration on Aging (AOA). (2014a). *Elder rights protection.* Retrieved from http://www.aoa.gov/AoARoot/AoA_Programs/Elder_Rights/index.aspx

Administration on Aging (AOA). (2014b). *Prevention of elder abuse, neglect, and exploitation (Title VII-A3).* Retrieved from http://www.aoa.gov/AoARoot/AoA_Programs/Elder_Rights/EA_Prevention/index.aspx

Agency for Healthcare Research and Quality (AHRQ). (2009). *Health care in urban and rural areas, combined years 2004–2006.* Retrieved from http://www.ahrq.gov/policymakers/health-initiatives/meps/chbook13up.html

Agency for Healthcare Research and Quality (AHRQ). (2011). *Rates of hospital emergency department use greater among women and low-income, older, and rural Americans.* Retrieved from http://www.ahrq.gov/news/newsletters /research-activities/jan11/0111RA23.html

Agency for Healthcare Research and Quality (AHRQ). (2012). *2012 National disparities report.* Retrieved from http://www.ahrq.gov/research/findings/nhqrdr/nhdr12 /index.html#

Agency for Healthcare Research and Quality (AHRQ). (2013a). *2012 National Healthcare Disparities Report.* Rockville, MD. Retrieved from http://www.ahrq.gov /research/findings/nhqrdr/nhdr12/index.html

Agency for Healthcare Research and Quality (AHRQ). (2013b). *Minority health: Recent findings.* Retrieved from http://www.ahrq.gov/research/minorfind.pdf

Agency for Healthcare Research and Quality (AHRQ). (2014). *Overview of emergency department visits in the United States, 2011: Statistical brief #174.* Retrieved from http://www .hcup-us.ahrq.gov/reports/statbriefs/sb174-Emergency -Department-Visits-Overview.jsp

American Association of Colleges of Nursing (AACN). (2008). *The essentials of baccalaureate education for professional nursing practice.* Washington, DC: Author.

American Association of Colleges of Nursing (AACN). (2013). *Public health: Recommended baccalaureate competencies and curricular guidelines for public health nursing.* Washington, DC: Author.

American Nurses Association. (2013). *Public health nursing: Scope and standards of practice* 2nd ed. Silver Spring, MD: Nursebooks.org.

American Public Health Association (APHA). (1991). *Healthy communities 2000: Model standards: Guidelines for community attainment of the year 2000 objectives.* Washington, DC: American Public Health Association.

American Public Health Association (APHA). (2014). *Public health nursing section.* Retrieved from http://www.apha .org/membergroups/sections/aphasections/phn/about/

Aspden, P., Wolcott, J., Bootman, J. L., & Cronenwett, L. R. (Eds.). (2006). *Preventing medication errors.* Washington, DC: National Academies Press.

Bolin, J. N., & Bellamy, G. (2014). *Rural healthy people 2020.* Retrieved from http://sph.tamhsc.edu/centers/srhrc /images/rhp2020

Centers for Disease Control and Prevention (CDC). (2010a). Data2010 focus area 01—access to quality health services: The Healthy People 2010 Database, January, 2010 ed. Retrieved from http://wonder.cdc.gov/data2010/

Centers for Disease Control and Prevention (CDC). (2011a). *Mean physically unhealthy days in last 30 by demographic characteristics, chronic disease conditions, and risk factors, adults >=18 years, BRFSS 2009.* Retrieved from http://www.cdc.gov/hrqol/data/tables/table4a.htm

Centers for Disease Control and Prevention (CDC). (2011b). *Mean recent activity limitation days in last 30 by demographic characteristics, chronic disease conditions, and risk factors, adults >=18 years, BRFSS 2009.* Retrieved from http://www.cdc.gov/hrqol/data/tables/table2a.htm

Centers for Disease Control and Prevention (CDC). (2012). *Health-related quality of life: Nationwide trend.* Retrieved from http://apps.nccd.cdc.gov/HRQOL /TrendV.asp?State=1&Category=3&Measure=2

Centers for Disease Control and Prevention. (2013a). *Health equity.* Retrieved from http://www.cdc.gov/chronicdisease /healthequity/index.htm

Centers for Disease Control and Prevention. (2013b). *Healthy people targets.* Retrieved from http://www.cdc.gov/aging /help/DPH-Aging/healthy-people.html

Centers for Disease Control and Prevention. (2013c). Conclusion and future directions: CDC health disparities and inequalities report—United States, 2013. *Morbidity and Mortality Weekly Report, Supplements 62*(03), 184–186. Retrieved from http://www.cdc.gov/mmwr/preview /mmwrhtml/su6203a32.htm?s_cid=su6203a32_w

Centers for Disease Control and Prevention. (2013d). *The state of aging and health in America.* Retrieved from http://www.cdc.gov/aging/help/DPH-Aging /state-aging-health.html

Centers for Disease Control and Protection Office of Minority Health and Health Equity (CDCOMHHE). (2014). *Minority health.* Retrieved from http://www.cdc.gov /minorityhealth/populations.html#REMP

CDC National Center for Health Statistics (CDCNCHS). (2014). *NCHS data on health insurance and access to care.* Retrieved from http://www.cdc.gov/nchs/fastats/ health-insurance.htm

CDC Office of Minority Health and Health Equity (CDC OMHHE). (2013). *About OMHHE.* Retrieved from http://www.cdc.gov/minorityhealth/OMHHE.html

CDC Office of Minority Health and Health Equity. (2013). *CDC health disparities and inequalities report.* Retrieved from http://www.cdc.gov/minorityhealth/CHDIReport.html

Centers for Medicare and Medicaid (CMS). (2013). *Medicare benefit policy manual Chapter 13 - Rural Health Clinic (RHC) and Federally Qualified Health Center (FQHC) services.* Retrieved from http://www.cms.gov /Regulations-and-Guidance/Guidance/Manuals/ Downloads/bp102c13.pdf

Collins, K. S., Hughes, D. L., Doty, M. M., Ives, B. L., Edwards, J. N., & Tenney, K. (2002). *Diverse communities, common concerns: Assessing health-care quality for minority Americans.* New York: The Commonwealth Fund.

DHHS National Partnership for Action. (2011). *Learn about the NPA.* Retrieved from http://minorityhealth.hhs.gov /npa/templates/browse.aspx?lvl=1&lvlid=11#mis

Federal Communications Commission (FCC). (2014). *Rural health care program.* Retrieved from http://www.fcc.gov /encyclopedia/rural-health-care

Federal Interagency Forum on Aging-Related Statistics. (2012). *Older Americans 2012: Key indicators of well-being.* Retrieved from http://www.agingstats.gov/agingstatsdotnet/Main _Site/Data/2012_Documents/Docs/EntireChartbook.pdf

Gamble, V. N., Stone, D., Ladenheim, K., Gibbs, B. K., et al. (2006). Special Issue: Comparative perspectives on health disparities. *Journal of Health Politics, Policy and Law, 31*(1), 1–9.

Health Resources Services Administration (HRSA). (2014). *Defining the rural population.* Retrieved from http:// www.hrsa.gov/ruralhealth/policy/definition_of_rural.html

Institute of Medicine (IOM). (2014). *Population health implications and the Affordable Care Act: Workshop summary.* Washington, DC: National Academy Press.

Kindig, D., & Stoddart, G. (2003). What is population health? *American Journal of Public Health, 93*, 380–383.

National Center on Elder Abuse. (2014). *Elder abuse prevalence and incidence.* Retrieved from http://www.ncea.aoa.gov/Main_Site/pdf/publication/FinalStatistics050331.pdf

National Domestic Violence Hotline. (2014). *The hotline.* Retrieved from http://www.thehotline.org/is-this-abuse/statistics/

National Institute on Aging. (2009). *Aging in the United States: Past, present, and future.* Washington, DC: U.S. Department of Commerce, Economics and Statistics Administration, Bureau of the Census.

National Institute on Aging. (2011). *Global health and aging* (NIH Pub. No. 111-7737). Retrieved from http://www.nia.nih.gov/sites/default/files/global_health_and_aging.pdf

National Prevention, Health Promotion, and Public Health Council. (2013). *Annual status report.* Retrieved from http://www.surgeongeneral.gov/initiatives/prevention/about/annual_status_reports.html

National Rural Health Association (NRHA). (2014a). *How is rural defined?* Retrieved from http://www.ruralhealthweb.org/go/left/about-rural-health/how-is-rural-defined

National Rural Health Association (NRHA). (2014b). *What's different about rural health care?* Retrieved from http://www.ruralhealthweb.org/go/left/about-rural-health/what-s-different-about-rural-health-care

Perot, R. T., & Youdelman, M. (2001). *Racial, ethnic, and primary language data collection in the health care system: An assessment of federal policies and practices.* New York: The Commonwealth Fund.

President's Advisory Commission on Consumer Protection and Quality in the Health Care Industry. (1998). *Quality first: Better health care for all Americans* (Final report to the President of the United States). Columbia, MD: Consumer Bill of Rights.

Rowe, J. W., & Kahn, R. L. (1987). Human aging: Usual and successful. *Science, 237,* 143–149.

Secretary's Advisory Committee on the National Health Promotion and Disease Prevention Objectives for 2020. (2008). *Phase I report: Recommendations for the framework and format of Healthy People 2020.* Washington, DC: Author.

Teutsch, S. M., Chokshi, D. A., Stine, N. W., & Fielding, J. E. (2013). *HALE—unificaion theory or clinical medicine and population health.* Washington, DC: Institute of Medicine. Retrieved from http://iom.edu/~/media/Files/Perspectives-Files/2013/Discussion-Papers/BPH-HALE.pdf

U.S. Department of Health and Human Services (USDHHS). (2000a). *Healthy People 2010: Volume 1* (2nd ed.). Washington, DC: Author

U.S. Department of Health and Human Services (USDHHS). (2000b). *Healthy People 2010: Volume 2* (2nd ed.). Washington, DC: Author.

U.S. Department of Health and Human Services (USDHHS). (2006a). *Objective 24–5 school or work days lost, asthma. Healthy People Midcourse Review.* Washington, DC: Author.

U.S. Department of Health and Human Services (USDHHS). (2006b). *Objective 25–5 human papillomavirus infection, viral STD illness and disability. Healthy People Midcourse Review.* Washington, DC: Author.

U.S. Department of Health and Human Services. (USDHHS, 2008). *The secretary's advisory committee on national health promotion and disease prevention objectives for 2020: Phase I report recommendations for the framework and format of Healthy People 2020.* Washington, DC: Author.

U.S. Department of Health and Human Services (USDHHS). (2014a). *About Healthy People.* Retrieved from http://www.healthypeople.gov/2020/about/default.aspx

U.S. Department of Health and Human Services (USDHHS). (2014b). *Disparities.* Retrieved from http://www.healthypeople.gov/2020/about/disparitiesAbout.aspx

U.S. Department of Health and Human Services (USDHHS). (2014d). *Healthy People 2020 leading health indicators: Social determinants.* Retrieved from http://www.healthypeople.gov/2020/LHI/HP2020_LHI_Soc_Determ.pdf

U. S. Department of Health and Human Services (USDHHS). (2014e). *Healthy People 2020 leading health indicators: Progress update.* Retrieved from http://www.healthypeople.gov/2020/LHI/progressUpdate.aspx

U.S. Department of Health and Human Services (USDHHS). (2014f). *Leading health indicators.* Retrieved from http://www.healthypeople.gov/2020/about/default.aspx

U.S. Department of Health and Human Services (USDHHS). (2014g). *Objective development and selection process.* Retrieved from http://healthypeople.gov/2020/about/objectiveDevelopment.aspx

White, F., Stallones, L., & Last, J. (2013). *Global public health.* New York: Oxford University Press.

World Health Organization. (2015). *Social determinants of health.* Retrieved from http://www.who.int/topics/social_determinants/en/

BIBLIOGRAPHY

Agency for Healthcare Research and Quality (AHRQ). (2013). *Minority health: Recent findings.* Retrieved from http://www.ahrq.gov/research/findings/factsheets/minority/minorfind/index.html

Centers for Disease Control and Prevention (CDC). (2000). *Measuring healthy days: Population assessment of health-related quality of life.* Atlanta, GA: Author. Retrieved from http://www.cdc.gov/hrqol/pdfs/mhd.pdf

Federal Interagency Forum on Child and Family Statistics. (2013). *America's children in brief: Key national indicators of well-being, 2013.* Washington, DC: U.S. Government Printing Office. Retrieved from http://www.childstats.gov/americaschildren/

Health Resources and Services Administration (HRSA). (2014). *The Affordable Care Act and Health Centers.* Retrieved from http://www.bphc.hrsa.gov/about/healthcenterfactsheet.pdf

Koh, H. K., Graham, G., & Glied, S. A. (2011). Reducing racial and ethnic disparities: The action plan from the Department of Health and Human Services. *Health Affairs, 30,* 1822–1829.

Institute of Medicine (IOM). (2009). *Race, ethnicity, and language data: Standardization for health care quality improvement.* Washington, DC: National Academies Press.

National Center for Health Statistics. (NCHS). (1999). *Healthy People 2000 review, 1998–99.* Hyattsville, MD: Public Health Service.

National Center for Health Statistics. (2012). *Healthy People 2010 final review.* Hyattsville, MD. Retrieved from http://www.cdc.gov/nchs/healthy_people/hp2010/hp2010_final_review.htm

Niew, M.A., & McEwen, M. (2015). *Community health nursing: Promoting the health of populations* (6th ed.). St. Louis, MO: Elsevier Saunders.

Public Health Agency of Canada. *What is the population health approach?* Retrieved from http://www.phac-aspc.gc.ca /ph-sp/approach-approche/index-eng.php

U.S. Department of Health and Human Services. (2011). *HHS action plan to reduce racial and ethnic health disparities: A nation free of disparities in health and health care.* Retrieved from http://www.minorityhealth.hhs.gov /npa/templates/content.aspx?lvl=1&lvlid=33&ID=285

U.S. Department of Health and Human Services, Office of Public Health and Science, Office of Disease Prevention and Health Promotion (USDHHS, OPHS). (2001). *Healthy people in healthy communities: A community planning guide using Healthy People 2010.* Washington, DC: U.S. Government Printing Office.

ONLINE RESOURCES

AARP: Caregiving
http://www.aarp.org/relationships/caregiving/

AHRQ
http://www.ahrq.gov/research/ruralix.htm

Administration on Aging
http://www.aoa.gov/

Administration for Community Living at
http://www.acl.gov/Index.aspx

CDC: Family Caregiving—The Facts
http://www.cdc.gov/aging/caregiving/facts.htm

CDC Office of Minority Health and Health Disparities
http://www.cdc.gov/omhd/
http://www.cdc.gov/minorityhealth/populations/atrisk.html #Geography

CDC Healthy Aging
http://www.cdc.gov/aging/
http://wonder.cdc.gov/
http://www.cdc.gov/features/agingandhealth/state_of_aging _and_health_in_america_2013.pdf

Family Caregiver Alliance
https://caregiver.org/about-fca

U.S. Department of Labor Family and Medical Leave Act at
http://www.dol.gov/whd/fmla/index.htm

Health Resources and Services Administration
http://www.hrsa.gov/ruralhealth/index.html

Healthy People 2020
http://www.healthypeople.gov/2020/about/default.aspx

Rural Health Centers
http://www.hrsa.gov/healthit/toolbox/RuralHealthI Ttoolbox/Introduction/ruralclinics.html

National Alliance for Caregiving
http://www.caregiving.org/

National Domestic Violence Hotline
http://www.thehotline.org

Home and Community Based Long-Term Care
http://www.aoa.acl.gov/AoA_Programs/HCLTC/Caregiver /index.aspx

Rural Health
http://www.ruralhealthweb.org/
http://ers.usda.gov/publications/eb-economic -brief/eb24.aspx

Rural Health Research Gateway database
http://www.ruralhealthresearch.org/

Rural Healthy People 2020
http://sph.tamhsc.edu/srhrc/rhp2020.html

USDHHS Office of Minority Health
http://minorityhealth.hhs.gov/

● Rose Kearney-Nunnery

15 Informatics and Documenting Outcomes

"There is a better way to do it; find it."

Thomas A. Edison

Chapter Objectives

On completion of this chapter, the reader will be able to:

1. Describe computer and informatics applications used in nursing practice, education, and research.
2. Define the basic terminology used in nursing informatics.
3. Describe the relationship between healthcare provision and health management information systems.
4. Define the specialty practice of nursing informatics and the integration of that role into the nursing services of a healthcare institution.
5. Identify opportunities for interdisciplinary collaboration from an informatics perspective.
6. Explain telehealth applications and their effect on patients and providers.
7. Describe nursing career opportunities in informatics.

Key Terms

Nursing Informatics
Health Information Systems
Electronic Health Record (EHR)
Standardized Nursing Language

Taxonomies
Nursing Management
  Minimum Data Set
  (NMMDS)

Electronic Prescribing (CPOE)
Office Applications
Handheld PCs
Telehealth

"**Nursing informatics (NI)** is a specialty that integrates nursing science with multiple information and analytical sciences to identify, define, manage, and communicate data, information, knowledge, and wisdom in nursing practice" (American Nurses Association [ANA], 2015b, pp. 1–2). Graves and Corcoran (1989) promoted nursing informatics as a specialty area, and it was quickly supported by several nursing graduate programs of study. Nursing informatics was recognized as a specialty for registered nurses by the American Nurses Association in 1992 and earned credibility through the offering of a certification examination by the American Nurses Credentialing Center. NI as a specialty grows and changes as quickly as the computer industry and the technology we use in daily life. This chapter addresses the use of informatics in practice, education, and research, as well as computer applications that support nursing activities.

OVERVIEW OF NURSING INFORMATICS

The primary interest of nursing informatics is to expand how data, information, and knowledge are used within practice. Those conducting research on informatics issues seek to identify and explain relationships between healthcare data and nursing care. However, as described by ANA (2015b), the definition of nursing informatics as a specialty was expanded from the science of information and knowledge acquisition to include the provision of wisdom. "Wisdom is defined as the appropriate use of knowledge to manage and solve human problems . . . . and an appreciation of the consequences of selected actions" (ANA, 2015b, p. 3). The actual work of informatics specialists varies with settings, according to organizational needs, individual practice interests, and specific research questions. The common element in all functions within informatics practice is the transformation of data to information and knowledge and, ultimately, to provide the wisdom that supports and advances nursing practice.

> The common element in all functions within the informatics practice is the transformation of data to information and knowledge and, ultimately, to provide the wisdom that supports and advances nursing practice.

Within healthcare delivery institutions such as hospitals, long-term care facilities, and home health agencies, the NI specialist could be involved with both the tasks of nursing and improvement of the quality of care. Carrington and Tiase (2013) describe nursing informatics as a "subdiscipline of health informatics that applies information technology to the skills and work of nurses in health care" (p. 136). Task-related NI activities include staffing and scheduling systems, effective implementation of the electronic health record, safety monitoring, real-time retrieval of patient information, and use of evidence-based practice information, telehealth applications, and interpretation of nursing needs for the interdisciplinary informatics team. Clinical performance measures initiatives as required and certification programs as promoted by the Joint Commission (2014a, 2014b) and the Centers for Medicare and Medicaid Services (CMS, 2013, n.d.) require the input and retrieval of data demonstrating

use of evidence-based practice guidelines. These guidelines are also available electronically (Box 15.1). The NI specialist is instrumental in creating communication standards and pathways to provide ease in accessing necessary information for reporting to these and other organizations. National benchmarking and accreditation databases and agencies now accept and return information only in electronic format.

Nursing informatics applications in academic settings have grown to include both the use of technology in the teaching process and the teaching of an informatics-focused curriculum. Many schools of nursing use a learning content management system (LCMS), such as BlackBoard or eCollege, to provide Web-enhanced or totally Web-based courses that include discussion boards, chat rooms, assignment drop boxes, online testing, and grade books, as well as areas to post interactive exercises and graphics presentations. Nursing and health science programs and orientation and residency programs in the practice setting are also using simulation activities in live classroom and laboratory settings. These activities include the use of human simulators like SimMan or MetiMan or the virtual patient in teaching simulations. The human simulators are programmed to present a variety of case scenarios and respond to the students' interventions in planned ways. Information can be downloaded from the simulators or video-recorded to provide feedback and debriefing opportunities on time management, decision making, and nursing competence. Students participate as active participants with the human simulators and as observers to the interventions of others. In a virtual patient situation, actors adhere to scripts in a class situation. Following the simulation, a group debriefing provides an opportunity for reflection and vicarious learning prior to the live patient situation. Both of these types of teaching activities enhance the learning process in a safe, simulated environment as a result of technological advances.

In addition to technology projects conducted within schools and colleges, electronic journals have made articles available online. These publications have gone through the peer review process of their print counterparts but are more accessible for readers. The *Online Journal of Nursing Informatics* and the *Online Journal of Issues in Nursing* were the first for nursing professionals. Because they are exclusively online, these journals differ from the electronically accessible versions of printed journals that may be accessed

---

BOX 15.1 **Evidence-Based Practice Electronic Resources**

National Guideline Clearinghouse
http://www.guidelines.gov/

Centers for Disease Control and Prevention
http://www.cdc.gov

Nursing Knowledge International
http://www.nursingknowledge.org

The Cochrane Collaboration
http://www.cochrane.org/

Agency for Healthcare Research and Quality
http://www.ahrq.gov

through major publishers, association Web sites, and subscribers to health science libraries. Online journals can give nurses an electronic format to share findings, experiences, perceptions, knowledge, and wisdom with nursing colleagues involved in all facets of their specialties. The intent is to exercise the power of technology to create an electronic nursing community that provides both virtually accessible and timely information about nursing globally. Online journals may also enhance the speed of peer review and communications through an expedited editorial process that provides rapid turnaround, publication, and availabilty of information. Downloading one copy of these electronically accessible articles is permitted for scholarly work, but proper citation is required. Other selected titles of electronic journals are listed in Box 15.2.

E-books, electronic versions of printed reports and books, are also now available both in libraries and for purchase. E-books and pdfs of national reports are convenient ways to access reference material. In addition, e-textbooks are available for purchase for a negotiated period of time and downloaded to your computer. Additional study resources may also accompany selected e-books. Many printed textbooks also come with electronic support in the form of a Web site (for access to additional learning resources, as with the site for this text) or DVDs to supplement the materials.

Given these advances in informatics, one might think that nursing is well evolved in the specialty. However, recall that the Institute of Medicine (IOM) formally identified utilizing informatics as one of the five competencies for all health professionals (Greiner & Kneibel, 2003). "Utilizing informatics" encompasses the responsibility to communicate, manage knowledge, mitigate error, and support decision making through the use of information technology.

Essential nursing informatics content in nursing education is a consideration as we address this imperative for safe and effective patient care. In a descriptive study of informatics competencies of both baccalaureate and graduate nursing students, Choi and DeMartinis (2013) found that students in both programs did not perceive themselves competent in applied computer skills and clinical informatics roles (p. 1974). However, in an earlier study, compared with prelicensure baccalaureate nursing students, both RN and BSN students perceived themselves as more competent in these roles, which the researcher attributed to experience in clinical practice (Choi, 2012, p. 7). To address competencies in undergraduate nursing education, the Canadian Association of Schools of Nursing (2012) identified specific nursing informatics competencies, with the overarching competency of "uses information and communication technologies to support information synthesis

in accordance with professional and regulatory standards in the delivery of patient/client care" (p. 5). In the *Essentials of Baccalaureate Education for Professional Nursing Practice* (AACN, 2008), "baccalaureate graduates are expected to ethically manage data, information, knowledge, and technology to communicate effectively; provide safe and effective patient care; and use research and clinical evidence to inform practice decisions" (p. 18).

Competencies in informatics and information technology are further supported in the American Association of Colleges of Nursing (AACN) in their Essentials for Baccalaureate, Master's and Doctoral Education in Nursing (AACN, 2008, 2011, 2006). The applications of informatics discussed in this chapter are derived from the specific informatics competencies described in the IOM reports and in the professional scope and standards of practice (ANA, 2015b). In addition, all nurses are expected to utilize informatics, whether beginning nurse, expert nurse, or specialty practitioner. Consider the informatics competencies for nurses identified in Box 15.3 that were part of the prior scope or practice (ANA, 2008). Since that time, a role delineation study by the American Nurses Credentialing Center (2013) resulted in refinements to the credentialing exam for the informatics nurse with baccalaureate preparation on current professional practice. However, with rapid enhancements to technology, including the implementation of the electronic health record across multiple settings and evidence of meaningful use, informatics competencies evolve and become expectations in practice. In the newly revised scope and standards of practice, basic computer competencies are an expectation for all nurses, including the novice nurse. However, a pathway from novice nurse, to aspiring informatics nurse with a minimum of 5 years in practice is recommended with graduate preparation for advanced specialty practice in nursing (ANA, 2015). In addition, the ANA (2015b) has identified further specialist competencies for the NI Specialist in practice areas of outcome identification, implementation, and evaluation and in standards of professional performance (ethics, education, evidence-based practice and research, quality of practice, leadership, collaboration, professional practice evaluation, resource utilization, and environmental health.

Nursing informatics is an evolving specialty area. Informatics and evolving technology are changing how nurses teach, deliver, communicate, and improve nursing care. Students and practitioners are able to learn more from home, creating new opportunities for formal and continuing education. Updating professional skills for those residing in isolated areas and accessing expert consultation from clinicians in distant geographic areas are two more reasons to embrace technology in nursing and healthcare.

BOX 15.2	Selected Online Journals

The Online Journal of Issues in Nursing
http://www.nursingworld.org/ojin/

Online Journal of Nursing Informatics
http://ojni.org/

Online Journal of Rural Nursing and Health Care
http://rnojournal.binghamton.edu/index.php/RNO

Online Brazilian Journal of Nursing
http://www.objnursing.uff.br/index.php/nursing

TRANSFORMATION OF DATA TO INFORMATION, KNOWLEDGE, AND WISDOM

The transformation of data into information, knowledge, and wisdom is essential in important informatics practice. A *datum* is a value placed on a variable. It exists without meaning or explanation. An example is the blood pressure (BP) measurement. The value of the BP, such as 90/54, is the datum for the BP. This value has little meaning until it is put into some context along with other data. For instance,

| BOX 15.3 | Informatics Competencies For Nurses |

Beginning nurses:
- Computer literacy skills for administration, communication, data access, documentation, education, monitoring, and basic desktop software
- Informatics knowledge on impact, privacy and security, and systems, and for patient safety

Experienced nurses:
- Computer literacy skills for communication, documentation, education, monitoring, basic desktop software, and systems
- Information literacy on evaluation, roles, and system maintenance
- Informatics knowledge on impact, privacy and security, systems, research, and organizational change management, and for patient safety

Informatics nurse specialists:
- Computer literacy for monitoring, desktop software, systems, quality improvement, research, and project management
- Informatics skills for evaluation, roles, system maintenance, analysis, data structures, design and development, implementation, management (including fiscal), programming, and system, agency, and agency requirements
- Informatics skills and knowledge for system, selection, testing and training, knowledge on impact, privacy and security, systems, regulations, usability, education, theoretical structures, taxonomies and classification systems, systems theory and operational change, and promotion of patient safety
- In addition, specific functional specialty areas have other expected competencies for those functional areas.

Source: Adapted from American Nurses Association. (2008). Nursing informatics: Scope and standards of practice. Silver Spring, MD: Nursesbooks.org.

if this were a 35-year-old adult, the BP might have one interpretation, but for a 10-year-old child, 90/54 would mean something very different. Age and BP may not be enough data to offer much information. You may also want to know the person's pulse and weight, which would allow you to understand the BP's significance better. Data viewed in association with one another provide meaning. Knowledge arises from using information, often from combined sources, to determine new meanings, make new discoveries, or expand understanding as wisdom. For example, patient diagnoses arise through the transformation of combined laboratory data, radiology data, symptomatology, and other information into a whole, the outcome of which is knowledge. Then, wisdom is the appropriate understanding and application of this knowledge to solve human problems (ANA, 2015b).

> An informatics nurse is someone who has a specialty practice in nursing, not simply a computer expert who happens to be working on a nursing-related problem.

Informatics nurses seek to create new knowledge and then wisdom by working first with data and then with information. Informatics specialists work as an integral part of an interdisciplinary team to support, promote, and advance the delivery of nursing care. They work toward informatics solutions, which may be an application, product, method, tool, workflow change, or other recommendation with competencies in both information literacy and management (ANA, 2015b, p. 46). Indeed, an informatics nurse is someone who has a specialty practice in nursing, not simply a computer expert who happens to be working on a nursing-related problem. Further, information nurse specialists with master's preparation analyze information for risk reduction and improvements in delivery and policy in practice while informatics specialists prepared at the doctoral level lead in the design, section and integration of technology systems (ANA, 2015b, p. 46).

In the past, nonintegrated health management systems were seen in larger health information management systems that hospitals, clinics, home health agencies, nursing homes, and health maintenance organizations to manage their various functions (Fig. 15.1). These systems often operated as separate, noncommunicating units, creating frustrations in the workplace and with the efficiency of care delivery. The goal is for these systems to operate seamlessly as we move toward full implementation of a totally computerized health record that allows for information capture, retrieval, and exchange. It is vital that nurses recognize that they are contributing data every time they carry out a nursing function. These data have the potential of providing powerful information when they are well understood within the environment of healthcare delivery (Hebda, Czar, & Mascara, 2008).

HEALTH INFORMATION SYSTEMS

Because few systems can address every component of healthcare and organizational management, there is generally an overriding information system with both clinical and administrative components, known as the **health information system**. Clinical systems include those functions that directly support patient care—documentation, order entry, and diagnostic reporting. Administrative systems address the financial, personnel, and managerial functions of the facility. Together, these systems use technology to process data into information for multiple uses.

Currently, no one health information system fits all organizations. However, the current use of certified electronic health records and the goals for portability have created the need for more common functioning. In 2010, the Department of Health and Human Services issued a regulation with standards and certification criteria that the electronic health record must meet (Blumenthal & Tavenner, 2010, p. 504).

The information system should accomplish two goals. First, it should support the way that nurses operate, giving them flexibility and permitting appropriate documentation. Second, the system should support and improve nursing practice through access to information and tools (Hebda et al.,

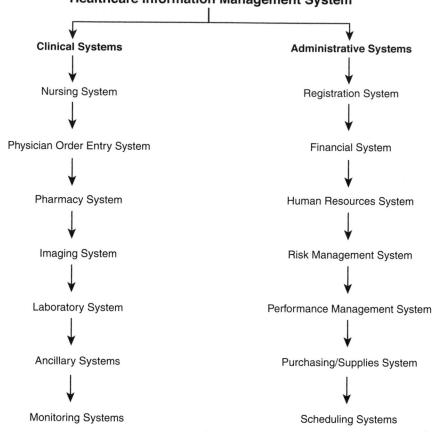

Figure 15.1 The Healthcare Information Management System.

2008). It is essential in an evidence-based practice environment to expect easy access to healthcare databases. Additionally, Intranet service often includes access to drug guides, policy and procedures, and patient teaching information. Box 15.4 describes how the integration of systems can help reduce medication errors.

Electronic Health Record

A major national effort to develop an **electronic health record (EHR)** has been under way for a number of years, and institutions have had challenges and some success in this area. The EHR is an electronic version of the patient record. As described in a report on the usability of the EHR for the Agency for Healthcare Research Quality (AHRQ), "EHRs are clinical support tools with the potential to reduce strains on clinician memory and cognition while improving efficiency in workflow and effectiveness in care quality and coordination (Armijo, McDonnell, & Werner, 2009, p. 2). Benefits of a fully functional and integrated EHR are listed in Box 15.5.

The purposes of creating EHRs are to improve the ability to share patient-specific information, create permanent lifelong health records, and have ready access to additional

---

BOX 15.4 System Integration to Reduce Medication Errors

1. The provider enters a medication order into the order entry system, eliminating confusion from handwriting and providing clinical decision support.
2. This information is transmitted to the pharmacy.
3. The pharmacy system checks for dosage, allergies, and potential interactions. Alerts are generated.
4. The medication order is filled by the pharmacy, using a barcode or robotic system.
5. The nurse checks the order against the electronic medication administration record and is alerted to administration times as well as any special considerations.
6. The nurse documents that the medication has been administered and notes the patient's response.
7. Reminders for reorders and 24-hour chart checks are generated automatically.

Adapted from: Cohen, M. R. (Ed.). (2007). *Medication errors* (2nd ed.). Washington, DC: American Pharmacists Association.

BOX 15.5 Benefits of a Fully Functional Electronic Health Record

- Patient access to own health information
- Better access to patient records by healthcare providers
- Decreased errors in health records
- Decreased unnecessary diagnostic testing and procedures
- More complete and accurate health records and data
- Improved longitudinal tracking of patients and patient groups
- Improved standards of care; reduction in medical errors
- Provision of research data to better inform clinical care, public health, and biomedical research
- Facilitation of better communication among patients and healthcare providers
- Facilitation of detection of healthcare fraud
- Improved tracking of healthcare costs and benefits for improvement in healthcare delivery and economics

Adapted from: JASON. (2014). *A robust health data infrastructure.* (AHRQ Publication No. 14-0041-EF). Retrieved from http://www.healthit.gov/sites/default/files/ptp13-700hhs_white.pdf

information that will improve the quality and safety of patient care. In 2009, passage of the American Recovery and Reinvestment Act provided major funding incentives to hospitals and eligible practitioners over the next several years to encourage the adoption and meaningful use of EHRs. CMS reported the identification of the "meaningful use" goals and standards, planned in three stages (Box 15.6). This incentive program could provide maximum payments over 5 years in excess of $43,000 for eligible providers that began participation in 2011 or 2012, with a reduction for starting in 2013 and no incentive payments for those starting after 2014. Eligible hospitals were similarly incentivized. The incentive payment is 75% of their Medicare-allowed charges up to a maximum annual cap, as long as their meaningful use requirements are met in their data reporting. Eligible providers included physicians, advanced practice registered nurses, dentists, therapists, and other qualified professionals who were not hospital based, with greater than 90% of services provided. And the program was with the individual provider, not a group practice. There were 90-day reporting periods, and the certified EHR provided the data for the objectives that had to meet a specified threshold. Reporting was required on core objectives, five menu objectives, and selected quality measures. Some exclusions could be claimed on some objective measures by certain providers who did not provide

BOX 15.6 Stages of Meaningful Use

Stage 1 (2011-2012): Data capture and sharing
Stage 2 (2014): Advanced clinical processes
Stage 3 (2017): Improved outcomes

Source: Centers for Medicare and Medicaid Services. (2014a). *EHR incentive programs.* Retrieved from http://www.cms.gov/Regulations-and-Guidance/Legislation/EHRIncentivePrograms/

the specified service. However, there were just reporting requirements on the quality measures in Stage 1.

The first stage began in 2011 with specific criteria to electronically capture health information to track key clinical conditions. Although this information could be used for care coordination for individual patients, the ultimate aim has also been to address population health with the reporting of clinical quality measures and public health information. Eligible providers and eligible hospitals could apply for the CMS Initiative Program if they could meet the requirements presented in core objectives (Table 15.1). CMS (2014b) reported that "between 2009 and 2012, EHR adoption nearly doubled among physicians and more than tripled among hospitals [and] nine in 10 eligible hospitals and eight in 10 eligible professionals had taken the initial step of registering for the Medicare or Medicaid EHR Incentive Programs as of October 2013" (p. 1). This program made more than $15.5 billion eligible to providers and hospitals (JASON, 2014, p. 2).

In Stage 2, most objectives were retained, with increased thresholds expected. Some objectives were combined or eliminated, as illustrated in Table 15.1. CMS (2012) expected that providers who reached Stage 2 would be able to demonstrate meaningful use of their EHR technology for an even larger portion of their patient population. Some new objectives were also introduced as menu objectives. However, as in Stage 1, exclusions could be claimed on some objective measures by certain providers who did not provide the specified service.

Stage 3 will be developed further based on data from Stage 2 but will focus on improvements in quality, safety, and efficiency; providing decision support for national high priority conditions; and improving population health. The IOM (2014) was charged with convening a committee to identify domains and measures that capture the social determinants of health to inform the development of recommendations for Stage 3 (p. S-2). The IOM addressed this charge in two phases; the Phase 1 report was issued in 2014 with the identification of sociodemographic, psychological, behavioral, individual social relationship, and neighborhood/community domains for inclusion in the EHR.

Advances in the development of large data repositories held within hospitals and other healthcare institutions allow linkages between an electronic patient record and administrative, bibliographic, clinical expertise, and research databases. Through these large data sets using common language and data values, trends and the basis for evidence-based practice can occur more readily. The domains identified were based on areas in which evidence was available on their association with health outcomes, with the goal of identifying measures in Phase 2 to develop strategies for improving health status of Americans (IOM, 2014, p. S-6).

Creating an EHR is far more difficult than may at first be apparent. Standardized language, data collection, record format, access, confidentiality, cost, and other ethical issues are but a few of the perceived barriers. To build an EHR that can be shared among institutions and providers, data must be collected and coded in a similar fashion. With the new certification requirements for EHRs, compatibility among systems and standards for vendors is the goal. JASON (2014), a research and advisory group for the federal government, reported that "the current inoperability among the data resources for EHRs is a major impediment

TABLE 15.1

Stage 1 Meaningful Use Requirements for Eligible Providers and Hospitals

Eligible Provider Core Objectives	Eligible Hospital Core Objectives
• Implement computerized provider order entry (CPOE) • Perform drug-drug and drug-allergy checks • Allow E-prescribing (eRx) • Record demographics • Maintain an up-to-date problem list of current and active diagnoses • Maintain active medication list • Maintain active medication allergy list • Record and chart changes in vital signs • Record smoking status for patients 13 years or older • Implement clinical decision support • Report ambulatory clinical quality measures to Centers for Medicare and Medicaid Services (CMS) and states • Provide patients with an electronic copy of their health information, on request • Provide clinical summaries for patients for each office visit • Allow exchange of key clinical information electronically (eliminated in 2013; not in Stage 2) • Protect electronic health information • Implement drug-formulary checks • Incorporate clinical laboratory test results as structured data • Generate lists of patients by specific condition for quality improvement • Send reminders to patients for preventative and follow-up care • Provide patients with timely electronic access to their health information (eliminated in 2014; not in Stage 2) • Identify specific patient education resources and provide these to the patient, if relevant • Perform medication reconciliation if patient received from another setting or provider, if appropriate • When transitioning patient to another care setting or provider, provide a summary of care record for each transition • Submit electronic data to immunization registries of systems • Submit electronic data on reportable laboratory test results to public health agencies	• Implement CPOE • Perform drug-drug and drug-allergy checks • Record demographics • Maintain an up-to-date problem list of current and active diagnoses • Maintain active medication list • Maintain active medication allergy list • Record and chart changes in vital signs, including body mass index and growth charts for children 2 to 20 years of age • Record smoking status for patients 13 years or older • Implement clinical decision support • Report ambulatory clinical quality measures to CMS and states • Provide patients with an electronic copy of their health information, on request • Provide patients with an electronic copy of their discharge instructions at time of discharge (eliminated in 2014; not in Stage 2) • Allow exchange of key clinical information among providers electronically (eliminated in 2013; not in Stage 2) • Protect electronic health information • Implement drug-formulary checks • Incorporate clinical laboratory test results as structured data • Generate lists of patients by specific condition for quality improvement • Identify specific patient education resources and provide these to the patient, if relevant • Perform medication reconciliation if patient received from another setting or provider, if appropriate • When transitioning patient to another care setting or provider, provide a summary of care record for each transition • Submit electronic data to immunization registries of systems • Submit electronic data on reportable laboratory test results to public health agencies and actual submission

Source: Centers for Medicare and Medicaid Services. (2014b). *EHR incentive programs.* Retrieved from http://www.cms.gov/
Regulations-and-Guidance/Legislation/EHRIncentivePrograms/

for the effective exchange of health care information" (p. 3). This group has made recommendations on the software architecture required for the effective exchange of health information among EHRs and systems. JASON (2014) also recommended the principle that the patient is the ultimate owner of the health record and that privacy issues be mapped into well-defined architectural elements in the data infrastructure (p. 4).

One issue regarding the EHR that will continue to be addressed is patient confidentiality. Fortunately, the Health Insurance Portability and Accountability Act (HIPAA) was implemented in 2003 in an effort to eliminate unnecessary, unwarranted, and inappropriate sharing of individual and personal information. In addition, one of the core requirements for *meaningful use* by eligible providers or hospitals is the protection of patient information in the EHR.

There are clear guidelines for when information can and cannot be shared and how to handle electronic communication (CMS, 2013a). Password protection for facility and personal computers is recommended for any patient, including name, age, gender, and Social Security number. However, consumers still have concerns, owing to the fear of identity fraud, that their records are not going to be protected, and that other personal information will be accessed. Encryption, passwords, audit trails, workstation security, and firewalls all serve to preserve the integrity of the EHR. Information for consumers on privacy and security is available at http://www.healthit.gov/patients-families/protecting-your-privacy-security.

Another consideration for implementation is the leadership required for the change. Getting people in the organization "on board" for the project requires committed and strong leadership. Various successful EHR implementation projects have been reported. Adler (2007) reported on an early successful implementation that required the three Ts: "*team* refers to people and organizational issues, *tactics* to specific techniques and choices made in design and setup, and *technology* to the software" (p. 33). Quality improvements, ease of communication, assistance with decision support, and enhanced safety are a few of the benefits with a successful implementation of an EHR.

The issue becomes the need for a common language to create a standard for the exchange, management, and integration of healthcare information. The goal is to create seamless systems that exchange information between and among each other to increase accessibility and safety for the healthcare patients.

Standardized Nursing Language

Common vocabulary, terminology, and usage are requirement for consistent understanding and application across nursing settings and practice environments with a **standardized nursing language**. A standardized nursing language benefits the profession and nursing practitioners, other colleagues, reimbursement practices, and patients. It provides a common basis and understanding. Rutherford (2008) has identified the following advantages of a standardized nursing language for the clinical nurse:

- Improved communication among nurses and other healthcare providers
- Increased visibility of nursing interventions
- Improved care for healthcare consumers
- Enhanced classification of data to evaluate nursing outcomes
- Greater adherence to standards of practice and care
- Facilitated assessment of nursing competency (p. 8)

The goal is for a common understanding and communication of what nurses do to affect patients' care and health outcomes. As a result, the profession has generated several **taxonomies**, or classification systems, for this common understanding and usage of terminology.

In 2012, the ANA recognized 12 terminologies or taxonomies that supported nursing practice. Subsequently, the ANA (2015a) focused further on the need for standardized terminologies to support the EHR. Perhaps the most widely known is the North America Nursing Diagnosis Association (NANDA), which expanded to an international taxonomy

with NANDA-I. Almost 30 years of experience in the identification and refinement of this classification system have been described by the president-elect of NANDA-I as follows:

The NANDA-I concepts support nurses in a clinical reasoning process to evaluate the holistic needs of patients, families, or communities, to make accurate decisions about care, and to document the health requests, patient safety risks, and the actual problems as "succinct" diagnostic concepts in the electronic health records and available for exchange between settings. (Brokel, 2010, pp. 184–185)

NANDA-I terminology and nursing diagnoses provide a standardized language that is evidence-based and that undergoes continual revision on a biannual basis based upon evidence in current practice. "The NANDA-I concepts include culturally sensitive concepts that have been translated into 10 languages—Spanish, German, Japanese, Portuguese, French, and others including third world countries" (Brokel, 2010, p. 185). Especially useful with this taxonomy is the identification of defining characteristics and related factors in addition to the diagnostic labels used to identify nursing diagnostic statements. This taxonomy is consistent with nursing's focus on functional health patterns as well as other nursing taxonomies. Thede and Schwiren (2011) discovered through survey research that most nurses are familiar with the NANDA taxonomy and less familiar with others.

The Center for Nursing Classification and Clinical Effectiveness (CNCCE), housed at the University of Iowa, has taken on the challenge of developing standardized nursing language and has published nursing interventions and outcomes (Appendix B) with definitions to be used in documentation systems. The Center also has collaborated with the NANDA-I to integrate these interventions and outcomes with nursing diagnosis language.

In the pursuit of comparability of data using common terminology, other classification systems have evolved over time, some specific to practice settings or expanded to other practice settings. A long-standing taxonomy used in nursing is the Omaha System (2013). This system was originally developed for home care but is now applicable to a wide range of settings with comparable data and language. SNOMED CT (Systematized Nomenclature of Medicine—Clinical Terms) is an interdisciplinary and international terminology system. In SNOMED CT each concept had a code for identification and a unique meaning used by more than 25 countries that are members of the International Health Terminology Standards Organisation (2014).

Another example of a taxonomy specific to nursing was developed and validated in the perioperative area. The Perioperative Nursing Data Set (PNDS) was developed by nurses to document the perioperative patient experience from preadmission through discharge, is recognized by the ANA, and is incorporated into SNOMED (AORN, 2013). This data set provides a platform for the evaluation of patient outcomes and also is the basis for evidence-based practices present and opportunities for further evaluation and research. (AORN, 2013).

For many years, we have also had the **Nursing Management Minimum Data Set (NMMDS)** in long-term care to categorize nursing care and patient care needs. Long-term care facilities are required to make electronic

ONLINE CONSULT

ANA Recognized Terminologies at
http://www.nursingworld.org/MainMenu
Categories/Policy-Advocacy/Positions-and
-Resolutions/ANAPositionStatements/Position
-Statements-Alphabetically/Inclusion-of
-Recognized-Terminologies-within-EHRs.html

International Council of Nurses Classification
for Nursing Practice at
http://www.icn.ch/pillarsprograms/international
-classification-for-nursing-practice-icnpr/

NANDA-I at
http://www.nanda.org/

Nursing Interventions Classifications (NIC) at
http://www.nursing.uiowa.edu/cncce/nursing
-interventions-classification-overview

Nursing Outcomes Classifications (NOC) at
http://www.nursing.uiowa.edu/cncce/nursing
-outcomes-classification-overview

Minimum Data Set (MDS) at
http://www.cms.gov/Medicare/Quality-Initiatives
-Patient-Assessment-Instruments/NursingHome
QualityInits/NHQIQualityMeasures.html

OMAHA System at
http://www.omahasystem.org

Perioperative Nursing Data Set (PNDS) at
http://www.aorn.org/syntegrity/

SNOMED CT at
www.ihtsdo.org/snomed-ct/

reports of the nursing MDS to CMS. Nurses must both assess residents on an ongoing basis and report this information using the electronic tools and standardized language. More than 16,000 long-term care facilities in the United States are required to comply with this reporting using this taxonomy.

The International Council of Nurses (ICN) has also been working on a language and taxonomy to improve communication of nursing activities across the globe as the International Classification for Nursing Practice (ICNP®). The vision for this classification system is focused on nursing to provide an infrastructure informing healthcare practice and policy to improve patient care worldwide (ICN, 2013).

Each of these classification systems must be useful in the identification and comparison of practice and be fully functional with the electronic health record. The critical concern for nursing is the consistent application of a terminology or classification system that is sensitive to measure and demonstrates the effectiveness of nursing care.

ONLINE CONSULT

AHRQ Health Information Technology at
http://healthit.ahrq.gov/

CMS EHR Incentive Program at
https://www.cms.gov/EHRIncentivePrograms/

Electronic Prescribing

An important component in the EHR for patient safety is **electronic prescribing** or computerized physician order entry (CPOE). The most sophisticated level of this technology is full integration with the EHR, has been shown to provide the highest degree of patient safety and the largest return on investment (AHRQ, 2013). Nursing personnel have found both positive and negative attributes of electronic prescribing. On the positive side, the provider must take responsibility for the patient care order and not rely upon the nurse for interpretation, assistance, or completion. The system cues the provider with correct spellings, dosages, and evidence-based guidelines, and alerts the provider to potential and known contraindications and interactions. The provider can view the patient's diagnostic results and initiate appropriate orders from home, office, or other Web-based settings. An electronic flag will appear in the patient's record, which indicates that a new electronic order has been entered for the patient; it has simultaneously been sent to the diagnostic or therapeutic department for processing. If a nurse does not acknowledge this electronic flag in a timely manner, the patient may have labs drawn before the nurse has time to inform the patient. The intent is to provide timely communication and intervention for the healthcare consumer through direct entry of orders, to eliminate careless errors, to improve efficiency in processes, and to reduce adverse events through medication management and an alert system for dosages, interactions, and contraindications. Providers who engage in this system generally become reliant upon this electronic tool as an adjunct for decisional support and for real-time modifications to the patient's plan of care. Cowan (2013) reports two human factors associated with errors and CPOE, namely work-arounds for the alerts generated and altered communication patterns between physicians and nurses due to the reliance on the technology. These become additional safety considerations.

In addition, medication reconciliation as another patient safety practice is now a requirement for all hospitals and other settings accredited by the Joint Commission. Medication histories must be current for each transition made by the patient, whether from the emergency department, to the intensive care unit, to the acute care unit, to home, or to a skilled care facility.

Computer Applications

Common **office applications**—word processing, spreadsheet, database, and presentation graphics—are useful in nursing practice, education, and research. Students in nursing programs are expected to submit papers using word processing, and sometimes electronically as attachments or in assignment drop boxes in Web-based courses. Oral or group presentations are accompanied with presentation graphics as a background. Spreadsheet and database management become increasingly important as nurses share in decision making and must understand the performance improvement data in order to contribute ideas to improve practice. Specialized applications have been created to improve management and dissemination of nursing information. In practice, nurses most commonly use computers to document care and access patient data. Documentation often involves selection of interventions and outcomes from a prepared list of appropriate terms, with little need for lengthy narrative comments. However, with a fully integrated EHR, there will be greater access to records and data files for a complete patient profile in the digital format.

Handheld Devices

Increasingly, reference materials accessible through the computer have become a necessary adjunct to effective care. Handheld computer devices in the form of smart phones and **handheld PCs** (personal computers) are quite popular with direct care providers since textbook publishers now provide many common references in this electronic format. Nursing students now have an array of reference materials electronically in the clinical setting. Clinical nurses no longer need to return to the nurse's station to review a drug guide or laboratory reference and are able to scroll through an electronic resources on a handheld PC in the patient's presence and answer his or her questions with confidence and competence. Password protection helps the nurse maintain confidentiality and compliance with HIPAA regulations. However, a word of caution when using the applications on a smart phone; consumers, observers, and colleagues may misinterpret that the smart phone is being used for personal communication. Use of a smart phone may be restricted to certain areas in some clinical settings.

Independent Learning Activities

Computers have become a popular way for nursing programs to provide independent learning activities; computer-assisted instruction (CAI) replaced the video, which replaced the audio-film strip. CAI consists of text, graphics, vignettes, and self-assessment quizzes. These can be loaded onto computers in a lab, played from a DVD, or downloaded from an account over the Internet. Although distance learning has been available since the first continuing education was provided by radio and then on special television stations, it has become now evolved into digital media and become a convenient way to complete continuing education requirements and for degree-seeking nurses.

For students, classes can be delivered via the Internet from a server on a campus or from a business through a LCMS. Students can access courses at times convenient to their individual schedules and have access to numerous resources linked to the course and real-time results through online assessments. A paperless system is created for the submission of reflective journals and assignments, group discussion can be conducted in a synchronous (live) or asynchronous (everyone at a different time) format. Searching for information on new medications and treatments, current information on obscure conditions, and national standards and guidelines can be easily accomplished using search engines. Registration for courses, records of educational compliance, and transcripts are managed by the college's learning management system. Many students are likely using a learning content management system to access information for the course supported by this textbook.

Noncredit continuing education activities are now readily available to assist active practitioners, whether for relicensure or recertification requirements or to enhance personal lifelong learning. These Web-based programs are available through various companies, professionals organizations, and select membership groups. There are also companies that assist professional by documenting their continuing education hours. However, hard copies of certificates of completion should be maintained throughout the licensure or certification period for audit purposes. Some nurses may also be required to enter this information electronically in the database of their respective state to renew their license.

Generally, nurses select to complete continuing education hours in their interest or specialty area. Some states have required as well as open content hours to meet the renewal requirements. Currency of content is a consideration, as well as the specific content. Some programs are time-limited for receiving credit. Remaining current in the area of nursing informatics is an option using this medium. However, in a study by Kleib, Sales, Lima, and Andrea-Baylon (2010), relatively low proportions of nurses reported continuing education in informatics, especially those working outside of hospitals or providing direct patient care (p. 329).

Evidence-Based Practice

As described in Chapter 5, evidence-based practice implies that nursing care is delivered on the basis of knowledge generated from research and documented evidence of efficacy. Demonstration of evidence-based practice is now a requirement in hospitals and other agencies for accreditations. Practicing nurses have access to this growing body knowledge and practice guidelines—and can enhance their practice using this knowledge—by simply searching for it. The National Guideline Clearinghouse is a product of the U.S. Department of Health and Human Services; nurses can search directly at its Web site or through their professional association Web sites to find the latest guidelines on topics such as pain management, continence care, and teaching protocols for congestive heart failure, to mention just a few. The Sigma Theta Tau product Nursing Knowledge International serves as a repository for clinical, research, career, and continuing education resources. This is a huge managed database with links to published, proprietary, and government resources. Using the speed and power of computer search engines, this database places accurate and current information in the hands of practitioners. Several evidence based practice resources are listed in Box 15.1.

Database Management

Access to data and databases has become increasingly important, especially in our global and electronic society. We search the Web for information on a question of interest when in the past we would wait until we could get to the library. In addition to e-commerce, online auctions, live chats, listservs, and other computer-based services, database management and access is a growing application for computers. A special tracking system through the Centers for Disease Control and Prevention (CDC) allows tracking of environmental effects (e.g., air and water quality) and specific conditions (e.g., asthma and cancers) in the different states. States can be compared on these measures as a result of this massive governmental database.

The National Healthy People initiative has progressed from identification of objectives and reports at the middle and end of the 10-year cycle to a searchable database of findings at any point in time. This database is provided by the CDC and the National Center for Health Statistics (NCHS) and provides practitioners, educators, planners, and the general public with current information on the state of the health of the nation and select groups and populations.

The National Database for Nursing Quality Indicators (NDNQI) is an example of an analysis and storage unit for nursing quality information. This is a proprietary database, and members can get reports comparing performance of their units to those of other similar facilities and can use the data about falls, skin breakdown, and nurse satisfaction to make decisions about organizational improvements (NDNQI, 2014).

These are just a few examples of the use of databases containing current information that provides opportunities for proactive decisions that cannot wait for published reports. But do make sure you verify the date of the last update to the database, which will probably be indicated at the top or bottom of the Web page.

Telehealth

Telehealth ranges from patient education television in a hospital room to analysis of urine in a smart toilet and transmission of the finding to a monitoring organization. In this age of healthcare provider shortages, the time it takes to travel to remote locations suggests that specialists such as mental health providers might better serve groups by hosting a net meeting where all participants can view each other and engage in the therapeutic discussion via a computer. One of the oldest telehealth applications is the transmission of pacemaker function via the telephone. By definition, **telehealth** is "the use of electronic information and telecommunications technologies to support long-distance clinical health care, patient and professional health-related education, public health and health administration [through] . . . videoconferencing, the Internet, store-and-forward imaging, streaming media, and terrestrial and wireless communications" (Health Resources and Services Administration [HRSA], 2014, p. 1).

HRSA wants to provide access to the underserved populations through telehealth in the following ways:

- Foster partnerships within HRSA, and with other federal agencies, states, and private sector groups to create telehealth projects.
- Administer telehealth grant programs.
- Provide technical assistance.
- Evaluate the use of telehealth technologies and programs.
- Develop telehealth policy initiatives to improve access to quality health services.
- Promote knowledge exchange about "best telehealth practices." (HRSA, 2014, p. 1)

The underserved populations are also those addressed in the *Healthy People* inititives, including the uninsured, underinsured, low-income, rural, and remote groups. Telehealth best practices can reach out to these groups with both primary and specialty care services. For example, an initiative in Ontario, Canada, has 24-hour access to a nurse using telehealth.

The National Council of State Boards of Nursing has recognized the challenges that practicing across state lines present and embarked upon a multistate regulation initiative called the Mutual Recognition Compact. In order to support telehealth and other interstate nursing practices, 24 states have joined the Compact, allowing registered nurses and licensed practical/vocational nurses to practice in all the listed states and thus provide long-distance services to patients (National Council of State Boards of Nursing, 2014). And pending legislation is present in additional states. However, the nurse must have a residence in a home state that is a member of the Compact and be granted a multi-state license and practice in accordance with the respective party states where he or she is granted the privilege to practice. There is also a compact for APRNs, but currently only two states are members of this APRN compact, given the current nature of the variability of practice regulations in advanced practice among the states.

Technologies currently in use include home monitoring with otoscopes, stethoscopes, and EKG monitors, which can transmit data to a home health agency. A digital image of a radiograph or ultrasound image can be conveyed to a radiologist or disease specialist in another location, even across the globe. Robotics can be used to perform skilled procedures when the skilled surgeon is in another location. The electronic ICU allows for experienced critical care nurses to monitor patients in partnership with remotely located critical care nurses. It is interesting to think about the monitoring that is provided through Homeland Security and the possibilities of knowing that an older adult has fallen or hasn't gotten out of bed for several days through previously surreptitious surveillance modes.

NURSING INFORMATICS: THE SPECIALTY

ANA (2015b) has identified that "the nursing informatics specialty and its constituent members contribute to achieving the goal of improving the health of populations, communities, groups, families, and individuals . . . [through] the identification of issues and the design, development, and implementation of effective informatics solutions and technologies within the clinical, administrative, educational, and research domains of practice" (p. 2). It is not unusual to see implementation of new technology and computer applications in the healthcare setting nearly every day. Without the aid of NI specialists, these applications might offer little improvement in patient care and create inefficiencies and errors. NI specialists can guide the collection, documentation, analysis, and aggregation of data with the intent of improving patient care, eliminating errors, and developing a body of knowledge based on evidence, as the wisdom we seek from their specialty practice.

Educators skilled in teaching informatics or NI specialists skilled in nursing applications are the best people to teach nurses how to use computer applications and other integrated technology. NI specialists possess the characteristics of a specialty (Box 15.7). The functional areas of NI practice include the following:

- Administration, leadership, and management
- Systems analysis and design
- Compliance and integrity management
- Consultation
- Coordination, facilitation, and integration
- Development of systems, products, and resources
- Educational and professional development
- Genetics and genomics
- Information management and operational architecture
- Quality and performance improvement
- Policy development and advocacy
- Research and evaluation
- Safety, security, and environmental health
- Telehealth and informatics (ANA, 2015b, pp. 18–36).

Nursing informatics is interested in phenomena of nursing: human beings, health, the environment, and nursing. However, interdisciplinary collaboration is a necessity to effectively provide knowledge and wisdom in informatics solutions that must be highly integrated for functionality. Nurses in clinical specialties tend to focus on the content of data and information. Currently, NI specialists are working to refine nursing's language, implement efficient telehealth systems, propagate NI educational programs, expand the use of NI in research, and address new and emerging technologies.

The standards of Nursing Informatics Practice were revised in 2015. As with the current scope and standards of nursing (ANA, 2010) described in Chapter 1, the Informatics Standards of Practice also contain standards of practice and standards of professional performance with measurement criteria. The standards of practice are also aligned with the nursing process, as follows:

- Assessment: skillful needs assessment toward the goal of informatics solutions using analytical models and standardized data measures
- Problem and issues identification: careful analysis and validation of the data with multiple stakeholders in the interdisciplinary environment
- Outcomes identification: the expected outcomes with additional criteria for the informatics nurse specialist,

who is expected to provide further wisdom as evolving evidence-based practice with clinical guidelines
- Planning and implementation: customization with the multiple stakeholders with consideration of regulatory requirements, financial implications, standardization, effective change strategies, safety, and continuous quality improvement
- Evaluation: informatics solutions (ANA, 2015)

Note that for this area of specialty practice, further implementation standards are specified with measurement criteria and additional measurement criteria for the NI specialist. The additional categories of implementation standards include coordination of activities; health teaching and health promotion, and consultation (ANA, 2015b). The evaluation standard contains two additional measurement criteria for the NI specialist and their leadership that will provide informatics solutions for further innovation and practice protocols and policy changes.

There are 10 standards of professional performance for the informatics nurse and the NI specialist, again similar roles to that of general nursing:

- Ethics
- Education
- Evidence-based practice and research
- Quality of practice
- Communication
- Leadership
- Collaboration
- Professional practice evaluation
- Resource utilization
- Environmental health (ANA, 2015b).

Within these role expectations, we see specialty practice emerge with directions for the future. Additional measurement criteria for the NI specialist are included with the standards for all of the performance areas listed above with the exception of communication. Again, the NI specialist is charged with taking a lead in development of innovative and interdisciplinary practices and the creation and promotion of evidence-based practices. As noted by Murphy (2010), as the practice of the NI specialist evolves, NI will not only support the process of care delivery, but also promote better patient outcomes and improvements in health (p. 205).

The NI specialty is represented by several professional associations, such as the American Nursing Informatics Association, a working group of the American Medical Informatics Association (AMIA), a group of the International Medical Informatics Association, and other international, regional, and local organizations. Although baccalaureate programs may have a requirement for competency in computers, some offer an elective in informatics. Specialization, however, is at the graduate level, with a master's degree in NI being offered first at the Universities of Maryland, Utah, and Colorado, and now by others, such as the University of Michigan, University of Iowa, and Excelsior University. Educational preparation for this specialty area can start with a nursing elective in a baccalaureate program to targeted continuing education opportunities to graduate preparation in either a degree or certificate program.

The American Nurses Credentialing Center (ANCC, 2014) offers certification in Nursing Informatics, with a baccalaureate in nursing or a related field and documented

---

BOX 15.7 **Attributes of a Specialty in Nursing Informatics**

- A differentiated practice
- A defined research program
- Organizational representation
- Educational programs
- A credentialing mechanism

Source: From Panniers, T. L., & Gassert, C. A. (1996). Standards of practice and preparation for certification. In M. E. Mills, C. A. Romano, and B. R. Heller (Eds.), Information management in nursing and health care. Philadelphia: Springhouse.

education and practice in NI. The designation reads RN-BC once awarded. Informatics nurses may also elect to pursue additional interdisciplinary certifications. When more candidates have been prepared at the specialty level of master's, an advanced practice test may be developed. Since a graduate degree is not yet a requirement for this certification opportunity, experience and education are required for the ANCC examination, which covers systems, ergonomics, technologies, information technology, management and generation of knowledge, theories, roles, and practice trends.

CAREERS IN NURSING INFORMATICS

The diversity of informatics projects and programs has led to tremendous professional career opportunities. Managers in the rapidly changing healthcare environment demand more and more information, patients receive care in many settings, and organizations have redesigned their services and care models. These changes mean continued growth for nursing and general health information systems and the creation of new positions in nursing informatics. In addition, a recent report by the Institute of Medicine (IOM, 2010) on the Future of Nursing: Leading Change, Advancing Health has the potential for the creation of future opportunities for NI specialists. Although the findings from this report will be discussed in greater detail in Chapter 19, one of the key messages was that "effective workforce planning and policy making require better data collection and an improved information infrastructure" (IOM, 2010, p. S-3). To this end, increased NI specialists will be needed in healthcare organizations, educational institutions, charitable organizations, and governmental and regulatory agencies.

Many of the future informatics jobs are yet to be defined. As the technology changes, so too will the work necessary to maintain and further the acquisition of information, knowledge, and wisdom for practice improvements. Currently, informatics nurses are working in healthcare organizations, for software and hardware vendors, in educational settings, and for insurance companies, to name only a few. In any position, the informatics specialist works closely with professionals from all other healthcare disciplines.

Positions in Healthcare Organizations

A variety of roles exist for the specialist in nursing informatics within hospitals, home health agencies, long-term care facilities, and other healthcare facilities. As organizations fully implement EHR, informatics nurses serve an important function in assessing the institution's information needs, evaluating available products and vendors, and assisting with product installations. The NI specialist may also serve to assist the organization in development and implementation of competency assessments and quality improvement initiatives. As communicator and interpreter, the NI specialist serves as a liaison between the nursing staff and the information systems people. When a system is ready for use (to "go live"), the NI specialist remains on site; later, the specialist is on call to provide expert assistance to staff, as coach and mentor. Once the system has been installed, modifications are made on the basis of user feedback, and the NI specialist is on to the next project. Informatics is a specialty that changes rapidly.

Electronic reporting is required in most regulated organizations in contemporary society. And the informatics nurse will be involved, if not leading this project, especially for data identification, coding, harvesting, and analysis. For example, long-term care facilities are required to make electronic reports to CMS of the MDS, an assessment tool for residents of long-term care facilities in which nurses must both assess residents on an ongoing basis and report this information using the electronic tools and standardized language. The vast numbers of these long-term care facilities that are required to comply with this reporting create many job opportunities for registered nurses. Quality improvement activities need NI competencies to navigate through the myriad of systems, reports, and guidelines that direct and document these improvement activities. Compliance offices require access to all the systems in a facility. The annual National Patient Safety Goals have created requirements for training staff for enhanced patient safety by improving, in part, data retrieval, management, and reporting. Performance improvement is concerned with national safety goals, clinical indicators of quality, and evidence-based practice guidelines. Informatics supports the achievement of these safety goals through providing information retrieval to support medication reconciliation, safe patient handoff, prevention of recording sound-alike/look-alike drugs, and accurately recording patient identifiers.

From safety reporting to reimbursement opportunities, informatics skills are necessary. And with the IOM (2010) recommendations for effective workforce planning and an improved information infrastructure, NI specialists will be essential to the success of this ambitious initiative.

Positions with Systems and Software Vendors

Producers of software and information systems seek to hire NI specialists. Nurses work to develop new products, market products and services, and install systems. Experience with documentation and standardized nursing language is an asset. Clinicians with enough patient care experience to predict barriers to implementation are extremely useful. NI experts serve as liaisons between the vendor and the healthcare organization, because they are able to comprehend and articulate the issues for both parties. Increasingly nurses with expertise are sought for these positions.

Positions in Educational Settings

With the expectation that beginning and experienced nurses must possess informatics competencies, the responsibilities of educators have grown. Whether it is expertise in instructional design to create a new and effective Web-based or Web-enhanced course or DVD, the effective use of electronic resources like e-books and handheld devices, or the effective use of simulation activities in the laboratory setting, this area presents many opportunities. While these are areas for the experienced nurse educator with a specialty in instructional design, the NI specialist is often consulted. The NI specialist can be an invaluable asset in the campus skills lab in implementing and revising scenarios to assist with the use of human simulator experiences. These laboratory experiences often require a faculty member to be working with the student group while another technician or lab assistant is running and revising the scenario for an effective learning experience. Part of the debriefing may also involve reviewing tapes of the student experience for review and commentary. In addition, recommendation of any required remediation activities may often require expertise in electronic resources and documentation of these activities.

Lifelong learning, changes in educational preparation, residency programs, interdisciplinary education, and workforce planning were important components of the IOM (2010) report on *The Future of Nursing: Leading Change, Advancing Health*. NI specialists will be of enormous assistance in all phases of analysis, planning, and reporting to address this national mandate.

Positions in Managed Care Organizations and Insurance Companies

As forms of managed care continue to develop, the demand for data and information will grow, as will the opportunities for informatics specialists. Informatics nurses are now working directly with care delivery institutions in developing data and information systems, as well as with the mechanisms involved in the internal reporting processes. New roles are emerging continuously, many of which have been designed and articulated by NI specialists as this new specialty continues to evolve.

For more information, search the various informatics association Web sites and read the *Online Journal of Nursing Informatics*. As with many nursing specialties, nurses should look for opportunities and then create the position that will best serve the organization.

DOCUMENTING OUTCOMES

We have looked at the evolving specialty practice in nursing informatics. These talented practitioners help us organize and make sense of the data and give us the wisdom to make changes in practice. They help us focus on the outcomes of care through standardized languages to avoid misunderstanding and to see the commonalities that create the evidence for quality practice. In doing so, they are assisting in the documentation of outcomes, whether on an EHR for a specific patient situation or in a database provided to a regulatory or accrediting agency. Their role in workforce analysis and monitoring is also critical for

addressing the challenges posed by the IOM (2011) on *The Future of Nursing: Leading Change*, Advancing Health. Consider for a moment informatics nurses' focus on outcomes of health care:

- Assist clinicians to "speak" the same language in documentation
- Assist students in understanding consistent language unique to the healthcare setting
- Analyze stated outcomes to ensure that they are measurable and reflect the clinical situation
- Work with interdisciplinary colleagues to ensure that there is a common understanding on the outcome that nurses wish to accomplish in collaboration with the patient
- Make sure that the databases have consistent and valid data
- Guarantee that administrative reports for regulatory and accrediting bodies have sufficient and quality data
- Monitor patient acuity and care requirements and workforce supply and demand considerations
- Provide valid databases for researchers who seek answers to questions of clinical concern
- Provide informatics solutions to new, novel, and complex technology issues ensuring that outcomes are documented in a retrievable format

And the list goes on.

What is apparent is the focus on documenting outcomes. The documentation of outcomes must be understandable to all, through the use of a common vocabulary. This vocabulary must be applicable to the various taxonomies to build on the body of knowledge and improve care for healthcare consumers. In the process, informatics solutions ensure efficient workflow and effective outcomes. The body of knowledge can be built on firm, comparable evidence. They do provide the wisdom to improve care through the evidence as documented outcomes of efficacy. So, it's all about quality outcomes.

ONLINE CONSULT

American Medical Informatics Association at
http://www.amia.org

American Nursing Informatics Association-Caring at
http://www.ania-caring.org

Alliance for Nursing Informatics at
http://www.allianceni.org/

Canadian Nursing Informatics Association at
http://www.cnia.ca/

Informatics Nurse Certification at
http://www.nursecredentialing.org
/NurseSpecialties/Informatics.aspx

Healthcare Information and Management Systems Society at
http://himss.org

International Medical Informatics Association, Nursing Informatics Special Interest Group at
http://www.imiani.org

EVIDENCE-BASED PRACTICE: *Consider this....*

You have noticed that the nurses on your unit are increasingly focused on the computer workstations, especially after you read last month's results from the patient satisfaction survey. You are searching for guidance on increasing effective nurse-patient interactions. You have just read a commentary that in their visits to healthcare institutions identified for leadership in the use of technology, Stead and Lin (2010) found that in one institution nurses reported only half of their time spent in direct patient care, with the rest of their time spent in documentation reportedly for regulatory or legal purposes rather than for improvements in care. In your role as the nurse manager for your unit, you consult with the nurse informatics specialist your hospital to increase both patient and nurse satisfaction with the use of electronic charting. Based on his recommendation, you both come up with a plan for a unit conference on documentation, standardized languages, and goals for improving quality of care that include patient involvement.

Question: How will you structure this clinical conference to encourage a focus on electronic documentation as a means or tool for improved patient care with both nurses and patients collaborating further on the content for documentation to allow further time for interaction and focus on care improvements?

Source: Stead, W. W., & Lin, H. S. (2010). New directions for health care information technology. National Quality Measures Clearinghouse. Retrieved from http://qualitymeasures.ahrq.gov/expert/expert-commentary.aspx?id=16453&search=health+care+information+technology

KEY POINTS

- "Nursing informatics (NI) is a specialty that integrates nursing science with multiple information and analytical sciences to identify, define, manage, and communicate data, information, knowledge, and wisdom in nursing practice" (ANA, 2015b, p. 1–2).

- Nursing informatics as a specialty grows and changes as quickly as telecommunications technologies.

- Few systems can address every component of healthcare, so there is generally an overriding information system with both clinical and administrative components.

- The EHR is an electronic version of the patient record used as a clinical support tool to assist clinicians and improving efficiency in workflow and effectiveness in care quality.

- Standardized languages offer common vocabulary, terminology, and usage and are a requirement for consistent understanding and application across nursing settings and practice environments.

- The Nursing Management Minimum Data Set (MDS) is used in long-term care to categorize nursing care and patient care needs.

- An important component in the EHR for patient safety is electronic prescribing. Full integration of e-prescribing with the EHR has been shown to promote patient safety and a return on investment (AHRQ, 2010).

- Telehealth has begun to explore the possible applications and innovations that could advance the provision of healthcare.

- Common office applications—word processing, spreadsheet, database, and presentation graphics—are useful in nursing practice, education, and research.

- The ANA (2015b) has identified that "the nursing informatics specialty and its constituent members contribute to achieving the goal of improving the health of populations, communities, groups, families, and individuals . . . [through] the identification of issues and the design, development, and implementation of effective informatics solutions and technologies within the clinical, administrative, educational, and research domains of practice" (p. 2).

- The NI specialty is represented by several professional associations, is supported by advanced education, and is credentialed through certification.

- The primary interest of nursing informatics is to expand how data, information, and knowledge are used to create wisdom within nursing practice.

- In practice, nurses most commonly use computers to document care and to access patient data. Yet, there are many applications for education and research.

- The diversity of informatics projects and programs has led to tremendous professional career and interdisciplinary opportunities.

Thought and Discussion Questions

1. Since you were initially licensed as an RN, identify some of the technological advances and changes you have observed in nursing practice and healthcare.

2. What would happen in your agency if the computer system "went down"? How would the failure affect patient care? What are the backup and redundant systems?

3. What is the representation of NI nurses in your facility?

4. How can handheld technology improve care for healthcare consumers?

5. What telehealth application would you like to invent to improve access to healthcare?

6. How would you explain the EHR and privacy to your patients? Be prepared to participate in an in-class or online discussion to be scheduled by your instructor.

7. Review the Chapter Thought on the first page of the chapter, and be prepared to discuss it online or in class.

Interactive Exercises

Go to the Intranet site and complete the exercises provided for this chapter.

REFERENCES

Adler, K. G. (2007). How to Successfully Navigate Your EHR Implementation. *Family Practice Management, 14*(2), 33–39.

Agency for Healthcare Research Quality (AHRQ). (2013). *Electronic prescribing.* Retrieved from http://healthit.ahrq.gov/key-topics/electronic-prescribing

American Association of Colleges of Nursing (AACN). (2006). *The essentials of doctoral education for advanced nursing practice.* Retrieved from http://www.aacn.nche.edu/publications/position/DNPEssentials.pdf

American Association of Colleges of Nursing (AACN). (2008). *The essentials of baccalaureate education for professional nursing practice.* Retrieved from http://www.aacn.nche.edu/education-resources/BaccEssentials08.pdf

American Association of Colleges of Nursing (AACN, 2011). *The essentials of master's education in nursing.* Retrieved from http://www.aacn.nche.edu/education-resources/MastersEssentials11.pdf

American Nurses Association (ANA). (2008). *Nursing informatics: Scope and standards of practice.* Silver Spring, MD: Nursesbooks.org.

American Nurses Association. (2010). *Nursing: Scope and standards of practice* (2nd ed.). Silver Spring, MD: Nursesbooks.org.

American Nurses Association (ANA). (2015a). *Inclusion of recognized terminologies within EHRs and other health information technology solutions.* Retrieved from http://www.nursingworld.org/MainMenuCategories/Policy-Advocacy/Positions-and-Resolutions/ANAPositionStatements/Position-Statements-Alphabetically/Inclusion-of-Recognized-Terminologies-within-EHRs.html

American Nurses Association (ANA). (2015b). *Nursing informatics: Scope and standards of practice* (2nd ed.). Silver Spring, MD: Nursesbooks.org.

American Nurses Credentialing Center (ANCC). (2013). *Nursing informatics role delineation study: National survey results.* Retrieved from http://www.nursecredentialing.org/Certification/NurseSpecialties/Informatics/RELATED-LINKS/Informatics-2013RDS.pdf

American Nurses Credentialing Center (ANCC). (2014). *Informatics nursing certification eligibility criteria.* Retrieved from http://www.nursecredentialing.org/Informatics-Eligibility.aspx

AORN. 2013 *AORN SYNTEGRITY* (R) *framework.* Retrieved from http://www.aorn.org/syntegrity/

Blumenthal, D., & Tavenner, M. (2010). The "meaningful use" regulation for electronic health records. *New England Journal of Medicine, 363*(56), 501–504. doi: 10.1056/NEJMp1006114. Retrieved from http://www.nejm.org/doi/pdf/10.1056/NEJMp1006114

Brokel, L. (2010). Moving forward with NANDA-I nursing diagnoses with Health Information Technology for Economic and Clinical (HITECH) Act legislation: News updates. *International Journal of Nursing Terminologies and Classifications, 21,* 182–185.

Carrington, J. M., & Tiase, V. L. (2013). Nursing informatics year in review. *Nursing Administration Quarterly, 37,* 136–143.

Centers for Medicare and Medicaid Services (CMS). (2012). *Stage 2 overall tipsheet.* Retrieved from http://www.cms.gov/Regulations-and-Guidance/Legislation/EHRIncentivePrograms/Downloads/Stage2Overview_Tipsheet.pdf

Centers for Medicare and Medicaid Services (CMS). (2013a). *HIPAA General Information: Overview.* Retrieved from http://www.cms.hhs.gov/HIPAAGenInfo/

Centers for Medicare and Medicaid. (2013b). *Progress on adoption of electronic health records.* Retrieved from http://www.cms.gov/eHealth/ListServ_Stage3Implementation.html

Centers for Medicare and Medicaid Services (CMS). (2014a). *2014 definition stage 1 of meaningful use.* Retrieved from http://www.cms.gov/Regulations-and-Guidance/Legislation/EHRIncentivePrograms/Meaningful_Use.html

Centers for Medicare and Medicaid Services. (2014b). *EHR incentive program: Stage 2.* Retrieved from http://www.cms.gov/Regulations-and-Guidance/Legislation/EHRIncentivePrograms/Stage_2.html

Centers for Medicare and Medicaid Services. (n.d.a). *An introduction to the Medicare EHR Incentive Program for Eligible*

Professionals. Retrieved from http://www.cms.gov/Regulations
-and-Guidance/Legislation/EHRIncentivePrograms/
downloads/Beginners_Guide.pdf

Centers for Medicare and Medicaid Services. (n.d.b). *Research, statistics, data, and systems.* Retrieved from http://www
.cms.gov/Research-Statistics-Data-and-Systems/Research-
Statistics-Data-and-Systems.html

Cohen, M. R. (Ed.) (2007). *Medication errors* (2nd ed.).
Washington, DC: American Pharmacists Association.

Cowan, L. (2013). Literature review and risk mitigation strategy for unintended consequences of computer order entry.
Nursing Economic$, 31(1), 27-31, 11.

Graves, J. R., & Corcoran, S. (1989). The study of nursing informatics. *Image: The Journal of Nursing Scholarship, 21,*
227–231.

Greiner, A. C., & Knebel, E. (Eds.). (2003). *Health professions education: A bridge to quality.* Washington, DC: Institute of
Medicine.

Health Resources and Services Administration (HRSA). (2014).
Telehealth. Retrieved from http://www.hrsa.gov/telehealth/

Hebda, T., Czar, P., & Mascara, C. (2008). *Handbook of informatics for nurses and health care professionals* (4th ed.). Upper
Saddle River, NJ: Prentice-Hall.

Institute of Medicine (IOM). (2011). *The future of nursing:
Leading change, advancing health.* Retrieved from http://
www.nap.edu/catalog/12956.html

Institute of Medicine. (2014). *Capturing social and behavioral domains in electronic health records: Phase 1.* Retrieved from
http://www.nap.edu/catalog.php?record_id=18709

International Council of Nurses (ICN). (2013). *About ICPN˚.*
Retrieved from http://www.icn.ch/what-we-do
/international-classification-for-nursing-practice-icnpr/

International Health Terminology Organisation. (2014).
SNOMED CT: Adding value to electronic health records.
Retrieved from www.ihtsdo.org/resource/resource/
16/SNOMED_CT/SnomedCt_Benefits_20140219.pdf

JASON. (April, 2014). *A robust health data infrastructure* (AHRQ
Publication No. 14-0041-EF). Retrieved from http://healthit
.gov/sites/default/files/ptp13-700hhs_white.pdf

Joint Commission. (2014a). *Improving America's hospitals:
The Joint Commission's annual report on quality and safety.*
Retrieved from http://www.jointcommission.org
/annualreport.aspx

Joint Commission. (2014b). *Top performance on key quality measures (R).* Retrieved from http://www.jointcommission
.org/accreditation/top_performers.aspx

Kleib, M., Sales, A. E., Lima, I., Andrea-Baylon, M., & Beaith,
A. (2010). Continuing education in informatics among regis-
tered nurses in the United States in 2000. *The Journal of
Continuing Education in Nursing, 41,* 329–336.

Lustig, T. A. (2012). *The role of telehealth in an evolving health care environment: Workshop summary.* Retrieved from
http://www.nap.edu/catalog.php?record_id=13466

Murphy, J. (2010). Nursing informatics: The intersection of
nursing, computer, and information sciences. *Nursing
Economic$, 28,* 204–207.

National Council of State Boards of Nursing (NCSBN).
(2014). *About Nurse Licensure Compact (NLC).* Retrieved
from https://www.ncsbn.org/nlc.htm

National Database of Nursing Quality Indicators (NDNQI).
(2014). About NDNQI. Retrieved from http://pressganey
.com/ourSolutions/performance-and-advanced-analytics
/clinical-business-performance/nursing-quality-ndnqi

Omaha System. (2013). *The Omaha System ICPN.* Retrieved from
http://www.omahasystem.org/overview.html

Rutherford, M. A. (2013). Standardized nursing language: What
does it mean for nursing practice? *Online Journal for Issues in
Nursing, 28*(1). doi: 10.3912/OJIN.Vol13No01PPT05
Retrieved from http://www.nursingworld.org/Main
MenuCategories/ANAMarketplace/ANAPeriodicals/OJIN
/TableofContents/vol132008/No1Jan08/ArticlePrevious
Topic/StandardizedNursingLanguage.html

Thede, L., & Schwiran, P. (February 25, 2011). Informatics:
The standardized nursing terminologies: A national survey
of nurses' experiences and attitudes–survey. *OJIN: The
Online Journal of Issues in Nursing, 16*(2). doi: 10.3912
/OJIN.Vol16No02InfoCol01. Retrieved from http://www
.nursingworld.org/MainMenuCategories/ANAMarketplace
/ANAPeriodicals/OJIN/TableofContents/Vol-16-2011
/No2-May-2011/Standardized-Nursing-Terminologies.html

BIBLIOGRAPHY

Centers for Medicare and Medicaid Services. (n.d.). *An introduction to the Medicare EHR Incentive Program for Eligible Professionals.* Retrieved from http://www.cms.gov/Regulations
-and-Guidance/Legislation/EHRIncentivePrograms
/downloads/Beginners_Guide.pdf

Eichner, J., & Dullabh, P. (2007). *Accessible health information technology (IT) for populations with limited literacy: A guide
for developers and purchasers of health IT* (AHRQ Pub. No.
08-0010-EF). Rockville, MD: Agency for Healthcare Research and Quality. Retrieved from http://healthit.ahrq.gov
/sites/default/files/docs/page/LiteracyGuide_0.pdf

Health Level 7 (2014). *About HL7.* Retrieved from http://www
.hl7.org/about/index.cfm?ref=nav

Herdman, T. H., & Kamitsuru, S. (Ed.). (2014). *Nursing diagnoses: Definitions and classifications 2015-2017* (10th ed.).
Oxford, UK: Wiley Blackwell.

Institute of Medicine. (2012). *The role of telehealth in an evolving health care environment: Workshop summary.* Retrieved
from http://www.nap.edu/download.php?record_id=13466

Moorhead, S., Johnson, M., Maas, M. L., & Swanson, E.
(eds.). (2008). *Nursing Outcomes Classification (NOC)*
(4th ed.). St. Louis: Mosby Elsevier.

Murphy, J. (2010). The journey to meaningful use of electronic
health records. *Nursing Economic$, 28,* 283–286.

Topaz, M. (2013). The hitchhiker's guide to nursing informatics theory: Using the data-knowledge-wisdom framework
to guide informatics research. *Online Journal of Nursing
Informatics, 17*(3). Retrieved from http://ojni.org/issues
/?p=2852

University of Iowa College of Nursing Centers (2014). *Center
for Nursing Classification and Clinical Effectiveness.* Retrieved
from http: //www.nursing.uiowa.edu/center-for-nursing
-classification-and-clinical-effectiveness

ONLINE RESOURCES

Agency for Healthcare Research and Quality
http://healthit.ahrq.gov/

American Medical Informatics Association
http://www.amia.org/

ANA Recognized Terminologies
http://www.nursingworld.org/Terminologies

http://www.nursingworld.org/MainMenuCategories/Policy
-Advocacy/Positions-and-Resolutions/ANAPosition
Statements/Position-Statements-Alphabetically
/Inclusion-of-Recognized-Terminologies-within
-EHRs.html

American Nursing Informatics Association
http://www.ania.org

British Computer Society: Health Informatics (Nursing)
Specialty Group
http://www.bcs.org/server.php?show=conWebDoc.1220

Canadian Nursing Informatics Association
http://www.cnia.ca/

CMS: EHR Incentive Program
https://www.cms.gov/EHRIncentivePrograms/

Informatics Nursing Certification
http://www.nursecredentialing.org/InformaticsNursing

International Council of Nurses Classification for Nursing
Practice at
http://www.icn.ch/icnp.htm

NANDA-I
http://www.nanda.org/NursingDiagnosisFAQ.aspx

Nursing Interventions Classifications (NIC)
http://www.nursing.uiowa.edu/cncce/nursing-interventions
-classification-overview

Nursing Outcomes Classifications (NOC) at
http://www.nursing.uiowa.edu/cncce/nursing-outcomes
-classification-overview

Omaha System
http://www.omahasystem.org

Online Brazilian Journal of Nursing
http://www.objnursing.uff.br/index.php/nursing

Online Journal of Issues in Nursing
http://www.nursingworld.org/ojin/

Online Journal of Nursing Informatics
http://ojni.org/

Online Journal of Rural Nursing and Health Care
http://rnojournal.binghamton.edu/index.php/RNO

Perioperative Nursing Data Set (PNDS)
http://www.aorn.org/syntegrity/

SNOMED CT
http://www.ihtsdo.org/snomed-ct/

● Rose Kearney-Nunnery   ● William Himmelsbach

16 Economics and Healthcare Policy

"I am an optimist. It does not seem too much use being anything else."

Winston Churchill, 1874–1965

Chapter Objectives

On completion of this chapter, the reader will be able to:

1. Demonstrate an understanding of the basic principles in healthcare economics and financing.

2. Characterize the history and processes used to provide healthcare to individuals and groups in the United States along with solutions proposed with the ACA.

3. Examine the major payment systems and access to healthcare coverage.

4. Discuss the major issues that nursing managers and leaders confront when healthcare coverage issues are addressed.

5. Evaluate policy issues and the role of professionals in clinical practice settings.

Key Terms

Economics
Healthcare Economics
Gross National Product (GNP)
Gross Domestic Product (GDP)
Patient Protection and Affordable Care Act (ACA)
Cost of Healthcare
Reimbursement
Payers

Prospective Payment System (PPS)
Fee-for-Service (FFS) Plan
Managed Care
Point-of-Service (POS) Plan
Preferred Provider Organization (PPO)
Medical Savings Account (MSA)
Accountable Care Organization (ACO)

Medicare
Health Maintenance Organization (HMO)
Medicaid
Children's Health Insurance Program (CHIP)
Health Equity
Fiscal Responsibility

We talk about the economy on a daily basis, whether comparing prices that have risen or the effect on people struggling to make mortgage payments or maintain business operations. However, consider the term **economics**, which is the study of production of a product or service along with issues of supply and demand and distribution of that product or service for the continuity or well-being of some entity. You may have taken courses in *macroeconomics* focusing on the decisions for national or global entities or *microeconomics* considering decisions of individuals or businesses on supply and demand in a defined marketplace. **Healthcare economics** has been defined as a specialty area of economics that analyzes how the different parts of the healthcare system work to supply and deliver healthcare services for patients (Miller, Chang, & Pfoutz, 2012, p. 309). This is not a simple issue of supplying services to meet the ongoing and increasingly complex health needs of individuals, families, and groups. Leaders and managers in the healthcare industry are challenged on a daily basis with regulatory requirements and restrictions, reimbursement considerations for continuity, professional boundary issues for service delivery, and ethical concerns for efficacy, equity, quality, and safety of patient outcomes. The healthcare leader using skills of vision, commitment, and empowerment or the manager focused on coordinating and directing resources for effective outcomes for both the organization and the patient are challenged far beyond the production of a discrete item to meet the demand of the consumer in a marketplace. Economic trends and the financing of healthcare are major considerations.

TRENDS IN HEALTHCARE ECOMOMICS

Everyone recognizes that healthcare is a big business and is viewed as costly. However, consider the trends in healthcare services and costs and the changes in the system that have occurred over time. The **gross national product (GNP)** is the goods and services produced in a nation and is measured on an annual basis. Alternately, you will see comparisons on the **gross domestic product (GDP)**, which is restricted to the goods and services produced within the nation, thus excluding business not located in the particular nation.

Annual per capital expenditures for healthcare in the United States is the highest in the world (Thomson, Osborn, Squires, & Jun, 2013, p. 134). Figure 16.1 illustrates healthcare expenditures by nation in 2011 and documents $8,507.60 per capita spending in the United States. We see the GDP used in comparisons on the rising costs of healthcare. Consider the trends in healthcare costs for the United States compared with other selected countries identified in Figure 16.1. As reported by the Organisation for Economic Cooperation and Development (OECD, 2013), in 2011, the United States spent 17.7 percent of its GDP on healthcare, nearly twice the average amount spent by other countries and significantly more than comparable industrial nations (Table 16.1). Consider the trends identified in Table 16.2. These costs include not only the provision of care to patients as goods and services but also physical resources, the preparation of practitioners across disciplines, research and development, and methods of financing all of these. In 2010, spending on healthcare in the United States was reported as $2.6 trillion, equating to $8,402 per person (Martin, Lassman, Washington, Catlin, & the National Health Expenditure Accounts Team, 2012, p. 208). And the upward trend has continued, although at a slower pace during the economic decline. Consider some of the differences in costs of healthcare for some of these countries illustrated in Table 16.3. For example, the United States and Canada have similar expenditures on inpatient care, with differences in percentage of expenditures for

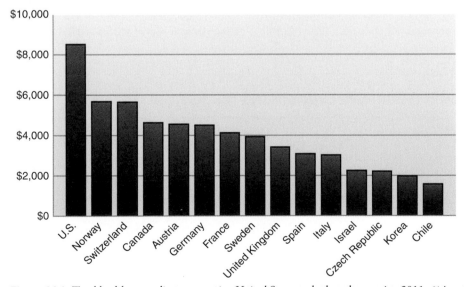

Figure 16.1 Total health expenditure per capita, United States and selected countries, 2011. *(Adapted from Organisation for Economic Cooperation and Development [OECD]. [2013]. Health at a glance 2013: OECD indicators. Retrieved from http://www.oecd-ilibrary.org/social-issues-migration-health/health-at-a-glance_19991312;jsessionid= 612e179lbg8ul.x-oecd-live-01; and OECD [2013]. Total expenditure on health per capita, Health: Key tables from OECD, no. 2. doi: 10.1787/hlthxp-cap-table-2013-2-en)*

TABLE 16.1

Expenditures on Health as a Percentage of Gross Domestic Product, 2005 versus 2011

Country	2005 (%)	2011 (%)
United States	15.8	17.7
Norway	9.0	9.3
Switzerland	10.9	11.0
Canada	9.8	11.2
Austria	10.4	10.8
Germany	10.8	11.3
France	11.0	11.6
Sweden	9.1	9.5
United Kingdom	8.3	9.4
Spain	8.3	9.3
Italy	8.7	9.2
Israel	7.9	7.7
Korea	5.6	7.4
Czech Republic	6.9	7.5
Chile	6.6	7.5

Source: Organisation for Economic Co-operation and Development (OECD). (2013). Total expenditure on health. *Health: Key tables from OECD*, no. 1. doi: 10.1787/hlthxp-total-table-2013-2-en.

outpatient and long-term care. The United States spends almost twice the amount on healthcare insurance and administration compared with Canada and more than the other nations listed except for France. However, the United States and France, as some of the highest spenders on healthcare, also see households financing a relatively small

share of the healthcare costs directly, with most spending made through public or private third-party arrangements (OECD, 2011a, p. 158).

An atypical trend has started to occur in the United States. Healthcare inflation has declined over the past 10 years from 10% to 4%. This line has gotten close to the overall inflation rate. If such a trend continues, or even flattens out, the implications are significant. For example, the Medicare Trust Fund projections may improve. In addition, state tax resources to fund the state's share of Medicaid may not be such a burden as it has been in the past. As reported in a 2014 poll conducted by the Kaiser Family Foundation (Henry J. Kaiser Family Foundation, 2014b) on the decline in healthcare expenditures trend, "when asked their perceptions of the cost of health care in the nation, half of the public says that over the past few years, costs have been going up faster than usual (50 percent), and only 8 percent say costs have been going up slower than usual" (p. 1). In addition for this period, researchers reported that "out-of pocket medical spending did not decline, which suggests that consumers began to bear more of the burden for medical care directly" (Herrera, Gaynor, Newman, Town, & Parente, 2013, p. 1721). The potential effect on the private insurance market (payers, employees, and individuals) is unsettled because implementation of the **Patient Protection and Affordable Care Act (ACA)** is not occurring as prescribed in the Act. Some of the decline in expenditures has been attributed to the downturn in the economy, with people delaying healthcare expenditures, especially preventative services. Nonetheless, future use of healthcare services is a factor as demand increases. This increased demand could be significant.

Financing healthcare in the United States, however, is more than simply a supply-and-demand equation. The four major factors driving healthcare costs are technology and prescription drugs, chronic disease, aging of the population, and administrative costs (Kimbuende, Ranji, Lundy, & Salganicoff, 2013, p. 550). Technology is increasing at a speed we can barely keep pace with, yet

TABLE 16.2

Differences in Healthcare Expenditures for Selected Countries, 1990–2011

	United States (%)	Ireland (%)	United Kingdom (%)	Netherlands (%)	France (%)	Mexico (%)	China (%)	OECD Countries Average (%)
1990	12.4	6.0	5.9	8.0	8.4	4.0	NA	
2000	13.7	6.1	7.0	8.0	10.1	4.5	4.6	
2009	17.4	9.5	9.8	12.0	11.8	<7.0	4.6	9.6
2010/ 2011	17.6	9.2	9.6	12.0	11.6	6.2	5.1	9.5

Sources: Organisation for Economic Co-operation and Development (OECD). (2013). *Health at a glance 2013: OECD indicators*. Retrieved from http://www.oecd-ilibrary.org/social-issues-migration-health/health-at-a-glance_19991312;jsessionid= 612e179lbg8ul.x-oecd-live-01; and Organisation for Economic Co-operation and Development (OECD). (2011). *Health at a glance 2011: OECD indicators*. Retrieved from http://www.oecd-ilibrary.org/social-issues-migration-health/health-at-a-glance-2011_health_glance-2011-en;jsessionid=60v7lrkqqook1.x-oecd-live-01.

TABLE 16.3

Differences in Healthcare Expenditures for Selected Countries, 2009

Country	Healthcare Expenditures on Inpatient Care (%)	Healthcare Expenditures on Outpatient Care (%)	Healthcare Expenditures on Long-Term Care (%)	Expenditures on Healthcare Insurance and Administration (%)
United States	19	51	6	7.0
Canada	20	33	15	3.7
Norway	32	26	27	0.8
Sweden	28	42	8	1.4
France	36	23	12	7.0
Germany	29	29	12	5.4
Japan	32	34	9	1.9

Source: Organisation for Economic Co-operation and Development (OECD). (2013). *Health at a glance 2013: OECD indicators.* Retrieved from http://www.oecd-ilibrary.org/social-issues-migration-health/health-at-a-glance_19991312;jsessionid=612e179lbg8ul.x-oecd-live-01.

afford. Prescription drugs are similarly multiplying as we chemically attempt to treat conditions as unique as the individuals themselves. And consumers are exposed to these new prescription drug options in the media on a daily basis. Chronic diseases and the aging of the population are well-documented trends as we now attempt to address population health and health promotion. And it is estimated that at least 7 percent of healthcare expenditures are for administrative costs, like marketing and billing (Kimbuende et al., 2013, p. 550). Financing healthcare has become a major challenge for consumers, employers, and payers.

HEALTHCARE FINANCING: A HISTORICAL CONTEXT

To address healthcare financing, we first consider the control of the money and resources to cover the cost of healthcare. Healthcare costs are generally covered in one of four ways: through health insurance, governmental healthcare coverage, individual or family assets, or charitable coverage.

As noted by Kovner and Knickman (2011), in the United States, the healthcare financing system has evolved continuously since the middle of the 20th century when health insurance began to be marketed (p. 49). Health insurance is obtained in two ways: through employer coverage or individual contracts. Employer coverage occurs as a component of a worker's compensation or benefit package as part of employment to provide for individual or family coverage. As part of a group plan, an economy of scale provides for coverage of a defined group. Risk-to-benefit ratios are an important part of this process, hoping for an employee population that uses a predictable amount of resources that is covered through premiums. However, increased costs to employers are considered as business and employee costs, with employers transferring some of this cost liability to employees through increased

individual employee premiums, copays, and deductibles. This cost shifting has affected individuals and families as usable income declines, even in a time of a stable income. Insurance companies address the issue of individuals using more healthcare services when covered than if they were not provided by insurance through deductibles and copayments. Unruh and Spetz (2012) describe this situation as a moral hazard that leads to greater demand for services and increased cost with use (p. 155).

As noted by Cowan and Hartman (2005), an increase in premiums resulted from increased costs and use, as well as the decline in manufacturing jobs and a resultant increase in service sector jobs, which occurred earlier in this decade and impacted worker benefits because service sector jobs are less likely to provide health insurance (p. 11). Employers contract through insurers to provide coverage for their employees. However, in recent years some major employers became their own insurers as the cost of group insurance premiums rose and coverage was questioned for cost-effectiveness or safety. Health insurance can also be obtained through personal funds, but this has often been cost prohibitive and has caused individuals and families to delay preventive healthcare when costs are considered part of the family monthly budget. Another coverage component is when a worker leaves, loses a position, or has a qualified event that allows for legal continuation of health insurance for a specified period of time through a group plan according to the Consolidated Omnibus Budget Reconciliation Act of 1985 (COBRA). However, this could still be a costly individual or family expense at a time with perhaps limited assets. As we will later see with the ACA, a focus on prevention, health promotion, and the development of insurance exchanges was the basis to address some of these issues.

Governmental healthcare coverage occurs through national, federal, or state provisions and entitlements. In the United States, federal programs are in place for special populations like active or retired members of the military or their dependents and the aging population. Other programs for children or disabled individuals are shared through federal, state, and local governments. We have seen how changes in plans and coverage have established reimbursement and coding plans that provide direction to reimbursement from the other sources. Further details on the initiatives associated with Medicare and Medicaid in the United States are presented in a later section.

Individual or family assets may be used to provide for healthcare, whether for insurance, copays, care, or private pay. In the past, individuals could seek private insurance or payment plans, but often at an increased cost without the purchasing power of numbers that occurs with a group plan. The Insurance Exchanges called for by the ACA were envisioned as a means to promote private insurance coverage through a federal or state "group" plan or insurance exchange.

Charitable coverage may be available in secular or religious communities by virtue of membership. Charitable coverage as uncompensated care may also occur on an episodic basis when an organization or institution "writes off" selected charges as a component of their contribution to the community, a tax liability, or an operational agreement, especially in the situation of uninsured or underinsured patients.

PRICE, COST, AND REIMBURSEMENT

The price and cost of healthcare are not the same when the issue of reimbursement is considered. The actual **cost of healthcare** is the price or the monetary amount of goods and services to cover the episode of care. On the other hand, **reimbursement** is the amount of money provided to pay for that particular episode of care based on an agreed or approved process. In healthcare, we have seen several accounting systems used for reimbursement because we are generally dealing with third-party payers. Providers usually do not know the true cost of providing their services.

Consider the **payers** for healthcare as first, second, and third parties. First-party payers are those seeking the healthcare service, whether an individual who is a private payer or a member of a group plan with specified copays or minimums to be met. The second-party payers are the providers, plan administrators, or employer who collects premiums, pays, or copays for a group of individuals. Third-party payers are the insurers who collect the premiums, assess and accept the risk of the group, and reimburse the providers for the service.

To pay for the healthcare service, several methodologies are used and have evolved as healthcare costs are addressed, whether in advance of the service, through prior anticipation or negotiation for the service, or after the service.

Retrospective payment plans were predominant before the middle 1980s and the introduction of diagnostic-related groups (DRGs). With the retrospective systems, hospitals and other providers were paid after services and treatments were performed through a complicated "cost-based" formula. Leading to the implementation of DRGs, a technical review committee noted that "until 1982,

Medicare employed a retrospective cost-based reimbursement approach whereby hospitals could recover from Medicare most of what they spent on Medicare beneficiaries . . . [with] little incentive to contain costs" and encouraged additional capacity, technologies, and complex services (Office of Technology Assessment, 1983, p. 3). DRGs were developed to address case load, costs, and reward structures for cost savings.

The **prospective payment system (PPS)** is a fixed payment method that is based on a predetermined amount for the usual care needed for a patient with a specific condition. If the care is more expensive, the provider must absorb the additional costs. If the cost of the patient care comes in at a lesser amount, the provider benefits. Providers would like to come in under budget to use the funds for systems maintenance and reinvestment, but safety and quality are vital and ethical considerations. Clinical or critical pathways and care maps have been used to standardize care for patients along expected trajectories and in line with evidence-based protocols and practice. Monitoring and evaluation are important components of this process that is alert for variations in patient conditions and care provisions.

Fee-for-service (FFS) plans are the traditional payment methods in which each service is charged separately, as with provider visits, laboratory tests, and supplies. Uninsured individuals are billed separately for each of these services. As a member of a group plan, individuals pay a premium based on risk assessments and historical use of services (typically 3 years), along with plan-associated deductibles and copays.

Managed care covers a variety of treatment and payment options. As noted by Chang, Price, and Pfoutz (2001), managed care combines the financing and delivery of services into a single entity (p. 88). Several forms of managed care have evolved and continue to address this concept, as with provider networks and selected plans. However, the ultimate goals are to maintain health and prevent disease and disability, thus reducing healthcare costs. A major concept in managed care is capitated payments, in which each enrollee is entered into the plan with a payment based on a risk ratio. The goal is to reduce the risk for high healthcare costs and to promote savings.

Point-of-service (POS) plans generally occur through a specified network of providers. The patient selects a primary care provider from this network. The primary care provider serves as a gatekeeper, and consultations with others must have prior approval for reimbursement. The patient may elect to go to providers outside the network, but that is a choice, and care can be more costly. Health, wellness, and illness prevention are goals for these plans to limit cost.

A **preferred provider organization (PPO)** is a provider or provider agency included as part of a network and agrees to negotiated rates for patients who use the PPOs listed. If the patient goes out of the network to another provider, additional and non-reimbursed patient charges will be incurred for that preference. An important consideration is the menu of negotiated rates and what may result in additional charges.

A **medical savings account (MSA)** is a federal tax incentive program used by employers or Medicare recipients in which a high deductible is agreed on with an amount provided in a nontaxable savings account to pay for initial care. Self-management of healthcare cost is a key feature, with payments made to the plan rather than insurance premiums. Money in the account will earn interest and can accumulate over the years until needed for a major medical expense. Tax liabilities are a consideration if the account funds are not used for approved expenses that reduce the deductible amount. After the deductible is met, services are provided without additional cost to the patient.

The **accountable care organization (ACO)** has evolved as a component of the ACA as a shared savings organization designed to promote accountability, risk management, and coordinated care. Beginning with pilot programs in 2012, care for minimum groups of Medicare FFS beneficiaries under Parts A, B, and D would be provided by selected groups of providers of services and care. The goals of these high-quality, efficient care coordination provider groups are to keep the Medicare recipients out of hospitals and encourage investment in infrastructure and redesigned care processes with quality reporting. As further described by the Centers for Medicare and Medicaid Services (CMS, 2013a), a provider that becomes an ACO "succeeds in both delivering high-quality care and spending health care dollars more wisely [and] will share in the savings it achieves for the Medicare program" (p. 1). However, of the 32 original ACOs selected

to participate in this program, a significant number subsequently withdrew from the program by 2014 based on the financials of the initiative.

MEDICARE, MEDICAID, AND THE CHILDREN'S HEALTH INSURANCE PROGRAM

In the United States, Medicare, Medicaid, and state Children's Health Insurance Programs (CHIP) are major governmental entities that provide healthcare for select populations. Medicare was the first program, beginning in 1965 with the Social Security Act under Title XVIII. Refer to Table 16.4 for major timelines for these federal programs.

As a refresher, consider the four parts of **Medicare:** A, B, C, and D. Recall that Medicare is available for Americans aged 65 years or older, those with certain disabilities, and those with end-stage renal disease. Medicare Part A provides for inpatient hospital, skilled rehabilitative, hospice, and home care services for enrolled individuals. Payment for this coverage occurred while working as employment taxes or may be provided through enrollment in Part B or through a documented disability. Coverage of charges depends on hospital admission and specific treatment orders. Medicare Part B

TABLE 16.4

Timelines on Medicare, Medicaid, and Children's Health Insurance Program

Medicare	1966	In excess of 19 million Americans 65 years and older to receive healthcare coverage
	1972	Medicare eligibility extended to selected individuals with disabilities
	1980	Home health services broadened and Medicare supplemental insurance available
	1983	Diagnostic-related groups (DRGs) implemented for all Medicare-participating hospitals
	1985	Emergency departments to provide screening and treatment stabilization (EMTALA)
	1987	Protections for nursing home residents (Omnibus Reconciliation Act)
	1988	Medicare Catastrophic Coverage Act (MCAA) for hospital/skilled facilities
		Spousal impoverishment costing with institutional and community living
	1989	MCCA repealed and new schedule of fees implemented
	1997	Managed care plan choices established to slow spending
	1999	Increased payments for some Medicare providers
	2000	Improved coverage for managed care
	2003	Prescription drug discounts and prevention coverage
	2006	Part D voluntary drug benefit and subsidies to retiree programs
		Part D premium differentials depending on incomes of beneficiaries
	2009	Establishment of Accountable Care Organizations (ACOs) and payments linked to quality outcomes as part of the Patient Protection and Affordable Care Act (ACA)

Continued

TABLE 16.4

Timelines on Medicare, Medicaid, and Children's Health Insurance Program—cont'd

Medicaid	1966	State phase-in process for children without parental support and their caregivers, and low-income individuals and individuals with disabilities
	1972	Eligibility extended for individuals with disabilities
	1981	Hospitals with high percentage of low-income patients received additional state support [Disproportionate share hospitals (DSH)]
	1986	State optional Medicaid coverage for pregnant women and infants
	1988	Mandated coverage for pregnant women and infants at 100% federal poverty level (FPL)
	1989	Coverage of pregnant women and children <6 years under 133% of FPL with expanded screening and treatment
	1990	Expanded coverage of children 6–16 years under 100% FPL and Medicaid Prescription Drug Rebate program established
	1991	Medicaid controls established
	1996	Welfare link to Medicaid reformed
	1999	Work incentives for Medicaid recipients and improved funding to hospitals and women's health services
	2000	Federal health and rural health clinics established
	2009	Exanded eligibility and funding as part of the ACA with specific requirements from 2014–2019
State Children's Health Insurance Program (CHIP)	1997	Program establishment under the Balanced Budget Act as Title XXI of the Social Security Act for uninsured children not eligible for Medicaid
	2007–2009	Program extended through March 2009; Reauthorized in 2009
	2009	States required to maintain eligibility through September 30, 2019 with funding increases from 2014–2019 under the ACA of 2009

Source: Adapted from: Centers for Medicare and Medicaid Services (CMS). (2005). Key milestones in Medicare and Medicaid history, selected years: 1965–2003. *Health Care Financing Review, 27*(2). Retrieved from http://www.cms.gov/Research-Statistics-Data-and-Systems/Research/HealthCareFinancingReview/downloads/05-06Winpg1.pdf

covers approved outpatient care, necessary and selected preventive services, and equipment, usually by virtue of an additional premium based on a prior year's annual income paid with Social Security. Medicare Part C is a selected "Advantage Plan" in which Part A and Part B services are provided by a FFS, PPO, **health maintenance organization (HMO)**, or a special plan selected by the participant, who follows the rules of the selected healthcare organization and pays the required premium. Medicare Part D is the optional prescription drug coverage plan. Monthly Part D premiums are based on the drug plan and the prior year's annual income and may be deducted from the monthly Social Security check.

The provision of Medicare Part D through the Medicare prescription Drug Improvement and Modernization Act of 2003 has been noted as the "the most significant improvement to senior health care in nearly 40 years" (CMS, 2013c, p. 1). In excess of 50 million Americans are covered by Medicare, but not all are enrolled in the optional Part D. As reported by the Henry J. Kaiser Family Foundation (2013a), at least 10 percent of Medicare beneficiaries do not have credible drug coverage despite the

fact that 39 million Medicare beneficiaries were enrolled in Medicare Part D, a Medicare Advantage Drug Plan, or an employee-sponsored retiree drug plan (p. 2). Subsidies are available and can be applied for, but outreach is an important consideration. One of the main issues with Part D is the "donut hole" that occurs when high users reach the maximum allowable amount and then must use personal resources to pay for medication until the next plateau for coverage is reached. Reducing this cost is one of the features of the ACA, which started in 2011 as a small rebate and then in 2014 became a reduction in the program feature.

Many Medicare recipients, however, carry supplemental insurance to pay for needed inpatient and outpatient expenses. "Due to Medicare's relatively high cost-sharing requirements, the vast majority of beneficiaries have some source of coverage that supplements Medicare, including nine million Medicare beneficiaries who purchase Medigap policies" (Jacobson, Huang, & Neuman, 2014, p. 1). This "Medigap" market has seen similar economic scrutiny as healthcare costs have escalated and measures have been directed at controlling Medicare spending for recipients, many of whom are on limited or fixed incomes and some who have additional supplementary retiree or federal coverage.

The **Medicaid** program was authorized under Title XIX of the Social Security Act in 1965 but was designed to be phased in as a joint program between federal, state, and local governments. Medicaid funding and programs at the state and local levels are provided by some federal funding and regulated through eligibility requirements. Primary recipients of Medicaid are pregnant women, children, parents and caregivers, seniors, and people with disabilities. However, Medicaid is the primary payer for long-term care services, with $257 billion spent in 2011 for long-term care for elders in nursing homes, for community diversion programs, and for assistance in payment of Medicare premiums (Henry J. Kaiser Family Foundation, 2013c, 2014c).

States address both federally mandated eligibility groups and other optional populations. For some groups, mandated eligibility requirements are based on 100 percent of the federal poverty level (FPL). The FPL is updated on an annual basis. For 2014, the FPL for a family of four was an annual income of between $23,850 and $27,430, depending on state of residence. Low income is only one test for Medicaid eligibility, and other financial resources have threshold levels determined by each state within the federal guidelines (Klees & Wolfe, 2013, p. 22). States can apply to increase the eligibility level, and many states provide benefits and care for pregnant women significantly above the minimum level. Additional eligibility requirements include state residency, immigration status, and documentation of citizenship. Optional populations include the medically needy, as identified by the state, and selected groups who earn above the minimum income requirement. In addition, the state can assess premiums or copayments to optional groups. The ACA provides additional eligibility for adults with the standard of 133 percent of the FPL beginning in 2014.

As noted by Cowan and Hartman (2005), "Medicaid accounts for the largest portion of State and local governments' health care expenditures" (p. 17). And this burden is increasing, especially given the additional eligibility with the ACA. But as these researchers continue to point out regarding the burden at the state and local levels, "unlike the Federal Government that can support deficit spending, almost all State governments must balance their budgets each year, making the pressure they face from rising State healthcare costs particularly acute" (Cowan & Hartman, 2005, p. 23). Promoting health and keeping residents healthy are less costly than chronic care, but this is still a controversial issue in many state governments. The ACA of 2009 gave states the option of expanding Medicaid eligibility in 2014 to 138 percent of the FPL. However, states were allowed to opt out of this requirement following a Supreme Court decision in 2012.

The **Children's Health Insurance Program (CHIP)** was originally enacted in 1997 as Title XXI of the Social Security Act for a 10-year period as SCHIP to provide health coverage for uninsured children who were not eligible for Medicaid. The program provides federal matching funds to states to provide this coverage. After the original 10-year period, it was extended for another 2 years and then reauthorized in April 2009 and renamed the CHIP program. To encourage state participation and to provide enhanced coverage for this program, the federal annual matching funds rate is higher than the Medicaid program. The CHIP program was further enhanced and extended through the ACA with funding to continue through fiscal year (FY) 2019 at increased levels, for example as follows:

FY 2012: $14,982,000,000
FY 2013: $17,406,000,000
FY 2014: $19,147,000,000
FY 2015: $18,211,000,000 (CHIP, 2011)

Further special CHIP initiatives are provided through the ACA. Although this program is jointly funded by the federal government and the individual states, the District of Columbia, and the territories, it is designed and delivered by the individual states in accordance with guidelines from the CMS. Some states, territories, and the District of Columbia use the federal program as an expansion of their Medicaid program, whereas other states treat CHIP as a separate program or a combination of the two. In addition to healthcare and health promotion services, benefits of the program include early detection and screening programs and dental care.

ONLINE CONSULT

The Centers for Medicare and Medicaid Services at:

http://www.medicare.gov/

http://www.medicaid.gov/

The Children's Health Insurance Program at

http://www.medicaid.gov/CHIP/CHIP-Program-Information.html

Coding and Comparisons

An important consideration for reimbursement is the coding of care for reimbursement or payment. As mentioned previously, the introduction of DRGs in 1982 provided a system of prospective reimbursement based on a typical case scenario in response to rapidly escalating hospital costs for Medicare recipients. Lack of cost controls with reimbursement methods and the expanding technology were blamed for dramatically increasing costs between 1967 (covering 19.5 million recipients at a cost of $4.7 million as 9.2 percent of healthcare expenditures) and 1985 (with 31.1 million Medicare recipients at a cost of $72.3 billion 16.9 percent of healthcare expenditures) (Office of Inspector General Office of Evaluation and Inspections Region IX, 2001, p. 2). In 1983, Medicare payments were capped, based on the diagnostic category on a per case basis. The effects of this system were not restricted to Medicare; private insurance reimbursements rapidly followed the lead with a PPS rather than a retrospective cost-based system or formula.

DRG categories "bundle" costs on a per case basis and include operating and delivery costs, such as care delivery, supplies, diagnostic studies, and equipment and technology. DRGs set the payment for a particular diagnosis, not for the costs of the actual services and care to the patient.

In the current DRG structure, more than 700 DRGs are identified and weighted. Claims for reimbursement for Medicare Part A inpatients were coded in accordance with International Classification of Diseases, initially under the ninth revision (ICD-9). DRGs are reimbursed for services considering certain "weighted" factors, such as case complexity as with case "outliers," geography (urban versus rural), labor costs, and special functions as with teaching hospitals and those hospitals caring for a larger proportion of low-income patients. In 2011, the three most frequently billed DRGs related to joint replacements, psychoses, and severe infection (Modern Healthcare, 2013). DRG classifications and weights and Medicare Part B premiums and deductibles are evaluated by CMS on an annual (calendar year [CY]) basis for reimbursement considerations. For example, the Medicare Part A inpatient deductible was $1,184 in 2013 and $1,216 in 2014 (Medicare Program, 2013).

Approved IDC codes lead to reimbursement for services and date back to their origin in 1899 when the focus was on causes of death. The first revision was IDC-1 and was in use from 1900 to 1909. With implementation of DRGs in the 1980s, IDC-9 codes were used from 1995 to 2011. In 2012, the ICD-9 system began the transition to ICD-10 with the deadline of October 1, 2015 for all diagnoses and inpatient procedures. There were nearly 5,000 classifications of disease in IDC-9, but this expands to nearly 8,000 in IDC-10, with increased details and focus on causes of morbidity (Moriyama et al., 2011). The IDC-10 uses three- to seven-digit codes and affects all diagnosis and inpatient coding for everyone covered by the Health Insurance Portability and Accountability Act (HIPAA).

In the case of coding for Medicare Part B (outpatient services), Current Procedural Terminology (CPT) codes are used. The CPT coding system is maintained by the American Medical Association and updated on an annual basis. The CPT coding system is used by practitioners to identify services and procedures provided for which they will bill private and public health insurance programs. To provide more transparency on this complex system, CMS (2014c) began providing a public data set on Medicare FFS beneficiaries, with information on services and procedures provided to Medicare beneficiaries by physicians and other healthcare professionals, including payment and submitted charges organized by the National Provider Identifier (NPI) and the Healthcare Common Procedure Coding System.

Coding and the use of the electronic health record have allowed for better data collection and comparison information. For example, the U.S. Department of Health and Human Services Office of Inspector General (USDHHS; 2014) reported that Medicare beneficiaries paid higher co-payments for outpatient services at critical access hospitals (CAHs). CAHs are certified to provide essential services to residents in rural areas and are reimbursed at higher rates for the provision of these needed services. However, it was found that Medicare beneficiaries paid between two and six times the amount in coinsurance than they would have paid for comparable services in acute care hospitals and with a demonstrated increase from 2009 to 2012 without this CAH designation (USDHHS, 2014). This report resulted in a recommendation for reform in the calculation of coinsurance for Medicare recipients.

HEALTHCARE POLICY AND REFORM

Healthcare reform efforts are not new. When Florence Nightingale transformed care for soldiers in the Crimea in the middle of the 19th century, her actions and initiatives transformed healthcare there and around the globe. Many examples, before and after, of her influence on the environment and hygiene can be identified as a reform initiative. More recent efforts in the Unites Stated include the initiation of Medicare in 1965 and DRGs in the 1980s. Political leaders have endeavored to address the needs of their constituents through attempts at legislation, some limited, with many efforts "dying" in committee.

Patient Protection and Affordable Care Act

The ACA was passed in 2010 with regulations and legal challenges that continued for several years, including a Supreme Court ruling in 2012. The legislation is widespread and far reaching and was designed for a phased-in implementation. The overall goals of the law were to expand healthcare coverage and improve the system, including attempts to control escalating costs. The law addresses quality, safe, and affordable care for people in the United States. Quality and accountability are key ingredients of the legislation that is designed to transform healthcare and stem the rising numbers of uninsured and underinsured individuals and families.

The text of the law is more than 1,200 pages in length and includes 10 sections. Benefits of the ACA have been categorized in three areas:

- Care and Access
  - Preventive care
  - Drug discounts for seniors
  - Choice of providers and access to emergency services
- Coverage and Costs
  - Coverage of adults younger than 26 years under patent's policy
  - Health insurance marketplace
  - Fraud protection
  - Tax credits for small businesses
- Consumer Protections
  - Elimination of exclusion for preexisting conditions
  - Consumer assistance
  - Removal of lifetime limits
  - Protection from unjustified premium increases (USDHHS, 2014.)

Initial provisions of the legislation began in 2011 with the insurance reforms, including the coverage of dependent children up to age 26 years and protections from cancellation of policies. Care coordination for individuals eligible for both Medicare and Medicaid was also a goal to make care more efficient. The "donut hole" for Medicare Part D was also a focus, with beginning plans to first offer a small rebate and then to slowly reduce the costs for high use of medications. Beginning in 2014, health insurance exchanges were implemented to assist individuals and employers to obtain insurance coverage. As noted previously, Medicaid coverage will be expanded for adults and families and especially for children thorough the CHIP program, depending on state policies.

Another key feature of the law is the encouragement of coordinated care models. New healthcare delivery models and projects began in 2012 with a focus on coordinated care linked to *reportable outcomes with a focus on quality and safety.* According to CMS (2013a), ACOs are groups of doctors, hospitals, and other healthcare providers that give coordinated high-quality care to Medicare patients. CMS further delineates three models of ACOs (Table 16.5).

As noted by Colpas (2013) on the analysis for the proposed ACO regulation, "Medicare could potentially save $960 million over three years" (p. 6). The efficacy of these models will depend on the data obtained to document the results of their innovations in care coordination and any resultant cost savings. "The high cost of being able to report the requisite quality metrics and to institute the information system plus clinical and financial management tools to improve performance over time were some of the main reasons many organizations decided not to become ACOs" (Nichols, 2012, pp. 711–712). Anderson and Hogan (2013) even address the concept of a "super ACO" for large systems that can expand geographic coverage, reduce competition, and garner the effects of economies of scale that smaller organizations could not address (p. 88). However, not all organizations can reinvent themselves as an ACO. As discussed by Hayen, van den Berg, Meijboom, and Westert (2013), "ACOs need to reconsider their provider configuration and make it capable of managing clinical and financial risk" (p. 517). The financial considerations being the reason for some ACO withdrawals in 2014. Further, Berry and Beckham (2014) emphasize the importance of a team-based model and of changing the culture for this emphasis.

Health promotion and prevention activities are highlighted with an enhanced focus on access, evidence-based practices, and system integrity and transparency through ACOs. Improved technology and system improvements for healthcare insurers and providers are key features. In the *Report to Congress: National Strategy for Quality Improvements in Health Care*, the national aims were specified as better care, healthy people/healthy communities, and affordable care (Healthcare.gov, 2011, p. 2). However, the effectiveness of ACOs has not yet been fully demonstrated, both clinically and in terms of cost.

In the inaugural year (2013–2014), health insurance exchanges received much attention and criticism. The U.S. Supreme Court upheld the regulation requiring health insurance coverage or the imposition of a penalty. The initial individual penalty would initially be applied on the 2015 income taxes, but this would increase in subsequent years. The penalty for those not covered in 2014 was $95 per adult and $47.50 per child, or 1 percent of the family income, whichever was higher. However, the penalty increases each year, as from $95 for a noncovered adult in 2014 to $325 in 2015, or 2 percent of the income, and higher in 2016. Insurance exchanges were either the federally facilitated marketplace for 26 states or the state-based marketplace. The accessibility of online access to the federal exchange was a major barrier because the original online system was not designed to handle the volume. Variable reports on registration goals were reported at the closing of the first enrollment period.

Initially, individual perception of "sticker shock" was reported, with consumers not expecting the cost required for the basic coverage. The exchanges provide basic, essential coverage but also have different levels of coverage (bronze, silver, gold, and platinum coverage). Although the exchanges were designed for "purchasing power," as opposed to the individual in the past attempting to obtain high-cost private health insurance, there is not an employer contribution to the cost of the premium. In addition, both individual risk scores (based on age, gender, and diagnoses)

TABLE 16.5

Accountable Care Organizations

Medicare Shared Savings	Advanced Payment Model	Pioneer Model
FFS for coordinated care, accountability, and encouraging investment in infrastructure and redesigned care processes. "The Shared Savings Program will reward ACOs that lower their growth in healthcare costs while meeting performance standards on quality of care and putting patients first" (CMS, 2013a, p. 1).	Upfront and monthly payments are made for coordinated care and investments in infrastructure for small and rural practices in an effort to demonstrate whether these advanced payments result in increased participation, improved care, and demonstrated Medicare savings.	Project involved 23 experienced, coordinated care healthcare organizations and providers to move to a population-based payment model. This model is designed to work in coordination with private payers by aligning provider incentives to improve quality and health outcomes and achieve cost savings.

Source: Centers for Medicare and Medicaid Services (CMS). (2013a). *Accountable care organizations.* Retrieved from http://www.cms.gov/Medicare/Medicare-Fee-for-Service-Payment/ACO/

and average risk scores for the individual plans are considerations. However, also consider the new ACA requirement that individuals could not be excluded for preexisting conditions. Insurance policies consider the "risk pool" and do not want to be at the higher end, resulting in more costs paid out. The ACA has another provision to encourage program participation and address the nonexclusion clause for prior existing conditions. The "temporary risk corridor program is intended to promote accurate premiums in the early years of the exchanges (2014 through 2016) by discouraging insurers from setting them high in response to uncertainty about who will enroll and what they will cost . . . by cushioning insurers participating in exchanges and marketplaces from extreme gains and losses" (Henry J. Kaiser Family Foundation, 2014a, pp. 7–8). With this program, targets were set for insurers at 80 percent of costs of healthcare and quality improvement. If the insurers fell below or above the allowable range, they would either be reimbursed or be required to reimburse the risk pool program. Note that this program targets both allowable costs and quality improvement initiatives. All of this requires a focus on access, quality improvement, and equity.

One of the goals of healthcare reform is to provide health equity and to promote population health. **Health equity** has been defined by the National Partnership for Action to End Health Disparities (2011) as follows:

> [T]he attainment of the highest level of health for all people. Achieving health equity requires valuing everyone equally with focused and ongoing societal efforts to address avoidable inequalities, historical and contemporary injustices, and the elimination of health and healthcare disparities. (p. 1)

The issue of health equity has an important role in healthcare reform and cost containment. Each organization will address this in its mission, policies, and procedures. Shared governance in nursing will also be a major contributor in this process.

ONLINE CONSULT

Patient Protection and Affordable Care Act at
http://www.hhs.gov/healthcare/rights/law/

Kaiser Family Foundation and Health Reform at
http://kff.org/health-reform/

Supreme Court Ruling at
http://www.supremecourt.gov/opinions/11pdf/
11-393c3a2.pdf

We discussed accountability and responsibility in Chapter 10 with delegation skills. Both of those concepts are also critical in terms of economics and healthcare policy. Accountability and responsibility mean we are answerable to our patients and the healthcare system for quality, cost-effective outcomes. The demonstration of these moral and ethical imperatives is provided in our commitment to evidence-based practices and the metrics we use to analyze and evaluate these practices. With the current initiative for transparency, this accountability is apparent to consumers, professionals, and society. **Fiscal responsibility** involves being answerable to our patients, our colleagues, and the healthcare system for quality, cost-effective outcomes. As Levine (2009) has observed on the topic of healthcare reform, "great savings could be achieved in two areas: administrative costs and unnecessary care" (pp. e16(1)–e16(2)). To do this requires ethical collaborative practice and involvement in healthcare policy and change. The American Nurses Association (2010) Standards of Professional Performance are particularly applicable here, especially evidence-based practice, quality of practice, communication, leadership, collaboration, and resource utilization. Involvement of nurses in policy making and politics is an imperative for professional practice, as we will discuss in Chapter 17.

EVIDENCE-BASED PRACTICE: *Consider this....*

Consider the issue of healthcare resources and the ability to benefit. The cost of healthcare services has escalated, with cost controls sought on a daily basis by both users and providers. Think about the amounts paid through the Medicaid program for long-term care. These costs include covering the elderly in both nursing homes and in the community. The goal is to keep elders in the community, and some states have implemented "diversion programs" to keep frail elders in the community rather than in nursing home settings. Review the conditions and eligibility for one Medicaid Diversion Program at http://elderaffairs.state.fl.us/doea/cares.php

Question: What are your thoughts about safety, cost-effectiveness, and health equity?

KEY POINTS

- Economics is the study of production of a product or service, along with issues of supply and demand and distribution of that product or service for the continuity or well-being of some entity. Healthcare economics is a specialty area of economics focused on the different parts of the healthcare system that supply and deliver services.

KEY POINTS—cont'd

- The gross national product (GNP) is the goods and services produced in a nation and is measured on an annual basis. The gross domestic product (GDP) is restricted to the goods and services produced within the nation.

- The cost of healthcare is the price or the monetary amount of goods and services to cover the episode of care.

- Reimbursement is the amount of money provided to pay for that particular episode of care based on an agreed or approved process.

- First-party payers are the individuals; second-party payers are the providers, plan administrators, or employers who collect the premiums; and third-party payers are the insurers who assess and assume the risks of the group and reimburse the healthcare providers for their services.

- The prospective payment system (PPS) is a fixed payment method that is based on a predetermined amount as the usual care needed for a patient with a specific condition.

- Fee-for-service (FFS) plans are the traditional payment methods in which each service is charged separately, as with provider visits, laboratory tests, and supplies.

- Managed care covers a variety of treatment and payment options, with the ultimate goals to maintain health and prevent disease and disability, thus reducing healthcare costs.

- Point-of-service (POS) plans generally occur through a specified network of providers, whereby the primary care provider serves as a gatekeeper and consultations with others must have prior approval for reimbursement.

- Preferred provider organizations (PPOs) are providers and provider agencies that are included as part of a network and agree to negotiated rates for patients who use the PPOs listed in the network.

- Health maintenance organizations (HMOs) are focused on managed care within a specified system, keeping capitated members healthy, and avoiding costs of expensive diagnostic and medical procedures.

- A medical savings account (MSA) is a federal tax incentive program used by employers or Medicare recipients for self-management of healthcare in which a high deductible is agreed on with an amount provided in a savings account to pay for initial care.

- Accountable care organizations (ACOs) have evolved as a component of the Patient Protection and Affordable Care Act (ACA) as shared savings organizations designed to promote accountability, risk management, and coordinated care.

- In the United States, Medicare, Medicaid, and state Children's Health Insurance Programs (CHIP) are major governmental entities that provide healthcare for select populations. Medicare was the first program, beginning in 1965 with the Social Security Act under Title XVIII. Refer to Table 16.4 for major timelines for these federal programs.

- Medicare is available for Americans aged 65 years or older, those with certain disabilities, and those with end-stage renal disease. Medicare Part A provides for inpatient hospital, skilled rehabilitative, hospice, and home care services. Medicare Part B covers approved outpatient care, necessary and selected preventive services, and equipment, usually by virtue of an additional premium. Medicare Part C is a selected "Advantage Plan" in which Part A and Part B services are provided by an FFS, PPO, HMO, or a special plan. Medicare Part D is the optional prescription drug coverage plan.

- The Medicaid program was authorized in 1965 under Title XIX of the Social Security Act with programs at the state and local levels provided by some federal funding and regulated through eligibility requirements.

- The Children's Health Insurance Program (CHIP), originally enacted in 1997 as Title XXI of the Social Security Act, provides health coverage for uninsured children who are not eligible for Medicaid.

- Health equity has been defined as "the attainment of the highest level of health for all people" (National Partnership for Action to End Health Disparities, 2011, p. 1).

- Fiscal responsibility involves being answerable to our patients, our colleagues, and the healthcare system for quality, cost-effective outcomes.

Thought and Discussion Questions

1. Discuss the values and demands for healthcare from the perspectives of:
   - An employer who is trying to choose a health plan
   - An employee who will be using the services of the health plan
   - An uninsured family who is seeking coverage through the state insurance exchange

2. From a public policy standpoint, can the U.S. healthcare system continue to reduce the number of uninsured while controlling demand and limiting overall costs with the current fragmented insurance structure? Would a single-payer system be better?

3. Describe how you would evaluate the clinical effectiveness and cost-effectiveness of strategies designed to limit costs. Provide examples of nursing-sensitive patient outcomes.

4. Discuss the financial implications of providing the following services in your community:
   - Ambulatory services
   - Hospital care
   - Preventative services
   - Rehabilitation

5. Review the Chapter Thought at the beginning of the chapter and be prepared to discuss its meaning in the context of the chapter.

Interactive Exercises

Go to the Intranet site and complete the interactive exercises provided for this chapter.

REFERENCES

American Nurses Association. (2010). *Nursing: Scope and standards of practice* (2nd ed.). Silver Spring, MD: Nursesbooks.org.

Anderson, D., & Hogan, N. (2013). Emerging 'super ACOs' fill unique needs. *Healthcare Financial Management, 67*(10), 88–94.

Berry, L. L., & Beckham, D. (2014). Team-based care at Mayo Clinic: A model for ACOs. *Journal of Healthcare Management, 59*(1), 9–13.

Centers for Medicare and Medicaid Services (CMS). (2005). Key milestones in Medicare and Medicaid history, selected years: 1965-2003. *Health Care Financing Review, 27*(2). Retrieved from http://www.cms.gov/Research-Statistics-Data-and-Systems/Research/HealthCareFinancingReview/downloads/05-06Winpg1.pdf

Centers for Medicare and Medicaid Services (CMS). (2013a). *Accountable care organizations.* Retrieved from http://www.cms.gov/Medicare/Medicare-Fee-for-Service-Payment/ACO/

Centers for Medicare and Medicaid Services (CMS). (2013b). *The IDC-10 transition: An introduction.* Retrieved from http://www.cms.gov/Medicare/Coding/ICD10/Downloads/ICD10Introduction20140819.pdf

Centers for Medicare and Medicaid Services (CMS). (2013c). *Prescription drug coverage: General information.* Retrieved from https://www.cms.gov/Medicare/Prescription-Drug-Coverage/PrescriptionDrugCovGenIn/index.html

Centers for Medicare and Medicaid Services (CMS). (2014). *Medicare provider utilization and payment data.* Retrieved from https://www.cms.gov/Research-Statistics-Data-and-Systems/Statistics-Trends-and-Reports/Medicare-Provider-Charge-Data/

Chang, C. F., Price, S. A., & Pfoutz, S. K. (2001). *Economics and nursing: Critical professional issues.* Philadelphia: F. A. Davis.

Children's Health Insurance Program (CHIP). (2011). Allotment methodology and states' fiscal years 2009 through 2015 CHIP allotments. 42 CFR § 457.

Colpas, P. (2013). Accountable care organizations help to coordinate care. *Health Management Technology, 34*(7), 6–9.

Cowan, C. A., & Hartman, M. B. (2005). Financing health care: Businesses, households, and governments, 1987–2003. *Health Care Financing Review Web Exclusive, 1*(2). Retrieved from https://www.cms.gov/HealthCareFinancingReview/Downloads/Cowan2.pdf.

Hayen, A. P., van den Berg, M. J., Meijboom, B. R., & Westert, G. P. (2013). Accountable care organizations: How to dress for success. *American Journal of Managed Care, 19*(6), 517–519.

Henry J. Kaiser Family Foundation. (2013a). *Fact sheet: The Medicare Part D prescription drug benefit.* Retrieved from http://kaiserfamilyfoundation.files.wordpress.com/2013/11/7044-14-medicare-part-d-fact-sheet.pdf

Henry J. Kaiser Family Foundation. (2013b). *Medicaid and its role in state/federal budgets and health reform.* Retrieved from http://kff.org/health-reform/fact-sheet/five-key-questions-and-answers-about-medicaid/

Henry J. Kaiser Family Foundation. (2013c). *Medicaid and the uninsured.* Retrieved from http://kaiserfamilyfoundation.files.wordpress.com/2012/05/8139-03.pdf

Henry J. Kaiser Family Foundation. (2014a). *Explaining health care reform: Risk adjustment, reinsurance, and risk corridors.* Retrieved from http://kff.org/health-reform/issue-brief/explaining-health-care-reform-risk-adjustment-reinsurance-and-risk-corridors/

Henry J. Kaiser Family Foundation. (2014b). *Kaiser health policy news index: January 2014.* Retrieved from http://kff.org

/health-reform/poll-finding/kaiser-health-policy-news-index
-january-2014/

Henry J. Kaiser Family Foundation. (2014c). *Visualizing health policy: A short look at long-term care for seniors*. Retrieved from http://kff.org/infographic/visualizing-health-policy-a -short-look-at-long-term-care-for-seniors/

Herrera, C-N., Gaynor, M., Newman, M., Town, R. J., & Parente, S. T. (2013). Trends underlying employer-sponsored health insurance growth for Americans younger than age sixty-five. *Health Affairs, 32*(10), 1715–1722.

Jacobson, G., Huang, J., & Neuman, T. (2014). Medigap reform: Setting the context for understanding recent proposals. *Kaiser Family Foundation Issue Brief*. Retrieved from http://kaiserfamilyfoundation.files.wordpress.com /2014/01/8235-02-medigap-reform-setting-the-context -for-understanding-recent-proposals1.pdf

Kimbuende, E., Ranji, U., Lundy, J., & Salganicoff, A. (2013). U.S. health care costs. In C. L. Estes, S. A. Chapman, C. Dodd, B. Hollister, & C. Harrington (Eds.), *Health policy crisis and reform* (6th ed., pp. 548–553). Burlington, MA: Jones & Bartlett.

Klees, B. S., & Wolfe, C. J. (2013). *Brief summaries of Medicare & Medicaid: Title XVIII and Title XIX of the Social Security Act as of November 1, 2013*. Washington, DC: Centers for Medicare and Medicaid. Retrieved from http://www.cms .gov/Research-Statistics-Data-and-Systems/Statistics-Trends -and-Reports/MedicareProgramRatesStats/Downloads /MedicareMedicaidSummaries2013.pdf

Kovner, A. R., & Knickman, J. R. (Ed.). (2011). *Health care delivery in the United States* (10th ed.). New York: Springer.

Levine, R. A. (2009). Fiscal responsibility and health care reform. *New England Journal of Medicine, 361*, e16(1)–e16(3).

Martin, A. B., Lassman, D., Washington, B., Catlin, A., & the National Health Expenditure Accounts Team. (2012). Growth in US health spending remained slow in 2010; health share of gross domestic product was unchanged from 2009. *Health Affairs, 31*(1), 208–219. Retrieved from http://content.healthaffairs.org/content/31/1/208

Medicare Program (2013). Inpatient Hospital Deductible and Hospital and Extended Care Services Coinsurance Amounts for CY 2014, 78 Fed. Reg. 2013-25595 (filed 10-28-13). Retrieved from http://www.gpo.gov/fdsys/pkg /FR-2013-10-30/pdf/2013-25595.pdf

Miller, L. M. P., Chang, C. F., & Pfoutz, S. K. (2012). Health-care economics. In R. Kearney-Nunnery (Ed.), *Advancing your career: Concepts for professional nursing* (5th ed., pp. 309–334). Philadelphia, PA: F.A. Davis.

Modern Healthcare (2013, October). Most frequently billed DRGs ranked by 2011 Medicare patient discharges. *Modern Healthcare, 32*.

Moriyama, I. M., Loy, R. M., Robb-Smith, A. H. T., Rosenberg, H. M., & Hoyert, D. L. (2011). *History of the statistical classification of diseases and causes of death*. Retrieved from http://www.cdc.gov/nchs/data/misc /classification_diseases2011.pdf

National Partnership for Action to End Health Disparities. (2011). *Health equity and disparities*. Retrieved from http:// www.minorityhealth.hhs.gov/npa/templates/browse.aspx?lvl =1&lvlid=34

Nichols, L. (2012). Accountable care organization pathways: Diverse but ultimately parallel. *Mayo Clinic Proceedings, 87*(8), 710–713.

Office of Inspector General Office of Evaluation and Inspections Region IX. (August 2001). Medicare Hospital Prospective Payment System How DRG Rates Are Calculated and Updated (OEI-09-00-00200). Retrieved from https://oig.hhs.gov/oei/reports/oei-09-00-00200.pdf

Office of Technology Assessment. (1983). Diagnostic related groups (DRGs) and the Medicare program: Implications for medical technology–a technical memorandum. Retrieved from http://www.fas.org/ota/reports/8306.pdf

Organisation for Economic Co-operation and Development (OECD). (2011a). *Health at a glance 2011: OECD indicators*. Retrieved from http://dx.doi.org/10.1787/health _glance-2011-en

Organisation for Economic Co-operation and Development (OECD). (2013). Total expenditure on health, *Health: Key tables from OECD*, no. 1. doi: 10.1787/hlthxp-total-table- 2013-2-en; http://www.oecd-ilibrary.org/social-issues -migration-health/health-at-a-glance_19991312;jsessionid =612e179lbg8ul.x-oecd-live-01

Thomson, S., Osborn, R, & Jun, M. (Eds.). (2013). *International profiles of health care systems, 2013*. The Commonwealth Fund. Retrieved from http://www.commonwealthfund. org/~/media/Files/Publications/Fund%20Report/2013/Nov /1717_Thomson_intl_profiles_hlt_care_sys_2013_v2.pdf

Unruh, L., & Spetz, J. (2012). A primer on health economics. In D. J. Mason, J. K. Leavitt, & M. W. Chaffee (Eds.), *Policy and politics in nursing and health care* (pp. 153–161). St. Louis, MO: Elsevier/Saunders.

U.S. Department of Health and Human Services. (2011). *Report to congress: National strategy for quality improvement in health care*. Retrieved from http://www.ahrq.gov /workingforquality/nqs/nqs2011annlrpt.htma

U.S. Department of Health and Human Services Office of Inspector General. (2014). *Medicare beneficiaries paid nearly half of the costs for outpatient services at Critical Access Hospitals*. Retrieved from http://oig.hhs.gov/oei/reports/oei -05-12-00085.pdf

BIBLIOGRAPHY

Agency for Healthcare Research and Quality (AHRQ). (2015). *Fact Sheet: Healthcare cost and utilization project (HCUP)*. Retrieved from http://www.ahrq.gov/research/data/hcup/

Centers for Medicare and Medicaid Services (CMS). (2012*). Your guide to Medicare medical savings account (MSA) plans*. Retrieved from http://www.medicare.gov/Publications /Pubs/pdf/11206.pdf

Centers for Medicare and Medicaid Services (CMS). (2013). *Critical access hospitals*. Retrieved from http://www.cms .gov/Medicare/Provider-Enrollment-and-Certification /CertificationandComplianc/CAHs.html

Centers for Medicare and Medicaid Services (CMS). (2013). *PPS overview*. Retrieved from http://www.cms.gov /ProspMedicareFeeSvcPmtGen/

Centers for Medicare and Medicaid Services (CMS). (2013). *Premiums, deductible, and coinsurance amounts*. Retrieved from http://www.cms.gov/Research-Statistics-Data -and-Systems/Statistics-Trends-and-Reports/Medicare ProgramRatesStats/PremiumsDeductiblesCoinsurance.html

Centers for Medicare and Medicaid Services (CMS). (2013). *Prospective payment systems general information:*

Overview. Retrieved from http://www.cms.gov/ProspMedicareFeeSvcPmtGen/

Centers for Medicare and Medicaid Services (CMS). (2014). *HIPPA general information: Overview.* Retrieved from https://www.cms.gov/MedHCPCSGenInfo/

Centers for Medicare and Medicaid Services (CMS). (2014). *Medicare and you.* Retrieved from http://www.medicare.gov/medicare-and-you/medicare-and-you.html

Centers for Medicare and Medicaid Services (CMS). (2014). *Medicare coverage general information: Overview.* Retrieved http://www.cms.gov/CoverageGenInfo/

Centers for Medicare and Medicaid Services (CMS). (n.d.). *Inpatient prospective payment system hospital and long term care hospital review and measurement fact sheet.* Retrieved from http://www.cms.gov/AcuteInpatientPPS/Downloads/InpatientReviewFactSheet.pdf

Centers for Medicare and Medicaid Services (CMS). (n.d.). *The Affordable Care Act: Helping providers help patients—a menu of options for improving care.* Retrieved from http://www.cms.gov/Medicare/Medicare-Fee-for-Service-Payment/ACO/Downloads/ACO-Menu-Of-Options.pdf

Democratic Policy Committee (DPC) Reports. (2009). Legislative bulletin: H.R. 3590, the legislative vehicle for the Patient Protection and Affordable Care Act of 2009. Retrieved from http://dpc.senate.gov/dpcdoc.cfm?doc_name=lb-111-1-151

Hogan, C., Lunney, J., Gabel, J., & Lynn, J. (2012). Medicare beneficiaries' costs of care in the last year of life. *Health Affairs, 20*(4), 188–195. Retrieved from http://content.healthaffairs.org/content/20/4/188.full

Hussey, P. S., Ridgely, M. S., & Rosenthal, M. B. (2011). The PROMETHEUS bundled payment experiment: Slow start shows problems in implementing new payment models. *Health Affairs, 30*(11), 2116–2124. Retrieved from http://content.healthaffairs.org/content/30/11/2116.full.html

Kaiser Family Foundation. (2014). Many Medicare outpatients pay more at rural hospitals, Federal report says. *KHN Kaiser Health News.* Retrieved from http://www.kaiserhealthnews.org/Stories/2014/October/08/Report-Finds-Higher-Outpatient-Costs-For-Many-Medicare-Patients-At-Rural-Hospitals.aspx

Martin, A. B., Hartman, M., Whittle, L., Catlin, A., & the National Health Expenditure Accounts Team. (2014). National health spending in 2012: Rate of health spending growth remained low for the fourth consecutive year. *Health Affairs, 33*(1), 67–77.

Organisation for Economic Co-operation and Development (OECD). (2011b). *Why is health spending in the United States so high?* Retrieved from http://www.oecd.org/dataoecd/12/16/49084355.pdf

Patient Protection and Affordable Care Act of 2009. Retrieved from http://democrats.senate.gov/pdfs/reform/patient-protection-affordable-care-act-as-passed.pdf

State Health Access Data Assistance Center. (2014). *For kids' sake: State-level trends in children's health insurance. A state-by-state analysis.* Retrieved from http://www.rwjf.org/content/dam/farm/reports/reports/2014/rwjf412274

Supreme Court of the United States. (2012). National Federation of Independent Business et al. *v.* Sebelius, Secretary of Health and Human Services, et al. No. 11–393. Retrieved from http://www.supremecourt.gov/opinions/11pdf/11-393c3a2.pdf

U.S. Department of Health and Human Services. (2014). *Read the law.* Retrieved from http://www.hhs.gov/healthcare/rights/law/index.html

ONLINE RESOURCES

Centers for Medicare and Medicaid Services
http://cms.gov

COBRA Insurance
http://cobrainsurance.com

The Henry J. Kaiser Family Foundation
http://kff.org/

Organisation for Economic Co-operation and Development
http://www.oecd.org/

Patient Protection and Affordable Care Act
http://www.hhs.gov/healthcare/rights/law/index.html

● Rose Kearney-Nunnery

The Politically Active Nurse: An Imperative

"There are risks and costs to a program of action, but they are far less than the long range risks and costs of comfortable inaction."

John F. Kennedy, 1917–1963

Chapter Objectives

On completion of this chapter, the reader will be able to:

1. Explain why it is important for nurses to possess political efficacy.

2. Discuss the process for the enactment of laws and associated regulations.

3. Identify the major committees at the federal and state levels, especially those that influence health policy.

4. Identify how nurses can influence the passing of legislation.

5. Analyze statutes and regulations governing nursing practice.

6. Examine the roles and activities of nurses and professional associations in influencing health policy decisions.

7. Demonstrate political involvement on a current health policy issue.

Key Terms

Political Efficacy
Government
Law
Bill
Committee Structure
Conference Committee

Regulations
Precedent
Nurse Practice Acts
Title Protection
Lobbying
Grassroots Effort

Political Action Committees (PACs)
Workplace Issues
Community or Civic Involvement
Professional Organizations
Voice of Agency

Hillary Rodam Clinton (2003) once observed,

A political life, I've often said, is a continuing education in human nature, including one's own. . . . In each place [of my involvement], I met someone or saw something that caused me to open my mind and my heart and deepen my understanding of the universal concerns that most of humanity share. (p. x)

Politics is a process for finding solutions to these universal concerns of humanity, one being the concern for public health and safety. Nurses likewise are engaged in finding solutions to problems of humanity on a daily basis. These problems are not restricted to a location or practice area. The nursing professional advocates for the health of people and policies aimed at health protection and promotion. This imperative for change requires a broader view of what is involved in making changes in public policy at the local, state, and national levels. Nurses have become increasingly interested in public policy, realizing that both their personal and their professional lives are significantly influenced by governmental policy and programs.

Nurses are effective in the political process when they understand the sources of power and are willing to be involved and make a difference. Interestingly, Wilson and Dilulio (2004) have defined **political efficacy** as having two components: internal political efficacy and external political advocacy. Internal political efficacy is personal competence or the "ability to understand and take part in political affairs" (Wilson & Dilulio, 2004, p. 93). External political advocacy is the "ability to make the system respond to the citizenry" (Wilson & Dilulio, 2004, p. 93). Nurses must develop their internal political efficacy by being increasingly able to take part in the political process. This will further the external political efficacy of the nursing profession. These two components are the political imperative of the profession. External political efficacy is possible by virtue of the number of nurses in the profession who are skillful in promoting change. In addition, we see the active involvement of nursing organizations in political initiatives to effect change in health policy. As described by Leininger (2002), "political aspects of nursing are now a dominant and frequent topic in hospitals and schools of nursing in the current era" (p. 189).

Both internal efficacy and external political efficacy are growing with the increasing involvement of nurses. As noted by Mason, Leavitt, and Chaffee (2011), healthcare is a political endeavor at all levels of government and influenced by healthcare institutions in the private sector. This is one area of influence for nursing professionals and their political efficacy. The first step in the development of political efficacy is understanding the political process in government.

STRUCTURE AND FUNCTION OF GOVERNMENT

When we think of the term **government**, different images may come to mind. We may be thinking of the federal structure with its three components, executive, legislative, and judicial. Or, at the local level, we may be envisioning the organizational, local, and state influences on the operation of the healthcare unit. Government is merely the controlling entity that has the authority to make decisions and regulations for the public good. Milstead (2013) describes government as an "iron triangle" of members of Congress, bureaucratic staff, and interest groups. Nursing has the responsibility to contribute to this process by providing the information needed and offering support for wise policy decisions that protect the public and the profession. To participate most effectively in the political process, one must understand the structure of government at each level. Because government structures do vary, it is essential to be familiar with your own local and state governing bodies.

Branches of Government

Each branch of government plays a significant role in the development and implementation of health policy. The federal government and most state governments have three branches: legislative, executive, and judicial. The powers of the three federal branches are vested in accordance with the U.S. Constitution.

Executive Branch

At the federal level, the executive branch consists of the president, the cabinet-level departments, and regulatory agencies. The executive branch is responsible for the administration of government and the laws enacted. The president sets the legislative agenda for Congress and the annual budget for the nation. The president's budget influences the funding available for healthcare programs, reimbursement, and education. In addition, the agenda set by the president determines what programs have a high priority for the administration. The president can recommend legislation and can approve or veto legislation passed by Congress. It is also the executive branch that makes appointments to government departments, courts, boards, and committees, as with the appointment of the surgeon general or the secretary of health and human services. The Constitution mandates that certain executive appointments be confirmed by the legislative branch.

Legislative Branch

The legislative branch comprises the two houses or chambers of the U.S. Congress, the Senate and the House of Representatives. Congress is responsible for lawmaking, representation, and administrative oversight, including oversight of the agencies of the executive branch. Congress also provides the operational funding for the administrative agencies. The composition of and qualifications for the U.S. Congress are listed in Table 17.1. Compare these qualifications with those for the president. Also consider the reelection cycle and how the priorities, policies, and laws can be influenced by executive and legislative agendas and majority control.

Judicial Branch

The judicial branch includes the Supreme Court, which interprets laws and, through its judicial review process, can

TABLE 17.1

Qualifications for Service in the U.S. Congress or Executive Office

	Senate	House of Representatives	Presidency
Number	100 senators (two from each state) Equal representation Senior senator (elected first) and junior senator	435 members Representation based on state population; minimum of one from each state with reapportionment every 10 years based on the U.S. census The House also includes delegates from the District of Columbia, Guam, the Virgin Islands, American Samoa, and Puerto Rico, who have voting rights in committees but not in matters before the full House	One; In the case of the inability of the president to fulfill his or her role, succession of power occurs as follows: vice president as second in line, then speaker of the house, and then president pro tempore of the Senate
Term	Elected for a term of six years, on alternate schedules	Elected for a term of two years	Elected for a term of four years
Reelection	Every two years, one third of senators face reelection	Entire membership is up for reelection every two years	Eligible for reelection once (two-term limit)
Qualifications	At least 30 years of age Citizen of United States for nine years Resident of the state represented when elected	At least 25 years of age Citizen of United States for seven years Resident of the state represented when elected	At least 35 years of age A natural-born citizen of the United States and a resident for at least 14 years

declare an act of Congress or the president unconstitutional. The nine federal Supreme Court Justices are appointed for life by the president after their selection has been confirmed by the Senate. The federal system also comprises lower courts and appellate or circuit courts. Federal judges are nominated by the executive branch and confirmed by the Senate. This system of checks and balances is designed to create equilibrium, vesting limited power in each branch with oversight by another branch.

State and Local Systems

State government structures are similar to those described at the federal level. They also receive their mandates from the U.S. Constitution, with which their respective state constitutions must abide. Like the president, the governor can sign legislation into law and use the power of the veto. State legislatures can also override a governor's veto. In some states, members of the state board of nursing, or other important health commissioners, are appointed by the governor. As with the federal government, some legislative branches must confirm selected executive appointments. State supreme courts and lower courts interpret the law and make decisions under their power of judicial review.

County government generally entails a board of supervisors or an elected board of commissioners and a county executive or county manager. Cities, towns, and villages also have a variety of elected officials similar to those of county government. Local health policies and politics must be consistent with state and federal law but can also have a profound influence on the health and welfare of a community, as with public utilities and local programs.

Although nurses are most often involved with the legislative branch of government, the executive branch and the judicial branch can also be of great importance to nursing and healthcare. It is essential that nurses understand the functions of the different branches of government and how laws and regulations are enacted and implemented.

HOW LAWS ARE MADE

A **law** is a mandate of prescribed conduct, grants certain rights, requires certain responsibilities, or a combination of these attributes. A law can come from a constitution, from the legislature, or from the courts. Administrative agencies promulgate regulations, which supplement and further interpret the laws. Consider the types of laws and regulations identified in Table 17.2.

The idea for a law may originate with an individual, a professional group, a legislator, or the executive branch. *Statutory law* is legislation that has been approved by both legislative houses of Congress and signed by the executive branch. The legislation starts as a **bill** or a proposal for a law authored or sponsored by either a representative or a senator, who introduces it after it has been written in appropriate

TABLE 17.2

Types of Law

Type	Description	Example
Constitutional	Specific guarantees granted by the U.S. Constitution	Freedom of speech
Statutory	Formal laws enacted by federal, state, and local legislative branches of government	Nurse practice acts
Administrative	Regulations created by administrative agencies under the direction of the executive branch of government	Regulations associated with nurse practice acts to assist with implementation
Court, case, or common law	Laws created from judicial decisions Judgments create a precedent on which future decisions are based	"Miranda Rights" must be read to an arrestee before he or she is taken into custody

language by the legislative counsel of either the House or the Senate. A bill may also be introduced from a legislative committee. A bill proposed in the Senate is designated "S." followed by a number, and a bill introduced in the House of Representatives is designated "H.R." followed by a number.

Congressional Committees

At the federal level, bills are referred to full committee and sometimes to a subcommittee, because of the thousands of bills introduced each year. The U.S. Senate has standing committees, with a variable number of associated subcommittees, depending on the scope and work of the committee, and select or special committees. The House of Representatives also has standing committees and additional special or select committees. There are also joint committees, staffed by both houses that focus on common oversight functions for taxation and economics.

It is within the **committee structure** that most of the work of Congress takes place, at both the federal and state levels. Committee action is perhaps the most important phase of the congressional process because it is at this phase that proposed measures are given the most intensive consideration and people have an opportunity to provide testimony for consideration and incorporation into the record. The committee or subcommittee level is where nursing can have a powerful impact. The subcommittee studies the issues contained in each bill carefully, holds hearings, and reports back to the full committee with recommendations. Each committee has jurisdiction over certain subjects. Some of the committees identified in Table 17.3 focus specifically on health-related issues.

Committee action is perhaps the most important phase of the congressional process, because it is at this phase that proposed measures are given the most intensive consideration.

States operate much like the federal government. In a particular state, there are also specific committees and subcommittees that handle selected topics. For example, in South Carolina, the Medical, Military, Public, and

ONLINE CONSULT

American Nurses Association at
http://nursingworld.org/MainMenu Categories/Policy-Advocacy

U.S. Government Web Portal at
http://firstgov.gov

THOMAS, U.S. Congress on the Internet at
http://thomas.loc.gov/home/thomas.php

Municipal Affairs Committee for the House and the Medical Committee of the Senate generally handle the topics of concern to nursing and healthcare. But state structures differ, and it is important to be aware of the differences and to know the committees in which the issues of major concern to nursing arise. Appointment to the committees is often based on congressional seniority or priority. Members often have special interests in an area. Because these members represent their constituents, it is important to know on which committees your congressperson serves and that they have valid information, resources, and background to address your concerns. Testimony, either written or in person, provides valuable information to the committee member, whether information from constituents, special interest groups, experts, or other public officials.

And visit your own state legislature online.

How a Bill Becomes a Law

Consider a bill, for instance, that has been sponsored by your legislator, a member of the House of Representatives. It has been sent to the applicable subcommittee or committee for review. After consideration by the full committee, several things may happen to this bill:

- It may be reported out of committee favorably and be scheduled for debate by the full House.
- It may be reported out favorably, but with amendments or "markups" to the bill.
- It may be reported out unfavorably or not acted upon at all; thus, it is "killed" or "dies in committee."

TABLE 17.3

Major Committees of the 114th U.S. Congress

House		Senate	
Standing committees (20)	Agriculture	Standing committees (16)	Agriculture, Nutrition, and Forestry
	Appropriations*		Appropriations*
	Armed Services		Armed Services
	Budget*		Banking, Housing, and Urban Affairs
	Education and Workforce		Budget*
	Energy & Commerce		Commerce, Science, and Transportation
	Ethics		Energy & Natural Resources
	Financial Services		Environment & Public Works*
	Foreign Affairs		Finance*
	Homeland Security*		Foreign Relations
	House Administration		Health, Education, Labor, & Pensions*
	Judiciary		Homeland Security and Governmental Affairs
	Natural Resources		Judiciary
	Oversight and Government Reform		Rules & Administration
	Rules		Small Business & Entrepreneurship
	Science, Space, and Technology		Veteran's Affairs*
	Small Business		
	Transportation and Infrastructure		
	Veteran's Affairs*		
	Ways and Means*		
Select, special, & other committees (2)	Intelligence	Select or special committees (4)	Aging*
	Special/Select event		Ethics
			Indian Affairs*
			Intelligence

Joint or Bicameral Congressional Committees	
	Economic
	Library
	Printing
	Taxation

*Frequently address health-related matters.

Generally, once the bill has been reported favorably out of a House committee, it goes to the Rules Committee, which schedules bills and determines (1) how much time will be spent on debate, and (2) whether amendments will be allowed. A written report is drafted, including a summary of the bill, along with impact statements. Impact statements are provided to project how the proposed legislation would affect existing laws and present and future resources. Bills are then placed on the calendar and scheduled for action. After a bill is debated under the procedural rules of the House, possibly amended, voted upon, and passed, it is sent to the Senate, where it goes through the same procedure. If the bill also passes the Senate without any changes, it is sent to the president or governor for signature. If minor changes were made in the Senate, it is referred back to the originating chamber (in this case the House of Representatives) for concurrence before submission to the executive branch. If significant changes were made to the bill in the Senate, the bill is sent to a **conference committee**, composed of representatives of both chambers, who reconcile differences and prepare a conference report for approval by both chambers. If it does not get approved, the bill dies. After the conference report, the bill must be accepted or rejected, because no further amendments can be made.

If the bill is approved in both houses, it goes to the executive branch. If the president or governor signs the bill, it becomes law, and Congress is notified. If the bill is vetoed, it is referred back to the House and Senate. A two-thirds vote by both chambers is required to override the veto. The bill may also become law if the president or governor fails to veto or return the bill to Congress with objections within a specified time. See Figure 17.1 for a description of the legislative process.

Once the bill is signed or passed, it becomes an act, and is *enacted* into law. Laws are enforceable if they do not violate the Constitution. Once a law is passed, it is assigned to the appropriate department of the executive branch of government, where the process of developing

1. Concerned party contacts legislator, bill drafted
2. Sponsors obtained, introduced to House and/or Senate
3. To committees for recommendation/amendments
4. Debate on floor
5. Vote and recommendation to other chamber
6. Consideration in a similar manner by the other chamber
7. Passage or to Conference Committee
8. Back to both houses for concurrence
9. If agreement by both chambers, to president or governor for signature
10. If executive veto, back to chambers for potential override with a 2/3 vote of Congress or the legislature

Figure 17.1 The legislative process.

regulations to interpret the law takes place. The department studies the law and drafts the regulations for implementation. Administrative agencies, governed by the executive branch, promulgate **regulations** or rules, which serve the purpose of detailing and applying the laws. For example, the Health Insurance Portability and Accountability Act (HIPAA) was enacted as Public Law 104–191 in 1996. The Department of Health and Human Services (HHS) published a final Privacy Rule in December 2000 with a general compliance date of April 14, 2003, and a compliance date of April 14, 2004, for small health plans. All of this activity involved detailing regulations for application of the law.

The legislative process can seem endless, especially when the bill stays in committee, perhaps during a recess or between legislative sessions. In addition, proposed regulations from the executive branch may require public hearings for input prior to finalization and enforcement. In the United States Congress, a legislative session spans a two-year period, with the 114th Congressional session running from January 1, 2015, through December 31, 2016. Variable legislative sessions occur in the different states; however, special sessions may be called for special circumstances.

Impact of Laws

Laws and regulations govern behavior and relationships with others in society. Consider the impact of laws that have been passed and their effect on nursing. When the federal government implemented diagnosis-related groups (DRGs) for Medicare reimbursement, patients began to be discharged from hospitals "sicker and quicker." Although this law applied only to Medicare patients, it set a precedent that other insurance carriers followed. In law, a **precedent** is a decision or verdict from a prior case that becomes the principle to follow in future cases. A precedent is more than an everyday custom to follow. If the precedent is set in a superior court, like the Supreme Court, it may become mandatory in lower court decisions.

Awareness of laws and regulations governing healthcare is essential in professional nursing practice so that nurses can help to influence the making of policy and laws.

Nurses can and do play a significant role at several points in the legislative process, whether through lobbying or providing testimony or information to legislators and regulatory bodies (Box 17.1).

REGULATING NURSING PRACTICE

Nursing practice and education are directly regulated by law. **Nurse practice acts** are contained in state statute (laws) and associated regulations that dictate practice parameters. As part of the statute, nursing education programs in different forms are regulated. For example, most states require a new, beginning nursing program to receive approval from the board of nursing according to specified standards before it can open. These standards ensure that the organization, curriculum, faculty, and

---

BOX 17.1 Nurses' Involvement in the Legislative Process

● Meeting with legislators, their aides or staff to influence the introduction of a bill as private citizens or as members of a professional organization
● Providing information to assist in drafting the bill and gathering support for legislators or bill sponsors on the proposed legislation
● Providing testimony in committee or subcommittee hearings about their position on the bill
● Contacting legislators to support or not support proposed legislation, both in the home district and the capitol
● Contacting either the president or the governor to sign or veto the proposed legislation
● Responding to requests for comments, either written or verbal testimony, by regulatory agencies or committees
● Submission of an *amicus curiae* (friend of the court) brief for consideration by the court

services are appropriate for preparation of students and protection of the public. Nursing education is further regulated indirectly through the accrediting bodies that are authorized by the Department of Education.

> The state boards of nursing and their associated practice acts define the scope of practice; establish the requirements for licensure, entry into practice, continuing competency, and advanced practice; create and empower a board of nursing; and identify grounds for disciplinary action.

Nurse Practice Acts

Nurse practice acts are developed by each state to protect the public health, safety, and welfare by regulating and overseeing nursing practice. The various state boards of nursing and their associated practice acts define the scope of practice; establish the requirements for licensure, entry into practice, continuing competency and advanced practice; create and empower a board of nursing; and identify grounds for disciplinary action. An important component in many practice acts is **title protection**. This is a part of the law that maintains the use of the title *nurse* only for the licensee authorized by the board. The term *nurse* is used in some contexts outside of professional practice, and more states are moving to protect the integrity and identity of this title.

Nurse practice acts can be revised or completely eliminated through a single legislative action, so the prospect of "opening the practice act" in the legislature can cause great anxiety. Although state practice acts (statute and regulations) are specific to the state, there is general content common to many state acts. For example, the National Council of State Boards of Nursing (NCSBN) has a model act and model rules that illustrate standard contents of the legislation and associated regulations for implementation (Box 17.2). In addition, in 1998 a mutual recognition model for interstate practice among the "compact states" was introduced. This mutual recognition model requires further specific language to be incorporated into state law to allow a nurse to have one license (in the state of residency) and to have practice privilieges in other states that are members of the compact. The nurse is required to practice in accordance with each state's specific practice law and regulations. There is also a national initiative for consensus to assist states in aligning their APRN regulation with the major elements of the Consensus Model for APRN Regulation within the four roles (clinical nurse specialist, nurse practitioner, nurse midwife, and nurse anesthetist) to include graduation from an accredited graduate nursing program, advanced certification, recognition of the four APRN roles, including by title and license, independent practice, and independent prescribing (NCSBN, 2014).

Appointments to a state board of nursing are often made by the governor. The state board should be composed of a variety of members who represent practice throughout all areas of nursing. In four states, there are separate boards for licensed practical nurses/licensed vocational nurses (LPNs/LVNs) and registered nurses

---

BOX 17.2 **Nurse Practice Acts**

General content for both statute and regulations:
- Title and purpose
- Definitions, scope, and standards of practice
- Board of nursing—authority and how it functions
- Application of other state statutes and the state's administrative law act
- Licensure
- Titles and abbreviations
- Nursing assistive personnel
- Approval of nursing education programs
- Violations and penalties
- Discipline and proceedings
- Emergency relief for public protection
- Reporting requirements
- Exemptions
- Revenue and fees
- Implementation of the statute and regulations

And if applicable to the particular state:
- Nurse licensure compact
- APRN scope of practice and APRN compact

(RNs), but the boards are combined in the remaining jurisdictions. RN boards generally address both professional nursing and advanced practice nurses (APRNs), although one state currently has separate RN and APRN Boards. APRN regulations may also be addressed in the respective practice acts of other health professions such as the board of medicine. In addition, boards of nursing may have advisory committees or practice committees that research issues for recommendations to the board on practice or policy issues. Review your state's practice act for the composition of members on the board or perhaps seek a seat on the board. In many cases, serving on a board of nursing is both a humbling and an enlightening experience, and allows you to serve your state and your profession.

Because changes proposed by a state board can lead to laws and rules that have the same force as laws, it is imperative for nurses to remain aware of the activities of the board that regulates practice within their state. The American Nurses Association (ANA) provides recent updates to practice acts and the status of proposed legislation on its Web site under the section on policy and advocacy. Trends in legislation are also tracked, for example, in the areas of title protection and staffing levels. In addition, some states issue advisory opinions; although such opinions do not have the same impact as law, they do guide acceptable standards of practice. Nurses are often unaware that changes are even being proposed. Some states distribute the state nurses association newsletter to all registered nurses, whether or not they hold membership in the ANA or the state association. Many of the newsletter issues (print or online) contain periodic informational alerts concerning changes in or interpretations to the statute or advisory opinions by the board.

State boards and their respective members are concerned about nurses' current understanding of their respective state law. To encourage and increase nurses' knowledge about their respective practice acts, some states award continuing education credits for specific courses. It is vital that nurses understand the content of their respective practice acts. This understanding must be ongoing, beyond the point of original licensure or title recognition. Put a bookmark in your computer's Internet browser with the Web site of your nursing board(s) to give yourself quick information and links to related resources.

Additional State and Federal Laws Affecting Nursing Practice

Laws have been passed on nursing practice issues, for example, allowing nurses to be directly reimbursed by patients or insurers. Legislation varies from state to state, but APRNs, particularly nurse anesthetists, nurse practitioners, and nurse midwives, are most commonly covered. The Bureau of Labor Statistics (2014) reported that there were 151,400 nurse anesthetists, nurse midwives, and nurse practitioners in practice in 2012, with more than 47,000 additional jobs projected by 2022. And these figures do not include the fourth APRN role of clinical nurse specialist.

State laws that affect practice can be passed with the support of nursing. Some states have passed laws to allow registered nurses to pronounce death. Others are addressing safe practice through staffing requirements, title protection, tort reform, environmental safety, and prohibitions on mandatory overtime. Still others are addressing delegation to assistive personnel. Public protection is a concern at all levels of government. In the area of advanced practice, for example, states differ in level of supervision or collaboration and prescriptive authority for advanced practice nurses. Several states allow independent APRN practice with proposals pending in other states. Nurses must be politically astute and must continue to develop their internal political efficacy and the external efficacy of the profession.

Also look for governmental affairs on Web sites of nursing specialty organizations.

INFLUENCING LEGISLATION

As mentioned previously, the idea for a law may originate from a concerned citizen or special interest group, a legislator, a professional group, or the executive branch to address a community problem or a public policy issue. Many laws originate from the legislature itself, which is composed of individuals who are elected by constituents with specific interests, needs, and concerns. Legislators' knowledge and recognition of particular needs and concerns come about through influence. For instance, special interest groups representing large numbers of the voting public can have a lot of influence on legislators. Special interest groups have

---

ONLINE CONSULT

ANA at
http://nursingworld.org/MainMenuCategories/
Policy-Advocacy

American Association of Colleges of Nursing:
Government Affairs at
http://www.aacn.nche.edu/Government
/index.htm

---

become more politically savvy at influencing the creation of public policy, and more controls have emerged, as with campaign financing reforms. Special interest groups influence legislators through lobbying activities, professional lobbyists, professional organizations, political action committees, and grassroots efforts. Each of these groups represents the dollars and votes of a particular special interest group, and each group uses expert communication and interpersonal skills to influence change.

Lobbying

Activities to influence legislators vary from formal to informal and often take the form of lobbying. **Lobbying** may be defined as attempting to persuade a legislator or legislative aide of the merits of your viewpoint in order to influence legislation. Individuals may lobby through face-to-face interviews, letter writing, telephone calls, faxes, e-mails, letters to the editor, and testimony (verbal or written). Valuable clues on and guidelines for letter writing are provided by professional associations that recognize the value of individual constituents' contacting their elected legislators. These professional organizations often provide special alerts or suggestions to the members to assist with lobbying activities. For example, some professional organizations provide an alert when members of Congress are on recess and should be contacted in their home states. Other organizations may include lobbying tips on their Web sites, along with background issues and talking points to assist in lobbying activities.

But there is definitely an art to getting your point across. The bottom line is that numbers mean something to the legislative aide or legislator, especially from constituents. There are other considerations, however, such as time. The impact of a well-composed, factual, meaningful, and succinct letter or e-mail far outweighs the form letter that has less impact or a letter that rambles on. Another consideration is the form of the correspondence. Postal delays or screenings cannot compete with the immediacy of e-mail, for instance. For a personal appointment, be aware of the congressional calendar, and do not be disappointed if you meet with a legislative aide. The aide may be more knowledgeable about your issue and can be persuaded to communicate the information to the legislator.

The professional lobbyist is a person on the staff of a professional association or hired consultant who has outstanding skills in persuasion, in-depth knowledge of the organization, and an acute sense of the intricacies of the political system. These professionals understand the legislators and their political agendas. The professional lobbyist is present at the appropriate time with the correct message, especially in the case of the undecided legislator. The role of the professional lobbyist is to provide the facts and the support base to persuade the legislator. The ANA has several professional lobbyists working at the federal level. A significant number of constituent state associations (CNAs) and specialty professional organizations also hire professional lobbyists.

Lobbying is especially effective when there is an associated strong **grassroots effort** that responds with mobilization of a group to provide additional correspondence and support on the position presented to the legislator or legislative aide. This approach has been used effectively by many professional organizations to influence public policy. Various nursing and other grassroots networks have been established to lobby in support of the legislative goals and objectives of the state nurses associations. There are specific channels of communication for response to a key issue. Key contacts for each legislator or legislative district must be active and ongoing.

Professional Organizations

Nurses have always had a great deal of potential power by virtue of numbers, but have now begun to use their power collectively. This is one important reason to join professional organizations. Only through united efforts will nurses be seen as a powerful group and will their voices be recognized in the policy arena. This has been demonstrated continually by many vocal and powerful organizations readily visible on Capitol Hill, on surrounding streets in Washington, DC, or in your state capitol, such as the American Medical Association (AMA) and the American Hospital Association (AHA). The ANA is also a visible and vocal organization in Washington, monitoring legislation and the initiatives of federal agencies, and presenting testimony to Congress or congressional committees on behalf of the nursing profession. And consider the number of professional nursing organizations with headquarters located in the Washington area (refer to the professional organizations listed on the Intranet site).

The ANA and its constituent state members are also associated with the Washington-area organizational affiliate members. The legislative or political arm of the ANA is known as its department of governmental affairs. It actively advocates for legislation and works with administrative agencies on regulations for implementation of laws and health policy. The ANA regularly monitors the work of more than a dozen federal agencies that affects healthcare policy. It monitors agencies like the Centers for Medicare and Medicaid Services (CMS) and the Agency for Health Research and Quality (AHRQ). The ANA Department of Governmental Affairs also publishes legislative and regulatory priorities and initiatives for each legislative session. Along with these priorities are informational documents on the issues. For example, for the 113th Congress, the ANA specified an advocacy agenda for nurses that focused on APRN practice, safe staffing, workplace health and safety, quality measures, patient safety and advocacy, mental health care, and the nursing shortage (ANA, 2014). These are broad-based initiatives with well-developed statements of the issue, background, and the ANA position.

The ANA's Department of Government Affairs also contains the political action unit N-STAT, made up of the grassroots lobbying network (Box 17.3) that functions through the activities of congressional district coordinators, Senate coordinators, and the ANA's political action committee (ANA-PAC).

Political Action Committees

As a result of campaign reform in the 1970s, restrictions were placed on contributions made by individuals or organizations to a candidate for a federal office. This

---

BOX 17.3 ANA Grassroots Political Action

ANA creates political action through grassroots efforts and successful lobbying. ANA's N-STAT is an example of this grassroots lobbying system. Established in 1993, N-STAT continues to grow, with more nurses providing a rapid response on legislative and policy issues. Information is provided on current topics as they move through Congress. Then, when the time to speak out on an issue will be most beneficial, nurses are assisted with electronic contact information and content for contacting their senators and representatives.

Nurses can register online, receive periodic alerts, and take an active step toward political efficacy. Sign up today, or periodically refer to the ANA Web site for particular national and state initiatives and legislative alerts at http://www.nursingworld.org (go to the Policy and Advocacy link or at http://www.rnaction.org/site/PageServer?pagename=nstat_take_action_home).

---

campaign financing reform also allowed for the creation of **political action committees (PACs)**, through which organizations could make openly reported contributions. Although any organization can form a PAC, most PACs are sponsored by corporations, labor groups, and special interest groups who want their message heard and promoted. It is a political reality that legislators are more likely to see and listen to a group of people who have contributed money to their campaign.

The ANA formed a PAC more than three decades ago to create power and influence for the nursing profession. Contributions to the ANA-PAC support candidates, current legislators, and legislation aligned with the ANA legislative agenda. It is bipartisan, supporting candidates of both national parties. The PAC is focused on the public office and the candidate for that office, whether incumbent or opponent. Endorsements and financial contributions are based on the candidates' support for the ANA legislative agenda and stance on health policy. In addition, some state constituents of ANA have separate state-associated PACs working on behalf of nursing issues in their particular states and at the federal level. Other specialty professional nursing organizations have PACs as well, representing issues critical to their respective missions.

GAINING SKILL IN POLITICAL EFFICACY

The initial step in developing political efficacy is understanding the process and having the willingness to be involved. But even more basic is possessing an understanding of people and policy needed for public health and welfare. This understanding of people and their healthcare needs is basic to nursing practice. The next prerequisite to political efficacy is an understanding of the issues involved. It is vital that nurses use their voices and individual power to empower nurses and nursing. As Abood (2007) observed, "as nurses interact with patients and families, they are often the first providers to see clearly when and how the healthcare system is not effectively meeting patient needs" (p. 1). This is your imperative for action. Nurses, particularly with their focus on health issues, can influence change in the workplace and health policy, in their communities, in professional organizations, and in government.

Workplace Issues

As illustrated with management in the organizational setting, the workplace is a significant area for nurses to promote policy changes, particularly regarding workplace advocacy and patient safety and advocacy. Nurses are highly regarded by patients and the public. In addition, they have the five general bases of power identified by Mintzberg (1983): control of resources, control of a technical skill, control of a body of knowledge, exclusive rights or privileges to impose choices (legal prerogatives), and access to people who have and can be relied on for the other four. To be influential, nurses must take an active role in institutional decision making, either at the unit level or by volunteering to serve on various committees. These opportunities are available in many hospital settings, especially those organizations demonstrating structural empowerment as a component for Magnet Recognition status. To contribute to policy decisions, nurses must remain current on health policy issues and must provide factual information. This involvement with **workplace issues** provides the basis for the improvements needed in the delivery of care and positive outcomes for both patients and the profession.

Community or Civic Involvement

A prime responsibility for all citizens is to be part of the electorate—to be registered and to vote in local, state, and national elections. Nurses have traditionally been involved in the community, whether serving on committees like the local school or hospital board or helping out with a local health fair. These activities constitute **community or civic involvement**. In the community, nurses can identify potential health hazards that require the attention of local officials or businesspersons, and can intervene in the case of health risks or hazards. Nurses are adept at understanding community issues, and active involvement of professional nurses in community or civic activities is truly an imperative.

Professional Organizations

Active involvement in **professional organizations** provides both constant development and valuable information. As illustrated with the governmental functions of the ANA, professional organizations offer policy analysis and updates, and they can lead effective campaigns to influence policy change. As already described, in their federal governmental affairs and state initiatives, ANA (2014b) addresses many policy areas that the ANA and the other professional organizations are committed to addressing. Nurses should remain knowledgeable about the positions of the professional organizations on issues that are likely to come before Congress. This awareness can assist with needed action on health policies and legislation through

participation in grassroots efforts of the organization. It can also lead to service in elected and appointed positions or opportunities to provide testimony on behalf of the organization.

Government

Be aware of who your legislators and other elected or appointed officials are, at local, state, and national levels. Keep yourself informed on how they support the issues, especially those related to health policy. Communicate with these officials. Nurses have the expertise in the care for patients and they witness the impact of health policy on a daily basis. Legislators want to hear the concerns of their nurse constituents and will appreciate the information you provide to help address the concerns of all their constituents. Often, legislators' only view of the healthcare arena is through the care they or a family member receives and the views imparted to them by their legislative aides and constituents. At times, this perspective can be narrow and very personal. The issues being confronted by federal, state, and local legislators on health policy can have long-term and wide-ranging effects on both the profession and care of patients. Nurses are serving in growing numbers in important roles to assist with the passage of health policy for the good of both the public and the profession.

At the state level, nurses have successfully lobbied to enact legislation that allows them to bill insurance companies directly for the care they provide. Prescriptive authority, interstate practice, amendments or revisions to practice acts, and safe staffing requirements are current issues in many state legislatures. To have legislation enacted, individual nurses or a nursing organization can seek a sponsor and cosponsors to introduce it. Once the legislation is introduced, nurses must lobby legislators to provide information on how passage of the bill will benefit the legislator's constituents. Nurses elected to leadership positions and appointed to serve on boards at the state government level are becoming more common, but there is a great need to increase the numbers who are willing and prepared to serve in these roles. Often it is through involvement at the local level that nurses gain the experience and confidence to move on to state positions.

To effectively influence policy, nurses must establish a relationship with legislators and their legislative aides whenever possible. These officials are elected to serve— and are concerned about the needs of their constituents. They expect constituents to inform them of their concerns. Watch the interactions that occur at your next community or state function attended by a legislator. It may not be an election year, but the legislator is present because the particular function is of importance to a group the legislator represents. A nurse's offer to serve as a personal resource is frequently welcomed by the legislator and his or her staff. This is particularly true at the local and state levels, at which legislators may not have extensive staff to assist with legislation involving health policy. Nurses can also be valuable in providing testimony for regulatory change. Practice and preparation are needed for developing proficiency, effectiveness, and ease in these activities, particularly in dealing with the media. Being knowledgeable and articulate in both subject matter and presentation is essential.

Nurses must be part of the process, whether providing needed facts and background on the issues or serving in an office. Buresh and Gordon (2006) have described this as the **voice of agency**, a strong and authentic voice talking about what you do as a nurse and being more visible and vocal as individuals and as members of organizations (p. 25). It is being the "agent" for both nursing and the consumer of nursing services. Nurses must increasingly be involved in advocating beyond the hospital or healthcare unit environment. We have unique insights and the knowledge base to effect change and improve healthcare

and health policy. This is the political imperative: Be informed, be involved, be active, continue to develop interpersonal and political skills, and continue to understand the evolving needs of people and the profession. As noted by Dodd (2013), "be polite, be persistent, be persuasive, and be polite" (p. 46). The issues for action with public policy are further discussed in Chapter 19. However, act now on current legislation and consider the information provided in Box 17.4 on tips for communicating with your legislator and Box 17.5 on tips for presenting testimony before a committee or regulatory body.

BOX 17.4 **Tips for Talking to Legislators**

- Before meeting with your legislator, get to know as much as possible about his or her background, special interests or initiatives, voting record, committee assignments, and involvement with health policy issues.
- Prepare your position, including a list of talking points to assist you during the discussion.
- Investigate both sides of the issue but stay focused on the facts.
- Request a meeting of at least 15 to 30 minutes.
- Practice your presentation with a friend or colleague to gain comfort with the content and to anticipate questions that may arise.
- If the legislator is not available, meet with the legislative aide or a staff member who has a good knowledge of the issues.
- Be on time, and be professional.
- Introduce yourself and thank the legislator or legislative aide for his or her time and interest.
- Be prepared to explain what you do as a nurse, your philosophy of care, and the impact of pending legislation on healthcare and care delivery for the legislator's constituents.
- Use concise and explicit examples from your practice to illustrate your position.
- Be prepared to offer additional information or solutions, but stick to the facts.
- If the legislator or legislative aide indicates support for your position, ask what you can do to reach other legislators or sponsors.
- Provide an opportunity to answer any questions and offer any additional assistance on the circumstances of the proposed legislation or regulation.
- Send a follow-up thank you note for the time spent, in which you restate your position.
- And you may even want to follow your interview with a well-worded letter on your position to the editor of the local newspaper—and perhaps gain further support among other constituents.

BOX 17.5 **Tips for Presenting Testimony**

- Be prepared, with:
    - A full, well-developed written statement and talking points.
    - An understanding of the committee process and regulatory structure.
    - An anticipation of any follow-up questions that may be asked of you.
- Be on time.
- Be confident in your abilities and knowledge base, and remain calm.
- Be flexible; you may not have the time for your presentation that you were told you would.
- Recognize the members of the body ("Mr./Madam Chairperson and members of the _____ Committee") and thank them for allowing you the opportunity to address them.
- Introduce yourself and be respectful.
- Do not read your written testimony; ask to have it placed in the record.
- Use the talking points to present your case and focus on the facts.
- Try to use concise and explicit examples from your practice to illustrate your position.
- Do not go over your allocated time.
- Leave time at the end of your presentation for any questions from the members.
- Thank the committee for the opportunity to present your testimony at the end.

EVIDENCE-BASED PRACTICE: *Consider this....*

The American Association of Critical Care Nurses (AACN) issued a practice alert on family presence during CPR and invasive procedures.

You are the nurse manager in an emergency department (ED). The vice president for patient care has come to you with a problem. Last night, a city council member complained that one of his constituents called him yesterday because she was not allowed to be with her spouse during CPR in the ED. Currently, the patient is in the intensive care unit (ICU) following a myocardial infarction in guarded condition. You are aware of the practice alert and have been trying to establish a policy in the ED and ICU. The vice president for patient care has asked that you meet with the council member and his constituent on this issue.

Question: Consider your plan for meeting with the council member and his constituent.

Source: American Association of Critical-Care Nurses. (AACN). (2014). *Family presence during CPR and invasive procedures.*
Retrieved from http://www.aacn.org/wd/practice/content/family-presence-practice-alert.pcms?menu=practice

KEY POINTS

- Internal political efficacy is personal competence or the "ability to understand and take part in political affairs," and external political advocacy is the "ability to make the system respond to the citizenry" (Wilson & Dilulio, 2004, p. 93).

- Laws are mandates based on the Constitution, enacted by federal or state legislatures, and interpreted by the courts. Administrative agencies, governed by the executive branch, promulgate regulations or rules, which serve the purpose of detailing and applying the laws.

- In the United States, the enactment of a law begins with introduction of the bill by the sponsoring legislator to either the House or the Senate. Then, it is referred to committee for recommendations and amendments.

- Common law is created by judicial decisions that form a precedent upon which future decisions are based.

- Nurse practice acts are statutory law with associated administrative regulations developed by each state to protect the public health, safety, and welfare. They define the scope of practice; establish requirements for licensure, entry into practice, continuing competency and advanced practice; create and empower a board of nursing to oversee licensees; and identify grounds for disciplinary action.

- Title protection is the part of the nursing practice act that protects and restricts the use of the term *nurse* to the licensee authorized to practice by the board.

- Activities to influence legislators vary from formal to informal. Lobbying may be defined as attempting to persuade a legislator or legislative aide of the merits of your viewpoint and to influence legislation.

- Lobbying is especially effective when there is an associated strong grassroots effort that provides additional correspondence and support on the issues.

- Special interest groups have become more politically savvy at influencing the creation of public policy, and more controls have emerged, as with campaign financing reforms. One form of a special interest group is the political action committee (PAC).

- Buresh and Gordon (2006) define a voice of agency as a strong and authentic voice talking about what you do as a nurse and being more visible and vocal as individuals and as members of organizations (p. 25). Nurses can influence change in the workplace, the community, professional organizations, and government.

Thought and Discussion Questions

1. Consider the campaign for consensus on the practice of APRNs at https://www.ncsbn.org/apm.htm. This initiative involves the changes in state laws (nursing practice acts). Discuss the processes that are required for changes in state laws.

2. Identify how you will demonstrate both internal and external political efficacy. Be prepared to participate in a discussion in class or online to be scheduled by your instructor.

3. Select a current issue of concern and develop an action plan to present your views to a legislator.

4. Review the Chapter Thought located on the first page of the chapter, and discuss it in the context of the contents of the chapter.

Interactive Exercises

Go to the Intranet site and complete the interactive exercises provided for this chapter.

REFERENCES

Abood, S. (2007). Influencing health care in the legislative arena. *Online Journal of Issues in Nursing, 12*(1). Retrieved from http://nursingworld.org/MainMenuCategories/ANAMarketplace/ANAPeriodicals/OJIN/TableofContents/Volume122007/No1Jan07/tpc32_216091.aspx

American Nurses Association. (2014a). *American Nurses Association Political Action Committee (ANA-PAC).* Retrieved from http://www.nursingworld.org/MainMenuCategories/PoliticalPower/ANAPAC.aspx

American Nurses Association. (2014b). *Federal governmental affairs.* http://www.nursingworld.org/MainMenuCategories/Policy-Advocacy/Federal

American Nurses Association. (2014c). *113th Congress federal legislative agenda.* Retrieved from http://www.nursingworld.org/MainMenuCategories/Policy-Advocacy/Federal/113th-Congress-Federal-Legislative-Agenda

Bureau of Labor Statistics. (2014). *Nurse anesthetists, nurse midwives, and nurse practitioners.* Retrieved from http://www.bls.gov/ooh/healthcare/nurse-anesthetists-nurse-midwives-and-nurse-practitioners.htm

Buresh, B., & Gordon, S. (2006). *From silence to voice: What nurses know and must communicate to the public* (2nd ed.). Ithaca, NY: Cornell University Press.

Clinton, H. R. (2003). *Living history.* New York: Simon & Schuster.

Dodd, C. J. (2013). Passing legislation requires more than good ideas and prayers. In C. L. Estes, S. A. Chapman, C. Dodd, B. Hollister, & C. Harrington, (Eds.), *Health policy: Crisis and reform* (pp. 39-54). Burlington, MA: Jones & Bartlett.

Leininger, M. (2002). Cultures and tribes of nursing, hospitals, and the medical culture. In M. Leininger & M. R. McFarland, *Transcultural nursing: Concepts, theories, research, and practice* (3rd ed.) (pp. 181–204). New York: McGraw-Hill.

Mason, D. J., Chaffee, M. W., & Leavitt, J. K. (2011). *Policy and politics in nursing and health care* (6th ed.). Philadelphia, PA: Elsevier/Saunders.

Milstead, J. A. (2013). *Health policy and politics: A nurse's guide* (4th ed.). Boston, MA: Jones & Bartlett.

Mintzberg, H. (1983). *Power in and around organizations.* Englewood Cliffs, NJ: Prentice-Hall.

Wilson, J. Q., & Dilulio, J. J. (2004). *American government: Institutions and policies* (9th ed.). Boston, MA: Houghton Mifflin.

BIBLIOGRAPHY

Estes, C. L., Chapman, S.A., Dodd, C., Hollister, B., & Harrington, C. (2013). *Health policy: Crisis and reform.* Burlington, MA: Jones & Bartlett.

Federal Election Commission. (2014). *Administering and enforcing federal campaign finance laws.* Retrieved from http://www.fec.gov

Johnson, C. W. (2007). *How our laws are made.* Retrieved from http://thomas.loc.gov/home/lawsmade.toc.html

U.S. Department of Health and Human Services. (2003). *Summary of the HIPAA Privacy Rule.* Retrieved from http://www.hhs.gov/ocr/privacy/hipaa/understanding/summary/

White, P., Olsan, T. H., Bianchi, C., Glessner, T., & Mapstone, P. (2010). Legislative: Searching for health policy information in the Internet: An essential advocacy skill. *Online Journal of Issues in Nursing, 15*(2). Retrieved from http://www.nursingworld.org/MainMenuCategories/ANAMarketplace/ANAPeriodicals/OJIN/Columns/Legislative/Health-Policy-Information-on-the-Internet.aspx

ONLINE RESOURCES

American Association of Colleges of Nursing: Government Affairs
http://www.aacn.nche.edu/Government/index.htm

American Nurses Association
http://nursingworld.org/MainMenuCategories/Policy-Advocacy/State

THOMAS, U.S. Congress on the Internet
http://thomas.loc.gov/home/thomas.php

U.S. Constitution
http://thomas.loc.gov/teachers/constitution.html

U.S. Government Web Portal
http://firstgov.gov

● Sister Rosemary Donley

18

Healthcare Reform and Global Issues

"Nursing in its broadest sense may be defined as an art and a science which involves the whole patient—body, mind, and spirit; promotes his spiritual, mental, and physical health by teaching and by example; stresses health education and health preservation, as well as ministration to the sick; involves the care of the patients' environment—social and spiritual as well as physical; and gives health service to the family and community as well as to the individual."

Sr. M. Olivia Gowan, founding Dean, The Catholic University of America School of Nursing, June 1944

Chapter Objectives

On completion of this chapter, the reader will be able to:

1. Describe the global and domestic issues that affect healthcare policy, healthcare delivery, and nursing education and practice.
2. Analyze three goals of the ACA that directly affect nursing education and practice.
3. Discuss how nurses' active participation in policy formulation can strengthen the profession and patient care outcomes.

Key Terms

Global Health
Health Policy
Patient Protection and Affordable Care Act (ACA)
Newly Insured Persons
Nursing Shortage

The 3 Ds: Workforce Diversity, Health Disparities, and Social Determinants of Health
Clinical Nurse Leader (CNL)
Doctor of Nursing Practice (DNP)
Social Justice

Evidence-Based Practice
Cost-Benefit-Burden Ratios
Market Justice
www.Healthcare.gov
Health Disparities

GLOBAL HEALTH, NURSING, AND THE NEW MILLENNIUM

Nursing, like all the health professions, faces exciting challenges in the 21st century because the world is interconnected and many factors other than disease affect global health. Demography, urbanization, migration, the economy, war, and terrorism influence well-being and human flourishing. What do students of nursing and nurses need to know about these significant health indicators? The American population is aging, becoming more diverse and more mobile. These demographic changes are not unique to the United States; they are the faces and patterns of people around the world. For example, Japan and many countries in Western Europe are seeing an increase in the number of people older than 65 years, whereas young people compose the populations in Iraq, Pakistan, Afghanistan, Colombia, Gaza, and Yemen, a phenomenon described as the *youth bulge*. Yet even with this youth bulge, it is estimated that by 2050, the global population older than 65 years will increase from 6.9 percent in 2000 to 16.3 percent (Central Intelligence Agency [CIA], 2001). This demographic picture has implications for healthcare, for the economy, and for world peace. In the future, the world's population will be less white and more urban. In 2015, for the first time in history, more people will live in some city in the world. Globally, people are also on the move. Internal and external migration has been stimulated by war, natural disasters, unstable currencies, and lack of work. Low fertility and the aging of local populations also stimulate migration. Illegal immigration is more common than legal entry into many countries; today one in every 40 persons is an immigrant living somewhere in the world (CIA, 2001). It is recognized that the economy plays a major role in health status.

People in the United States are slowly recovering from the crises in the housing and financial markets. The stock market has rebounded, and there are fewer foreclosures and public auctions of family homes. This stabilization is reflected in the world's economy, although experts say that debt and unemployment are still too high and economic growth is too low both in the United States and around the world (Boccia, 2013). In the United States, unskilled, blue-collar, and white-collar workers have lost jobs and their benefits because the companies for which they worked declared bankruptcy, contracted for work outside the country, downsized, or went out of business. Long-term unemployment has caused some American workers to give up searching for jobs (Hollander, 2014). Some observers consider this phenomenon a response to the recent economic recession; others say it is a structural problem brought on by a mismatch between worker skills and job demands (Mitchell, 2013). Although technological development requires a more educated workforce, degrees no longer assure employment in the job of one's dreams after graduation. In the United States, it may be necessary to leave home to find work. There have been long and costly wars in Afghanistan and Iraq. Everywhere in the world, there is palpable fear of violence and terrorism. Worldwide travel coupled with technological innovation and instant communication via television, the Internet, and social media blur the distance between countries and peoples. The global nature of the workforce influences health; old assumptions about the geography of disease lack validity (CIA, 2001).

Communicable diseases once found only in developing countries are spread rapidly by air travel and immigration. Chronic illnesses occur everywhere in the world. The World Health Organization *Kampala Declaration and Agenda for Global Action* (Global Health Workforce Alliance, 2008), recognizing the worldwide effects of HIV/AIDS, the burdens of chronic and communicable diseases, accidents, and injuries, asserts that health issues have delayed progress in meeting the Millennium Development Goals (Global Health Workforce Alliance, 2008). Any factor that influences health and human development, taken alone, has the potential to alter health status in a person or a community. Together, these influences pose threats to **global health** and challenge nurses and other health professionals to work collegially and cooperatively at the bedside and at policy tables around the world. Preparing nurses to practice in the 21st century is a sacred trust. Teaching students to become engaged in the policy process is a primary responsibility of educators, leaders in nursing, professional organizations, and practicing nurses.

NURSING AND HEALTH POLICY

Nurses want seats at the policy tables. Nursing's efforts to prepare health system advocates and policymakers are bearing fruit. During the past 40 years, American nurses have been educated about **health policy** and have become interested and more engaged in policy decisions, especially those that affect their patients and their practices. Schools of nursing teach courses in health policy and arrange trips to lobby members of state or federal governments. Some schools of nursing offer semester-long internships with state legislators or members of Congress. Professional and specialty nursing organizations monitor federal and state legislation and regulations, provide information to legislators, give testimony about health and nursing issues, lobby, make financial contributions to candidates, join political action committees (PACs), participate in get-out-the-vote campaigns, and educate their own members and the public about nursing's legislative and policy agenda (Abood, 2007).

One example of a professional effort to influence health policy is the Nurse in Washington Internship (NIWI) program. NIWI brings leaders from professional and specialty organizations to an immersion experience on Capitol Hill. Prepared by briefings and discussions with health policy experts, nurse leaders bring the perspectives of their organizations and the views of their patients to members of Congress (Nursing Organizations Alliance, 2014). It is also affirming that six nurses currently serve in the Congress of the United States (American Nurses Association, 2014). Not only have nurses been elected to positions that determine policy, they have also been appointed to direct important work in federal and state governments. Most notable is Mary Wakefield's 2009 appointment as the Director of the Health Resources and Services Administration (HRSA, 2014b).

Despite progress, however, organized nursing is perceived to yield little influence on health policy. The validity of the decade-old observations of Mechanic and Reinhard (2002) about the influence of American physicians in policy literature and policy making prevails. That nurses' voices are not heard in American halls of power is also conveyed by quips. One familiar saying is that although nurses are underrepresented at policy tables, nursing is on the menu. It is too soon to tell whether major changes in federal health priorities and the **Patient Protection and Affordable Care Act (ACA)** efforts to emphasize prevention as well as treatment will shift the balance of power. The irony and injustice of excluding nurses from meaningful policy debates is astonishing because registered nurses are the largest group of health professionals, now numbering about 3.1 million (USDHHS, 2010a). Beyond these impressive statistical data, the overwhelming majority of registered nurses are on the ground, at the bedside, and in the community. Anyone who has been ill, especially patients treated in acute care hospitals, can provide testimony that nurses positively influence their healthcare outcomes (Aiken, Clarke, & Sloan, 2002; Aiken et al., 2014; DeCuccio, 2014).

Unfortunately, these positive findings about nursing are threatened by the nursing shortage and poor staffing ratios. Studies, especially in acute care hospitals, report that the quality of care varies across the country and the world (Aiken et al., 2014; Kalish, Tshannen, Lee, & Friese, 2011). These data also highlight the impact of inadequate staffing and the limited education of registered nurses on patient care outcomes; these issues must be addressed not only in local institutions but also through national policy and political venues. All nurses need to engage directly or indirectly in health policy.

American nurses are watching the implementation of the ACA. They express concern about their ability to care for the growing number of senior citizens and chronically ill persons, their availability to work aggressively to prevent illness as well as treat it, and their capacity to address the healthcare needs of **newly insured persons** (Abrams, Nuzum, Mika, & Lawlor, 2011; Benner, Sutphen, Leonard, & Day, 2010; Smedley, Stith, & Nelson, 2003; The Future of Nursing, 2010). At a micro level, nurses are affected by the impact of the staffing crisis on safety and patient expectations. Another recurring theme is the lack of respect that nurses experience in the workplace (Wong, 2012). Although advanced practice registered nurses applaud the ACA's recognition of their capabilities, they are very aware of resistance to expanding their roles in care management (Brassard & Smolenski, 2011). Some medical groups continue to influence state legislators to block expansion of nurse practice acts (The Future of Nursing, 2010).

Global issues such as war, terrorism, trade agreements, the economy, and immigration have been added to nursing's policy agenda. These complex and far-reaching issues overshadow and compete for funding with the issues that have dominated nursing's policy agenda. Yet global issues evoke new awareness and interest in intraprofessional collaboration and reveal the force that world events and global governments exert on health status and on health professionals. Knowledge of health policy also calls attention to the lack of diversity in the American nurse workforce and healthcare team (Aiken et al., 2014). In the 21st century, policy competence is increasingly identified as an essential behavior of professional nurses. Illustrative of this goal is the American Association of Colleges of Nursing (AACN, 2004b) description of advanced practice:

Any form of nursing intervention that influences health care outcomes for individuals or populations, including the direct care of individual patients, management of care for individuals and populations, administration of nursing and health care organizations, and the development and implementation of health policy. (p. 2)

How can nurses be savvy representatives of their profession and contribute meaningfully to policy debates? This chapter examines nursing's policy agenda, particularly issues of workforce shortage and role transformation and the changing delivery system. It also presents the impact of the ACA on the uninsured, unsafe healthcare practices, and health disparities. If nurses are to be recognized as citizens of the world, they must be grounded in how health policies affect them, their practices, their patients, and the health system.

THE NURSING SHORTAGE AND CHANGING WORKFORCE

Nursing is an exciting, meaningful, and socially relevant profession. The U.S. Department of Labor (USDL, 2012) data indicate that nursing will remain the top occupation for job growth until 2020. Yet American nursing has failed to sustain a relevant image of professional practice and career opportunities (Nurses for a Healthier Tomorrow, n.d.). Consequently, stereotypes and myths about nursing are passed on: nursing is too demanding, too dangerous, and too undervalued. In the United States, the **nursing shortage** represents a recurring paradox of failures and successes in recruitment and retention (Donley et al., 2002). This suggests that factors other than the value of the profession influence decisions to become or remain a nurse. The shortage of nurses is described by the International Council of Nurses (ICN) as a global crisis (Oulton, 2006). Yet in the face of a worldwide nursing shortage, the United States continues to recruit nurses from other countries by promises of good salaries and opportunities for them and their families, an action that is observed, sometimes negatively, around the world. One positive effort to stabilize the global nurse force is the European Union's plan to enhance graduate education and research across Europe (Carney, 2005; Chaguturu & Vallabhaneni, 2005; Davies, 2008). The American nursing community has increased its enrolment in 4-year programs and designed accelerated BSN degree programs and bridge programs as RN to BSN, RN to MSN, or BSN to PhD or DNP (AACN, 2010a). It has also created new online and hybrid nursing programs. However, nursing has not successfully addressed the faculty shortage, inadequate faculty salaries, and limited clinical space for additional students (AACN, 2010b, 2014c). Although the global demand for nurses is fueled by the economy, aging populations, and urbanization, American nurses have new responsibilities, care of newly insured persons (AACN, 2010b). Even the most optimistic observer does not expect nursing to meet its manpower projections.

Recognizing that good will does not resolve projected shortage, federal and state governments have allocated additional funding to stimulate enrollment and to encourage more nurses to go back to school (Juraschek, Zhang, Ranganathan, & Lin, 2011). The ACA also supports expanding the nursing workforce by providing new funds for program development and scholarships, low-interest loans, and loan-forgiveness programs for graduate students who prepare to be teachers or nurse practitioners (Patient Protection and Affordable Care Act [ACA], 2010). The Health Resources and Services Administration (HRSA) initiatives also emphasize programs that address **the "3 Ds": workforce diversity, health disparities, and social determinants of health** (White, Zangaro, Kepley, & Camacho, 2014). HRSA funds demonstration projects to support nurse practitioners' collaborative engagement in primary care teams and in the development of more nurse-managed clinics (*Affordable Care Act bolters,* 2010; HRSA, 2014a). The Veterans Administration has partnered with the HRSA to improve the care of returning veterans and also provide career opportunities for veterans. They are funding schools of nursing to recruit, retain, and support veterans in accelerated BSN programs (Bureau of Health Professions, 2013). Recently there has been another call for the Veterans Administration Health Services to form new partnerships with schools of nursing and to develop new Veterans Affairs Nursing Academies (U.S. Department of Veterans Affairs, 2013). The federal government provides scholarships and loans for students who agree to work in underserved areas after graduation. These funds also support the education of disadvantaged or minority students and help educate more teachers of nursing and advanced practice registered nurses, especially nurse practitioners (AACN, 2014c; ACA, 2010). Other programs offer loan forgiveness of up to 60% of the loan if new RN or NP graduates work for a period of time (usually 2 years) within the state or, in the case of federal grants, in some critical shortage facility (NURSECORPS, 2014). States have also joined the federal government in addressing the nursing shortage. Maryland, Illinois, and Kansas have awarded grants to schools of nursing to increase the nurse workforce in their states. Some state legislatures in Massachusetts, Kansas, Connecticut, and Pennsylvania have initiated special initiatives to encourage nurses to return to school and become teachers (AACN, 2006).

There is renewed private sector emphasis on the retention of practicing nurses. Nurse leaders are actively collaborating with the the Robert Wood Johnson Foundation, the American Association of Retired Persons, and the Johnson & Johnson Foundation to advance the public image of nursing and to promote leadership and advanced practice (The Future of Nursing, 2014).

EVOLVING NURSING ROLES

Another response to the shortage of nurses is the creation of new career pathways. Almost a decade ago, The American Association of Colleges of Nursing (AACN, 2004b) proposed new roles: **clinical nurse leader (CNL)** and **doctor of nursing practice (DNP)**. The CNL, prepared at the master's level, is educated to assume clinical, managerial,

and leadership roles, particularly in hospitals. These students are not educated for advanced practice registered nurse roles as clinical specialist, nurse practitioner, midwife, or nurse anesthetist. Rather, their preparation is directed toward improving the quality of patient care (AACN, 2011).

Although the CNL degree has evoked less attention than the DNP, the AACN reports that 104 CLN programs exist in 38 states (AACN, 2014b).

The DNP program educates nurses who seek a practice rather than a research-oriented degree, a DNP rather than a PhD. The AACN envisions that by 2015, the DNP will be the standard educational preparation for nurses in advanced practice roles. The 2014 AACN data show that 241 DNP programs of study are available in 49 states and the District of Columbia (AACN, 2014a). Supporters of practice doctorates argue that clinical care is increasingly complex and that advanced practice registered nurses are disenfranchised because they lack the education and the credentials enjoyed by other health team practitioners: physicians, pharmacists, physical therapists, and social workers (AACN, 2014a). Opponents think that the new doctoral degree will contribute to an already confusing pattern of academic credentialing and weaken research-oriented PhD degrees (Meleis & Dracup, 2005).

Although the DNP was proposed as an academic pathway to advanced practice, faculty members now conceptualize the DNP degree as preparation for advanced practice, management of patients and health systems, policy development, and clinical teaching. This conceptualization better reflects the AACN description of advanced practice:

Any form of nursing intervention that influences healthcare outcomes for individuals or populations, including the direct care of individual patients, management of care for individuals and populations, administration of nursing and healthcare organizations, and the development and implementation of health policy. Preparation at the practice doctorate level includes advanced preparation in nursing, based on nursing science, and is at the highest level of nursing practice. (p. 3)

The American Medical Association (AMA) has been a vocal opponent of the practice doctorate, a position expressed in 2006 by Resolution 211 (AMA, 2015). Organized medicine has argued that patients will confuse the DNP with the doctor of medicine degree.

As noted, major campaigns encourage RNs to earn baccalaureate degrees and remain competitive in the workforce. Nursing promotes baccalaureate education with the slogan, "80% by 2020" as it increases program offerings and enrollment in traditional, hybrid, and online programs (The Future of Nursing, 2010).

THE HEALTHCARE DELIVERY SYSTEM: PRIVATIZATION, MARKET JUSTICE, AND THE BUSINESS OF HEALTHCARE

Privatization of Health Care

In the United States, healthcare is more than human service. It contributes significantly to the economic well-being of the country. America has developed a unique model of private and public (government) collaboration around healthcare delivery, the education of health professionals, and the licensing and accrediting of health institutions. This unique American model enables people whose care or education is paid for by the government to receive healthcare or education in the private sector. In the case of healthcare, doctors and nurses, who are not employees of the government, provide this care. Students of nursing earn degrees in schools operated by state and county governments or by private institutions, some of which are for-profit enterprises. Federal government scholarships and loans are given to all students in the private and public sector. This public-private model is different from the way that other nations provide or pay for health or education. Global health systems and health education programs operate from a political philosophy that supports governments' responsibility to provide and pay for healthcare and education of health professionals. These different philosophies around healthcare delivery and manpower development invite comparisons of cost and outcomes, discussions that are informative, are provocative, and produce evidence. For example, the United States spent more than 17.7 percent of its gross domestic product (GDP) on healthcare in 2011; American health spending almost doubled the spending of countries such as France and Sweden and was two and one half times greater than the average spending of Organisation for Economic Cooperation and Development (OECD) countries in 2011 (OECD, 2013b). The worldwide recession caused many countries to lessen or slow their spending on healthcare; the 2011 data show no immediate change in healthcare indicators in these OECD countries (OECD, 2013a). Significant public health indicators, especially mortality, the burden of disease, and infant mortality, still show that U.S. outcomes fall behind those of countries in Western Europe and Canada that spend less money on healthcare (Rubenstein, 2013). These data embarrass and distress American public health experts and policymakers.

Even with these findings, supporters of private sector involvement in healthcare observe that the U.S. healthcare system not only contributes to the economy but also is the envy of the world. America's innovative technology is exported to many countries; its medical and nursing schools and hospitals are training sites for multinationals. The United States is also a major developer of new drugs and technologies; its biomedical researchers collaborate with and contribute to scientific advancement throughout the world. Closer to home, hospitals, colleges, and universities are large employers in their communities, providing jobs to workers with wide-ranging educational backgrounds and skills. The U.S. Bureau of Labor Statistics reported that health careers compose 12 of the 20 fastest-growing occupations in the United States (USDL, 2012). Health careers are sought after; places in nursing, medical, and pharmacy schools are coveted; and jobs in the healthcare sector remain stable even in periods of recession (*Ten recession-proof jobs*, 2014). Hospitals and universities are also major purchasers of goods and contribute to the economic and political development in their communities.

Influence of Business on Healthcare

The goal of the private health and educational sectors is to make these enterprises financially viable, competitive, and attractive to patients, doctors, insurers, students, donors, and investors. However, both profit and nonprofit health and education sectors find that a focus on business can transcend or filter out other values. The influence of business on healthcare is evident in the language of the health community. It is not uncommon for patients to be described as consumers, market shares, or covered lives and for nursing service to be labeled a product line. Some schools view their students as customers. Writers label this transformation in the conceptualization of contemporary nursing, medicine, and healthcare as the *commoditization of healthcare* (Budetti, 2008, p. 93). This commoditization creates a market in which any vendor can provide health services or education and in which decisions about where to purchase services or where to attend school are based on convenience, cost, and response to successful marketing of programs. Nurses have experienced the influence of business in their practices, language, and education. Some nurses have learned or adapted to the market model. Nurses have also joined unions or advocated through professional organizations for legislation to mandate safer practices, such as establishing staffing ratios in acute care hospitals (Buerhaus & Needleman, 2000; Wallis, 2013). Others practice what they believe is important to patients and more reflective of caring behavior and **social justice** (Donley, 2010). A positive impact of market forces on American healthcare and professional education is visible in **evidence-based practice,** insistence that outcomes are more important than processes, and in renewed emphasis on success in the NCLEX and advanced practice certification examinations.

Social justice principles are also integrated into **cost-benefit-burden ratios** (Shi & Singh, 2010). These principles emphasize the importance of patients' perceptions and wishes about diagnostic testing and therapeutic interventions. Social justice puts patients and their wellbeing at the center of clinical decision making. Advocates of both market and social justice want healthcare outcomes to show demonstrable benefits to patients and positive cost-benefit ratios to society. Both modes of practice are concerned about the rising costs of education and healthcare. The United States invests about 18 percent of its GDP on healthcare and spends on average $8,233 per person for healthcare each year (Kane, 2012). As noted previously, this is twice what is spent in European countries. It is not surprising that one major goal of the ACA is cost reduction. However, lowering health costs will require major changes in payment and delivery modes. Current payment incentives in both fee-for-service and managed care methodologies encourage overtreatment. Both the federal government and private insurers are considering new payment methodologies based on performance and outcomes rather than payment based on the number of diagnostic or treatment modalities. Payment for performance and value relies on evidence-based practice and rewards positive outcomes of care. Malpractice claims also influence the cost of healthcare by raising insurance premiums, threatening professional reputations, and triggering more diagnostic procedures and treatment. Defensive medicine is rare in other countries because patients and families do not sue their healthcare providers. On the delivery side, the ACA encourages providers to be cost conscious in their use of treatment sites. Preference is given to ambulatory or community settings. Providers are asked to watch and wait rather than to intervene, to prevent illness, and to avoid or minimize complications.

As noted, the U.S. health system is characterized by competition among and between physicians, nurses (especially advanced practice registered nurses), hospitals, healthcare systems, and insurers. Today, pharmacies, supermarkets, and ambulatory clinics also compete for insurance contracts, healthcare professionals (especially nurse practitioners), and the right to practice primary care. Hospitals and physician groups have opened neighborhood clinics and surgi-centers and urgi-centers in shopping malls. The availability of diagnostic and informational technology, changes in reimbursement (which will be accelerated after ACA is fully implemented), and the pressure to limit admissions and lengths of stay in hospitals favor primary care settings. Hospitals have downsized, merged, and closed. Kodner and Spreeuwenberg (2002) describe another delivery system, called an *integrated delivery system*, that brings together diagnostic and primary care services in women's health, geriatric care, or sports medicine. The *medical home* is another effort to assure continuity and cost-effective care for persons with limited incomes, providing comprehensive care to children, adults, and families (Fisher, 2008). Integrated systems and medical homes bring together a range of services under one operating network. In true marketplaces, competition drives down prices and allows the most competent and efficient institutions and providers to prosper (Feldstein, 2011). Yet no one engaged in American-style healthcare notices that healthcare is not the best example of a competitive marketplace. Illness is the decision maker; lack of information and uncertainty about insurance benefits interfere with free market choices. It is difficult to assess the "best buy" in gallbladder surgery or to select the most qualified and experienced surgeon, even for well-informed and Internet-savvy patients and families. Regulation, originally designed to ensure patient safety, also restricts competition. For example, mandated nurse-patient staffing ratios in California limit hospitals' ability to market and use their nurse-to-patient ratios to attract patients and nurses. Political influences inhibit competition. As noted, medical societies oppose revisions of state nurse practice acts when studies continue to demonstrate the competence, cost-effectiveness, and positive outcomes of care given by nurse practitioners (ACA, 2010; Adams, 2001; Laurent et al., 2005).

Market justice is the term used to name the individualism, self-interest, and profit orientation of healthcare in the United States. Market forces can overshadow concern for the common good and blur public responsibility for the underserved (Budetti, 2008).

The Patient Protection and Affordable Care Act of 2010

The latest effort to transform healthcare delivery and reduce rising health costs became law in 2010. The ACA or "Obama Care" is designed to make health insurance accessible and affordable. Its entry in the marketplace was slowed because software glitches delayed online enrollment. Although the law has supporters and opponents, it will be at least 5 to 10 years before anyone will know if the ACA achieves its ambitious goals: reductions in the number of uninsured people; control over healthcare costs; improved access to health services; more favorable healthcare outcomes; increased use of preventive health services; and a more effective primary care workforce (*Preventive care under the Affordable Care Act*, 2014). Significant questions revolve around the real cost of implementing the ACA. It is unusual that any large federal program conforms to it early budget projections; the affordability of ACA will be discussed for many years. Members of Congress and the public have expressed their unwillingness to extend governmental investment in healthcare. They fear that more governmental intervention will affect their interests, diminish their insurance coverage, and increase their insurance premiums and taxes. Americans are also wary of a single-payer system, like that found in Canada, or any insurance system that can be labeled *socialized medicine*. Yet people like and depend on Medicare, Medicaid, the state Children's Health Insurance Programs (CHIPs), and the military and veterans healthcare systems. Whether the ACA will achieve a place on the list of valued government health programs is an open question. In the interim, energy, money, and time have been dedicated to encourage people, especially the young and those who are underinsured or uninsured, to go online and explore **www.healthcare.gov**. This Web site brings users into a healthcare exchange in which they can view and compare benefits and costs of various insurance products in their state. They can also sign up for the insurance program that meets their healthcare needs and their budget. If they cannot afford to purchase an insurance policy, government subsidies are available to them (Healthcare.gov, 2013). Several options embedded in the ACA make enrollment attractive: Young adults can remain covered under their parents' health plans until they are 26 years old; persons with preexisting conditions can obtain health coverage and not be charged extraordinary rates; preventive health services are part of each plan; and the poverty index under Medicaid has been raised to 133 percent of the poverty level (ACA, 2010). The least attractive provision of ACA mandates that uninsured individuals and employers with more than 50 workers must purchase health insurance or pay fines. When the enrollment period ended on March 31, 2014, 7.5 million people had signed up for health insurance. Even with this positive response, the Congressional Budget Office estimates that by 2020, 30 million nonelderly Americans will still be uninsured (Bier, 2013). This group will include those who are in the United States without proper documents and people who did not sign up for programs for which they or their children are eligible.

Although healthcare reform is the cornerstone of the Obama Administration, lack of insurance is only one barrier to receiving healthcare. Persons with health insurance face cultural, linguistic, informational, and bureaucratic hurdles that limit their access to care. The Institute of Medicine (IOM) 2004 report on being without insurance describes the consequences of lack of access to healthcare services. More than 30 million working-age people, one in seven workers, received too little medical care; received it too late; were sicker; died sooner; and received poorer care even when hospitalized for trauma (Committee on the Consequences of Uninsurance, 2004).

Health Disparities

Health disparities is a term that describes one consequence of inadequate access to healthcare. The Surgeon General's Report, *Healthy People 2020,* highlights health disparities associated with age and developmental states, quality and safety, and preparedness for natural and manmade disasters and terrorism (USDHHS, 2010b). The importance of addressing global health is emphasized in this report by naming infections associated with well-recognized illnesses as health disparities: tuberculosis, malaria, HIV/AIDs, and vaccine-preventable diseases. The Surgeon General's list also includes emergent infectious diseases, SARS, H1N1 virus, influenza virus, and foodborne illnesses (*Healthy People 2020,* 2011; USDHHS, 2010b).

Safety

Almost 15 years ago, a trilogy of studies by the IOM alerted the public, Congress, and providers about the frequency, seriousness, and cost of medical error. Failure to protect sick people, especially those who are hospitalized, imposes unnecessary burdens on individuals and costs to the entire health system. Medical error can be classified as a health disparity. The first IOM study, *To Err Is Human: Building a Safer Health System* (Kohn, Corrigan, & Donaldson, 2000), addressed the importance of developing a culture of safety in contemporary healthcare systems. The second IOM study, *Crossing the Quality Chasm: A New Health System for the 21st Century* (Committee on Quality Health Care, 2001), presented recommendations to reduce error and enhance quality. The third study in the series, *Patient Safety: Achieving a New Standard of Care* (Committee on Data Standards for Patient Safety, 2004), endorsed the need for a national infrastructure on patient safety information. The government, accreditors, and health systems have directed dollars and written standards to improve patient safety and decrease error, especially medication and transcription errors (The Joint Commission, 2014). However, more than a decade after the IOM published its last study, medical error continues to increase the burden of illness and healthcare costs.

EVIDENCE-BASED PRACTICE: *Consider this....*

Review the Medicaid CHIP enrollments in your state at State at www.Medicaid.gov. and at http://www .medicaid.gov/Medicaid-CHIP-Program-Information/By-State/By-State.html.

Question: What is the current Medicaid enrollment in your state, and how has your state responded to the ACA provision to increase eligibility for Medicaid?

Source: State Medicaid and CHIP policies for 2014. Medicaid.gov. Retrieved from www.medicaid.gov and http://www. medicaid.gov/Medicaid-CHIP-Program-Information/By-State/By-State.html.

KEY POINTS

- Healthcare in the United States is a partnership between the public and private sectors and is a model of collaboration around health delivery, finance, and professional educators.

- American-style healthcare emphasizes expensive acute care rather than cheaper prevention or primary care.

- The influence of business is evident in the language and ethics of healthcare. Two positive influences from the business community are a focus on outcomes rather than processes and the value placed on evidence-based practice.

- Some critics of the public/private American plan blame rising healthcare costs and the failures to achieve good outcomes on the involvement of business in healthcare and the desire for efficiency and economic gain above the care of patients.

- Hospitals have merged and formed systems to ensure economies of scale, access to capital for expansion, and acquisition of physician practices.

- The simplicity and availability of technology, changed reimbursement, and the pressure to lower healthcare costs encourage surgi-centers, urgi-centers, and community-based clinics.

- *Medicare,* a federal health insurance program that serves the elderly and disabled people who receive Supplemental Social Security, has four Parts (A, B, C, and D), each offering different benefits and financing mechanisms.

- *Medicaid* is a means-tested federal/state health program that pays for medical and long-term care for five indigent groups: pregnant women, adults in families with dependent children, children, persons with disabilities, and the poor elderly. Under the ACA, Medicaid will be expanded.

KEY POINTS—cont'd

- *CHIP* is a federal health insurance program designed for children who live in working-class families above the federal poverty level.

- The nursing shortage represents a failure in both recruitment and retention. The shortage of nurses, nurse practitioners, and nurse educators prompted Congress to integrate provisions from the Nurse Reinvestment Act into the ACA.

- Legislation to mandate staffing ratios has been introduced in the Congress and several states to ensure that a sufficient number of nurses are available to care for patients.

- The AACN has promoted new educational pathways, the *clinical nurse leader* (CNL) and the *doctor of nursing practice* (DNP), and has encouraged schools of nursing to build and bridge programs from RN to BSN or MSN and from BSN to PhD or DNP.

- Uninsured or underinsured Americans have limited access to care and suffer greater health disparities.

- Competence in health policy is within the reach of each nurse and student of nursing.

Thought and Discussion Questions

1. A student, who is not a nursing major, asks you whether she should buy health insurance from the government's healthcare Web site or pay a fine that is less costly than the insurance premium. She is 24 years old and is healthy. Everyone in her family is healthy.
   - How would you advise the student?
   - Give reasons for your advice, citing the benefits of the ACA.

2. What populations are most at risk for health disparities? Is your fellow student at risk?

3. How do health disparities affect access, outcomes, and cost?

4. Identify three factors associated with recruitment and retention in nursing.

5. Discuss two advantages and two disadvantages of new educational pathways for nurses.

Interactive Exercises

Go to the Intranet site and complete the interactive exercises provided for this chapter.

REFERENCES

Abood, S. (2007). Influencing health care in the legislative arena. *Online Journal of Issues in Nursing, 12*(1):3.

Abrams, M., Nuzum, S., Mika, S., & Lawlor, G. (2011, January). *Realizing health reform's potential: How the Affordable Care Act will strengthen primary care and benefit patients, providers and payers.* New York: Commonwealth Fund. Retrieved from http://www.commonwealthfund.org/Publications/Issue-Briefs/2011/Jan/Strengthen-Primary-Care.aspx

Adams, D. (2001, October 15). Maryland examines doctors' influence. *AMA MedEd Update. Affordable Care Act bolsters the primary care workforce in medically underserved communities, 2010.* Retrieved from http://www.businesswire.com/news/home/20101122006098/en/Affordable-Care-Act-Bolsters-Primary-Care-Workforce#.VUUiPflViko

Aiken, L. H., Clarke, S., & Sloane, D. (2002). Hospital staffing, organization and quality of care: Cross national findings. *Nursing Outlook, 50*(5), 187–194.

Aiken, L. H., Sloane, D. M., Bruyneel, L., Van den Heede, K., Griffiths, P., Busse, R., Diomidous, M., Kinunen, J., Kozka, M., Lesaffre, E., McHugh, M. D., Moreno-Casbas, M. T., Rafferty, A. M., Schwendimann, R., Scott, P. A., Tishelman, C., van Achterberg, T., & Sermeus, W. (2014). Nurse staffing and education and hospital mortality in nine European countries: A retrospective observational study. *The Lancet, 383*(9931), 1824–1830. doi:10.1016/50140-6736(13)62631-8.

American Association of Colleges of Nursing (AACN). (2004a). *Leading initiatives: CLN programs.* Retrieved from http://www.aacn.nche.edu/cnl/about/cnl-programs

American Association of Colleges of Nursing (AACN). (2004b). *Position statement on the practice doctorate in nursing.* Retrieved from http://www.aacn.nche.edu/publications/position/DNP positiontatement.pdf

American Association of Colleges of Nursing (AACN). (2006). *State legislative initiatives to address the nursing shortage.* Retrieved from http://www.aacn.nche.edu/aacn-publications/issue-bulletin/state-legislative

American Association of Colleges of Nursing (AACN). (2010a). *New AACN data show that enrollment in baccalaureate nursing programs expands for the 10th consecutive year.* Retrieved from http://www.aacn.nche.edu/news/articles/2010/bacc-growth

American Association of Colleges of Nursing (AACN). (2010b). *Nursing faculty shortage.* Retrieved from http://www.aacn.nche.edu/media-relations/Faculty ShortageFS.pdf

American Association of Colleges of Nursing (AACN). (2011). *CNL programs.* Retrieved from http://www.aacn.nche.edu/cnl/about/cnl-programs

American Association of Colleges of Nursing (AACN). (2014a). *DNP fact sheet.* Retrieved from http://www.aacn.nche.edu/media-relations/fact-sheets/dnp

American Association of Colleges of Nursing (AACN). (2014b). *Leading initiatives.* Retrieved from http://www.aacn.nche.edu/cnl/about/cnl-programs

American Association of Colleges of Nursing (AACN). (2014c). *Special survey on vacant faculty positions for academic year 2013–2014.* Retrieved from www.aacn.nche.edu

American Medical Association (AMA). (2006). *Need to expose and counter nurse doctoral programs (NDP) misrepresentation. Resolution 211(A-06).* Retrieved from https://www.ama-assn.org/ssl3/ecomm/PolicyFinderForm.pl?site=www.ama-assn.org&uri=/resources/html/PolicyFinder/policyfiles/HnE/H-35.972.HTM

American Nurses Association. (2014). *Nurses currently serving in Congress.* Retrieved from http://www.nursingworld.org/MainMenuCategories/Policy-Advocacy/

Benner, P., Sutphen, M., Leonard, V., & Day, L. (2010). *Educating nurses: A call for radical transformation.* San Francisco, CA: Jossey-Bass.

Bier, J. P. (2013, June 4). *CBO: Obamacare will leave 30 million uninsured.* Retrieved from http://cnsnews.com/news/article/cbo-obamacare-will-leave-30-million-uninsured

Boccia, R. (2013, February 12). *How the United States' high debt will weaken the economy and hurt Americans.* The Heritage Foundation. Retrieved from http://www.heritage.org/research/reports/2013/02/how-the-united-states-high-debt-will-weaken-the-economy-and-hurt-americans

Brassard, A., & Smolenski, M. (2011, September). *Removing barriers to advanced practice registered nurse care: Hospital privileges. AARP Public Institute Insight on the Issues.* Retrieved from http://www.aarp.org/health/doctors-hospitals/info-10-2011/Removing-Barriers-to-Advanced-Practice-Registered-Nurse-Care-Hospital-Privileges.html

Budetti, P. (2008). Market justice and US health care. *Journal of the American Medical Association, 299*(1), 92–94.

Buerhaus, P., & Needleman, J. (2000). Policy implications of research on nurse staffing and quality of patient care. *Policy, Politics, & Nursing Practice, 1*(1), 5–15.

Bureau of Health Professions (BHP). (2013). *Helping veterans become nurses.* Retrieved from http://bhpr.hrsa.gov/veterans/nurses.html.

Bureau of Labor Statistics. (2012). Fastest growing occupations. *Occupational Outlook Handbook.* Retrieved from http://www.bls.gov/ooh/fastest-growing.htm

Carney, B. (2005, November–December). The ethics of recruiting foreign nurses. *Health Progress, 86*(6), 31–35.

Central Intelligence Agency (CIA). (2001, July). *Long term global demographic trends: Reshaping the geopolitical landscape.* Retrieved from https://www.cia.gov/library/reports/general-reports-1/Demo_Trends_For_Web.pdf

Chaguturu, S., & Vallabhaneni, S. (2005). Aiding and abetting: Nursing crisis at home and abroad. *New England Journal of Medicine, 553*, 1761–1763.

Committee on Data Standards for Patient Safety. (2004). *Patient safety: Achieving a new standard of care.* Washington, DC: National Academies Press.

Committee on Quality Health Care. (2001). *Crossing the quality chasm: A new health system for the 21st century.* Washington, DC: National Academies Press.

Committee on the Consequences of Uninsurance (CCU). (2004). *Insuring America's health: Principles and recommendations.* Washington, DC: National Academies Press.

Davies, R. (2008). The Bologna process: The quiet revolution in nursing higher education. *Nurse Education Today, 28,* 935–942.

DeCuccio, M. H. (2014, March). The relationship between patient safety culture and patient outcomes: A systematic review. *Journal of Patient Safety,* 1–8.

Donley, R. (2010). Nursing, social justice and the marketplace. *Health Progress, 91*(5), 35–37.

Donley, R., Flaherty, M. J., Sarsfield, E., Taylor, L., Maloni, H., & Flanagan, E. (2002). The nursing shortage: What does the Nurse Reinvestment Act mean to you? *Online Journal of Issues in Nursing, 8*(1), Manuscript 5. Retrieved from http://nursingworld.org/MainMenuCategories/ANAMarketplace/ANAPeriodicals/OJIN/TableofContents/Volume82003/No1Jan2003/ArticlesPreviousTopics/NurseReinvestmentAct.html

Feldstein, P. (2011). *Health care economics* (7th ed.). New York: Delmar.

Fisher, E. B. (2008). Building a medical neighborhood for the medical home. *New England Journal of Medicine, 359,* 1202–1205.

Global Health Workforce Alliance, World Health Organization. (2008). *The Kampala Declaration and Agenda for Global Action.* Retrieved from http://www.who.int/workforcealliance/knowledge/resources/kampala_declaration/en/

Healthcare.gov. (2013). Retrieved from www.healthcare.gov/families/

Healthy People 2020. (2011). Retrieved from http://healthypeople.gov/2020/default.aspx

Health Resources and Services Administration (HRSA). (2014a). *Advanced nursing education.* Retrieved from http://bhpr.hrsa.gov/nursing/grants/ane.html

Health Resources and Services Administration (HRSA). (2014b). *Mary Wakefield biography.* (2014). Retrieved April 3, 2014, from http://www.hrsa.gov/about/organization/biowakefield.html

Hollander, C. (2014, March 20). Study: Long-term unemployed, if they get a job, more likely to leave than settle into labor force. *National Journal.* Retrieved from http://www.nationaljournal.com/economy/study-long-term-unemployed-if-they-get-a-job-more-likely-to-leave-than-settle-into-labor-force-20140320

Juraschek, S. P., Zhang, X., Ranganathan, V., & Lin, V. (2011, November 19). United States registered nurse workforce report card and shortage forecast. *American Journal of Medical Quality.* doi: 10.1177/1062860611416634.

Kalisch, B. J., Tschannen, D., Lee, H., & Friese, C. R. (2011). Hospital variation in missed nursing care. *American Journal of Medical Quality, 26*(4), 291–299.

Kane, J. (2012, October 22). Health costs: How the U.S. compares with other countries. PBS NewsHour. Retrieved from http://www.pbs.org/newshour/rundown/health-costs-how-the-us-compares-with-other-countries/?utm_source=UCSF+Center+for+Healthcare+Value+List&utm_campaign=7be2f6f4

9b-Center+for+Healthcare+Value+-+Aug+Update&utm_medium=email

Kodner, D. L., & Spreeuwenberg, C. (2002). Integrated care: Meaning, logic, applications and implications, a discussion paper. *International Journal of Integrated Care*. Retrieved from http://www.ncbi.nlm.nih.gov/pmc/articles/PMC1480401

Kohn, L., Corrigan, J., & Donaldson, M. (Eds.). (2000). *To err is human: Building a safer health system*. Washington, DC: National Academies Press.

Laurent, M., Reeves, D., Hermans, R., Braspenning, J., Grol, R., & Sibbald, B. (2004). Substitution of doctors by nurses in primary care. *Cochrane Database of Systematic Reviews, July 2005, Issue 3*.

Mechanic, D., & Reinhard, S. C. (2002). Contributions of nurses to health policy: Challenges and opportunities. *Nursing and Health Policy Review, 1*(1), 7–15.

Meleis, A., & Dracup, K. (2005). *The case against the DNP: History, timing, substance, and marginalization*. Retrieved from http://www.nursingworld.org/MainMenuCategories/ANAMarketplace/ANAPeriodicals/OJIN/TableofContents/Volume102005/No3Sept05/tpc28_216026.html

Mitchell, J. (2013). *Who are the long-term unemployed?* The Urban Institute. Retrieved from http://www.urban.org/uploadedpdf/412885-who-are-the-long-term-unemployed.pdf

NURSECORPS. (2014). *Loan Repayment program*. Retrieved from http://www.hrsa.gov/loanscholarships/repayment/nursing/nursecorpsloanrepaymentfactsheet.pdf

Nurses for a Healthier Tomorrow. (n.d.). *Campaign news*. Retrieved from http://www.nursesource.org/campaign_news.html

Nursing Organizations Alliance. (2014). *Nurse in Washington Internship (NIWI)*. Retrieved from http://www.nann.org/advocacy/content/niwi.html

Organisation for Economic Co-operation and Development (OCED). (2013a). *Health at a glance 2013*. Retrieved from http://www.oecd.org/els/health-systems/Health-at-a-Glance-2013.pdf

Organisation for Economic Co-operation and Development (OCED). (2013b). *OCED Health Data 2013. How does the United States compare?* Retrieved from http://www.oecd.org/unitedstates/Briefing-Note-USA-2014.pdf

Oulton, J. J. (2006). The global nursing shortage: An overview of issues and actions. *Policy Politics Nursing Practice, 7*, 34S.

Patient Protection and Affordable Care Act of 2010 (ACA). (2010). Retrieved from http://burgess.house.gov/UploadedFiles/hr3590_health_care_law_2010.pdf

Preventive care under the Affordable Care Act/HealthCare (2014). Retrieved from https://www.healthcare.gov/preventive-care-benefits/

Rubenstein, G. (2013, January). New health rankings: Of 17 nations, U.S. is dead last. *The Atlantic*. Retrieved from http://www.theatlantic.com/health/archive/2013/01/new-health-rankings-of-17-nations-us-is-dead-last/267045

Shi, L., & Singh, D. (2010). *Essentials of the U.S. health system* (2nd ed.). Sudbury, MA: Jones & Bartlett.

Smedley, B. D., Stith, A. Y., & Nelson, A. R. (Eds.). (2003). *Unequal treatment: Confronting racial and ethnic disparities in health care*. Washington, DC: National Academies Press.

Ten recession-proof jobs. (2014). Retrieved from http://www.salary.com/Articles/ArticleDetail.asp?part=par1098

The Future of Nursing. (2010). *Leading change, advancing health*. Washington, DC: National Academies Press.

The Future of Nursing. (2014). *Campaign for action*. Retrieved from http://campaignforaction.org/

The Joint Commission. (2014). *Infection control*. Retrieved from http://www.jointcommission.org/topics/patient_safety.aspx

U.S. Department of Health and Human Services (USDHHS). (2010a). *Registered nurse population: Findings from the 2008 National Sample of Registered Nurses*. Rockville, MD: Health Resources and Services Administration, Bureau of Health Professions, Division of Nursing.

U.S. Department of Health and Human Services (USDHHS). (2010b). *Healthy People 2020*. Retrieved from http://www.healthypeople.gov

U.S. Department of Labor (USDL). (2012). *Bureau of Labor Statistics' employment projections, 2010–2020*. Retrieved from http://www.bls.gov/news.release/ecopro.t06.htm

U.S. Department of Veteran Affairs (USDVA). (2013). *VA nursing academic partnerships*. Retrieved from http://www.va.gov/oaa/vanap/default.asp

Wallis, L. (2013, August). Nurse-patient staffing ratios. *American Journal of Nursing, 113*(8), 222.

White, K. M., Zangaro, G., Kepley, H. O., & Camacho, A. (2014). The Health Resources and Services Administration Data Collection. *Public Health Reports Supplement 2: Nursing in 3D: Workforce diversity, health disparities, social determinants of health increase*. Retrieved from http://www.publichealthreports.org/issueopen.cfm?articleID=3082

Wong, M. (2012, July 11). 3 big problems facing nursing today. *Health Careers*. Retrieved from www.healthcareers.com/article/3-big-problems-facing-nursing-today/170629

ONLINE RESOURCES

The Patient Protection and Affordable Care Act
www.hhs.gov/healthcare/rights

Medicaid and Children's Health Insurance Program
http://www.medicaid.gov/Medicaid-CHIP-Program-Information/By-State/By-State.html

American Association of Colleges of Nursing
http://www.aacn.nche.edu

Healthy People 2010 and *Healthy People 2020*
http://www.healthypeople.gov

● Rose Kearney-Nunnery

19

Expanding the Vision

*"Success comes to those who are
too busy to be looking for it."*

Henry David Thoreau, 1817–1862

Chapter Objectives

On completion of this chapter, the reader will be able to:

1. Evaluate trends in professional practice.
2. Continue to evaluate her or his personal philosophy.
3. Envision personal competencies in professional nursing practice.
4. Develop personal strategic initiatives for future contributions to professional nursing practice.

Key Terms

Competencies   Continued Competence
Collaboration   Involvement

We have seen nursing and healthcare change radically in recent years. With restructuring of healthcare, nursing professionals have responded with refinements, advancements, and innovations. Nursing has moved from the functional service mode of the mid-1900s to a cost-, community-, quality-, evidence-based–, and consumer-focused orientation. It is no longer the nursing care plan for the patient, but is now the collaborative care plan of the patient. And this care must be framed in the context of safety and patient involvement in an environment with shortages of healthcare providers in increasingly diverse settings.

To address the health of people, all health professions are now faced with the challenges of transformation, innovation, and collaboration. We have opportunities and challenges ahead. Collaboration must extend beyond the structural walls of a single institution or the boundaries of a community. In a global society, we can reach out to colleagues and patients physically or electronically. Shared best practices are no longer restricted by geography. Evidence-based practices are a mandate limited only by the needs of the patient population. Critical components of professional practice continue to expand and be enhanced through technology. And we continually strive to envision the challenges ahead. It is now time to expand the vision and address these challenges.

HEALTHCARE PROFESSIONALS IN THE 21ST CENTURY

Several initiatives have led to the changes in practice, in the nursing profession, and throughout the health professions during the last decades that frame the opportunities we face.

The Pew Health Professions Commission

The Pew Charitable Trust Foundation established the Pew Health Professions Commission, which worked from 1989 to 1999 to address issues of healthcare reform and health policy across the professions. At that time, the healthcare industry was in the midst of redesigning services and roles and containing costs with declining resources. The commission identified 21 specific competencies for health professionals for the year 2005. These competencies addressed ethics, critical thinking and evidence-based practice, primary and preventative healthcare, access, diversity and health disparities, consumer empowerment and outcomes, the use of informatics and interdisciplinary practice, quality and continuous improvement, leadership and public policy, and continued learning. **Competencies** are those qualities that illustrate effectiveness and appropriateness in our respective professional roles. In 1995, reports from the commission produced strong reactions and responses throughout the professional communities, with predictions for redesign needed in education and healthcare and for a rapid transformation in the health professions workforce. The four *r*'s were redesign, re-regulate, right-size, and restructure. The view of the healthcare system presented by the commission was market-driven and integrated with more managed and primary care. In addition, this healthcare system and its professionals would be more accountable to the public and responsive to consumers. Recommendations directed at the profession of nursing involved public accountability, recognition of our assets, the need for clarity in our roles and functions, and the need to meet the demands of the marketplace.

As a result of the findings of the commission and the associated reactions from different professional groups, O'Neil (1998) identified strategic directions for nursing that included addressing differentiated practice, curricula changes, core competencies, a commitment to research, the creation of strategic partnerships, and enhanced leadership. Later that year, however, the focus changed from the future competencies of health professionals to a call for immediate attention to patient safety.

The Institute of Medicine Quality Chasm

As we have discussed previously, the health professions came under fire with the release of reports from the Institute of Medicine (IOM) of the National Academies on the high incidence of medical errors, changing the focus from the future of healthcare to the current need to improve safety for patients and healthcare consumers. The IOM is a nonprofit organization designed to provide science-based advice as a public service. Its reports, whether self-initiated or as mandated from the U.S. Congress, are published after rigorous research, careful deliberation from professionals from healthcare and other scientific and professional disciplines, and a peer review process (IOM, 2013, p. 1). The 2001 report from the IOM, *Crossing the Quality Chasm*, proposed rules for the health system in the 21st century for quality healthcare that were the basis for six overall aims—that care should be safe, effective, patient-centered, timely, efficient, and equitable (IOM, 2001). A further report after a Health Professions Education Summit led to the identification of the five core competencies for all health professionals:

● Provide patient-centered care.
● Work in interdisciplinary teams.
● Employ evidence-based practice.
● Apply quality improvement.
● Utilize informatics. (Greiner & Knebel, 2003)

Patient safety and effectiveness of outcomes became major national objectives and directed additional attention to nursing. Research by the Agency for Healthcare Research and Quality (AHRQ) focused on expanding the knowledge base on how the quality of the healthcare workplace affects the quality of healthcare provided, especially in the areas of workload and working conditions, effects of stress and fatigue, reducing adverse events, and the organizational climate and culture. Patient outcomes were now being investigated, along with nursing-sensitive indicators and factors that promote safe and effective practice.

In late 2003, nursing itself was the focus of the IOM in their report, *Keeping Patients Safe: Transforming the Work Environment of Nurses*. The IOM's Committee on the Work Environment and Patient Safety provided specific recommendations to both acute care and long-term care organizations on issues of management practices, workforce capability, work design, and the organizational safety culture (Page, 2004, p. 3). The following risk factors were identified for patient safety in nursing work environments:

- More acutely ill patients
- Shorter hospital stays
- Redesigned work
- Frequent patient turnover
- High staff turnover
- Long work hours
- Rapid increases in new knowledge and technology
- Increased interruptions and demands on nurses' time (Page, 2004, pp. 37–45)

Although these facts were no surprise, their identification as risk factors to patients was significant. Nurses have been reporting these factors, but now they were included in a major national report. This committee also documented the national shortages of both nurses and nursing assistants. Recommendations to nursing leadership and management on how to address the deficiencies in the documented work environments called attention to the following areas:

- Leadership, communication skills, collaborative decision making, and resources
- Emphasis on safety goals along with productivity and financial goals
- Management practices promoting safety, trust, change, engagement, and learning collaboratives
- External support for evidence-based management practices

In addition, at the staff level, the committee found "strong evidence that nurse staffing levels, the knowledge and skills level of nursing staff, and the extent to which workers collaborate in sharing their knowledge and skills affect patient outcomes and safety" (Page, 2004, p. 161). This finding provides further support for the need to incorporate the five core competencies into professional nursing practice on a consistent basis. Nurses consistently strive to provide patient-centered care, but, for positive patient outcomes, this must also be done in light of the other core competencies, given the nature of the healthcare environment. Evolving technologies, evidence-based collaborative practice, and continued competence are essential components for quality improvement in the delivery of healthcare to consumers.

In subsequent years, the IOM investigated health disparities, the role of the government (including Medicare), rural health, healthcare reimbursement practices, and mental health conditions among other quality improvement initiatives, including the objectives for *Healthy People 2020*. Of particular note were two studies mandated by the United States Congress, on insurance and reimbursements and preventing medication errors. In July 2006, the IOM report on *Preventing Medication Errors* presented information available on the incidence of medication errors in acute care settings, long-term care, and in ambulatory care—including errors in the homes of consumers—in an effort to develop an agenda for the nation to reduce preventable errors and adverse drug events

and enhance medication safety. Although the incidence rates were approximated based on the data, the report did emphasize that these rates were most likely underestimates, based on available and reportable data and the incidence of adverse events. It was reported, however, that at least 25 percent of all harmful adverse drug events are *preventable* (Aspden, Wolcott, Bootman, & Cronenwett, 2006, p. 4).

Based on the rules from the earlier *Quality Chasm* Report in 2001, the IOM (Aspden et al., 2006) recommended the transformation of the entire system to a patient-centered, integrated-use system with specific action agendas to support consumer-provider partnership. The seven recommendations provided by the IOM (Aspden et al., 2006) focused further on:

- Consumer empowerment for self-medication management
- Improvement and standardization of resources by governmental agencies
- Implementation of patient-information and decision-support technologies nationwide
- Improved labeling, packaging, and distribution, including studies on use of samples
- Establishment of standards for drug information technologies, including design and alert systems
- Broad, federally funded research on safe and appropriate medication use across settings, focused on error prevention
- Use of legislation, regulation, accreditation, payment mechanisms, and the media for adoption of practices, technologies, and professional behaviors focused on safety and error reduction

Collaborative efforts among professionals, governmental agencies, suppliers, educators, and regulators with the consumer involved in the process were a mandate. The IOM Committee on the Work Environment and Patient Safety (Page, 2004) identified necessary patient safeguards in the environment (Box 19.1).

However, in a report 10 years later on these recommendations (RWJF, 2014), the following areas were noted

---

BOX 19.1 **Necessary Patient Safeguards in the Work Environment**

- Governing boards that focus on safety
- Leadership and evidence-based management structures and processes
- Effective nursing leadership
- Adequate staffing
- Organizational support for ongoing learning and decision support
- Mechanisms that promote interdisciplinary collaboration
- Work design that promotes safety
- Organizational culture that continually strengthens patient safety

Source: Page, A. (Ed.). (2004). *Keeping patients safe: Transforming the work environment of nurses.* Washington, DC: National Academies Press.

with positive progress but also with recommendations for further transformation in the workplace:

- Creating work environments that promote patient safety
- Ensuring adequate nurse staffing
- Curbing unprofessional and disruptive behaviors
- Harnessing nurse leadership
- Fostering interprofessional collaboration (p. 2)

Evidence-based practice is the standard, with a focus on safety, positive patient outcomes, and the used of known and evolving technologies. Changes in the practice environment have received serious attention, with the focus on safety and patient outcomes.

A Call for Change and Leadership by Nursing

In 2008, a two-year collaborative initiative between the IOM and the Robert Wood Johnson Foundation (RWJF) started looking at the nursing profession and the need for more than change, but *transformation*. The report by the committee was released in October 2010 with four key messages and eight recommendations (Table 19.1). However, as voiced in one of the follow-up briefings to the public, this was not to be a report to sit on a shelf but rather a call to action.

The key messages focus on more consistency of advanced practice nurse (APRN) practice among the states and licensing jurisdictions, the development of residency programs across settings and practice areas, seamless and ongoing education for nurses, active nursing involvement in redesign of the healthcare system, and better workforce data systems. Their report also supported implementation of the *APRN Consensus Model* (APRN Consensus Work Group & the National Council of State Boards of Nursing APRN Advisory Committee, 2008) and the National Council of State Boards of Nursing (NCSBN) *Nurse Licensure Compact* (NCSBN, 2014). The recommendations provide directives

ONLINE CONSULT

Agency for Healthcare Research and Quality (AHRQ) at
http://www.ahrq.gov

Institute of Medicine (IOM) at
http://www.iom.edu

to the federal and state governments, regulatory bodies, accrediting agencies, healthcare providers, funding agencies, educational programs, and individual nurses. As stated by the IOM (2011), "together, these groups have the power to transform the healthcare system to provide seamless, affordable, quality care that is accessible to all, patient-centered, and evidence-based and leads to improved health outcomes" (p. S-13). These recommendations call for leadership, collaboration, and action.

The Professional Nursing Practice Environment

Leadership, collaboration, and action in the practice environment are essential for patient safety but also for the satisfaction, involvement, and commitment of dedicated healthcare professionals. One area that is receiving serious consideration at the national and state levels is adequacy of staffing. In addition, the American Nurses Association (ANA) has been actively looking at the roles of both the employer and the nurse to promote healthy work hours and consider the effect of fatigue on safety for both patients and nurses. The focus on productivity and appropriate staffing has led to a renewed emphasis on quality outcomes. Indicators that are nursing sensitive, such as infection rates, patient satisfaction, and nursing hours per patient day, are being studied in relation to staffing. As noted by Clark et al. (2005), we cannot simply tell staff to do more, "rather, we need to create systems that support staff in their

TABLE 19.1

IOM and RWJF Report on the Future of Nursing

Key Messages	Committee Recommendations
1. Nurses should practice to the full extent of their education.	1. Remove scope of practice barriers.
2. Nurses should achieve higher levels of education and training through an improved education system that promotes seamless academic progression.	2. Expand opportunities for nurses to lead and diffuse collaborative improvement efforts.
	3. Implement nurse residency programs.
	4. Increase the proportion of nurses with a baccalaureate degree to 80 percent by 2020.
3. Nurses should be full partners, with physicians and other healthcare professionals, in redesigning healthcare in the United States.	5. Double the nurses with a doctorate by 2020.
	6. Ensure that nurses engage in lifelong learning.
	7. Prepare and enable nurses to lead change to advance health.
4. Effective workforce planning and policy-making require better data collection and an improved information infrastructure.	8. Build an infrastructure for the collection and analysis of interprofessional healthcare workforce data.

Source: Institute of Medicine (IOM). (2011). *The future of nursing: Leading change, advancing health.* Retrieved from http://www.nap.edu/catalog.php?record_id=12956

efforts and set them up for success" (p. 8). In addition to staffing numbers, a body of research has evolved from Linda Aiken and her associates and others on educational preparation and patient complexity and nurse sensitive measures. The complexity of the environment, the acuity of the patients, and the distractions nurses face are serious factors in contemporary healthcare settings. In addition to current concerns on adequacy of staffing to meet the patient acuity needs are the projections of nursing shortages in the future with deferred retirements taking place along with an increased demand for nursing professionals. In addition, in the 10-year follow-up report to *Keeping Patients Safe*, ensuring adequate nurse staffing was one of the areas identified for further transformation, and the report stated that "staffing adequacy is a function of the composition as well as the size of the nursing workforce and concerted efforts are now underway to increase the education level of nurses" (RWJF, 2014, p. 4). An increase in baccalaureate-prepared nurses is further supported by the American Association of College of Nursing (AACN, 2014a), which has documented "the unique value that baccalaureate-prepared nurses bring to the practice setting" (p. 1).

The American Association of Colleges of Nursing (AACN) has identified selected characteristics of work environments that support professional nursing practice (AACN, 2002):

● Magnet status
● Preceptorships and residencies
● Differentiated practice
● Interdisciplinary collaboration

Recognition as a Magnet hospital requires that applicant healthcare organizations meet specific eligibility criteria, including strong nursing leadership in line with national standards of practice. From the original model that identified 14 forces of magnetism, a revised model for the Magnet Recognition Program° was introduced in 2008 and contained the following five components:

● Transformational Leadership
● Structural Empowerment
● Exemplary Professional Practice
● New Knowledge, Innovation, and Improvements
● Empirical Quality Results (ANCC, 2014)

These five components contain the 14 Forces of Magnetism and guide the self-assessment requirement for the institution applying for Magnet recognition Retention and appropriate staffing are characteristics of Magnet organizations. The Joint Commission (2013) identified that its accreditation standards, the Baldrige quality standards, and the AACN Magnet Recognition Model components contain many parallels that share the following characteristics:

● Were developed using a consensus-building approach
● Are built on a set of core values and principles
● Use a framework of important functions that cross internal organizational structures
● Recognize organizations as systems
● Focus on continuous improvement in outcomes and organization performance
● Do not prescribe specific structures
● Promote the use of organization self-assessment (p. 1)

Retention is enhanced when professionals have had an opportunity to expand their knowledge base and skills with a rapidly changing practice environment through preceptorships for students and residencies for graduates. The implementation of residency programs for new nurses from prelicensure programs and advanced practice programs, as well as when transitioning to a new clinical practice area, was one of the recommendations from the IOM (2011). Finkelman and Kenner (2012) describe effective residency programs with "graduated patient care responsibilities, additional educational experiences and competency development, professional socialization, and support for the critical transition during the first post graduation year" (pp. 72–73). Mentorship is also an important component to advance the skills of the neophyte and of the seasoned clinician. Matching the knowledge and skills of the professionals with the requirements of the position is an ongoing consideration. This can be promoted through mentorship programs and activities for continuing education, competency, and differentiated practice.

Differentiated nursing practice, the third characteristic identified by AACN in the supportive practice environment, is illustrated through advancement structures in the organization based on experience, additional education, certification, or other identified indicators of excellence (AACN, 2002, pp. 6–7). Implementation of differentiated practice has historically been difficult; the combination of skills matched to the position requirements must be delineated. As Nelson (2002) proposed more than a decade ago, it is not feasible to try to differentiate practice along current educational points of entry when the roles have not been translated into the practice setting (p. 7). And this remains the case, as clinical ladders are inconsistent and diverse. However, the need for lifelong learning and a seamless educational system have been highlighted by the IOM (2011).

Interdisciplinary collaboration, illustrated through teamwork, trust, shared responsibility, and respect, also enhances patient outcomes. The AACN (2002) proposed eight hallmarks of excellence in the professional nursing practice environment. Consider how these hallmarks for the practice environment (Table 19.2) also address the core competencies for all health professionals identified by the IOM. Note the focus on quality care for patients, collaboration, competency, and leadership throughout. Again, we see collaboration and leadership in collaborative improvement efforts in healthcare settings in the recent recommendations from the IOM (2011).

COLLABORATION

Essential activities of contemporary practice include strategic partnerships, leadership, and collaboration. As stated by the AACN (2011), "in a redesigned health system a greater emphasis will be placed on cooperation, communication, and collaboration among all health professionals in order to integrate care in teams and assure that care is continuous and reliable" (p. 22). However, collaboration and collegiality must both occur within the profession and be interdisciplinary. The initial step in collaboration and collegiality is valuing our colleagues who

TABLE 19.2

Hallmarks of Professional Practice and Core Competencies

Hallmarks of the Professional Nursing Practice Environment*	Core Competencies for Health Professionals†			
	Provide Patient-Centered Care	Work in Interdisciplinary Practice Teams	Employ Evidence-Based Practice	Apply Quality Improvement
Manifest a philosophy of clinical care emphasizing quality, safety, interdisciplinary collaboration, continuity of care, and professional accountability.	✓	✓	✓	✓
Recognize contributions of nurses' knowledge and expertise to clinical care quality and patient outcomes.	✓	✓	✓	✓
Empower nurses' participation in clinical decision making and organization of clinical care systems.	✓	✓	✓	✓
Promote executive-level nursing leadership.	✓	✓	✓	✓
Maintain clinical advancement programs based on education, certification, and advanced preparation.	✓	✓	✓	✓
Demonstrate professional development support for nurses.	✓	✓	✓	✓
Create collaborative relationships among members of the healthcare provider team.	✓	✓	✓	✓

*Source: American Association of Colleges of Nursing (AACN). (2002). *Hallmarks of the professional nursing practice environment.* Washington, DC: Author.

†Source: Greiner, A. C., & Knebel, E. (Eds.). (2003). *Health professions education: A bridge to quality.* Washington, DC: Institute of Medicine.

provide clinical nursing care, medical care, specialty care, advanced clinical practice, education, administration, or research. Collaboration and collegiality are both intradisciplinary, within the discipline of nursing, and interdisciplinary, among other healthcare professionals.

The healthcare team should be an ideal example of collaboration, especially for effective communication (see Chapter 6). **Collaboration** involves actively working together to meet some identified goal, such as the patient's treatment goals. Within the discipline, nurses from each area of nursing would contribute to that goal—the admission nurse or discharge planner, the student in a clinical rotation, the operative nurse, the acute care nurse practitioner, and other professional nurses providing care to raise the patient's level of well-being. However, as noted by Weston (2006), this sense of teamwork may be particularly challenging for the four different generations of nurses in practice—veterans, baby boomers, generation Xers, and millennials—with their different characteristics and perspectives that can either enhance or traumatize the

practice environment. And the complexity increases with the addition of clinicians from other healthcare disciplines. Collaboration must also extend beyond the discipline of nursing for effective, efficient, and patient-centered care. In times of limited staffing and growing responsibilities, seeing the broader picture with collaboration is necessary to ensure effective patient outcomes. As noted by the IOM (2013), "healthcare delivery organizations should develop organizational cultures that encourage continuous improvement by incentivizing the incorporation of best practices, transparency, open communication, staff empowerment, coordination, teamwork, and mutual respect" (p. 6).

A cooperative spirit with collaboration will bring more efficient achievement of goals and greater personal reward for both colleagues and patients. Questions of authority and responsibility arise with this cooperative or collaborative spirit, such as who is the leader of the team and who is responsible for ensuring quality patient outcomes. This ownership of responsibility must be shared in a true collaborative relationship rather than create "turf" issues in a more competitive environment. The goal is the effectiveness of the patient outcomes with collaboration as the means to reach the goal. Effective communication and clinical skills, along with trust, leadership, and collegiality, are important attributes of the healthcare professional collaborating with other healthcare professionals. Consider the lessons for collaboration described by Gardner (2005) that are listed in Box 19.2.

Suppose that you are on an acute care unit one morning when the pulmonologist arrives to see his patient with COPD hospitalized with respiratory complications. You know that the respiratory therapist is currently working with the patient on a treatment. How will you capitalize on this opportunity for interdisciplinary collaboration for home care since you know all parties involved, the patient's wife is present but concerned about at-home compliance, and there is a need for good follow-up and discharge teaching? How can you get all parties involved and create a win-win situation for all, focused on the efficacy of treatment for this patient? These skills are critical for the efficient use of scarce human and physical resources in a consumer environment that must be focused on effectiveness of patient outcomes and overall safety.

Although collaboration involves actively working together to meet some identified goal, *collegiality* is sharing responsibility and authority to achieve a goal or prescribed outcome. Power and responsibility for outcomes related to patients' health and well-being are invested in more than one person. Mutual respect and collaboration are important components of a collegial relationship. All colleagues contribute to the intended goals and are accountable for the outcomes.

Collaboration is specified by the American Nurses Association as a standard of professional performance in its document *Nursing: Scope and Standards of Practice*. Recall that this document contains six standards of practice

reflective of the nursing process and ten standards of professional performance as expected professional behaviors, with objectives and measurement criteria for all of the standards (ANA, 2010a). Collaboration is demonstrated by virtue of partnerships with the healthcare consumer along with other healthcare providers for positive patient outcomes and includes effective communication, consultation, group process, negotiation and conflict management skills, documentation, referrals within and outside the nursing discipline, and effective teamwork. Additional measurement criteria have been added for the advanced practice nurse and specialty nurse to accommodate the additional expectations in their respective leadership roles in interdisciplinary practice.

Nursing professionals are responsible for promoting collaboration and collegiality among the professions. As described throughout this text, healthcare delivery systems are becoming more and more integrated and interdisciplinary. In our present multidisciplinary healthcare system, collaboration must be effective among all members of the various health professions and care disciplines.

Almost 20 years ago, the President's Advisory Commission on Consumer Protection and Quality in the Healthcare Industry (1998) reported that "the challenge for industry leaders is to harness the tremendous talent, energy, and commitment of the 10 million people who have been drawn to work in the healthcare industry because of its strong sense of mission" (p. 197). Since then, the IOM report *Keeping Patients Safe* has recommended that healthcare organizations "should take action to support interdisciplinary collaboration by adopting such interdisciplinary practice mechanisms as interdisciplinary rounds, and by providing ongoing formal education and training in interdisciplinary collaboration for all healthcare professionals on a regularly scheduled, continuous basis" (Page, 2004, p. 216). Then, in 2010, the IOM recommendations for nursing went even further:

Private and public funders, healthcare organizations, nursing education programs, and nursing associations should expand opportunities for nurses to lead and manage collaborative efforts with physicians and other members of the healthcare team to conduct research and to redesign and improve practice environments and healthcare systems. (IOM, 2011, p. S-9)

Following this recommendation from the IOM in the *Future of Nursing: Leading Change, Advancing Health* has been the call for educational revisions and enhanced interprofessional education and collaboration. The American Association of Colleges of Nursing and the American Organization of Nurse Executives (2012) developed guiding principles for academic-practice relationships to include nursing and other professions, corporations, governmental entities, and foundations (p. 1). Mutual goals, shared vision, joint efforts, transparency, commitment, communication, and lifelong learning were common threads in the eight principles. Thibault (2013) further identifies the following six areas for reform in the education of all health professionals:

- Increased interprofessional education
- Clinical education that is longitudinal and community based

---

BOX 19.2 Characteristics for Collaboration

- Know yourself—your biases, values, and goals.
- Value and manage diversity.
- Develop constructive conflict resolution skills.
- Create win-win situations.
- Demonstrate clinical competence, cooperation, and flexibility.
- Allow time and practice for skills in collaboration
- Use all multidisciplinary opportunities for building partnerships.
- Appreciate that collaboration can occurspontaneously.
- Be reflective, seek feedback, and admit mistakes for autonomy and unity.
- Understand that collaboration is not required in all situations.

Source: Adapted from Gardner, D. B. (2005). Ten lessons in collaboration. *Online Journal of Issues in Nursing*. Retrieved from http://www.nursingworld.org/MainMenuCategories/ANAMarketplace/ANAPeriodicals/OJIN/TableofContents/Volume102005/No1Jan05/tpc26_116008.html

- In addition to biological sciences, greater awareness of systems, quality improvement, safety, economics, and population health
- Competency-based education and ensuring lifelong learning
- Greater incorporation of new educational technologies including online and simulation experiences
- Faculty development for educational innovation (pp. 1929–1931)

Previously, the IOM also identified two necessary precursors to collaboration—individual clinical competence and mutual trust and respect—and the following four characteristics of collaboration:

- Shared understanding of goals and roles
- Effective communication
- Shared decision making
- Conflict management. (Page, 2004, pp. 212–213)

In addition to these characteristics is the necessary ingredient of continued competence to maintain safety and quality care for the patient and effective interdisciplinary practice.

COMPETENCE

The issue of competence is vital to all professionals. Although not restricted to nursing, professional competence has received greater attention after the reports from both the Pew Health Professions Commission and the IOM. Professional competence is of great concern to health professionals, their regulatory bodies, and consumers. It is an issue of definition, ownership, policy development, and demonstration. Regulatory bodies are required to assure the public of safe and competent professional practice by the professionals they regulate. But definitions vary by statute, and measurement issues are complex. Consider two different ways in which competence can be measured: by continuing practice and through continuing education. But then the following question arises: Is the continuing practice safe and effective in meeting appropriate patient outcomes using evidence-based practice? Or, in the case of continuing education, are the programs or sessions directed at the area of practice to improve and enhance practice or merely counting hours toward license renewal without a focus on patients and responsible professional practice? For registered nurses, some states or jurisdictions require continuing education in the nurses' practice area, and some specify required content in addition to self-selected topical areas. Other states or jurisdictions provide a selection of options that can be pursued in a selected time frame. And still other states are silent on the demonstration of competence in the renewal requirement. In fact, measurement issues are further complicated by the different levels of practice that must be regulated—new graduate, continued practice, and advanced practice.

Entry into practice occurs through licensure on the basis of performance on a psychometrically sound instrument, the National Council Licensure Exam (NCLEX-RN). Advanced practice is regulated differently but often through advanced education and the certification process. But how should the regulators monitor continued professional competence for the clinician not governed by specialty practice certification, and what about variable requirements for recertification? And consider the role of both the nurse and the employer in monitoring continued professional competence.

The issue of **continued competence** is not restricted to state and federal regulatory bodies. As described in *Nursing's Social Policy Statement* (ANA, 2010b), regulation of practice also includes the following:

- Professional regulation, including a professional code of ethics, standards of practice, educational and specialty certification requirements, and a defined scope of practice
- Legal regulation, through statutory and regulatory requirements
- Institutional policies and procedures for safe, effective, and evidence-based practice
- Self-regulation, in terms of personal accountability and demonstration of continued competence

Continued competence is an issue of both a professional responsibility within each of the core competencies and one of patient safety. In 1996, the National Council of State Boards of Nursing (NCSBN) illustrated a collaborative model for continued competence that included the individual nurse, the employer, the regulatory body, the educator, and the consumer of nursing care (NCSBN, 2005a), but further work and understanding of best practices continues for a system that is reliable, valid, and feasible. In some Canadian provinces and in other countries like New Zealand, a portfolio system to document their continued competence has been required of individual nurses. This system requires critical reflection and assessment of continued competence by the nurse with documentation of evidence in a portfolio, often including some form of peer review in the process. The International Council of Nurses (2006) encourages reflective practice and believes that individual nurses are responsible and accountable for their practice and for maintaining continued competence but also identifies the following key stakeholders as contributing to the continued competence of the nurse:

- Public and patients
- Government
- Regulatory bodies
- The individual nurse
- The employer
- The education community
- National nursing associations (pp. 1–2)

Although continued competence is ultimately the professional responsibility of the individual clinician, the professional education level must be appropriate to the defined scope of practice and professional standards, the healthcare employer must ensure the competence in the practice setting, and the patients must be assured (and should assure themselves) of safe and effective practice. As noted by the NCSBN (2005b), "responsibility for interpreting and enforcing nursing scopes of practice, including the determination of the appropriate education, training and experience necessary to support a given scope of practice, rests solely with the boards of nursing" (p. 1). However, in the case of advanced practice with disparities of scope and supervision requirements among the states, the IOM (2011) has recommended that "states with unduly restrictive regulations should be urged to amend them to allow advanced practice registered nurses to provide care to patients in all circumstances in which they are qualified to do so" (p. S-9). Still, there will be concerns raised as to continued competence.

The professional performance standard of education of the *Scope and Standards of Practice* states that for continued competence, "the nurse attains knowledge and competency that reflects current nursing practice" (ANA, 2010a, p. 49). In addition, nurses are expected to perform appropriate to the situation, setting, resources, and the person, along with engagement in lifelong learning and ongoing assessment of competencies (ANA, 2010b, p. 13). Ongoing educational activities occur through continuing education (CE)—formal, noncredit, and on-the-job. Interestingly, in research conducted by the NCSBN, respondents "rated contributions of work experience, initial professional education, and mentors above the contributions of CE in assisting them to their current levels of ability" (Smith, 2003, p. 25). Concerning continued learning in the work environment, the IOM report *Keeping Patients Safe* recommended that healthcare organizations should "dedicate budgetary resources equal to a defined percentage of the nursing payroll to support nursing staff in their ongoing acquisition and maintenance of knowledge and skills" (Page, 2004, p. 210). Further, the concept of a learning environment is extended beyond its start in an educational setting to one that is encouraged in the practice setting and that must address interdisciplinary practice. But budgetary considerations have resulted in associated cuts in funding education departments and programs in some agencies. A learning environment in the practice setting supports the core competencies and ongoing professional competence. The individual professional must determine, seek, request, and utilize resources to maintain his or her continued competence in the safe and effective performance of nursing practice activities. In addition, the IOM (2011) recently recommended an increase in the proportion of nurses with both baccalaureate and doctoral degrees, along with a separate recommendation on "lifelong learning to gain the competencies needed to provide care for diverse populations across the lifespan" (p. S-11).

> Although continued competence is ultimately the professional responsibility of the individual clinician, the professional education level must be appropriate to the defined scope of practice and professional standards, the healthcare employer must ensure the competence in the practice setting, and the patient must be assured of safe and effective practice.

Competent practice in the unique environment addresses the metaparadigm concepts of nursing: human beings, health, environment, and nursing. The individual nurse is responsible and accountable for the demonstration of competent practice. However, assurance of this competence to the consumer is a shared responsibility. As stated

ONLINE CONSULT

American Nurses Association (ANA) at
http://www.nursingworld.org

American Nurses Credentialing Center (ANCC)
http://www.nursecredentialing.org/default.aspx

IOM at
http://iom.edu/Reports/2010/The-Future-of-Nursing-Leading-Change-Advancing-Health.aspx

International Council of Nurses at
http://www.icn.ch/publications/position-statements/

NCSBN at
https://www.ncsbn.org/index.htm

in their Position Statement on Professional Role Competence, the ANA (2008) has stated:

> *Assurance of competence is the shared responsibility of the profession, individual nurses, professional organizations, credentialing and certification entities, regulatory agencies, employers, and other key stakeholders. (p. 1)*

The demonstration of competence requires skillful, effective, and evidence-based practice in both nursing and interdisciplinary endeavors, with a view of the core competencies and the challenges ahead.

Both professional and personal contributions are the ingredients of your professional career. Skills, though, which are the ingredients of professional nursing practice, require ongoing refinement. The International Council of Nurses (ICN, 2007) states that "individual nurses have a responsibility to plan and develop their careers through continuous self-assessment and goal setting" (p. 1). This includes personal and professional development to remain flexible, analytical, reflective, and innovative. As noted by the ICN (2013), nurses need appropriate ongoing education as well as lifelong learning to practice competently within their scope of practice (p. 2). Your skills and abilities will be enhanced through ongoing knowledge development for evidence-based practice and by your views on practice, human beings, the environment, health, and nursing.

TAKING THE LEAD

The recommendations and changes in the healthcare environment present all nurses with additional career opportunities and responsibilities, whether they are in acute, ambulatory, home, or long-term care settings or in a nontraditional setting as a clinician, case manager, researcher, administrator, consultant, educator, advanced practice nurse, or nurse entrepreneur.

The AACN (2008a) *Essentials of Baccalaureate Education for Professional Nursing Practice* are designed to prepare the generalist nurse with a broad preparation to address many of these career opportunities. From a firm foundation in liberal education, experiences throughout a baccalaureate nursing curriculum focus on patient-centered care that addresses quality improvement, safety, ethical principles, leadership and management, and evidence-based practice within a complex and changing healthcare system. Leadership development and a focus on health promotion and disease prevention for individuals and groups prepare the nurse for practice challenges. As described by AACN (2008a), the baccalaureate-prepared nurse understands and respects the variations of care, the increased complexity, and the increased use of healthcare resources inherent in caring for patients (AACN, 2008a). Building on the baccalaturate, the AACN (2011) *Essentials of Master's Education in Nursing* provide graduates with an advanced level of understanding of nursing and relevant sciences, so that they can then integrate this knowledge into practice in both direct and indirect care components in our evolving healthcare systems (pp. 1–2). And even further leadership in nursing science and practice is provided by nurses prepared at the doctoral level through curriculum guides by the AACN (2006) *Essentials of Doctoral Education for Advanced Nursing Practice* through programs offering the practice (Doctor of Nursing Practice [DNP]) doctorate. There are two types of doctorates in nursing. As described by AACN (2006), the research-focused doctorate (DNS, DSN, or DNSc) is designed to prepare nurse scientists and scholars, whereas the practice-focused doctorate (DNP) places greater emphasis on practice that is innovative and evidence-based, reflecting the application of credible research findings (p.3).

The challenges in your future are dynamic and evolve daily as we address the themes of safety, quality outcomes, evolving technology, and interdisciplinary practice. Consider the implications of the following challenges in the workforce or in a specific delivery setting:

- A culture supportive of safe and quality patient outcomes
- Appropriate staffing patterns and skill mixes
- Appropriate delegation activities
- Training and supervision of unlicensed assistive personnel
- Competencies and continued knowledge development of professionals
- Ongoing education and skill attainment and refinement
- Coordination of care across practice settings
- Changes in populations and healthcare needs
- Strategies to improve health and eliminate health disparities
- Cost containment
- Evidence-based interdisciplinary practice
- Consumer satisfaction
- Using information technologies and quality-based indicators
- Providing leadership on system change and redesign

The challenges in your future truly depend on you, your practice environment, colleagues, and future initiatives. Consider how individual colleagues and groups can challenge the status quo for positive change.

Nursing Education

The majority of baccalaureate and graduate programs in nursing are guided by the three *Essentials* documents published by AACN (2006, 2008a, 2010). Generalist practice occurs following baccalaureate program completion. Advanced generalist or specialty practice is the outcome of graduate education in nursing. And then there is the opportunity for specialty practice as an advanced practice nurse (APRN). Consider the APRN practice roles of nurse practitioner, clinical nurse specialist, nurse anesthetist, or nurse midwife. As the knowledge base grows, evidence-based practice is guided by the specialty area. Nevertheless, while we are experiencing an uneven shortage of nurses active in generalist staff practice settings, there have been predictions that shortages will increase drastically as retirements in the current workforce occur. Even more significant is the critical shortage of nursing faculty. Although we have seen an increase in the numbers of nurses prepared at the master's and doctoral levels, graduate education in the 1990s was directed at APRN clinical practice in four areas: nurse practitioner, clinical nurse specialist, nurse anesthetist, and nurse midwife.

Since the 1980s, education tracks in graduate programs declined with nurses pursuing APRN roles, and the average age of nursing faculty continues to rise. And impending retirements of nurse educators looms to create an even greater shortage of educators. The AACN (2011) recognizes the preparation of clinical educators at the master's level but has endorsed the Carnegie Foundation Report recommending the preparation of the clinical educator in both a clinical specialty and in principles of education, including curriculum design and teaching and evaluation methods. "Consistent with academy expectations, faculty with primary responsibility for the oversight of courses in baccalaureate, master's, and doctoral nursing programs will have doctoral preparation [and] doctoral graduates who will be involved in an academic role will have preparation in educational methods and pedagogies" (AACN, 2008b, p. 1). The shortage of nursing faculty has been documented. For several years, AACN (2014b) has documented that faculty shortages are limiting student capacity in nursing programs related to budget constraints, an aging faculty, a limited pool of faculty, and noncompetitive salaries compared with positions in practice settings. So, in addition to an area of specialization and clinical skill, skills in curriculum development and evaluation, teaching and learning, and interdisciplinary education are required in the nurse educator role. Although the AACN (2005) reported on the demographics, stressors, and competing demands along with the changes in the student population, it was observed that the "faculty shortage offers nurse educators an unique opportunity to challenge past norms and think collaboratively and nontraditionally to meet the future" (p. 12). However, doctoral education is the expected level of preparation for the full academic role and preparation of nurse researchers and scientists. The IOM (2011) has further recommended that the number of nurses with doctoral degree be doubled by 2020 (p. S-11).

The overriding challenges ahead in professional practice are ongoing professional development and involvement for engagement in the delivery of patient-centered care with a focus on safety, efficacy, and quality through the use of informatics, and evidence-based practice and leadership in the interdisciplinary practice setting. This involvement reflects the core competencies of health professionals and advances practice, patient outcomes, and the profession.

INVOLVEMENT

When we think of **involvement**, we often think of our function as advocates and healthcare providers for our patients. These functions represent one form of involvement. Our professional involvement focuses on the individual attributes of, needs of, and outcomes for our patients, the consumers of nursing and healthcare. This involvement, as individual professionals with the patients and families who are the consumers of evidence-based, quality nursing care, must address all core competencies.

Our involvement is also as members of the healthcare team. Collaboration and collegiality have been described in relation to nursing and interdisciplinary practice. This book also discussed the importance of group dynamics and group skills, and the art of negotiation in leading and managing. All of these functions relate to active involvement with a defined group to attain specified goals for the consumers of healthcare.

A third form of professional involvement is as a member of the professional group. This form of involvement requires time and commitment for advancement of the profession. Professional contributions result from participation in professional organizations, research, publications, theory evaluation, and promotion of the further development of the profession. Personal contributions in professional practice occur through your education, competency, ethical behaviors, use of theory and evidence-based interventions, and communication, political efficacy, patient advocacy, and leadership.

REVISITING YOUR PHILOSOPHY OF NURSING

Now is the time to reflect on your personal contributions to and philosophy of nursing. Nurses are talented, creative, and visionary—when they allow themselves to be. They are frequently viewed as leaders and risk takers as they advocate for the perceived good of their patients. But what skills required of professionals do we need to refine? Step back and think of the vital and basic skills needed to demonstrate our professional competencies. These skills are what we continually strive to refine:

- Knowledge base
- Critical thinking skills
- Technical skills
- Interpersonal skills
- Articulation skills
- Leadership skills
- Policy and advocacy skills

Clinical practice requires these skills for provision of patient-centered care, involvement in interdisciplinary and evidence-based practice, and the use of informatics and emerging technologies for quality improvement and effective patient outcomes. These skills are enhanced through the professional attributes of collaboration, collegiality, continued competence, and leadership in the health promotion of society. Concern for the health of people, whether individual patients, families, communities, or groups in their environment, is the core of professional nursing. Individuals like you are dedicated and exemplify those characteristics of a professional described here. Your philosophy of nursing will evolve and develop, just as you do as a professional.

EMBRACING CHANGE

The recent focus on the health professions and the evident shortages of professionals has had the beneficial effect of opening up the discussion for needed changes in the healthcare system and the professions. Discussions have been held at national, state, and local meetings, and debate and discussion on the issues continue in professional newsletters and journals as well as online. And the calling to action became even more resounding with the recent IOM (2011) report calling for more leadership by nursing in healthcare reform. Communication and critical thinking are taking place. The restraining and driving forces of change are present. We see that practice and education can no longer serve the needs of the consumers without change. Interdisciplinary collaboration and practice are essential. All professionals are shareholders in the process of improving the health of the population.

Technology continues to expand our horizons and challenge our practice. Improved equipment and technologies are developing at a rapid pace. Information is available immediately. Colleagues readily communicate at a distance using e-mail, instant messaging, listservs, and news groups. Computer-adaptive testing for licensure and certification is a given. Reengineering has become a common occurrence in practice settings, as have cost containment, measurement of patient outcomes, evidence-based practice, care coordination, and a focus on consumer satisfaction.

The topics that you have embraced through this book have presented you with some of the issues involved in this time of rapid change in the profession and in practice. Facing the responsibilities inherent in professional practice is a way of revisiting our present roles and considering how they meet the needs of our patients and contribute to the future of our profession. The student role provides the setting for analyzing information related to current practices. Theories that guide practice continue to be tested and refined as appropriate to their utility in practice, education, and research. Communication and critical thinking are vital components of this activity as we operate as leaders, managers, and care providers in organizations, communities, and globally. We function as change agents, teachers, coordinators, and group leaders in practice settings. Evidence-based practices must be used in all situations, provision of direct and indirect care, administration, and education. Knowledge of research and the political process give us direction, as change agents, for addressing policy changes needed for a healthier society. The focus remains on healthcare consumers, their safety, needs, and healthful outcomes.

Current healthcare initiatives must be evaluated for applicability, acceptability, and appropriateness for meeting the needs of the population, with due consideration given to economic, linguistic, cultural, and quality indicators. All of these issues are addressed within the ethical parameters of professional nursing practice.

The information presented here has been designed to address the challenge of the book's title, *Advancing Your Career: Concepts of Professional Nursing*. We are all challenged to advance our professional practice.

EVIDENCE-BASED PRACTICE: *Consider this....*

As your hospital is preparing for application for the Magnet Recognition Program®, you notice that one of the five components of the Magnet Recognition Model is new knowledge, innovation, and improvements:

Magnet organizations have an ethical and professional responsibility to contribute to patient care, the organization, and the profession in terms of new knowledge, innovations, and improvements . . . [which] includes new models of care, application of existing evidence, new evidence, and visible contributions to the science of nursing (ANCC, 2014).

Question: Considering your career development and career path, what contributions can be identified to you or your unit to provide evidence of this component? What are your plans for the future?

Source: American Nurses Credentialing Center (ANCC). (2014). *Magnet Recognition Program® Model.* Retrieved from http://nursecredentialing.org/Magnet/ProgramOverview/New-Magnet-Model

KEY POINTS

- Competencies are those qualities that illustrate effectiveness and appropriateness in our respective professional roles. The Health Professions Education Summit led to the identification of five core competencies for all health professionals:
  - Provide patient-centered care.
  - Work in interdisciplinary teams.
  - Employ evidence-based practice.
  - Apply quality improvement.
  - Utilize informatics. (Greiner & Knebel, 2003)
- The IOM's Committee on the Work Environment and Patient Safety identified the following necessary patient safeguards in the practice environment (Page, 2004):
  - Governing boards that focus on safety
  - Effective nursing leadership
  - Adequate staffing
  - Organizational support for ongoing learning and decision support
  - Mechanisms that promote interdisciplinary collaboration
  - Work design that promotes safety
  - Organizational culture that continually strengthens patient safety
- The IOM (2011) recommended transformation and leadership by nursing with the identification of four key messages and eight recommendation directed at government, regulation, education, administration, and practice including the statement that nurses should practice to the full extent of their education and continue with the necessity for lifelong learning.
- The AACN (2002) has proposed hallmarks of excellence in the professional nursing practice environment based on selected characteristics of work environments that support professional nursing practice.
- Collaboration involves actively working together to meet some identified goal, such as the patient's treatment goals, while collegiality is the sharing of responsibility and authority to achieve a goal or prescribed outcome.
- Continued competence is of great concern to health professionals, their regulatory bodies, employers, and consumers. As described in their Position Statement on Professional Role Competence the ANA (2008) assurance of competence is the shared responsibility.

Continued

KEY POINTS—cont'd

- A nurse's involvement as a professional takes three forms:
  - As an individual professional with patients, families, and communities who are the consumers of nursing care
  - As a group member or leader of an interdisciplinary healthcare team
  - As an active member of the professional group
- Professional contributions result from participation in professional organizations, research, publications, theory evaluation, and promotion of the further development of the profession.
- Vital and basic skills needed and continually refined by professionals include expanding one's knowledge base, critical thinking, and technical, interpersonal, articulation, leadership, and policy and advocacy skills.

Thought and Discussion Questions

1. Identify three additional challenges for improvements in the delivery of quality healthcare.

2. Design a nurse residency program for a new graduate with yourself in the role of the mentor. Now, design a residency program for yourself if you were changing practice area, for example from an acute care surgical unit to an intensive care unit or hospice setting.

3. Describe your plans for two specific personal contributions to professional nursing practice that you will accomplish during the next 10 years.

4. Develop three personal goals to be met in your professional nursing practice during the next five years.

5. Think about the characteristics you would desire in a mentor to assist in the development of your career. List these characteristics and describe how you would identify and request the assistance of a mentor. Be prepared to participate in a class or online discussion to be scheduled by your instructor.

6. Review the Chapter Thought located on the first page of the chapter, and discuss it in the context of the contents of the chapter.

Interactive Exercises

Go to the Intranet site and complete the interactive exercises provided for this chapter.

REFERENCES

American Association of Colleges of Nursing (AACN). (2002). *Hallmarks of the professional nursing practice environment.* Retrieved from http://www.aacn.nche.edu/publications/white-papers/hallmarks-practice-environment

American Association of Colleges of Nursing (AACN). (2005). *Faculty shortages in baccalaureate and graduate nursing programs: Scope of the problem and strategies for expanding the supply.* Retrieved from http://www.aacn.nche.edu/publications/white-papers/faculty-shortages

American Association of Colleges of Nursing (AACN). (2006). *The essentials of doctoral education for advanced nursing practice.* Retrieved from http://www.aacn.nche.edu/DNP/pdf/Essentials.pdf

American Association of Colleges of Nursing (AACN). (2008a). The *essentials of baccalaureate education for professional nursing practice.* Retrieved from http://www.aacn.nche.edu/education/pdf/BaccEssentials08.pdf

American Association of Colleges of Nursing (AACN). (2008b). *Preferred vision for the professoriate in baccalaureate and graduate nursing programs.* Retrieved from http://www.aacn.nche.edu/publications/position/preferred-vision

American Association of Colleges of Nursing (AACN). (2011). *The essentials of master's education in nursing.* Retrieved from http://www.aacn.nche.edu/education-resources/MastersEssentials11.pdf

American Association of Colleges of Nursing (AACN). (2014a). *Fact sheet: The impact of education on nursing practice.* Retrieved from http://www.aacn.nche.edu/media-relations/EdImpact.pdf

American Association of Colleges of Nursing (AACN). (2014b). *Fact sheet: Nursing faculty shortage.* Retrieved from http://www.aacn.nche.edu/media-relations/FacultyShortageFS.pdf

American Association of Colleges of Nursing (AACN) and the American Organization of Nurse Executives (AONE). (2012). *AACN-AONE Task Force on Academic-Practice Partnerships: Guiding principles.* Retrieved from

http://www.aacn.nche.edu/leading-initiatives/academic
-practice-partnerships/GuidingPrinciples.pdf

American Nurses Association (ANA). (2008). *Position statement: Professional role competence.* Retrieved from http://gm6 .nursingworld.org/MainMenuCategories/Policy-Advocacy /Positions-and-Resolutions/ANAPositionStatements /Position-Statements-Alphabetically/Professional-Role -Competence.html

American Nurses Association (ANA). (2010a). *Nursing: Scope and standards of practice* (2nd ed.). Silver Spring, MD: Nursesbooks.org.

American Nurses Association (ANA). (2010b). *Nursing's social policy statement* (2010 ed.). Silver Spring, MD: Nursesbooks.org

American Nurses Credentialing Center (ANCC). (2014). *The Magnet recognition program* model.* Retrieved from http://nursecredentialing.org/Magnet/ProgramOverview /New-Magnet-Model

APRN Consensus Work Group & the National Council of State Boards of Nursing APRN Advisory Committee. (2008). *Consensus model for APRN regulation: Licensure, accreditation, certification & education.* Retrieved from https://www.ncsbn.org/Consensus_Model_for_APRN_ Regulation_July_2008.pdf

Aspden, P., Wolcott, J., Bootman, L., & Cronenwett, L. R. (eds.). (2006). *Preventing medication errors.* Washington, DC: National Academies Press.

Clark, P. A., Davis, M., Drevs, K., Fuerbringer, P., Gloss, M., & Spite, D. (2005). The healthcare landscape. In P. A. Clark and M. P. Malone, *Making it right: Healthcare service recovery tools, techniques, and best practices.* Marblehead, MA: HCPro.

Finkelman, A., & Kenner, C. (2012). *Teaching IPM: Implications of the Institute of Medicine reports for nursing education* (3rd ed.). Silver Spring, MD: Nursesbooks.org.

Gardner, D. B. (2005). Ten lessons in collaboration. *Online Journal of Issues in Nursing.* Retrieved from http:// nursingworld.org/MainMenuCategories/ANAMarketplace /ANAPeriodicals/OJIN/TableofContents/Volume102005 /No1Jan05/tpc26_116008.aspx

Greiner, A. C., & Knebel, E. (Eds.). (2003). *Health professions education: A bridge to quality.* Washington, DC: Institute of Medicine.

Haas, S., Swan, B. A., & Haynes, T. (2013). Developing ambulatory care registered nurse competencies for care coordination and transition management. *Nursing Economic$, 31*(1), 43–49.

Institute of Medicine (IOM). (2001). *Crossing the quality chasm: A new health system for the 21st century.* Retrieved from http://www.iom.edu/Reports/2001/Crossing-the-Quality -Chasm-A-New-Health-System-for-the-21st-Century.aspx

Institute of Medicine (IOM). (2011). *The future of nursing: Leading change, advancing health.* Retrieved from http://www.nap .edu/catalog/12956.html

Institute of Medicine (IOM). (2013). *Informing the future: Critical issues in health* (7th ed.). Retrieved from http://www .iom.edu/About-IOM/~/media/Files/About%20the% 20IOM/ITF_seventh.pdf

International Council of Nurses. (2006). *Position statement: Continuing competence as a professional responsibility and public right.* Retrieved from http://www.icn.ch/images /stories/documents/publications/position_statements /B02_Continuing_Competence.pdf

International Council of Nurses. (2007). *Position statement: Career development in nursing.* Retrieved from http://www.icn.ch /images/stories/documents/publications/position_statements /C02_Career_Development_Nsg.pdf

International Council of Nurses. (2013). *Position statement: Scope of nursing practice.* Retrieved from http://www.icn.ch /images/stories/documents/publications/position _statements/B07_Scope_Nsg_Practice.pdf

Joint Commission. (2013). *Comparison between Joint Commission standards, Malcolm Baldrige National Quality Award Criteria, and Magnet Recognition Program components.* Retrieved from http://www.jointcommission.org/assets/1/6/Comparison _Document2013.pdf

National Council of State Boards of Nursing (NCSBN). (2005). *Meeting the ongoing challenge of continued competence. 2005 continued competence concept paper.* Retrieved from https://www .ncsbn.org/Continued_Comp_Paper_TestingServices.pdf

National Council of State Boards of Nursing (NCSBN). (2014). *Nurse Licensure Compact (NLC).* Retrieved from https://www .ncsbn.org/nlc.htm

Nelson, M. A. (2002). Education for professional nursing practice: Looking backward into the future. *Online Journal of Issues in Nursing* (Manuscript 3), *7*(3), 1–13. Retrieved from http://nursingworld.org/MainMenuCategories/ ANAMarketplace/ANAPeriodicals/OJIN/TableofContents /Volume72002/No2May2002/EducationforProfessional NursingPractice.html

O'Neil, E. (1998). Nursing in the next century. In E. O'Neil & J. Coffman (Eds.), *Strategies for the future of nursing* (pp. 211–224). San Francisco, CA: Jossey-Bass.

Page, A. (ed.). (2004). *Keeping patients safe: Transforming the work environment of nurses.* Washington, DC: National Academies Press.

President's Advisory Commission on Consumer Protection and Quality in the Health Care Industry. (1998). *Quality first: Better health care for all Americans* [Final report to the President of the United States]. Columbia, MD: Consumer Bill of Rights.

Robert Wood Johnson Foundation (RWJF). (2014). Ten years after keeping patients safe: Have nurses' work environments been transformed? *Charting Nursing's Future: Reports on Policies That Can Transform Patient Care.* Retrieved from http://www.rwjf.org/content/dam/farm/reports/issue_briefs /2014/rwjf411417

Smith, J. (2003). *Report of findings: Exploring the value of continuing education mandates.* Chicago, IL: National Council of State Boards of Nursing.

Thibault, G.E. (2013). Reforming health professions education will require culture change and closer ties between classroom and practice. *Health Affairs, 32,* 1928–1932. doi: 10.1377/hlthaff.2013.0827

Weston, M. J. (2006). Integrating generational perspectives in nursing. *Online Journal of Issues in Nursing.* Retrieved from http://nursingworld.org/MainMenuCategories /ANAMarketplace/ANAPeriodicals/OJIN/TableofContents /Volume112006/No2May06/tpc30_216074.html

BIBLIOGRAPHY

Aiken, L. H., Clarke, S. P., Cheung, R. B., Sloane, D. M., & Sibler, J. H. (2003). Education levels of hospital nurses and surgical patient mortality. *Journal of the American Medical Association, 290,* 1617–1623.

Aiken, L. H., Clarke, S. P., Sloane, D. M., Lake, E. T., & Cheney, T. (2008). Effects of hospital care environment on patient mortality and nurse outcomes. *Journal of Nursing Administration, 38,* 223–229.

Aiken, L. H., Sloane, D. M., Bruyneel, L., Van den Heede, K., Griffiths, P., Busse, R., . . . Sermeus, W. (2014). Nurse staffing and education and hospital mortality in nine European countries: A retrospective observational study. *Lancet, 383,* 1824–1830. Retrieved from http://dx.doi.org /10.1016./S0140-6736(13)62631-8

Amer, K. S. (2013). *Quality and safety for transformational nursing: Core competencies.* Boston, MA: Pearson.

American Association of Colleges of Nursing (AACN). (1999). *Position statement on defining scholarship for the discipline of nursing.* Retrieved from http://www.aacn.nche.edu/ Publications/positions/scholar.htm

American Association of Colleges of Nursing (AACN). (2004). *Position statement on the practice doctorate in nursing.* Retrieved from http://www.aacn.nche.edu/publications /position/DNPpositionstatement.pdf

American Association of Colleges of Nursing (AACN). (2006). *AACN statement of support for clinical nurse specialists.* Retrieved from http://www.aacn.nche.edu/publications /position/DNPpositionstatement.pdf

American Association of Critical-Care Nurses. (2005). *AACN standards for establishing and sustaining healthy work environ-ments.* Retrieved from http://www.aacn.org/WD/HWE/ Content/hwehome.content?menu=hwe

American Nurses Association (ANA). (2014). *The national database for nursing quality indicators (NDNQI).* Retrieved from http://www.nursingquality.org/

Benner, P., Stuphen, M., Leonard, V., & Day, L. (2009). *Educating nurses: A call for radical transformation.* San Francisco, CA: Jossey-Bass.

Corrigan, M. S., Donaldson, M. S., Kohn, L. T., Maguire, S. K., & Pike, K. C. (2001). *Crossing the quality chasm: A new health system for the 21st century.* Washington, DC: National Academy Press.

Donley, R. (2005). Challenges for nursing in the 21st century. *Nursing Economics, 23,* 312–318.

Federal Trade Commission. (2014). *Policy perspective: Competi-tion and the regulation of advanced practice nurses.* Retrieved from http://www.ftc.gov/system/files/documents/reports /policy-perspectives-competition-regulation-advanced -practice-nurses/140307aprnpolicypaper.pdf

Lamb, G. (Ed.). (2014). *Care coordination. The game changer: How nursing is revolutionizing quality care.* Silver Spring, MD: Nursebooks.org.

National Council of State Boards of Nursing. (2009). *Changes in healthcare professions' scope of practice: Legislative considerations.* Retrieved from https://www.ncsbn.org/ScopeofPractice _09.pdf

National Council of State Boards of Nursing (NCSBN). (2011). *Fact sheet: Licensure of nurses and state boards of nursing.* Retrieved from https://www.ncsbn.org/Fact _Sheet_Licensure_of_Nurses_and_State_Boards_of _Nursing.pdf

North Carolina Board of Nursing. (2014). *Continued compe-tence requirements.* Retrieved from https://www.ncbon.com /dcp/i/licensurelisting-renewalreinstatement-continuing -competence-requirements

Nursing Council of New Zealand. (2014). *Continuing compe-tence.* Retrieved from http://nursingcouncil.org.nz/Nurses /Continuing-competence

O'Neil, E. H., & Pew Health Professions Commission. (1998). *Recreating health professions practice for a new century: Fourth report of the Pew Health Professions Commission.* San Francisco: Pew Health Professions Commission.

Pew Health Professions Commission. (1995). *Critical chal-lenges: Revitalizing the health professions for the twenty-first century.* San Francisco: UCSF Center for the Health Professions.

Registered Nurses Association of Northwest Territories and Nunavat. (2003). *Continuing competence (PDP).* Retrieved from http://www.rnantnu.ca/?page_id=28

Safriet, B .J. (2002). Closing the gap between can and may in health care providers' scopes of practice: A primer for policy makers. *Yale Journal on Regulation, 19*(2), 301–334.

Texas Board of Nursing. (2013). *Education: Continuing nursing education and competency.* Retrieved from http://www.bon .texas.gov/education_continuing_education.asp

Virginia Board of Nursing. (2014). Regulations governing the practice of nursing, 18 VAC 90-20-10 et seq. Retrieved from https://www.dhp.virginia.gov/nursing/

Washington State Board of Nursing and Washington State Nurses Association. (2010). *Position paper: Continuing competence in nursing.* Retrieved from http://www.wsna .org/practice/publications/documents/pp.continuing competence.pdf

Washington State Nurses Association. (2014). *Continuing competency.* Retrieved from http://www.wsna.org/Topics /Continuing-Competency/

Weinberg, D. B., Cooney-Miner, D., & Perloff, J. N. (2012). Analyzing the relationship between nursing education and patient outcomes. *Journal of Nursing Regulation, 3*(2), 4–10.

ONLINE RESOURCES

Agency for Healthcare Research and Quality (AHRQ)
http://www.ahrq.gov

American Nurses Association (ANA)
http://www.nursingworld.org

American Nurses Credentialing Center (ANCC)
http://www.nursecredentialing.org/default.aspx

Institute of Medicine
http://iom.edu
http://books.nap.edu/catalog/12956.html

International Council of Nurses
http://www.icn.ch/publications/position-statements/

National Council of State Boards of Nursing
https://www.ncsbn.org/index.htm

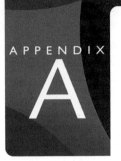

Professional Nursing Organizations

Academy of Medical-Surgical Nurses (AMSN)
https://www.amsn.org/practice-resources

Academy of Spinal of Spinal Cord Injury Professionals, Inc. (ASCIP)
http://www.academyscipro.org/

Accreditation Commission for Education in Nursing (ACEN)
http://www.acenursing.org/

Air & Surface Transport Nurses Association (ASTNA)
http://www.astna.org

American Academy of Ambulatory Care Nursing (AAACN)
http://www.aaacn.org

American Academy of Nurse Practitioners (AANP)
http://www.aanp.org

American Academy of Nursing (AAN)
http://www.aannet.org

American Assembly for Men in Nursing (AAMN)
http://www.aamn.org

American Association of Colleges of Nursing (AACN)
http://www.aacn.nche.edu

American Association of Critical-Care Nurses (AACN)
http://www.aacn.org

American Association for the History of Nursing (AAHN)
http://www.aahn.org

American Association of Legal Nurse Consultants (AALNC)
http://www.aalnc.org

American Association of Managed Care Nurses (AAMCN)
http://www.aamcn.org

American Association of Neuroscience Nurses (AANN)
http://www.aann.org

American Association of Nurse Anesthetists (AANA)
http://www.aana.com

American Association of Nurse Attorneys (TAANA)
http://www.taana.org

American Association of Occupational Health Nurses (AAOHN)
http://www.aaohn.org

American College of Healthcare Executives (ACHE)
http://www.ache.org

American College of Nurse-Midwives (ACNM)
http://www.midwife.org/

American Holistic Nurses Association (AHNA)
http://www.ahna.org

American Medical Informatics Association (AMIA)
http://www.amia.org

American Nephrology Nurses' Association (ANNA)
http://www.annanurse.org

American Nurses Association (ANA)
http://www.nursingworld.org

American Nurses Credentialing Center (ANCC)
http://www.nursecredentialing.org

> **Certification Center**
> http://www.nursecredentialing.org/Certification
>
> **Magnet Recognition Program**
> http://www.nursecredentialing.org/Magnet
>
> **Pathway to Excellence Program**
> http://www.nursecredentialing.org/Pathway

American Nurses Foundation (ANF)
http://www.anfonline.org

American Nursing Informatics Association (ANIA)
https://www.ania-caring.org

American Organization of Nurse Executives (AONE)
http://www.aone.org

American Psychiatric Nurses Association (APNA)
http://www.apna.org

American Society for Parenteral and Enteral Nutrition (ASPEN)
http://www.nutritioncare.org

American Society of PeriAnesthesia Nurses (ASPAN)
http://www.aspan.org

American Thoracic Society (ATS): Nursing Assembly
http://www.thoracic.org/assemblies/nur/index.php
https://www.ania.org/

Association of Camp Nurses (ACN)
http://www.acn.org

Association of Nurses in AIDS Care (ANAC)
http://www.nursesinaidscare.org

Association for Nursing Professional Development
http://www.anpd.org/

Association of periOperative Registered Nurses (AORN)
http://www.aorn.org

Association of Pediatric Hematology/Oncology Nurses (APHON)
http://www.aphon.org

Association for Professionals in Infection Control and Epidemiology (APIC)
http://www.apic.org

Association for Radiologic and Imaging Nursing (ARIN)
http://www.arinursing.org/

Association of Rehabilitation Nurses (ARN)
http://www.rehabnurse.org

Commission on Collegiate Nursing Education (CCNE)
http://www.aacn.nche.edu/accreditation

Commission on Graduates of Foreign Nursing Schools (CGFNS)
http://www.cgfns.org

Dermatology Nurses' Association (DNA)
http://www.dnanurse.org

Developmental Disabilities Nurses Association (DDNA)
http://www.ddna.org

Emergency Nurses Association (ENA)
http://www.ena.org

Gerontological Advanced Practice Nurses Association (GAPNA)
https://www.gapna.org

Health Ministries Association (HMA)
http://www.hmassoc.org

Home Healthcare Nurses Association (HHNA)
http://www.hhna.org

Hospice and Palliative Nurses Association (HPNA)
http://hpna.advancingexpertcare.org/

Infusion Nurses Society (INS)
http://www.ins1.org

International Association of Forensic Nurses (IAFN)
http://www.iafn.org

International Council of Nurses (ICN)
http://www.icn.ch

International Nurses Society on Addictions (INTNSA)
http://intnsa.org

International Society of Nurses in Genetics (ISONG)
http://www.isong.org

International Society of Psychiatric-Mental Health Nurses (ISPN)
http://www.ispn-psych.org

International Transplant Nurses Society (ITNS)
http://www.itns.org

National Association of Clinical Nurse Specialists (NACNS)
http://www.nacns.org

National Association of Directors of Nursing Administration in Long Term Care (NADONA/LTC)
http://www.nadona.org

National Association of Hispanic Nurses (NAHN)
http://www.thehispanicnurses.org

National Association of Neonatal Nurses (NANN)
http://www.nann.org

National Association of Nurse Massage Therapists (NANMT)
http://www.nanmt.org

National Association of Orthopaedic Nurses (NAON)
http://www.orthonurse.org

National Association of Pediatric Nurse Practitioners (NAPNAP)
http://www.napnap.org

National Association of School Nurses (NASN)
http://www.nasn.org

National Black Nurses Association (NBNA)
http://www.nbna.org

National Council of State Boards of Nursing (NCSBN)
http://www.ncsbn.org

National League for Nursing (NLN)
http://www.nln.org

National Organization of Nurse Practitioner Faculties (NONPF)
http://www.nonpf.com

North American Nursing Diagnosis Association International (NANDA-I)
http://www.nanda.org

Nurses Organization of Veterans Affairs (NOVA)
http://www.vanurse.org

Nurse Practitioner Associates for Continuing Education (NPACE)
http://www.npace.org

Nurse Practitioners in Women's Health (NPWH)
http://www.npwh.org

Oncology Nursing Society (ONS)
http://www.ons.org

Pediatric Endocrinology Nursing Society (PENS)
http://www.pens.org

Philippine Nurses Association (PNA)
http://www.pna-ph.org

Preventive Cardiovascular Nurses Association (PCNA)
http://www.pcna.net

Respiratory Nursing Society (RNS)
http://www.respiratorynursingsociety.org

Sigma Theta Tau International (STTI)
http://www.nursingsociety.org

Society of Gastroenterology Nurses and Associates (SGNA)
http://www.sgna.org

Society of Trauma Nurses (STN)
http://www.traumanurses.org

Society of Urologic Nurses and Associates (SUNA)
http://www.suna.org

Society for Vascular Nursing (SVN)
http://www.svnnet.org

Transcultural Nursing Society (TCNS)
http://www.tcns.org

Wound, Ostomy, and Continence Nurses Society (WOCN)
http://www.wocn.org

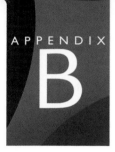

Nursing Interventions Classification (NIC) and Nursing Outcomes Classification (NOC) Systems

NURSING INTERVENTIONS CLASSIFICATION (NIC)

Abuse Protection Support
   Child
   Domestic Partner
   Elder
   Religious
Acid-Base Management
   Metabolic Acidosis
   Metabolic Alkalosis
   Respiratory Acidosis
   Respiratory Alkalosis
Acid-Base Monitoring
Active Listening
Activity Therapy
Acupressure
Admission Care
Airway Insertion and Stabilization
Airway Management
Airway Suctioning
Allergy Management
Amnioinfusion
Amputation Care
Analgesic Administration
   Intraspinal
Anaphylaxis Management
Anesthesia Administration
Anger Control Assistance
Animal-Assisted Therapy
Anticipatory Guidance
Anxiety Reduction
Area Restriction
Aromatherapy
Art Therapy
Artificial Airway Management
Aspiration Precautions
Assertiveness Training
Asthma Management
Attachment Promotion
Autogenic Training
Autotransfusion
Bathing
Bed Rest Care
Bedside Laboratory Testing
Behavior Management
   Overactivity/Inattention
   Self-Harm
   Sexual

Behavior Modification
   Social Skills
Bibliotherapy
Biofeedback
Bioterrorism Preparedness
Birthing
Bladder Irrigation
Bleeding Precautions
Bleeding Reduction
   Antepartum Uterus
   Gastrointestinal
   Nasal
   Postpartum Uterus
   Wound
Blood Products Administration
Body Image Enhancement
Body Mechanics Promotion
Bottle Feeding
Bowel Incontinence Care
   Encopresis
Bowel Irrigation
Bowel Management
Bowel Training
Breast Examination
Breastfeeding Assistance
Calming Technique
Capillary Blood Sample
Cardiac Care
   Acute
   Rehabilitative
Cardiac Precautions
Caregiver Support
Case Management
Cast Care
   Maintenance
   Wet
Cerebral Edema Management
Cerebral Perfusion Promotion
Cesarean Section Care
Chemical Restraint
Chemotherapy Management
Chest Physiotherapy
Childbirth Preparation
Circulatory Care
   Arterial Insufficiency
   Mechanical Assist Device
   Venous Insufficiency
Circulatory Precautions
Circumcision Care

Code Management
Cognitive Restructuring
Cognitive Stimulation
Communicable Disease Management
Communication Enhancement
    Hearing Deficit
    Speech Deficit
    Vision Deficit
Community Disaster Preparedness
Community Health Development
Complex Relationship Building
Conflict Mediation
Constipation/Impaction Management
Consultation
Contact Lens Care
Controlled Substance Checking
Coping Enhancement
Cost Containment
Cough Enhancement
Counseling
Crisis Intervention
Critical Path Development
Culture Brokerage
Cutaneous Stimulation
Decision-Making Support
Defibrillator Management
    External
    Internal
Delegation
Delirium Management
Delusion Management
Dementia Management
    Bathing
Deposition/Testimony
Developmental Care
Developmental Enhancement
    Adolescent
    Child
Dialysis Access Maintenance
Diarrhea Management
Diet Staging
Discharge Planning
Distraction
Documentation
Dressing
Dying Care
Dysreflexia Management
Dysrhythmia Management
Ear Care
Eating Disorders Management
Electroconvulsive Therapy (ECT) Management
Electrolyte Management
    Hypercalcemia
    Hyperkalemia
    Hypermagnesemia
    Hypernatremia
    Hyperphosphatemia
Electrolyte Monitoring
Electronic Fetal Monitoring
    Antepartum
    Intrapartum
Elopement Precautions

Embolus Care
    Peripheral
    Pulmonary
Embolus Precautions
Emergency Care
Emergency Cart Checking
Emotional Support
Endotracheal Extubation
Energy Management
Enteral Tube Feeding
Environmental Management
    Attachment Process
    Comfort
    Community
    Home Preparation
    Safety
    Violence Prevention
    Worker Safety
Environmental Risk Protection
Examination Assistance
Exercise Promotion
    Strength Training
    Stretching
Exercise Therapy
    Ambulation
    Balance
    Joint Mobility
    Muscle Control
Eye Care
Fall Prevention
Family Integrity Promotion
    Childbearing Family
Family Involvement Promotion
Family Mobilization
Family Planning
    Contraception
    Infertility
    Unplanned Pregnancy
Family Presence Facilitation
Family Process Maintenance
Family Support
Family Therapy
Feeding
Fertility Preservation
Fever Treatment
Financial Resource Assistance
Fire-Setting Precautions
First Aid
Fiscal Resource Management
Flatulence Reduction
Fluid/Electrolyte Management
Fluid Management
Fluid Monitoring
Fluid Resuscitation
Foot Care
Forensic Data Collection
Forgiveness Facilitation
Gastrointestinal Intubation
Genetic Counseling
Grief Work Facilitation
    Perinatal Death
Guided Imagery

Guilt Work Facilitation
Hair Care
Hallucination Management
Health Care Information Exchange
Health Education
Health Literacy Enhancement
Health Policy Monitoring
Health Screening
Health System Guidance
Heat/Cold Application
Heat Exposure Treatment
Hemodialysis Therapy
Hemodynamic Regulation
Hemofiltration Therapy
Hemorrhage Control
High-Risk Pregnancy Care
Home Maintenance Assistance
Hope Inspiration
Hormone Replacement Therapy
Humor
Hyperglycemia Management
Hypervolemia Management
Hypnosis
Hypoglycemia Management
Hypothermia Induction
Hypothermia Treatment
Hypovolemia Management
Immunization/Vaccination Management
Impulse Control Training
Incident Reporting
Incision Site Care
Infant Care
Infection Control
    Intraoperative
Infection Protection
Insurance Authorization
Intracranial Pressure (ICP) Monitoring
Intrapartal Care
    High-Risk Delivery
Intravenous (IV) Insertion
Intravenous (IV) Therapy
Invasive Hemodynamic Monitoring
Journaling
Kangaroo Care
Labor Induction
Labor Suppression
Laboratory Data Interpretation
Lactation Counseling
Lactation Suppression
Laser Precautions
Latex Precautions
Learning Facilitation
Learning Readiness Enhancement
Leech Therapy
Limit Setting
Lower Extremity Monitoring
Malignant Hyperthermia Precautions
Massage
Mechanical Ventilation Management
    Invasive
    Noninvasive
Mechanical Ventilator Weaning

Medication Administration
    Ear
    Enteral
    Eye
    Inhalation
    Interpleural
    Intradermal
    Intramuscular
    Intraosseous
    Intraspinal
    Intravenous
    Nasal
    Oral
    Rectal
    Skin
    Subcutaneous
    Vaginal
    Ventricular Reservoir
Medication Management
Medication Prescribing
Medication Reconciliation
Medication Facilitation
Memory Training
Milieu Therapy
Mood Management
Multidisciplinary Care Conference
Music Therapy
Mutual Goal Setting
Nail Care
Nausea Management
Neurologic Monitoring
Newborn Care
Newborn Monitoring
Nonnutritive Sucking
Normalization Promotion
Nutrition Management
Nutrition Therapy
Nutritional Counseling
Nutritional Monitoring
Oral Health Maintenance
Oral Health Promotion
Oral Health Restoration
Order Transcription
Organ Procurement
Ostomy Care
Oxygen Therapy
Pacemaker Management
    Temporary
    Permanent
Pain Management
Parent Education
    Adolescent
    Childrearing Family
    Infant
Parenting Promotion
Pass Facilitation
Patient Contracting
Patient-Controlled Analgesia (PCA) Assistance
Patient Rights Assistance
Peer Review
Pelvic Muscle Exercise
Perineal Care

Peripheral Sensation Management
Peripherally Inserted Central (PIC) Catheter Care
Peritoneal Dialysis Therapy
Pessary Management
Phlebotomy
    Arterial Blood Sample
    Blood Unit Acquisition
    Cannulated Vessel
    Venous Blood Sample
Phototherapy
    Mood/Sleep Regulation
    Neonate
Physical Restraint
Physician Support
Pneumatic Tourniquet Precautions
Positioning
    Intraoperative
    Neurologic
    Wheelchair
Postanesthesia Care
Postmortem Care
Postpartal Care
Preceptor
    Employee
    Student
Preconception Counseling
Pregnancy Termination Care
Premenstrual Syndrome (PMS) Management
Prenatal Care
Preoperative Coordination
Preparatory Sensory Information
Presence
Pressure Management
Pressure Ulcer Care
Pressure Ulcer Prevention
Product Evaluation
Program Development
Progressive Muscle Relaxation
Prompted Voiding
Prosthesis Care
Pruritus Management
Quality Monitoring
Radiation Therapy Management
Rape-Trauma Treatment
Reality Orientation
Recreation Therapy
Rectal Prolapse Management
Referral
Relaxation Therapy
Religious Addiction Prevention
Religious Ritual Enhancement
Relocation Stress Reduction
Reminiscence Therapy
Reproductive Technology Management
Research Data Collection
Resiliency Promotion
Respiratory Monitoring
Respite Care
Resuscitation
    Fetus
    Neonate

Risk Identification
    Childbearing Family
    Genetic
Role Enhancement
Seclusion
Security Enhancement
Sedation Management
Seizure Management
Seizure Precautions
Self-Awareness Enhancement
Self-Care Assistance
    Bathing/Hygiene
    Dressing/Grooming
    Feeding
    Instrumental Activities of Daily Living (IADL)
    Toileting
    Transfer
Self-Efficacy Enhancement
Self-Esteem Enhancement
Self-Hypnosis Facilitation
Self-Modification Assistance
Self-Responsibility Facilitation
Sexual Counseling
Shift Report
Shock Management
    Cardiac
    Vasogenic
    Volume
Shock Prevention
Sibling Support
Skin Care
    Donor Site
    Graft Site
    Topical Treatments
Skin Surveillance
Sleep Enhancement
Smoking Cessation Assistance
Social Marketing
Socialization Enhancement
Specimen Management
Spiritual Growth Facilitation
Spiritual Support
Splinting
Sports Injury Prevention: Youth
Staff Development
Staff Supervision
Subarachnoid Hemorrhage Precautions
Substance Use Prevention
Substance Use Treatment
    Alcohol Withdrawal
    Drug Withdrawal
    Overdose
Suicide Prevention
Supply Management
Support Group
Support System Enhancement
Surgical Assistance
Surgical Precautions
Surgical Preparation
Surveillance
    Community

Late Pregnancy
Remote Electronic
Safety
Sustenance Support
Suturing
Swallowing Therapy
Teaching
   Disease Process
   Foot Care
   Group
   Individual
   Infant Nutrition 0–3 Months
   Infant Nutrition 4–6 Months
   Infant Nutrition 7–9 Months
   Infant Nutrition 10–12 Months
   Infant Safety 0–3 Months
   Infant Safety 4–6 Months
   Infant Safety 7–9 Months
   Infant Safety 10–12 Months
   Infant Stimulation 0–4 Months
   Infant Stimulation 5–8 Months
   Infant Stimulation 9–12 Months
   Preoperative
   Prescribed Activity/Exercise
   Prescribed Diet
   Prescribed Medication
   Procedure/Treatment
   Psychomotor Skill
   Safe Sex
   Sexuality
   Toddler Nutrition 13–18 Months
   Toddler Nutrition 19–24 Months
   Toddler Nutrition 25–36 Months
   Toddler Safety 13–18 Months
   Toddler Safety 19–24 Months
   Toddler Safety 25–36 Months
   Toilet Training
Technology Management
Telephone Consultation
Telephone Follow-Up
Temperature Regulation
   Intraoperative
Therapeutic Play
Therapeutic Touch
Therapy Group
Thrombolytic Therapy Management
Total Parenteral Nutrition (TPN) Administration
Touch
Traction/Immobilization Care
Transcutaneous Electrical Nerve Stimulation (TENS)
Transfer
Transport
   Interfacility
   Intrafacility
Trauma Therapy: Child
Triage
   Disaster
   Emergency Center
   Telephone
Truth Telling
Tube Care
   Chest
   Gastrointestinal
   Umbilical Line

   Urinary
   Ventriculostomy/Lumbar Drain
Ultrasonography: Limited Obstetric
Unilateral Neglect Management
Urinary Bladder Training
Urinary Catheterization
   Intermittent
Urinary Elimination Management
Urinary Habit Training
Urinary Incontinence Care
   Enuresis
Urinary Retention Care
Validation Therapy
Values Clarification
Vehicle Safety Promotion
Venous Access Device (VAD) Maintenance
Ventilation Assistance
Visitation Facilitation
Vital Signs Monitoring
Vomiting Management
Weight Gain Assistance
Weight Management
Weight Reduction Assistance
Wound Care
   Burns
   Closed Drainage
Wound Irrigation

Nursing Specialty Core Interventions Areas

Additions Nursing
Ambulatory Nursing
Anesthesia Nursing
Chemical Dependency Nursing
Child/Adolescent Psychiatric Nursing
College Health Nursing
Community Public Health Nursing
Correctional Nursing
Critical Care Nursing
Dermatology Nursing
Developmental Disability Nursing
Emergency Nursing
End-of-Life Care Nursing
Flight Nursing
Forensic Nursing
Gastroenterological Nursing
Genetics Nursing
Gerontological Nursing
Holistic Nursing
Infection Control/Epidemiological Nursing
Intravenous Nursing
Medical-Surgical Nursing
Midwifery Nursing
Neonatal Nursing
Nephrology Nursing
Neuroscience Nursing
Obstetric Nursing
Occupational Health Nursing
Oncology Nursing
Ophthalmic Nursing
Orthopedic Nursing
Otorhinolaryngology and Head/Neck Nursing

Pain Management Nursing
Parish Nursing
Pediatric Nursing
Pediatric Oncology Nursing
Perioperative Nursing
Psychiatric/Mental Health Nursing
Radiological Nursing
Rehabilitation Nursing
School Nursing
Spinal Cord Injury Nursing
Urologic Nursing
Vascular Nursing
Women's Health Nursing

Source: Bulechek, G. M., Butcher, H. K., Dochterman, J. M., & Wagner, C. (Eds.). (2013). *Nursing Interventions Classification (NIC)* (6th ed.). St. Louis: Mosby Elsevier. Reprinted with permission.

NURSING OUTCOMES CLASSIFICATION (NOC)

Abuse Cessation
Abuse Protection
Abuse Recovery
    Emotional
    Financial
    Physical
    Sexual
Abusive Behavior: Self-Restraint
Acceptance: Health Status
Activity Tolerance
Acute Confusion Level
Adaptation to Physical Disability
Adherence Behavior
    Healthy Diet
Aggression Self-Control
Agitation Level
Alcohol Abuse Cessation Behavior
Allergic Response
    Localized
    Systemic
Ambulation
    Wheelchair
Anxiety Level
Anxiety Self-Control
Appetite
Aspiration Prevention
Asthma Self-Management
Balance
Blood Coagulation
Blood Glucose Level
Blood Loss Severity
Blood Transfusion Reaction
Body Image
Body Mechanics Performance
Body Positioning: Self-Initiated
Bone Healing
Bowel Continence
Bowel Elimination
Breast Feeding Establishment
    Infant
    Maternal

Breastfeeding Maintenance
Breastfeeding Weaning
Burn Healing
Burn Recovery
Cardiac Disease Self-Management
Cardiac Pump Effectiveness
Cardiopulmonary Status
Caregiver Adaptation to Patient Institutionalization
Caregiver Emotional Health
Caregiver Home Care Readiness
Caregiver Lifestyle Disruption
Caregiver-Patient Relationship
Caregiver Performance
    Direct Care
    Indirect Care
Caregiver Physical Health
Caregiver Role Endurance
Caregiver Stressors
Caregiver Well-Being
Child Adaptation to Hospitalization
Child Development
    1 Month
    2 Months
    4 Months
    6 Months
    12 Months
    2 Years
    3 Years
    4 Years
    5 Years
    Middle Childhood
    Adolescence
Circulation Status
Client Satisfaction
    Access to Care Resources
    Caring
    Care Management
    Communication
    Continuity of Care
    Cultural Needs Fulfillment
    Functional Assistance
    Pain Management
    Physical Care
    Physical Environment
    Protection of Rights
    Psychological Care
    Safety
    Symptom Control
    Teaching
    Technical Aspects of Care
Cognition
Cognitive Orientation
Comfort Status
    Environment
    Physical
    Psychospiritual
    Sociocultural
Comfortable Death
Communication
    Expressive
    Receptive
Community Competence
Community Disaster Readiness

Community Disaster Response
Community Health Status
   Immunity
Community Risk Control
   Chronic Disease
   Communicable Disease
   Lead Exposure
   Violence
Community Violence Level
Compliance Behavior
   Prescribed Diet
   Prescribed Medication
Concentration
Coordinated Movement
Coping
Decision Making
Depression Level
Depression Self-Control
Development
   Late Adulthood
   Middle Adulthood
   Young Adulthood
Diabetes Self-Management
Dignified Life Closure
Discharge Readiness
   Independent Living
   Supported Living
Discomfort Level
Distorted Thought Self-Control
Drug-Abuse Cessation Behavior
Electrolyte and Acid/Base Balance
Elopement Occurrence
Elopement Propensity Risk
Endurance
Energy Conservation
Fall Prevention Behavior
Falls Occurrence
Family Coping
Family Functioning
Family Health Status
Family Integrity
Family Normalization
Family Participation in Professional Care
Family Resiliency
Family Social Climate
Family Support During Treatment
Fatigue Level
Fear Level
   Child
Fear Self-Control
Fetal Status
   Antepartum
   Intrapartum
Fluid Balance
Fluid Overload Severity
Gastrointestinal Function
Grief Resolution
Growth
Health Beliefs
   Perceived Ability to Perform
   Perceived Control
   Perceived Resources
   Perceived Threat

Health Orientation
Health Promoting Behavior
Health Seeking Behavior
Hearing Compensation Behavior
Heedfulness of Affected Side
Hemodialysis Access
Hope
Hydration
Hyperactivity Level
Identity
Immobility Consequences
   Physiological
   Psycho-Cognitive
Immune Hypersensitivity Response
Immune Status
Immunization Behavior
Impulse Self-Control
Infection Severity
   Newborn
Information Processing
Joint Movement
   Ankle
   Elbow
   Fingers
   Hip
   Knee
   Neck
   Passive
   Shoulder
   Spine
   Wrist
Kidney Function
Knowledge
   Arthritis Management
   Asthma Management
   Body Mechanics
   Breastfeeding
   Cancer Management
   Cancer Threat Reduction
   Cardiac Disease Management
   Child Physical Safety
   Conception Prevention
   Congestive Heart Failure Management
   Depression Management
   Diabetes Management
   Diet
   Disease Process
   Energy Conservation
   Fall Prevention
   Fertility Promotion
   Health Behavior
   Health Promotion
   Health Resources
   Hypertension Management
   Illness Care
   Infant Care
   Infection Management
   Labor and Delivery
   Medication
   Multiple Sclerosis Management
   Ostomy Care
   Pain Management
   Parenting

Personal Safety
Postpartum Maternal Health
Preconception Maternal Health
Pregnancy
Pregnancy and Postpartum Sexual Functioning
Prescribed Activity
Preterm Infant Care
Sexual Functioning
Substance Use Control
Treatment Procedure
Treatment Regimen
Weight Management
Leisure Participation
Loneliness Severity
Maternal Status
    Antepartum
    Intrapartum
    Postpartum
Mechanical Ventilation Response: Adult
Mechanical Ventilation Weaning Response: Adult
Medication Response
Memory
Mobility
Mood Equilibrium
Motivation
Multiple Sclerosis: Self-Management
Nausea and Vomiting Control
Nausea and Vomiting: Disruptive Effects
Nausea and Vomiting Severity
Neglect Cessation
Neglect Recovery
Neurological Status
    Autonomic
    Central Motor Control
    Consciousness
    Cranial Sensory/Motor Function
    Peripheral
    Spinal Sensory/Motor Function
Newborn Adaptation
Nutritional Status
    Biochemical Measures
    Energy
    Food and Fluid Intake
    Nutrient Intake
Oral Hygiene
Ostomy Self-Care
Pain: Adverse Psychological Response
Pain Control
Pain: Disruptive Effects
Pain Level
Parent-Infant Attachment
Parenting
    Adolescent Physical Safety
    Early/Middle Childhood Physical Safety
    Infant/Toddler Physical Safety
Parenting Performance
Parenting: Psychosocial Safety
Participation in Healthcare Decisions
Personal Autonomy
Personal Health Status
Personal Resiliency
Personal Safety Behavior

Personal Well-Being
Physical Aging
Physical Fitness
Physical Injury Severity
Physical Maturation
    Female
    Male
Play Participation
Postpartum Maternal Health Behavior
Post-Procedure Recovery
Prenatal Health Behavior
Pre-Procedure Readiness
Preterm Infant Organization
Psychomotor Energy
Psychosocial Adjustment: Life Change
Quality of Life
Respiratory Status
    Airway Patency
    Gas Exchange
    Ventilation
Rest
Risk Control
    Alcohol Use
    Cancer
    Cardiovascular Health
    Drug Use
    Hearing Impairment
    Hyperthermia
    Hypothermia
    Infectious Process
    Sexually Transmitted Diseases (STDs)
    Sun Exposure
    Tobacco Use
    Unintended Pregnancy
    Visual Impairment
Risk Detection
Role Performance
Safe Home Environment
Safe Wandering
Seizure Control
Self-Care Status
Self-Care
    Activities of Daily Living (ADL)
    Bathing
    Dressing
    Eating
    Hygiene
    Instrumental Activities of Daily Living
      (IADL)
    Non-Parenteral Medication
    Oral Hygiene
    Parenteral Medication
    Toileting
Self-Direction of Care
Self-Esteem
Self-Mutilation Restraint
Sensory Function
    Cutaneous
    Hearing
    Proprioception
    Taste and Smell
    Vision

Sexual Functioning
Sexual Identity
Skeletal Function
Sleep
Smoking Cessation Behavior
Social Interaction Skills
Social Involvement
Social Support
Spiritual Health
Stress Level
Student Health Status
Substance Addiction Consequences
Substance Withdrawal Severity
Suffering Severity
Suicide Self-Restraint
Swallowing Status
   Esophageal Phase
   Oral Phase
   Pharyngeal Phase
Symptom Control
Symptom Severity
   Perimenopause
   Premenstrual Syndrome (PMS)
Systemic Toxin Clearance: Dialysis
Thermoregulation
   Newborn
Tissue Integrity: Skin and Mucous Membranes
Tissue Perfusion
   Abdominal Organs
   Cardiac
   Cellular
   Cerebral
   Peripheral
   Pulmonary
Transfer Performance
Treatment Behavior: Illness or Injury
Urinary Continence
Urinary Elimination
Vision Compensation Behavior
Vital Signs
Weight: Body Mass
Weight Gain Behavior
Weight Loss Behavior
Weight Maintenance Behavior
Will to Live
Wound Healing
   Primary Intention
   Secondary Intention

Core Outcomes for Nursing Specialty Areas

Air and Surface Transport
Ambulatory Care
Anesthesia
Cardiac Rehabilitation
Chemical Dependency
Community Health
Critical Care
Dermatology
Emergency Care
Gastroenterology
Genetics
Gerontology
Home Healthcare
Hospice and Palliative Care
Intravenous Therapy
Medical-Surgical
Neonatology
Nephrology
Neuroscience
Nurse Practitioner
Oncology
Operating Room
Ophthalmology
Orthopaedics
Otorhinolaryngology and Head-Neck
Pain Management
Parish Nursing
Pediatrics
Pediatric Oncology
Perianesthesia
Postoperative Care
Psychiatric-Mental Health
Radiology
Rehabilitation
School Health
Spinal Cord Injury
Urology
Vascular
Women's Health and Obstetrics

Source: Moorhead, S., Johnson, M., Maas, M. L., & Swanson, E. (Eds.). (2013). *Nursing Outcomes Classification (NOC)* (5th ed.). St. Louis: Mosby Elsevier. Reprinted with permission.

REFERENCES

Bulechek, G. M., Butcher, H. K., Dochterman, J. M., & Wagner, C. (eds.). (2013). *Nursing Interventions Classification (NIC)* (6th ed.). St. Louis: Mosby Elsevier.

Moorhead, S., Johnson, M., Maas, M. L., & Swanson, E. (eds.). (2013). *Nursing Outcomes Classification (NOC)* (5th ed.). St. Louis: Mosby Elsevier.

INDEX

Note: Page numbers followed by an "f" indicate a figure, page numbers followed by a "b" indicate a box, and page numbers followed by a "t" indicate a table.

A